Cardiorespiratory Fitness in Cardiometabolic Diseases

Peter Kokkinos • Puneet Narayan
Editors

Cardiorespiratory Fitness in Cardiometabolic Diseases

Prevention and Management in Clinical Practice

Springer

Editors
Peter Kokkinos
Veterans Affairs Medical Center
Georgetown University School of Medicine
Rutgers University Department of Kinesiology and Health
University of South Carolina Arnold School of Public Health
George Washington University School of Medicine and Health Sciences
Washington
DC
USA

Puneet Narayan
Clinical Research Institute of Northern Virginia
Burke
VA
USA

ISBN 978-3-030-04815-0 ISBN 978-3-030-04816-7 (eBook)
https://doi.org/10.1007/978-3-030-04816-7

Library of Congress Control Number: 2019932846

This Springer imprint is published by the registered company Springer Nature Switzerland AG
The registered company address is: Gewerbestrasse 11, 6330 Cham, Switzerland

This book is dedicated to Evangeline, spouse, friend, and mother, and to my sons Nicholas and John Peter, who make life a wonderful journey!

Peter Kokkinos

This book is dedicated to my Parents for instilling us with their values of hard work, dedication and sacrifice with endless support and love.

Puneet Narayan

Preface

Physical activity is the most underutilized medical intervention in prevention and management of cardiovascular disease. This despite the fact that it is inexpensive, relatively low risk, and easily incorporated in most lifestyles. The link between physical activity and health was recognized by Hippocrates in the fifth century BC. Hippocrates stated that a sedentary lifestyle renders the body liable to disease and premature aging. Conversely, moderate physical activity promotes health and slows the aging process. Scientific scrutiny of this concept began in the early 1950s with the landmark work of Morris and coworkers reporting that mortality rates were approximately 50% lower in civil servants with jobs requiring more physical activity versus those serving in more sedentary positions. For more than half a century now, a plethora of evidence has accumulated from large, long-term epidemiological studies that support a strong, inverse, and independent association between physical activity, cardiorespiratory fitness, and cardiovascular and overall mortality in apparently healthy individuals and in patients with documented chronic disease. In addition, similar associations have been observed between incidence of chronic disease and fitness.

The exercise-related health benefits are related in part to favorable modulations in both the traditional and novel cardiovascular risk factors that have been observed with increased physical activity patterns or structured exercise programs. The primary reason for this protection is the innate capacity of the body to adapt to an imposed demand. Specifically, the increased energy requirements during physical activity (work) place a greater demand on all biological systems involved to meet this demand. Consequently, acute changes occur to meet the increased metabolic demand. Moreover, if the demand (exercise) is adequate and chronic (over several weeks), the adaptations made are also chronic and designed to make the systems involved in the task more efficient and, ultimately, more resilient to injury and disease. Specific mechanisms modulating these adaptations and the protection against disease and death have also been defined in recent years.

The overwhelming evidence on the link between cardiorespiratory fitness, chronic diseases, and mortality risk has shifted attention of the medical profession to seriously consider fitness status as part of the patient's medical profile and to encourage patients to increase their daily physical activity.

Accordingly, this book provides a comprehensive overview on exercise-related cellular, cardiovascular, and metabolic chronic adaptations in healthy and diseased populations and, in addition, an extensive review of the literature on the preventive and therapeutic aspects of physical activity, exercise, and cardiorespiratory fitness on cardiovascular risk factors and cardiometabolic diseases.

Washington, DC, USA Peter Kokkinos
Burke, VA, USA Puneet Narayan

Contents

Contributors

Elizabeth Anderson Department of Exercise Science, Norman J. Arnold School of Public Health, University of South Carolina, Columbia, SC, USA

Mark A. Chapman Department of Physiology and Pharmacology, Karolinska Institutet, Solna, Sweden

Department of General Engineering, University of San Diego, San Diego, CA, USA

Costas Chryssanthopoulos Department of Physiology, Medical School, National and Kapodistrian University of Athens, Athens, Greece

Louise de Lannoy Queen's University, School of Kinesiology and Health Studies, Kingston, ON, Canada

George Dimitriadis Second Department of Internal Medicine-Research Institute and Diabetes Center, "Attikon" University Hospital, Medical School, National and Kapodistrian University of Athens, Athens, Greece

Cleyton C. Domingues Department of Medicine, George Washington University, Washington, DC, USA

Michael Doumas 2nd Propedeutic Department Internal Medicine, Hippokration Hospital, Thessaloniki, Greece

J. Larry Durstine Department of Exercise Science, Norman J. Arnold School of Public Health, University of South Carolina, Columbia, SC, USA

Jonathan K. Ehrman Department of Internal Medicine, Division of Cardiovascular Medicine, Preventive Cardiology, Henry Ford Medical Group, Detroit, MI, USA

Charles Faselis Veterans Affairs Medical Center, Washington, DC, USA

Barry A. Franklin Preventive Cardiology and Cardiac Rehabilitation, Department of Cardiovascular Diseases, Beaumont Health and Wellness Center, Royal Oak, MI, USA

Oakland University William Beaumont School of Medicine, Rochester, MI, USA

Shruti M. Gandhi Department of Endocrinology, Washington D.C. VA Medical Center, Washington, DC, USA

Eva-Karin Gidlund Department of Physiology and Pharmacology, Karolinska Institutet, Solna, Sweden

Steven P. Hooker College of Health and Human Services, San Diego, CA, USA

Konstantinos P. Imprialos 2nd Propedeutic Department Internal Medicine, Hippokration Hospital, Thessaloniki, Greece

Sergey Kachur Graduate Medical Education, Ocala Regional Medical Center, Ocala, FL, USA

Peter Kokkinos Veterans Affairs Medical Center, Georgetown University School of Medicine, Rutgers University Department of Kinesiology and Health, University of South Carolina Arnold School of Public Health, George Washington University School of Medicine and Health Sciences, Washington, DC, USA

Michael Koutsilieris Department of Physiology, Medical School, National and Kapodistrian University of Athens, Athens, Greece

Anubhav Kumar Clinical Research Institute of Northern Virginia, Burke, VA, USA

Nabanita Kundu Department of Medicine, George Washington University, Washington, DC, USA

Raj Lakshman Veterans Affairs Medical Center and George Washington University School of Medicine, Washington, DC, USA

Michael J. LaMonte Department of Epidemiology and Environmental Health, University at Buffalo – SUNY, School of Public Health, Buffalo, NY, USA

Carl J. Lavie Department of Cardiology, Ochsner Medical Center, New Orleans, LA, USA

Hayley V. MacDonald Department of Kinesiology, The University of Alabama, Tuscaloosa, AL, USA

Maria Maridaki Department of Sports Medicine & Biology of Physical Activity, Faculty of Physical Education and Sport Science, National and Kapodistrian University of Athens, Athens, Greece

Mary M. McDermott Northwestern University, General Internal Medicine and Geriatrics, Chicago, IL, USA

Michelle N. McDonnell School of Health Sciences, University of South Australia, Adelaide, SA, Australia

Jonathan Myers Department of Cardiology, VA Palo Alto Health Care System/Stanford University, Palo Alto, CA, USA

Puneet Narayan Clinical Research Institute of Northern Virginia, Burke, VA, USA

Michelle Phuong Nguyen UCF/HCA Graduate Medical Education - Internal Medicine, Ocala Regional Medical Center, Ocala, FL, USA

Eric S. Nylén Department of Endocrinology, VAMC and George Washington University School of Medicine, Washington, DC, USA

Linda S. Pescatello Department of Kinesiology, University of Connecticut, Storrs, CT, USA

Anastassios Philippou Department of Physiology, Medical School, National and Kapodistrian University of Athens, Athens, Greece

Andreas Pittaras Department of Cardiology, GW University, Veteran Affairs Medical Center, Washington, DC, USA

Ryan R. Porter Department of Exercise Science, Norman J. Arnold School of Public Health, University of South Carolina, Columbia, SC, USA

Kyra E. Pyke Queen's University, School of Kinesiology and Health Studies, Kingston, ON, Canada

Robert Ross Queen's University, School of Kinesiology and Health Studies, Kingston, ON, Canada

Labros S. Sidossis Rutgers University, Department of Kinesiology and Health, New Brunswick, NJ, USA

Konstantinos D. Tambalis Department of Nutrition and Dietetics, Harokopio University, Athens, Kallithea, Greece

Joshua C. Tremblay Queen's University, School of Kinesiology and Health Studies, Kingston, ON, Canada

Apostolos Tsimploulis Department of Cardiology, Stony Brook University Hospital, Stony Brook, NY, USA

Sabyasachi Sen Department of Medicine, George Washington University, Washington, DC, USA

Konstantinos Stavropoulos 2nd Propedeutic Department Internal Medicine, Hippokration Hospital, Thessaloniki, Greece

Carl Johan Sundberg Department of Physiology and Pharmacology, Department of Learning, Informatics, Management and Ethics, Karolinska Institutet, Stockholm, Sweden

Xuewen Wang Department of Exercise Science, Norman J. Arnold School of Public Health, University of South Carolina, Columbia, SC, USA

1 Physical Activity, Cardiorespiratory Fitness, and Health: A Historical Perspective

Peter Kokkinos and Jonathan Myers

Introduction

Survival for the primitive man depended on his ability to hunt, carry the prey back to his family, and at times fight fiercely to keep it. As ancient civilizations began to develop, the importance of physical strength and endurance in the battlefield was recognized, leading to the development and implementation of rigid training programs solely for the military purposes and ultimately for the expansion of the empire [1, 2].

A clear departure from this concept for the first time in history was observed in ancient Greece, particularly Athens. No other ancient civilization has held fitness in such high regard. Greeks viewed the development of a strong and enduring body not only as part of a military doctrine but also, and even more important, as an integral part in the pursuit of physical and mental health. The enduring concept of the harmonious existence between mind and body and the importance of equally cultivating both are also eloquently echoed later by the philosopher Plato in the following statement:

> Physical activity is not merely necessary to the health and development of the body, but to balance and correct intellectual pursuits as well. The mere athlete is brutal and philistine, the mere intellectual unstable and spiritless. The right education must tune the strings of the body and mind to perfect spiritual harmony.

These concepts provided the basis for athletics—from the Greek "athlos" meaning competition requiring physical attributes for ultimate achievement—the development of certain sports that are still practiced (running, discus and javelin throwing, decathlon, pentathlon, boxing, etc.), the spirit of competition, and, finally, the Olympics.

Physical Activity and Health Connection

In addition to athletics, the overall health benefits of physical activity and fitness was recognized by founding medical practitioners including Hippocrates and Galen [3]. The most systematic

P. Kokkinos (✉)
Veterans Affairs Medical Center, Department of Cardiology, Washington, DC, USA

Georgetown University School of Medicine, Washington, DC, USA

Department of Kinesiology and Health, Rutgers University, New Brunswick, NJ, USA

George Washington University School of Medicine and Health Sciences, Washington, DC, USA

University of South Carolina, Department of Exercise Science, Arnold School of Public Health, Columbia, SC, USA
e-mail: peter.kokkinos@va.gov

J. Myers
Department of Cardiology, VA Palo Alto Health Care System/Stanford University, Palo Alto, CA, USA

Stanford University, Stanford, CA, USA

P. Kokkinos, P. Narayan (eds.), *Cardiorespiratory Fitness in Cardiometabolic Diseases*,
https://doi.org/10.1007/978-3-030-04816-7_1

recordings of observations, concepts, and statements describing health benefits attributed to physical activity are from ancient Greek physicians and philosophers. These concepts had a great influence on Western civilization and provided the basis for our modern views in the association between physical activity and health.

More importantly, it is the precise statements and details that emphasize not only the connection between fitness and health but also the implementation of fitness to a large population, something we also struggle with today. For example, the Greek physician Hippocrates states:

> Speaking generally, all parts of the body which have a function, if used in moderation and exercised in labors to which each is accustomed, become thereby healthy and well developed and age slowly; but if unused and left idle, they become liable to disease, defective in growth, and age quickly.

Within that short statement, Hippocrates introduces two major and essential concepts regarding fitness and health. First, he emphasizes the importance of moderation in the pursuit of health through increased physical activity, something that was documented only recently after years of research. Second, Hippocrates makes the connection between physical inactivity, the incidence of disease, and premature aging. In another profound statement, Hippocrates is more direct:

> Walking is a man's best medicine.

Today, after years of research, most authorities on the subject agree that walking is the safest and the most effective form of exercise that can be implemented in large populations to foster health.

And then:

> If we could give every individual the right amount of nourishment and exercise, not too little and not too much, we would have found the safest way to health.

In addition to combining diet and physical activity, Hippocrates in the later statement touches upon another important concept. He emphasizes the "right amount, not too little and not too much…" This statement clearly indicates that Hippocrates was keenly aware that only the proper amount will yield health benefits. Too much is likely to cause harm, and not enough will be ineffective.

Galen followed in the footsteps of Hippocrates. Overall, Galen viewed hygiene as an important part of medicine and exercise as a key branch of hygiene. Accordingly, in his text *On Hygiene*, Galen emphasized the need for physical activity in all ages. He also explains that for exercise to yield health benefits, it must be of certain vigor, enough to increase respiration, and that movements which do not alter the respiration are not called exercise. He viewed hygiene as an important part of medicine and exercise as a key branch of hygiene. He viewed health as not just the absence of disease but a physiological state that can be optimized by regimental exercise. He wrote "The term 'health' applies to a certain state; the term 'good condition' to excellence within the state, and to its stability." Galen states that the healthiest body is a "well-conditioned" and concludes that "the 'well-conditioned' is the healthiest arrangement, and the goal of all men" [4, 5].

Interestingly, Galen did not view athletes kindly. He accuses them of violating the concept "Παν μέτρον άριστον" (moderation in all is best) that prevailed in the ancient Greek world. Galen further suggests that athletes "exceed the proper measure in exertion, are in miserable pain," and when they stop competing, most parts of their bodies become deformed. As discussed later, Galen's view of athletes had lasting influence on Western medicine well into the late nineteenth century [4, 5].

Following the decline of Hellenism, the Romans, despite their admiration for the Greek civilization and their attempt to emulate it, the Athenian concept of fitness as an integral part of a healthy individual and a healthy vibrant society perished, and physical conditioning was, once again, used strictly for military purposes [6]. Fitness levels of the general Roman population declined as individuals became enamored with wealth and entertainment, such as the gladiator battles. Materialistic acquisition and excess became higher priorities than physical condition. The historian Dr. Pierre Cagniart states and sums up the difference between Greek and Roman attitude toward sports in the following statement: "a Greek would throw a javelin for distance whereas a Roman would throw at a target." Eventually, the lavish lifestyle and decadence of the Romans led to a decline of interest in fitness and physical decay ensued. Some historians believe that this decay leads to the downfall of the Roman civilization to the physically superior barbarian tribes from Northern Europe [7]. The lifestyle of these tribes consisted of hunting and gathering food, and once again, physical activity and fitness became a prerequisite for survival [8].

During the Renaissance, a renewed interest in the human body emerged. Physical education programs expanded within emerging nations of Europe, especially Germany, Denmark, Sweden, and Great Britain. Educators such as Per Henrik Ling of Sweden used science and physiology to better understand the importance of fitness. Per Henrik Ling and Archibald Maclaren, a medical student in England, also advocated that exercise programs should be tailored based on individual differences [9, 10].

Physical Activity in the United States

In the 1800s United States, fitness to some extent was influenced by European concepts. Benjamin Franklin and Thomas Jefferson recognized the importance of regular physical activity for good health and encouraged physical activity for all Americans [11]. President Thomas Jefferson acknowledged the necessity for fitness and advocated no less than 2 h a day should be devoted to exercise regardless of weather.

Galen's unfavorable view of athletics was shared by many physicians of the nineteenth century as they witnessed athletes enduring severe injuries related to participation in college and professional sports. Following the civil war, a number of scholars and physicians with vision believed that physical education programs should be developed and promote exercise that would improve health-related fitness, not sports and games. They founded and led the "physical education" movement and were the proponents of moderate exercise for all, focusing on bodily development and health instruction. However, the popularity of sports was increasing. Consequently, the majority of physical education programs focused on sports and games. Physical education gradually became associated with sports skills, and those who taught physical education classes were generally coaches. Accordingly, they focused on highly skilled students and neglected the less athletically inclined majority.

The debate between health-related fitness and skill-related fitness physical education programs continued to exist [12]. Harvard educator Dudley Allen Sargent was motivated to understand how exercise prescription could make the weak strong and the strong well and ensure a course of action that would attack the incipient forms of diseases. While Sargent was not an exercise physiologist, he was a physical educator and conducted seminal observational studies using physical examinations, strength assessments, and anthropometric measurements to assess human performance. His work framed questions related to understanding how individuals varied in size, strength, and development compared to the mean values for the same age and sex. He developed simple tests such as the Sargent vertical jump test and the 40-yard dash which have been used for decades to assess power, explosive strength, and speed. Clearly, one can appreciate the diversity in body types, or somatotypes, ranging from ectomorph to mesomorph to endomorph. However, physical fitness was not promoted in the United States as was in Europe and, despite the attempts of scholars such as Dr. J.C. Warren and Catherine Beecher, remained missing from the public education system for the better part of the nineteenth century [10].

In 1887, the physician, J. William White, a faculty member at the University of Pennsylvania, wrote: "Let it be understood that the main object and idea of exercise is the acquirement or preservation of health; that it is by far the most important therapeutic and hygienic agency at the command of the physician of today; that it can be prescribed on as rational a basis with as distinct reference to the correction of existing troubles or the prevention of threatened ones as any of the drugs of the pharmacopeia" [13]. By 1900, all states required instruction in the "Laws of Health," which became part of the curriculum of "physical education." The earliest books about physical fitness were "*Health, Strength and Power*", written by Harvard M.D. Dudley Sargent in 1904 [14] and *Exercise in Education and Medicine*, published in 1909 by R. Tait McKenzie, a University of Pennsylvania physician and physical educator [15].

At the beginning of the twentieth century, the decadence of the twenties and the great depression that followed shifted the nations' emphasis elsewhere, and up to World War II, fitness was ignored [10, 16, 17]. During this time, two reports prompted action towards emphasis on fitness. First, The World War II statistics gathered on draftees revealed a gloomy picture on the physical fitness of young men. Of the nine million registrants, almost three million were not qualified to serve for physical and mental reasons [16, 18]. Shortly after, the finding of muscular fitness of schoolchildren released in 1954 was equally disturbing. The Kraus-Weber test consisted of six simple movements of key muscle groups was administered to US children. Almost 58% of the children failed the test compared to only 8.7% of European children [19]. These findings prompted President Eisenhower to call for a special White House Conference, held in 1956. As a result of this, the President's Council on Youth Fitness and the President's Citizens Advisory Committee on the Fitness of American Youth were formed.

An important departure from the random approach to physical activity and fitness also came during the 1940s. Dr. Thomas K. Cureton at the University of Illinois introduced the application of research to fitness. Dr. Cureton recognized the numerous benefits of regular exercise and strived to answer questions concerning on the type and volume of exercise required to achieved health. He also developed fitness tests for muscular strength and flexibility and cardiorespiratory endurance. His research resulted in multiple recommendations for the improvement of cardiorespiratory fitness, including the identification of exercise intensity guidelines necessary for improved fitness levels. His suggestions became the fundamental basis behind future exercise programs. This is an enormous contribution because it propelled physical activity, human performance, and health from the hearsay to a discipline governed by scientific principles.

In 1954, the American College of Sports Medicine (ACSM) was formed. Perhaps this is the most important and a pivotal event in the history of physical activity and health. Throughout its history, ACSM has established position stands on various exercise-related issues based on scientific research. The College has been one of the premier organizations in the promotion of health and fitness to the American society and worldwide and provides merit and legitimacy to the coming fitness movement [12].

In the 1960s, President John F. Kennedy was a major proponent of fitness and its health-related benefits to the American people. Kennedy spoke openly about the need for American citizens to improve their fitness levels including writing an article in *Sports Illustrated* entitled "The Soft American." He said, "We are under-exercised as a nation; we look instead of play; we ride instead of walk" [20, 21]. Kennedy prompted the federal government to become more involved in national fitness promotion and started youth programs. In a statement that is reminiscent of ancient Greek philosophical concepts on fitness and health, Kennedy said that "For physical fitness is not only one of the most important keys to a healthy body; it is the basis of dynamic and creative intellectual activity. The relationship between the soundness of the body and the activities of the mind is subtle and complex. Much is not yet understood. But we do know what the Greeks knew: that intelligence and skill can only function at the peak of their capacity when the body is healthy and strong; that hardy spirits and tough minds usually inhabit sound bodies" [20, 21].

Perhaps the most influential individual for the popularity and promotion of exercise and fitness in the United States and around the world was Dr. Kenneth Cooper. He is generally credited with encouraging more individuals to exercise than any other individual in history. The publication of his first book entitled *Aerobics* in 1968 expended the concept of fitness beyond the high school or college gyms. Almost overnight exercise and fitness became popular. He coined the word "aerobics" for activities such as running, biking, swimming, and walking and proclaimed that such activities are the best exercises to promote fitness. In addition, the book sent a powerful message to the American people to prevent the development of chronic diseases, exercise regularly, and maintain high fitness levels throughout life. Cooper advocated a philosophy that shifted away from disease treatment to one of disease prevention.

Physical Activity, Exercise Capacity, and Health

The fifties marked the beginning of the scientific scrutiny of the association between physical activity and health. In 1953, a landmark study was published in the distinguished British medical journal *The Lancet* [22]. In this study, Dr. Morris and his co-workers observed that mail handlers who walked to deliver the mail and bus conductors who climbed up and down the stairs of the double-decker busses were dying from cardiovascular disease at half the rate of bus drivers and postal workers with desk jobs. This finding sparked an interest worldwide. A number of scientific investigations followed from different countries reached the same conclusion: The death rate for physically active individuals was about half compared to that of sedentary.

In the 1970s, several studies published by Professor Paffenbarger and his co-workers assessed mortality risk related to occupational physical work of longshoremen and leisure time physical activity of Harvard alumni [23–26]. These studies concluded that increased physical activity was associated with lower risk of coronary mortality [longshoremen] and the risk of fatal and nonfatal myocardial infarctions. Several important findings of these studies had public health relevance. First, reduction in risk was only evident if physical activity was maintained throughout life. Those who played varsity sports but did not maintain a physically active lifestyle had higher mortality rate compared to those who maintained a physically active lifestyle in adulthood. Moreover, those who avoided athletics in college but subsequently took up a more active lifestyle also had similarly low rates of mortality [25]. Second, there was a consistent, inverse, and graded association toward lower all-cause mortality rate; as physical activity-related caloric expenditure increased from 500 Kcal to 2000 Kcal per week, the mortality rate decreased. Third, the investigators speculated that physical activity accounted for approximately 1–2 years of additional life. Finally, for the first time, there was evidence suggesting excessive exercise may be harmful. The investigators observed that an increase, although slight, in mortality risk in those expending more than 3500 Kcal per week [25, 26]. This will be equivalent to about 30–35 miles of jogging per week.

The Aerobic Center Longitudinal Study, a prospective, observational cohort study, was designed to examine the effects of physical activity and fitness on various health outcomes. Over the years, this study, under the direction of Professor Steven Blair, has provided a wealth of epidemiologic evidence to support the association and benefits of regular exercise and health. Dr. Blair's work clearly demonstrated that most of the exercise-related health benefits are realized at moderate-intensity physical activities such as brisk walking most days a week for approximately 30–40 min per session. This was

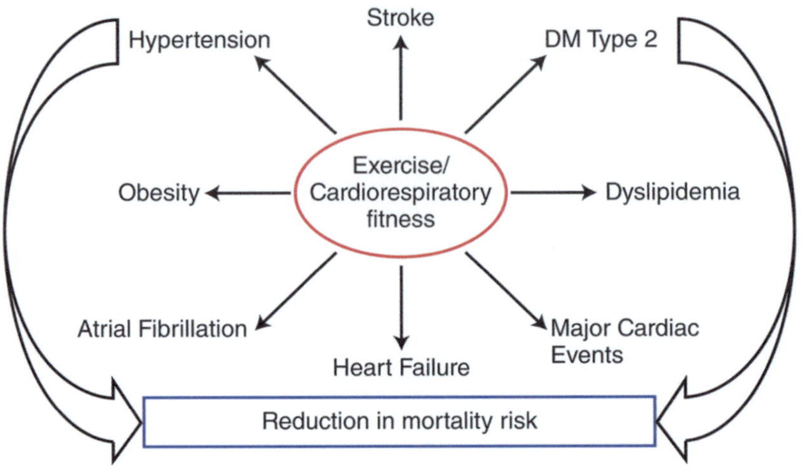

Fig. 1.1 Exercise effects on chronic illness and mortality

of enormous public health significance as this level of physical activity is well tolerated by most middle-aged and older individuals. It was also a paradigm shift for the concept of high-intensity exercise that prevailed during the decade of the 1970s and 1980s [27, 28].

As a wealth of scientific evidence accumulated over the years, it became increasingly more convincing that physical activity is the cheapest and perhaps the single most powerful deterrent for a number of chronic diseases that plague the human race. In general, their findings are based on middle-aged and relatively healthy cohorts. In addition, many of these cohorts lack comorbidities and medications of the participants.

At the beginning of the twenty-first century, a number of relatively large prospective epidemiologic studies assessed the cardiorespiratory fitness (CRF) and health association in US veterans from two Veterans Affairs Medical Centers in Washington, DC (Drs. Peter Kokkinos and Charles Faselis), and Palo Alto, CA (Dr. Jonathan Myers) with multiple cardiac risk factors, and chronic disease referred for an exercise tolerance test for clinical reasons. In general, these studies have strongly supported a strong, inverse, and graded association between the incidence of chronic disease (hypertension, type 2 DM, atrial fibrillation, major cardiac events, heart failure, etc.) and the risk of all-cause mortality (Fig. 1.1). In addition, these studies provided strong evidence that the cost of health care is significantly reduced by small gains in CRF [29–50].

The unique contributions of these studies are noteworthy. First, the cohort consisted of middle-aged or older black and white males with multiple comorbidities. Second, detailed information on the medication used to treat chronic illness of the participants allowed investigators to assess the interaction between CRF and certain medications [44, 49, 50]. Finally, equal access to health care independent of financial status and the electronic health records that exist in the Veterans Affairs Healthcare System minimized the influence of disparities in medical care and also enabled the investigators to account for prior history and alterations in health status and the interactions between certain medications and CRF.

A Call to Action

Despite the overwhelming evidence on the impact of CRF on human health, the alarming increase of obesity in both adults and children, and the related health consequences, efforts to foster a physically active lifestyle nationwide have been sporadic and with questionable success.

In 1992, physical inactivity was declared an independent risk factor for the development of CHD equal in status to the traditional risk factors of HTN, DM, dyslipidemia, and smoking [51]. In 1996, the Surgeon General's Report on Physical Activity and Health [52], the Center for Disease Control, the American Heart Association, and a number of other health agencies have declared physical inactivity as a health hazard for all people. It is now recognized by authorities that increasing physical activity is an important public health objective of equal importance as sound nutrition, the use of seat belts, and the prevention of adverse health effects of tobacco use. The main message that the government and health organizations want to get across is that "People can substantially improve their health and Quality of life by including moderate amounts of physical activity in their daily lives." The report continues by stating the amount of physical activity and recommended that every US adult should accumulate 30 min of moderate-intensity physical activity on most, preferably all, days of the week.

In the summer of 2007, the American Heart Association and the American College of Sports Medicine issued two reports on exercise recommendations for the public [53, 54]. The central message of these reports is that all adults should participate in daily physical activity. The reports also clearly quantify the recommended amount of exercise needed for health (150 min of moderate-intensity aerobic physical activity for a minimum of 30 min on 5 days each week and aerobic activity for a minimum of 20 min on 3 days each week). Resistance exercises (weight training) are also recommended to maximize strength development, flexibility, and exercise to improve balance for older adults. In 2013, the AHA Scientific Meeting, the AHA Global Congress All Hearts Need Exercise: A Global Call to Action by The American Heart Association. Finally, several publications by prominent scientists have emphasized the need to consider physical activity and CRF as part of the patient's evaluation [55].

Final Note

Despite the indisputable evidence of the association between exercise, CRF, and health benefits, it is difficult to find any progress in our fitness status as a nation since the Surgeon General's report in 1996. On the contrary, all indications are that we are becoming fatter and less fit by the day. In fact, the epidemic proportions of obesity that is sweeping across the United States and the galloping increase in the prevalence of type 2 diabetes, even in children as young as 10 years, are directly and indirectly related to the physical inactivity epidemic that is prevailing throughout the country. Approximately 55–60% of US adults are classified as overweight, and approximately 25% of these individuals are obese. Even more alarming is that children are becoming overweight and obese at progressively younger age. This trend in childhood obesity raises concerns of an even greater preponderance of adult obesity and chronic health problems. Still, many businesses allow or at least tolerate multiple "breaks" throughout the day for smoking. However, few allocate time for exercise. Perhaps it is time to give equal time to those who wish to walk as we give to those who wish to smoke.

Attempts to reverse this trend have begun on the national level. Although this is a welcoming and long overdue approach, it falls short of a long-lasting solution. We, as a nation, need to change our attitude toward fitness, sports, and diet. For several decades now, there is a debate whether physical education programs should emphasize sports or health-related fitness. This should have never been debated. The two should and must coexist, for each complements the other. Our pursuit of sports and athletics should be inspired more by the olive wreath of ancient Olympians and less by the sword of ancient gladiators.

References

1. Wuest DA, Bucher CA. Foundations of physical education and sport. St. Louis: Mosby; 1995.
2. Green P. Classical bearings: interpreting ancient history and culture. London: Thames and Hudson; 1989.

3. Grant MA. Short history of classical civilization. London: Weidenfeld and Nicolson; 1991.
4. Berryman JW. The art of medicine motion and rest: Galen on exercise and health. Lancet. 2012;380:210–1.
5. Berryman JW. Exercise is medicine: a historical perspective. Curr Sports Med Rep. 2010;9(4):1–7.
6. Grant M. The birth of Western civilization: Greece and Rome. New York: McGraw-Hill; 1964.
7. Harris HA. Sport in Greece and Rome. Ithaca: Cornell University Press; 1972.
8. Randers-Pehrson JD. Barbarians and Romans: the birth struggle of Europe, A.D. 400–700. Norman: University of Oklahoma Press; 1993.
9. Matthews DO. A historical study of the aims, contents, and methods of Swedish, Danish, and German gymnastics. Proceedings National College Physical Education Association for Men 1969.
10. Welch PD. History of American physical education and sport. 2nd ed. Springfield: Charles C. Thomas; 1996.
11. Karolides NJ, Karolides M. Focus on fitness. Santa Barbara: ABC-CLIO; 1993.
12. Barrow HM, Brown JP. Man and movement: principles of physical education. 4th ed. Philadelphia: Lea & Febiger; 1988.
13. White JW. A physician's view of exercise and athletics. Lippincott's 1887;39:1008–33.
14. Sargent DA. Health, strength & power. Boston: H.M. Caldwell; 1904.
15. RT MK. Exercise in education and medicine. Philadelphia: W.B. Saunders; 1909.
16. Rice EA, Hutchinson JL, Lee M. A brief history of physical education. New York: The Ronald Press Co; 1958.
17. Jenkins PA. History of the United States. New York: St. Martin's Press; 1997.
18. Nieman DC. Fitness and sports medicine: an introduction. Palo Alto: Bull Publishing Co; 1990.
19. Kraus H, Hirschland R. Minimum muscular fitness tests in school children. Res Q. 1954;25:178.
20. Kennedy, J.F. The soft American. Sports Illustrated 1960;13:15–17.
21. Kennedy, J.F. The vigor we need. Sports Illustrated 1962;17:12–15.
22. Morris JN, Heady JA, Raffle PA, Roberts CG, Parks JW. Coronary heart-disease and physical activity of work. Lancet. 1953;265(6796):1111–20.
23. Paffenbarger RS, Hale WE. Work activity and coronary heart mortality. N Engl J Med. 1975;292(11):545–50.
24. Paffenbarger RS Jr, Wing AL, Hyde RT. Physical activity as an index of heart attack risk in college alumni. Am J Epidemiol. 1978;108(3):161–75.
25. Paffenbarger RS Jr, Hyde RT, Wing AL, Hsieh CC. Physical activity, all-cause mortality, and longevity of college alumni. N Engl J Med. 1986;314(10):605–13.
26. Paffenbarger RS Jr, Hyde RT, Wing AL, Lee IM, Jung DL, Kampert JB. The association of changes in physical-activity level and other lifestyle characteristics with mortality among men. N Engl J Med. 1993;328(8):538–45.
27. Blair SN, Kampert JB, Kohl HW, Barlow CE, Macera CA, Paffenbarger RS, et al. Influences of cardiorespiratory fitness and other precursors on cardiovascular disease and all-cause mortality in men and women. JAMA. 1996;276(3):205–10.
28. Blair SN, Kohl HW, Paffenbarger RS Jr, Clark DG, Cooper KH, Gibbons LW. Physical fitness and all-cause mortality. A prospective study of healthy men and women. JAMA. 1989;262(17):2395–401.
29. Blair SN, Kohl HW, Barlow CE, Paffenbarger RS Jr, Gibbons LW, Macera CA. Changes in physical fitness and all-cause mortality. A prospective study of healthy and unhealthy men. JAMA. 1995;293(14):1093–8.
30. Kokkinos P, Myers J. Exercise and physical activity: clinical outcomes and applications. Circulation. 2010;122:1637–48.
31. Faselis C, Doumas M, Kokkinos JP, Panagiotakos D, Kheirbek R, Sheriff HM, et al. Exercise capacity and progression from prehypertension to hypertension. Hypertension. 2012;60:333–8.
32. Kokkinos P, Faselis C, Myers J, Sui X, Zhang J, Tsimploulis A, et al. Exercise capacity and risk of chronic kidney disease in US veterans: a cohort study. Mayo Clin Proc. 2015;90:461–8.
33. Faselis C, Kokkinos P, Tsimploulis A, Pittaras A, Myers J, Lavie CJ, et al. Exercise capacity and atrial fibrillation risk in veterans. A Cohort Study Mayo Clin Proc. 2016;91:558–66.
34. Kokkinos PF, Faselis C, Myers J, Narayan P, Sui X, Zhang J, et al. Cardiorespiratory fitness and incidence of major adverse cardiovascular events in US veterans: a cohort study. Mayo Clin Proc. 2017;92:39–48.
35. Myers J, Kokkinos P, Chan K, Dandekar E, Yilmaz B, Nagare A, et al. Cardiorespiratory fitness and reclassification of risk for incidence of heart failure: the veterans exercise testing study. Circ Heart Fail. 2017;10:e003780.
36. Myers J, Prakash M, Froelicher V, Do D, Partington S, Atwood JE. Exercise capacity and mortality among men referred for exercise testing. N Engl J Med. 2002;346:793–801.
37. Kokkinos P, Myers J, Kokkinos JP, Pittaras A, Narayan P, Manolis A, et al. Exercise capacity and mortality in black and white men. Circulation. 2008;117:614–22.
38. Kokkinos P, Myers J, Nylen E, Panagiotakos DB, Manolis A, Pittaras A, et al. Exercise capacity and all-cause mortality in African American and Caucasian men with type 2 diabetes. Diabetes Care. 2009;32:623–8.
39. Kokkinos P, Manolis A, Pittaras A, Doumas M, Giannelou A, Panagiotakos DB, et al. Exercise capacity and mortality in hypertensive men with and without additional risk factors. Hypertension. 2009;53:494–9.
40. Kokkinos P, Doumas M, Myers J, Faselis C, Manolis A, Pittaras A, et al. A graded association of exercise capacity and all-cause mortality in males with high-normal blood pressure. Blood Press. 2009;18:261–7.
41. Kokkinos P, Myers J, Doumas M, Faselis C, Manolis A, Pittaras A, Kokkinos JP, Singh S, Fletcher

RD. Exercise capacity and all-cause mortality in prehypertensive men. Am J Hypertens. 2009;22:735–41.
42. Kokkinos P, Myers J, Faselis C, Doumas M, Kheirbek R, Nylen E. BMI-mortality paradox and fitness in African American and Caucasian men with type 2 diabetes. Diabetes Care. 2012;35:1021–7.
43. Kokkinos P, Faselis C, Myers J, Kokkinos JP, Doumas M, Pittaras A, et al. Statin therapy, fitness, and mortality risk in middle-aged hypertensive male veterans. Am J Hypertens. 2014;27:422–30.
44. Kokkinos PF, Faselis C, Myers J, Panagiotakos D, Doumas M. Interactive effects of fitness and statin treatment on mortality risk in veterans with dyslipidaemia: a cohort study. Lancet. 2013;381:394–9.
45. Kokkinos P, Faselis C, Myers J, Pittaras A, Sui X, Zhang J, McAuley P, Kokkinos JP. Cardiorespiratory fitness and the paradoxical BMI-mortality risk association in male veterans. Mayo Clin Proc. 2014;89:754–62.
46. Kokkinos P, Faselis C, Myers J, Sui X, Zhang J, Blair SN. Age-specific exercise capacity threshold for mortality risk assessment in male veterans. Circulation. 2014;130:653–8.
47. McAuley PA, Kokkinos PF, Oliveira RB, Emerson BT, Myers JN. Obesity paradox and cardiorespiratory fitness in 12,417 male veterans aged 40 to 70 years. Mayo Clin Proc. 2010;85:115–21.
48. Myers J, Lata K, Chowdhury S, McAuley P, Jain N, Froelicher V. The obesity paradox and weight loss. Am J Med. 2011;124:924–30.
49. Nylen ES, Faselis C, Kheirbek R, Myers J, Panagiotakos D, Kokkinos P. Statins modulate the mortality risk associated with obesity and cardiorespiratory fitness in diabetics. J Clin Endocrinol Metab. 2013;98:3394–401.
50. Kokkinos P, Faselis C, Narayan P, Myers J, Nylen E, Sui X, et al. Cardiorespiratory fitness and incidence of type 2 diabetes in United States veterans on statin therapy. Am J Med. 2017;130:1192–8.
51. American Heart Association Position Statement. Circulation. 1992;86(1):340–4.
52. United States Department of Health and Human Services: a report by the Surgeon General. 1996.
53. Haskell WL, Lee IM, Pate RR, et al. Physical activity and public health: updated recommendation for adults from the American College of Sports Medicine and the American Heart Association. Circulation. 2007;116(9):1081–93.
54. Williams MA, Haskell WL, Ades PA, et al. Resistance exercise in individuals with and without cardiovascular disease: 2007 update: a scientific statement from the American Heart Association Council on clinical cardiology and council on nutrition, physical activity, and metabolism. Circulation. 2007;116(5):572–84.
55. Ross R, Blair SN, Arena R, et al. Importance of assessing cardiorespiratory fitness in clinical practice: a case for fitness as a clinical vital sign: a scientific statement from the American Heart Association. Circulation. 2016;134(24):e653–99.

Exercise, Gene Regulation, and Cardiometabolic Disease

2

Mark A. Chapman and Carl Johan Sundberg

Abbreviations

CMD	Cardiometabolic disease
miRNA	MicroRNA
RISC	RNA-induced silencing complex
PGC-1α	Peroxisome proliferator-activated receptor gamma coactivator 1-alpha
T2D	Type II diabetes
OXPHOS	Oxidative phosphorylation
HATs	Histone acetyltransferases
HDACs	Histone deacetylases

Introduction

This chapter deals with the regulation of gene activity in cardiometabolic disease (CMD) and how exercise/physical activity can alter gene expression to ameliorate CMD. The definition of physical activity is "bodily movement produced by skeletal muscles that results in energy expenditure," encompassing all types, intensities, and domains [1]. Exercise is defined as "physical activity that is planned, structured, repetitive, and designed to improve or maintain physical fitness, physical performance, or health" [1].

The adaptations that follow regular exercise training over weeks, months, and years are induced by cellular signaling events, including protein modifications and changes in gene activity in various tissues. In connection with each exercise session, the internal environment is affected. Some of these changes, often referred to as stimuli, are biophysical, e.g., increased body temperature, lowered O_2 pressure, increased vascular wall shear stress (friction) resulting from higher blood flow, and mechanical tension in the heart, skeletal muscles, and tendons. Additionally, biochemical stimuli include changes in cytoplasmic calcium concentrations, pH, adenosine monophosphate/adenosine triphosphate (AMP/ATP) ratio, and reactive oxygen species (ROS) abundance. Furthermore, physiological stimuli during exercise constitute the release of growth factors and cytokines, enhanced immune cell activity, hormone level changes, acetylcholine release from α-motor neuron activation, and the arrival of blood-borne substrates. The level of change of specific stimuli depends on exercise type (e.g., endurance or strength) and dose (intensity, duration, and frequency), which influences the nature and magnitude of the training response.

M. A. Chapman
Department of Physiology and Pharmacology, Karolinska Institutet, Solna, Sweden

Department of Integrated Engineering, University of San Diego, San Diego, CA, USA
e-mail: markchapman@sandiego.edu

C. J. Sundberg (✉)
Department of Physiology and Pharmacology, Department of Learning, Informatics, Management and Ethics, Karolinska Institutet, Stockholm, Sweden
e-mail: Carl.J.Sundberg@ki.se

P. Kokkinos, P. Narayan (eds.), *Cardiorespiratory Fitness in Cardiometabolic Diseases*, https://doi.org/10.1007/978-3-030-04816-7_2

The exercise-induced stimuli described above result in gene expression changes that, in turn, cause adaptation in numerous tissues within the body. Additionally, physical inactivity, obesity, and type II diabetes are all associated with changes in gene expression patterns. The altered gene expression states in these disorders arise, in part, from elevated blood glucose levels, insulin resistance, and inflammatory factors [2, 3]. As a way to better understand how physical activity can be beneficial for cardiometabolic disease risk factors and symptoms, this chapter will specifically discuss gene regulation in metabolically active tissues implicated in cardiometabolic diseases and how physical activity has the potential to improve health via alterations in gene expression. Before we specifically discuss gene regulation in cardiometabolic disease, it is important to discuss gene regulation in general.

Gene Regulation

The control of gene expression takes place at various levels between the original gene sequences in DNA and the production of a functional protein. Despite the various levels of gene expression control, perhaps the most important step, and the one that will be the focus of this chapter, is transcriptional control. Transcription is the first step in gene expression where DNA is transcribed into various forms of RNA transcripts [4]. Numerous processes take place to either prevent or promote the transcription of genes. Among these processes are the binding of gene regulatory proteins (i.e., transcription factors) to DNA, local chromatin structure reorganization via covalent histone modifications, and covalent modifications directly on DNA nucleotides. These covalent alterations affecting gene expression are termed epigenetic modifications. In addition to these processes that regulate gene transcription, this chapter will touch on some processes that affect the presence and stability of mature mRNA transcripts.

Transcription Factor Binding

Gene regulatory proteins, or, more commonly, transcription factors, bind to DNA in order to either positively or negatively regulate gene expression [4]. Sections of genes called enhancers and promoters are particularly important for gene regulation because protein binding at these two sites is critical for the initiation of transcription [4]. Transcription factors bind and assemble at the gene promoter – a region upstream of the gene to be transcribed. Additional proteins bind, including RNA polymerase, and the RNA polymerase is maneuvered into position between DNA strands [4]. This group of transcription factors, RNA mediator proteins, and RNA polymerase is called the transcription initiation complex. Once the transcription initiation complex is assembled, activator proteins bound to an area upstream of the promoter (the enhancer region) make contact with the transcription initiation complex, causing transcription initiation [4]. Gene regulation at the point of transcription initiation is a common way that gene expression is controlled. Specifically, the presence or absence of transcription factors plays a large role in the activation or silencing of genes. As this chapter will highlight, several transcription factors and the corresponding gene expression are associated with cardiometabolic disease. Additionally, physical activity has the ability to alter the presence of various transcription factors and potentially influence the gene expression profile in tissues important in cardiometabolic disease.

Epigenetic Control: Histone Modifications

In order to understand the role of histone modifications on gene expression, it is important to understand how DNA is organized within the nucleus of our cells. DNA is tightly packed around a group of eight core histone proteins called a nucleosome. The nucleosome is composed of a group of four core histone proteins (H2A, H2B, H3, and H4) grouped together as two H2A/H2B dimers and an H3/H4 tetramer [4]. Generally, DNA in contact with the nucleosome is inaccessible for protein binding, and thus, gene transcription is inhibited. Alternatively, DNA can unravel from nucleosomes, making it available for transcription to occur. Histones within nucleosomes can be covalently modified resulting in DNA rearrangement around histones, histone protein removal, or histone insertion to either promote or inhibit gene expression. These histone modifications are diverse and include methylation, acetylation, ubiquitylation, phosphorylation, SUMOylation, citrullination, and ADP-ribosylation [4].

The complex of DNA and histones is termed chromatin and is found in either the "transcriptionally available" state of euchromatin or "transcriptionally unavailable" state of heterochromatin [4]. The covalent modifications mentioned above play a large role in dictating whether the chromatin is in the euchromatic or heterochromatic state. The most common histone modifications that dictate chromatin state, and the ones to be discussed throughout this chapter, are acetylation and methylation. Specifically, acetylation of histone proteins H3 and H4 and di- and trimethylation of lysine 4 on the H3 protein subunit, denoted as H3K4me2 (dimethylated) or H3K4me3 (trimethylated), correspond to a euchromatic region open for transcription. However, transcriptionally repressed heterochromatic regions are associated with minimal acetylation and methylation of H3K9 and H3K27 [5, 6].

Epigenetic Control: DNA Methylation

In addition to covalent modifications on histones that affect gene transcription, methyl groups can bind directly to DNA itself to influence gene expression. Generally, DNA methylation in gene promoters is associated with gene silencing. This gene silencing is thought to block the binding of proteins to DNA important for transcription initiation. Furthermore, there is a set of proteins that specifically bind to methylated DNA thereby blocking other proteins from binding [4]. DNA methylation primarily occurs in CpG islands of the genome, which are areas dense in cytosine bases followed by a guanine nucleotide. These CpG islands typically correspond with promoter regions of genes, especially near common housekeeping genes [4]. Cytosine methylation is an effective way to silence genes that are not expressed in a particular cell type. Simply put, since every cell nucleus contains the entire genome, DNA methylation is a way to silence genes that are not required for a particular cell type. For example, a cardiomyocyte does not need genes for the production of bile, so these genes would be silenced. In addition to epigenetically silencing genes that are not important for a particular cell's function, DNA methylation also functions to transcriptionally regulate genes in response to environmental changes [6]. In this way, DNA methylation acts to acutely regulate gene expression via methylation and demethylation of particular nucleotides.

miRNA

In addition to transcriptional control, gene expression can also be altered once a fully functional mRNA transcript is created. This is accomplished in various ways, but this chapter will focus on microRNAs (miRNA). miRNA decreases or completely inhibits translation by first binding to a group of proteins to create an RNA-induced silencing complex (RISC) [7]. The assembled RISC then binds to complementary nucleotide sequences in the mRNA transcript. RISC binding on mRNA transcripts in eukaryotes typically leads to inefficient translation and a degradation of the poly-A tail on the mRNA transcript [4]. This destabilization of the transcript ultimately leads to its degradation and inhibition of protein translation.

Gene Regulation in CMD

Prior to discussing the genetic and epigenetic alterations that occur with exercise training, it is important to first understand the genetic and epigenetic landscape of cardiometabolic disease. Recently, a significant amount of work has been done examining gene regulation in individuals with cardiometabolic disease in an effort to understand the underlying mechanisms of the disease. Here, we will outline some of the major recent findings that examine how CMD influences the expression of genes critical for maintaining a healthy efficient metabolism.

Transcription Factors and Co-regulators

Perhaps the most important regulator in metabolism is peroxisome proliferator-activated receptor gamma coactivator 1-alpha (PGC-1α). PGC-1α is a transcriptional coactivator that binds to a diverse array of transcription factors to regulate gene expression related to mitochondrial biogenesis, glucose/fatty acid metabolism, and fiber-type switching in skeletal muscle [8, 9]. Unlike transcription factors, coactivators, such as PGC-1α, do not bind directly to DNA. Instead they bind to transcription factors to influence gene expression. PGC-1α binds to a diverse array of transcription factors, making it a potent activator of the genes associated with those transcription factors. The transcription factors that PGC-1α binds to and the subsequent activation of associated genes have been extensively described in comprehensive reviews and thus will not be discussed in full detail here [8, 9]. In short, there are several transcription factors that PGC-1α targets, a majority of which influence the transcription of genes encoding mitochondrial proteins, namely, NRF-1, NRF-2, PPARα, PPARδ, ERRα, and TR [8, 10, 11]. These transcription factors go on to stimulate the expression of various genes associated with ATP production, specifically genes associated with fatty acid beta-oxidation, the Krebs cycle, and oxidative phosphorylation [8]. In addition to its role in mitochondrial gene expression, PGC-1α also has been shown to play a large role in CMD.

Given the important role that PGC-1α has in maintaining a healthy metabolism, one should not be surprised that its expression is affected in CMD. In type II diabetes (T2D), there is a large body of evidence demonstrating a coordinated downregulation in genes that are stimulated by PGC-1α [12–15]. Specifically, these studies examined skeletal muscle from individuals with T2D using microarrays to examine the genes expressed in each biopsy. Interestingly, these studies showed a systemic downregulation of genes associated with oxidative phosphorylation (OXPHOS) in diabetic muscle compared with muscle from individuals with normal glucose control. Furthermore, Mootha et al. identified a co-regulated subset of OXPHOS-associated genes (OXPHOS-CR) that are controlled by PGC-1α, which demonstrated a significantly lower expression in T2D compared with nondiabetic humans [12]. Following the identification of these OXPHOS-CR genes, this study went on to find a relationship ($r^2 = 0.22$, $P = 0.0012$) between the expression level of these genes and overall metabolic performance as measured by VO_2 max [12]. This study demonstrates that the control of these OXPHOS-CR genes by PGC-1α is critical for proper metabolic health and function of skeletal muscle. Since the identification of PGC-1α as a major influencer of mitochondrial biogenesis and controller of metabolism, numerous studies have shown that with the downregulation of PGC-1α, there is a decrease in transcription of genes associated with metabolism and mitochondrial health [8, 16, 17]. This decreased gene expression then leads to decreased OXPHOS, lipid oxidation, accumulation of lipids in skeletal muscle, and ultimately insulin resistance, obesity, and diabetes [13]. It should be pointed out though that a causal relationship is difficult to prove – that is, is the downregulation of PGC-1α and its effectors a cause or the consequence of metabolic disease? It is likely that the majority of patients with T2D are also rather physically inactive and have lower aerobic fitness than a control population.

As described above, the consequences of PGC-1α downregulation in the skeletal muscle of patients with CMD are severe. However, CMD is also associated with altered PGC-1α gene expression in other metabolically active tissues (i.e., liver and pancreas). PGC-1α expression levels in the liver are generally much lower than in skeletal muscle, but they rise significantly in the fasted state [18]. Increased PGC-1α expression in the liver results in the activation of the fatty acid oxidation pathway. Additionally, PGC-1α activates genes involved in gluconeogenesis, which is normally important for avoiding hypoglycemia during fasting [8, 18]. However, PGC-1α is also highly expressed in the non-fasted liver of diabetic and obese people, which then can lead to hyperglycemia [18]. Furthermore, elevated PGC-1α levels in the liver can promote insulin resistance by induction of TRB-3, which inhibits Akt, a major player in the insulin pathway. Similar to the liver, pancreatic islet cells have elevated levels of PGC-1α in animal models of T2D and obesity [18, 19]. Additionally, insulin secretion is inhibited by the overexpression of PGC-1α in islet cells, suggesting an avenue in which PGC-1α can induce or exacerbate the diabetic condition [20]. Interestingly, in diabetic or obese humans, the exact opposite PGC-1α expression pattern is found [21]. A causal link was also shown in the same study where decreased PGC-1α expression was experimentally induced using siRNA knockdown of PGC-1α in healthy human islet cells. Decreased insulin secretion was seen in the cells with PGC-1α knockdown, confirming the findings seen in diabetic patients.

Up until this point, we have shown that PGC-1α expression and the genes it regulates are significantly reduced in individuals with CMD, but how exactly is the expression of PGC-1α decreased in CMD? To answer this question, many recent studies have focused on the epigenetic regulation of PGC-1α and found there to be significant alterations in the methylation patterns in the regions regulating PGC-1α [16, 17, 21–25]. These data beg the question – is it the methylation patterns causing these changes, or is it obesity, lifestyle, and diabetes that cause these methylation changes? In an attempt to answer this question, researchers recruited 20 young healthy men with no family history of T2D to examine the effects of 10 days of bedrest on insulin sensitivity and muscle gene expression [16]. The goal behind this study was to determine the mechanisms behind how inactivity can lead to metabolic disease through alterations in gene expression. Interestingly, insulin sensitivity decreased in response to bedrest, and this was accompanied by dramatic changes in muscle gene expression, including decreased PGC-1α expression. The decreased expression of PGC-1α was accompanied with a corresponding increase in methylation of the promoter region of PGC-1α, which is in line with other studies showing decreased PGC-1α expression with increased promoter methylation [17, 21]. The results from that study begin to shed light on how lifestyle choices, such as inactivity, can lead to insulin resistance and, eventually, T2D. It also highlights the fact that, in healthy humans not predisposed to T2D, a new epigenetic landscape develops with inactivity that leads to changes in gene expression and ultimately to a metabolic syndrome phenotype.

In a separate study attempting to link epigenetic alterations and CMD, Wahl and colleagues identified 187 CpG sites in the genome that are associated with body mass index (BMI) [26]. The study measured genome methylation from blood samples from over 5000 individuals to identify CpG sites associated with adiposity. Interestingly, through causality analyses, the authors were able to show that the altered methylation with adiposity was actually a consequence, and not the cause, of increased BMI. That study provided further evidence that the disease state is able to influence the epigenome and thus gene expression in CMD. Researchers in the field suggest that in addition to BMI influencing "classic" markers of CMD, such as hypertension, we should be aware that disease can be caused by an alteration in gene expression initiated from lifestyle choices [27].

Transgenerational Epigenetics

In addition to epigenetics influencing how our own genes are expressed, evidence has been found highlighting the possibility of transgenerational epigenetics [28–33]. Epigenetic alterations were once thought to not be inherited from previous generations because during development the entire genome is cleansed of all epigenetic modifications [34]. Despite this reprogramming of the epigenome, new evidence shows that some epigenetic patterns can indeed be inherited. In mice, for example, it has been shown that offspring with prediabetic fathers have an increased likelihood of developing diabetes [31]. This inherited metabolic condition was hypothesized to be linked to epigenetic patterns present in sperm that are passed down to the next generation. These epigenetic patterns are preserved, potentially through the presence of spermatozoal RNAs, and passed on to the next generations [29]. In addition to factors following egg fertilization that influence epigenetic patterns in offspring, there is also evidence that diet and exercise influence the epigenetic landscape of a developing embryo [28]. This is a newly developing field with primarily epidemiological data, and more research into the mechanisms behind transgenerational epigenetics is necessary to prove definitive links.

Inflammation and CMD

Another large player in CMD is the presence of chronic inflammatory markers in individuals with CMD. "Classic" inflammatory markers such as C-reactive protein (CRP), interleukin 6 (IL-6), resistin, tumor necrosis factor-α (TNF-α), interleukin 1−β (IL-1β), and nuclear factor kappa-B (NF-κB) among others are increased in CMD [35–39]. It is clear that the gene expression of these inflammatory markers is elevated in diabetic, insulin-resistant, and obese patients, but the question is, how do these inflammatory proteins affect metabolic health [40, 41]? TNF-α production and secretion by adipose tissue play a pivotal role in the development/continuation of T2D, obesity, and insulin resistance [35]. TNF-α in adipose tissue stimulates IL-6 expression in adipose tissue and blood mononuclear cells, which then goes on to systemically stimulate gene expression of numerous inflammatory cytokines, including CRP [35]. These inflammatory factors are largely stimulated by obesity and high-fat diets as well as elevated blood levels of insulin, leptin, and glucose common in metabolic syndrome [36, 41]. Additionally, the persistent presence of these inflammatory factors is implicated in insulin resistance [2, 3, 42]. Similar to PGC-1α in the previous paragraphs, gene expression of these important inflammatory factors has recently been linked to epigenetic regulation.

The epigenetic links between metabolic disease and inflammatory factors show that the changes that occur are a consequence of the condition and not the cause. For instance, in a study examining the activation of TNF-α expression, it was found that high levels of glucose in culture media result in the acetylation of histones in the promoter region of TNF-α in cultured human myocytes [43]. Acetylation of histone proteins, as described previously, is associated with an "open" euchromatic chromatin structure which allows for transcription factor binding and, ultimately, expression of the gene. In addition to that study, it has been shown in other studies that an elevated blood glucose level can influence the activity of histone acetyltransferases (HATs) and histone deacetylases (HDACs) which then go on to influence the transcriptional availability of inflammatory genes related to metabolic diseases [44]. Persistent high blood sugar seen in diabetic patients could then, in theory, maintain the euchromatic chromatin configuration in regions coding for inflammatory genes, resulting in a chronic inflammatory state. The continual expression of these inflammatory genes then results in insulin resistance, increased plasma fatty acid levels, and a positive feedback loop that promotes continual inflammatory gene expression [2, 45].

miRNA and CMD

In addition to increased inflammatory gene expression in CMD, there is also an alteration in miRNA expression that posttranscriptionally regulates many metabolic processes [7, 30, 38, 46–49]. As mentioned previously, miRNAs do not regulate gene expression transcriptionally, but instead modify the stability of existing mRNA transcripts. A review article detailing numerous miRNA families involved in metabolic disease was recently published and, thus, will not be discussed in extensive detail here [48]. To keep the discussion focused, we will just describe various miRNAs that have been examined in CMD as well as in response to exercise (to be discussed in further portions of this chapter). This discussion will result in a comprehensive understanding of how exercise-associated miRNA can potentially ameliorate the metabolic phenotype seen in CMD. With regard to CMD, miRNAs regulate various aspects of obesity and diabetes, including genes involved in insulin signaling and inflammation [48]. Unfortunately, the causal relationship between miRNAs and health has been difficult to prove – at the moment, in miRNA studies, it has been possible to detect disease-induced alterations in miRNA levels, but difficult to deduce *how* exactly they are acting [48, 50]. As such, miRNA levels can serve as markers for disease or health, but more research is clearly necessary in this relatively new and exciting field.

In terms of skeletal muscle-specific miRNA implicated in insulin resistance, the major player is miR-133a, which was found to be significantly reduced in T2D [51]. Additionally, miR-133a was found to be negatively correlated with fasting glucose levels as well as with HbA1c (percent glycosylated hemoglobin) and 2-hour glucose tolerance. It should be highlighted that an exact mechanism of action behind how miR-133a's downregulation could influence insulin resistance in skeletal muscle could not be found. In a separate study examining miRNA expression in skeletal muscle of monozygotic twins (one with T2D and the other without), it was found that glucose tolerance was related to miRNA expression [47]. In that study, 20 miRNAs were found to be significantly downregulated in the diabetic twin compared with the nondiabetic twin. Interestingly, no miRNAs were shown to be upregulated. The miRNA-15 family of miRNAs showed the most highly significant downregulation in the diabetic population compared with nondiabetic controls. There are numerous predicted mRNA targets (>900) for this miRNA family, but the most significantly affected ingenuity canonical pathway implicated was insulin signaling [47]. Again, it is important to point out that only some relationships between miRNA expression and insulin signaling genes were found and no significant effects on insulin signaling were found upon inhibition of the miRNA-15 family in vitro. Given this, further studies aimed at finding a conclusive link between miRNA levels and their influence on metabolic signaling.

Treatments for CMD to Alter Gene Expression

Although efforts have been made to treat CMD in ways that attempt to alter the aberrant gene expression patterns described above, they have seen mixed results. For instance, histone deacetylase inhibitors (HDACi), in theory, could be used to alter the acetylated state of histones to affect expression of gene associated with insulin resistance [52]. In fact, valproate, a branch-chain amino acid with HDAC inhibitor functionality, has been shown to alter insulin release, but the mechanism of action is unclear. It could stem from its HDAC inhibition properties or another mechanism. This area of research is still developing, but exercise mimetics altering gene expression via epigenetic mechanisms could potentially alter the CMD disease state. That being said, it is unlikely that such therapies could recapitulate the wide-ranging effects of exercise training. In this regard, research is showing that physical activity and exercise can actually have a broad and effective influence on gene expression to prevent/treat CMD.

Gene Regulation with Exercise

Physical activity has the ability to dramatically and robustly alter gene expression in response to both acute and long-term exercise [53, 54]. These profound gene expression changes induced by exercise alter a variety of processes in the body, including mitochondrial biogenesis, angiogenesis, and muscle hypertrophy to name a few.

However, for the interest of this chapter, we will focus on exercise-induced gene expression changes that can positively influence CMD.

As stated in the previous sections, PGC-1α is a major regulator of metabolic health in humans. It is well established that PGC-1α gene expression rapidly rises in skeletal muscle following a bout of exercise [55–58]. The implications of increased PGC-1α expression are far reaching and influence the expression of numerous genes, as described above, to promote exercise adaptation and cellular ATP production. The processes positively regulated by PGC-1α following exercise oppositely mirror the processes that occur with PGC-1α downregulation seen with CMD. Upon PGC-1α expression in muscle, gene expression of mitochondrial genes associated with biogenesis and respiration are increased [59]. In addition, increased PGC-1α expression following exercise helps to mediate the process by which cells increase expression of the glucose transporter GLUT4 [55]. Increased expression of GLUT4 corresponds to increased glucose uptake in skeletal muscle and thus improved systemic glucose control in response to both endurance and resistance training [60, 61]. Increased mitochondrial biogenesis, improved glucose control, and insulin sensitivity resulting from both aerobic and resistance training highlight the effectiveness of physical activity on CMD [46].

Just as PGC-1α expression was downregulated by epigenetic alterations in CMD, the same mechanisms are at play with physical activity to promote expression of PGC-1α. The ability for exercise to alter DNA methylation patterns was shown for the first time following an acute bout of cycling exercise [62]. In contrast to the epigenetic patterns seen in CMD discussed previously, acute exercise induced an overall hypomethylation in genes involved in mitochondrial biogenesis and energy usage, including PGC-1α. Until quite recently, epigenetic alterations to the DNA were thought to accrue over long periods of time to influence gene expression, so these findings that one acute bout of exercise could influence DNA methylation were somewhat unexpected and groundbreaking. Additionally, the researchers found that methylation at the PGC-1α promoter region preceded an increase in mRNA expression, thus strongly indicating an inverse relationship between promoter methylation and gene expression. A separate study examined the role of long-term aerobic training on the epigenetic landscape of skeletal muscle and found there to be alterations at 4000 sites in the genome, primarily in the enhancer regions of genes as opposed to the promoter regions [54]. Not only does the methylation state of healthy individuals change with exercise, but a study also found that an exercise program (composed primarily of endurance training) resulted in altered DNA methylation state [63]. Thus, although high glucose levels have the power to alter the methylation of important metabolic genes, there is strong evidence that this can be combatted with exercise training. The epigenetic response to exercise is clearly robust, and it is currently an active area of research. A vast majority of studies have performed observational studies (i.e., comparing the DNA methylation status of differently trained individuals), so a more thorough study of direct influences of training on epigenetics and pathways of metabolic disease is warranted [64].

Not only does physical activity affect the epigenetic landscape in muscle, but methylation patterns are also affected in adipose tissue. In a 6-month intervention study, the methylation status of adipose tissue from physically inactive healthy men was investigated [65]. In contrast to skeletal muscle studies, endurance exercise primarily induced an increase in DNA methylation (139 sites increased methylation; 4 decreased methylation) and a decrease in the corresponding mRNA transcript levels. Some of these changes occurred at sites known to be genes implicated in either obesity or diabetes [65]. Those data show the systemic effects that exercise has on the body and that metabolic adaptation to exercise does not only occur in skeletal muscle.

Inflammation and Exercise

Inflammation plays a large role in the adaptation process to exercise. Following an acute exercise bout, various pro-inflammatory and anti-inflammatory cytokines are released [66]. Over the long term, however, the chronic effects of exercise are anti-inflammatory in nature [35, 66]. Many of the same cytokines that are elevated in CMD, such as resistin, CRP, and TNF-α, are decreased in response to chronic exercise [35]. The mechanism by which this occurs has been suggested to be IL-6-induced. Interestingly, while IL-6 promotes inflammation in CMD, it does the opposite when released as a myokine from skeletal muscle [35]. IL-6's anti-inflammatory properties stem from its ability to inhibit the expression of TNF-α and its stimulation of IL-1ra and IL-10. Both IL-1ra and IL-10 serve to inhibit downstream pro-inflammatory cytokines including IL-1β, TNF-α, and the IL-1 receptor complex [35]. As previously discussed, since the epigenetic alterations seen in CMD with regard to inflammation are a consequence of the disease condition, they are reversible with exercise training. Indeed, following an endurance training program, various inflammatory cytokines were decreased in patients with CMD [67]. Interestingly, many genes associated with inflammatory processes were demethylated, thus demonstrating an influence of exercise on the epigenetic regulation of inflammatory genes [54]. These studies all show the potential for regular exercise to decrease the chronic low-grade inflammation that is so prominent with CMD.

miRNA

As discussed previously, miRNAs serve to post-translationally regulate gene expression. Similar to miRNA research in CMD, the studies examining miRNA expression in response to exercise are predominantly correlative. Numerous miRNAs have been shown to be exercise responsive, and many of these show opposite expression patterns when compared with CMD [50]. For instance, miRNA-133a was upregulated in serum 3 hours following an acute bout of cycling. As downregulation of miRNA-133a is associated with poor glucose handling, its upregulation following exercise could serve to improve metabolic health. The same trends for increased expression following acute exercise are seen with the miRNA-15 family [68, 69]. Kilian et al. demonstrated that circulating miR-16 was upregulated following 90 min of high-volume endurance cycling exercise, while Radom-Aizik et al. showed upregulation of circulating mir-15a following 20 min of cycling. Both of these studies also documented the upregulation of a vast array of miRNAs linked to exercise adaptation, such as vascular remodeling. Although those studies show that miRNAs downregulated in CMD are upregulated with exercise, a definitive link between their presence and healthy metabolism is lacking. As discussed previously, the current state of research primarily relegates miRNAs to biomarkers of health or disease as researchers have difficulties determining definitive roles for these molecules.

Variability in Training Response

Despite the large amount of data that suggest metabolism and fitness improve with exercise training due to alterations in gene expression, it is known that the effect size of a standardized type and dose of exercise are not uniform between individuals, i.e., there is a substantial interindividual variability in responsiveness to exercise with some individuals responding strongly ("high responders") and others less so ("low responders") [70–72]. Some of the response variability could depend on differences in pre-training status, adherence to the exercise training protocol, intake of alcohol or other drugs, and injuries or diseases but also on measurement errors and day-to-day variations [73]. High responders seem to activate key genes to a greater extent than low responders [74, 75]. Approximately 50% of the heritability for training responsiveness is explained by genetic variability [70]. Sequence differences (single-nucleotide polymorphisms, SNPs) in individual genes explain a very small fraction of the response variability, whereas sets of gene variants may explain a larger part [72, 75–77].

In an analysis of 1687 people from 5 separate studies, it was concluded that only a small fraction of people exposed to regular exercise training seem to respond poorly in the disease risk factors that were measured (blood pressure, high-density lipoprotein cholesterol, triglycerides, insulin, and cardiorespiratory fitness) [78]. In each individual, regular exercise does not influence all disease risk factors in the same way (i.e., certain risk factors will react to an exercise program, while others may not be altered). This indicates that the gene networks involved that influence disease risk factors are somewhat independent. It has also been shown that endurance training in people with T2D, irrespective of improvement in cardiorespiratory fitness, leads to significant reductions in HbA1c, waist circumference, and body fat percentage [79]. There are studies that refute the notion that there are individuals that do not respond to exercise – if the training regimen is optimized, everyone seems to improve [80].

Conclusions

Various diseases can be traced to the aberrant regulation of gene expression. As was described in this chapter, CMD is not an exception. Several metabolic abnormalities found in CMD can be linked to the misregulation of mitochondrial, metabolic, and inflammatory genes. Interestingly, many of the same processes that are negatively affected in CMD show an opposite effect with exercise training. Given this, there is strong evidence that physical activity and exercise can prevent the development of CMD as well as reverse existing cases of CMD in individuals.

References

1. Caspersen CJ, Powell KE, Christenson GM. Physical activity, exercise, and physical fitness: definitions and distinctions for health-related research. Public Health Rep. 1985;100(2):126–31.
2. Esposito K, Giugliano D. The metabolic syndrome and inflammation: association or causation? Nutr Metab Cardiovasc Dis. 2004;14:228–32.
3. Ndisang JF, Rastogi S. Cardiometabolic diseases and related complications: current status and future perspective. Biomed Res Int. 2013;2013:1–3.
4. Alberts B, Johnson A, Lewis J, Raff M, Roberts K, Walter P. Molecular biology of the cell. 5th ed. New York: Garland Science; 2008.
5. Li B, Carey M, Workman JL. The role of chromatin during transcription. Cell. 2007;128(4):707–19.
6. Portela A, Esteller M. Epigenetic modifications and human disease. Nat Biotechnol. 2010;28(10):1057–68.
7. Muhonen P, Holthofer H. Epigenetic and microRNA-mediated regulation in diabetes. Nephrol Dial Transplant. 2009;24(4):1088–96.
8. Lin J, Handschin C, Spiegelman BM. Metabolic control through the PGC-1 family of transcription coactivators. Cell Metab. 2005;1(6):361–70.
9. Liang H, Ward WF. PGC-1a: a key regulator of energy metabolism. Adv Physiol Educ. 2006;30:145–51.
10. Kelly DP, Scarpulla RC. Transcriptional regulatory circuits controlling mitochondrial biogenesis and function. Genes Dev. 2004;314:357–68.
11. Puigserver P, Spiegelman BM. Peroxisome proliferator-activated receptor-γ coactivator 1α (PGC-1α): Transcriptional coactivator and metabolic regulator. Endocr Rev. 2003;24(1):78–90.
12. Mootha VK, Lindgren CM, Eriksson K-F, Subramanian A, Sihag S, Lehar J, et al. PGC-1α-responsive genes involved in oxidative phosphorylation are coordinately downregulated in human diabetes. Nat Genet. 2003;34(3):267–73.
13. Patti ME, Butte AJ, Crunkhorn S, Cusi K, Berria R, Kashyap S, et al. Coordinated reduction of genes of oxidative metabolism in humans with insulin resistance and diabetes: Potential role of PGC1 and NRF1. Proc Natl Acad Sci. 2003;100(14):8466–71.
14. Attie AD, Kendziorski CM. PGC-1 alpha at the crossroads of type 2 diabetes. Nat Genet. 2003;34(3):244–5.
15. Mootha VK, Handschin C, Arlow D, Xie X, St. Pierre J, Sihag S, et al. Err and Gabpa/b specify PGC-1 -dependent oxidative phosphorylation gene expression that is altered in diabetic muscle. Proc Natl Acad Sci. 2004;101(17):6570–5.
16. Alibegovic AC, Sonne MP, Højbjerre L, Jacobsen S, Nilsson E, Færch K, et al. Insulin resistance induced by physical inactivity is associated with multiple transcriptional changes in skeletal muscle in young men. Am J Physiol Endocrinol Metab. 2010;299(5):752–63.
17. Barrès R, Osler ME, Yan J, Rune A, Fritz T, Caidahl K, et al. Non-CpG methylation of the PGC-1α promoter through DNMT3B controls mitochondrial density. Cell Metab. 2009;10(3):189–98.
18. Finck BN, Kelly DP. PGC-1 coactivators: inducible regulators of energy metabolism in health and disease. J Clin Invest. 2006;116(3):615–22.
19. Liu C, Lin JD. PGC-1 coactivators in the control of energy metabolism. Acta Biochim Biophys. 2010;43(4):248–57.
20. Yoon JC, Xu G, Deeney JT, Yang S, Rhee J, Puigserver P, et al. Suppression of Beta Cell Energy Metabolism and Insulin Release by PGC-1 _. Dev Cell. 2003;5:73–83.
21. Ling C, Del Guerra S, Lupi R, Rönn T, Granhall C, Luthman H, et al. Epigenetic regulation of PPARGC1A

in human type 2 diabetic islets and effect on insulin secretion. Diabetologia. 2008;51(4):615–22.
22. Sharples AP, Stewart CE, Seaborne RA. Does skeletal muscle have an "epi"-memory? The role of epigenetics in nutritional programming, metabolic disease, aging and exercise. Aging Cell. 2016;15(4):603–16.
23. Barres R, Kirchner H, Rasmussen M, Yan J, Kantor F, Krook A, et al. Weight loss after gastric bypass surgery in human obesity remodels promoter methylation. Cell Rep. 2013;3(4):1020–7.
24. Zhao J, Goldberg J, Bremner JD, Vaccarino V. Global DNA methylation is associated with insulin resistance: a monozygotic twin study. Diabetes. 2012;61(2):542–6.
25. Sookoian S, Rosselli MS, Gemma C, Burgueno AL, Gianotti TF, Castano GO, et al. Epigenetic regulation of insulin resistance in nonalcoholic fatty liver disease: impact of liver methylation of the peroxisome proliferator–activated receptor gamma coactivator 1alpha promoter. Hepatology. 2010;55:1992–2000.
26. Wahl S, Drong A, Lehne B, Loh M, Scott WR, Kunze S, et al. Epigenome-wide association study of body mass index, and the adverse outcomes of adiposity. Nature. 2017;541(7635):81–6.
27. Holmes MV, Pulit SL, Lindgren CM. Genetic and epigenetic studies of adiposity and cardiometabolic disease. Genome Med. 2017;9(82):1–4.
28. Barrès R, Zierath JR. The role of diet and exercise in the transgenerational epigenetic landscape of T2DM. Nat Rev Endocrinol [Internet]. 2016;12(8):441–51. Available from: https://doi.org/10.1038/nrendo.2016.87.
29. Schagdarsurengin U, Steger K. Epigenetics in male reproduction: effect of paternal diet on sperm quality and offspring health. Nat Rev Urol. 2016;13(10):584–95.
30. Ordovas JM, Smith CE. Epigenetics and cardiovascular disease. Nat Rev Cardiol. 2010;7(9):510–9.
31. Wei Y, Yang C, Wei Y, Zhao Z, Hou Y, Schatten H, et al. Paternally induced transgenerational inheritance of susceptibility to diabetes in mammals. Proc Natl Acad Sci. 2014;111:1873–8.
32. Morgan DK, Whitelaw E. The case for transgenerational epigenetic inheritance in humans. Mamm Genome. 2008;19:394–7.
33. Kaati G, Bygren LO, Edvinsson S. Cardiovascular and diabetes mortality determined by nutrition during parents ' and grandparents ' slow growth period. Eur J Hum Genet. 2002;10:682–8.
34. Dean W, Santos F, Reik W. Epigenetic reprogramming in early mammalian development and following somatic nuclear transfer. Semin Cell Dev Biol. 2003;14:93–100.
35. Petersen AMW, Pedersen BK. The anti-inflammatory effect of exercise. J Appl Physiol. 2005;98(4):1154–62.
36. Tsiotra PC, Boutati E, Dimitriadis G, Raptis SA. High insulin and leptin increase resistin and inflammatory cytokine production from human mononuclear cells. Biomed Res Int. 2013;2013:1–10.
37. Gleeson M. Immune function in sport and exercise. J Appl Physiol. 2007;103(2):693–9.
38. Reddy MA, Natarajan R. Epigenetic mechanisms in diabetic vascular complications. Cardiovasc Res. 2011;90(3):421–9.
39. Barnes PJ, Karin M. Nuclear Factor-kB – a pivotal transcription factor in chronic inflammatory diseases. N Engl J Med. 1997;336:1066–71.
40. Gray S, De Meyts P. Role of histone and transcription factor acetylation in diabetes pathogenesis. Diabetes Metab Res Rev. 2005;21:416–33.
41. Shoelson SE, Lee J, Goldfine AB. Inflammation and insulin resistance. J Clin Invest. 2006;116:1793–801.
42. Ndisang JF. Role of heme oxygenase in inflammation, insulin-signalling, diabetes and obesity. Mediators Inflamm. 2010;2010:1–18.
43. Miao F, Gonzalo IG, Lanting L, Natarajan R. In vivo chromatin remodeling events leading to inflammatory gene transcription under diabetic conditions. J Biol Chem. 2004;279(17):18091–7.
44. Villeneuve LM, Reddy MA, Natarajan R. Epigenetics: deciphering its role in diabetes and its chronic complications. Clin Exp Pharmacol Physiol. 2011;38(7):401–9.
45. Monteiro R, Azevedo I. Chronic inflammation in obesity and the metabolic syndrome. Mediators Inflamm. 2010;2010:1–10.
46. Zanuso S, Sacchetti M, Sundberg CJ, Orlando G, Benvenuti P, Balducci S. Exercise in type 2 diabetes: genetic, metabolic and neuromuscular adaptations. A review of the evidence. Br J Sports Med. 2017;0:1–8.
47. Bork-jensen J, Scheele C, Christophersen DV, Nilsson E, Friedrichsen M, Fernandez-twinn DS, et al. Glucose tolerance is associated with differential expression of microRNAs in skeletal muscle : results from studies of twins with and without type 2 diabetes. Diabetologia. 2015;58:363–73.
48. Deiuliis JA. MicroRNAs as regulators of metabolic disease: pathophysiologic significance and emerging role as biomarkers and therapeutics. Int J Obes. 2016;40:88–101.
49. Poy MN, Eliasson L, Krutzfeldt J, Kuwajima S, Ma X, MacDonald PE, et al. A pancreatic islet-specific microRNA regulates insulin secretion. Nature. 2004;432(7014):226–30.
50. Zacharewicz E, Lamon S, Russell AP. MicroRNAs in skeletal muscle and their regulation with exercise, ageing, and disease. Front Physiol. 2013;4:1–11.
51. Gallagher IJ, Scheele C, Keller P, Nielsen AR, Remenyi J, Fischer CP, et al. Integration of microRNA changes in vivo identifies novel molecular features of muscle insulin resistance in type 2 diabetes. Genome Med. 2010;2:1–18.
52. Christensen DP, Dahllöf M, Lundh M, Rasmussen DN, Nielsen MD, Billestrup N, et al. Histone deacetylase (HDAC) inhibition as a novel treatment for diabetes mellitus. Mol Med. 2011;17:378–90.
53. Stepto NK, Coffey VG, Carey AL, Ponnampalam AP, Canny BJ, Powell D, et al. Global gene expression in skeletal muscle from well-trained strength

and endurance athletes. Med Sci Sports Exerc. 2009;41(3):546–65.
54. Lindholm ME, Marabita F, Gomez-Cabrero D, Rundqvist H, Ekström TJ, Tegnér J, et al. An integrative analysis reveals coordinated reprogramming of the epigenome and the transcriptome in human skeletal muscle after training. Epigenetics. 2014;9(12):1557–69.
55. Baar K, Wende AR, Jones TE, Marison M, Nolte LA, Chen MAY, et al. Adaptations of skeletal muscle to exercise : rapid increase in the transcriptional coactivator PGC-1. FASEB J. 2002;16:1879–86.
56. Pilegaard H, Saltin B, Neufer PD. Exercise induces transient transcriptional activation of the PGC-1a gene in human skeletal muscle. J Physiol. 2003;546:851–8.
57. Norrbom J, Sundberg CJ, Ameln H, Kraus WE, Jansson E, Gustafsson T. PGC-1a mRNA expression is influenced by metabolic perturbation in exercising human skeletal muscle. J Appl Physiol. 2004;96:189–94.
58. Irrcher I, Adhihetty PJ, Sheehan T, Joseph A, Hood DA. PPARg coactivator-1a expression during thyroid hormone- and contractile activity-induced mitochondrial adaptations. Am J Physiol Cell Physiol. 2003;284:C1669–77.
59. Fernandez-marcos PJ, Auwerx J. Regulation of PGC-1 a, a nodal regulator of mitochondrial biogenesis. Am J Clin Nutr. 2011;93:884–90.
60. Richter EA, Hargreaves M. Exercise, glut4, and skeletal muscle glucose uptake. Physiol Rev. 2013;93:993–1017.
61. Holten MK, Zacho M, Gaster M, Juel C, Wojtaszewski JFP, Dela F. Strength training increases insulin-mediated glucose uptake, GLUT4 content, and insulin signaling in skeletal muscle in patients with type 2 diabetes. Diabetes. 2004;53:294–305.
62. Barrès R, Yan J, Egan B, Treebak JT, Rasmussen M, Fritz T, et al. Acute exercise remodels promoter methylation in human skeletal muscle. Cell Metab. 2012;15(3):405–11.
63. Nitert MD, Dayeh T, Volkov P, Elgzyri T, Hall E, Nilsson E, et al. Impact of an exercise intervention on DNA methylation in skeletal muscle from first-degree relatives of patients with type 2 diabetes. Diabetes. 2012;61(12):3322–32.
64. Voisin S, Eynon N, Yan X, Bishop DJ. Exercise training and DNA methylation in humans. Acta Physiol. 2015;213(1):39–59.
65. Rönn T, Volkov P, Davegårdh C, Dayeh T, Hall E, Olsson AH, et al. A six months exercise intervention influences the genome-wide DNA methylation pattern in human adipose tissue. PLoS Genet. 2013;9(6):1–16.
66. Gjevestad GO, Holven KB, Ulven SM. Effects of exercise on gene expression of inflammatory markers in human peripheral blood cells: a systematic review. Curr Cardiovasc Risk Rep. 2015;9(34):1–17.
67. Adoglou N, Perrea D, Iliadis F, Angelopoulou N, Liapis C, Alevizoa M. Exercise reduces resistin and inflammatory cytokines in patients with type 2 diabetes. Diabetes Care. 2007;30(3):719–21.
68. Kilian Y, Wehmeier UF, Wahl P, Mester J, Hilberg T, Sperlich B. Acute response of circulating vascular regulating micrornas during and after high-intensity and high-volume cycling in children subjects and ethics statement. Front Physiol. 2016;7:1–9.
69. Radom-aizik S, Zaldivar F, Leu S, Adams GR, Oliver S, Cooper DM. Effects of exercise on microrna expression in young males peripheral blood mononuclear cells. Clin Transl Sci. 2012;5(1):32–8.
70. Bouchard C, Antunes-Correa LM, Ashley EA, Franklin N, Hwang PM, Mattsson CM, et al. Personalized preventive medicine: genetics and the response to regular exercise in preventive interventions. Prog Cardiovasc Dis. 2015;57(4):337–46.
71. Vollaard NBJ, Constantin-Teodosiu D, Fredriksson K, Rooyackers O, Jansson E, Greenhaff PL, et al. Systematic analysis of adaptations in aerobic capacity and submaximal energy metabolism provides a unique insight into determinants of human aerobic performance. J Appl Physiol. 2009;106:1479–86.
72. Bouchard C, An P, Rice T, Skinner JS, Wilmore JH, Gagnon J, et al. Familial aggregation of VO2max response to exercise training: results from the HERITAGE Family Study. J Appl Physiol. 1999;87:1003–8.
73. Sarzynski MA, Ghosh S, Bouchard C. Genomic and transcriptomic predictors of response levels to endurance exercise training. J Physiol. 2017;595(9):2931–9.
74. Timmons JA, Larsson O, Jansson E, Fischer H, Gustafsson T, Greenhaff PL, et al. Human muscle gene expression responses to endurance training provide a novel perspective on Duchenne muscular dystrophy. FASEB J [Internet]. 2005;19(7):750–60. Available from: http://www.ncbi.nlm.nih.gov/pubmed/15857889.
75. Timmons JA, Jansson E, Fischer H, Gustafsson T, Greenhaff PL, Ridden J, et al. Modulation of extracellular matrix genes reflects the magnitude of physiological adaptation to aerobic exercise training in humans. BMC Biol. 2005;3(19):1–10.
76. Timmons JA, Knudsen S, Rankinen T, Koch LG, Sarzynski M, Jensen T, et al. Using molecular classification to predict gains in maximal aerobic capacity following endurance exercise training in humans. J Appl Physiol. 2010;108:1487–96.
77. Bouchard C, Sarzynski MA, Rice TK, Kraus WE, Church TS, Sung YJ, et al. Genomic predictors of the maximal O2 uptake response to standardized exercise training programs. J Appl Physiol. 2011;110:1160–70.
78. Bouchard C, Blair SN, Church TS, Earnest CP, Hagberg JM, Jenkins NT, et al. Adverse metabolic response to regular exercise: is it a rare or common occurrence? PLoS One. 2012;7(5):e37887.
79. Pandey A, Swift DL, Mcguire DK, Ayers CR, Neeland IJ, Blair SN, et al. Metabolic effects of exercise training among fitness- nonresponsive patients with type 2 diabetes: the HART-D study. Diabetes Care. 2015;38:1494–501.
80. Montero D, Lundby C. Refuting the myth of non-response to exercise training: "non-responders" do respond to higher dose of training. J Physiol. 2017;11:3377–87.

Exercise and the Mitochondria 3

Eva-Karin Gidlund

Abbreviations

AMPK	AMP-dependent protein kinase
ATP	Adenosine triphosphate
CaMK	Ca^{2+}-calmodulin-dependent protein kinase
CFCM	Cross-fiber connection mitochondria
CVDs	Cardiovascular diseases
D-loop	Displacement loop
ERR	Estrogen-related receptors
ETC	Electron transport chain
FPM	Fiber parallel mitochondria
HIF-1	Hypoxia inducible factor
HIIT	High-intensity interval training
HS1/HS2	Heavy strand 1/heavy strand 2
IBM	I-band mitochondria
IFM	Intrafibrillar mitochondria
IMJs	Intermitochondrial junctions
IMS	Intermembrane space
LKB1	Liver kinase B1
MDP's	Mitochondria-derived peptides
MOTS-c	Mitochondrial open reading frame of the 12S rRNA-c
mtDNA	Mitochondrial DNA
MTERFs	Mitochondrial transcription termination factors
mtSSB	Mitochondrial single-stranded DNA-binding protein
NRF-1	Nuclear respiratory factor 1
NUMTs	Nuclear genome insertions of mitochondrial origin
OH	Origin of heavy-strand replication, a.k.a OriH
OL	Origin of light-strand replication site
OXPHOS	Oxidative phosphorylation system
p53	Tumor protein p53
PGC-1α	Peroxisome proliferator-activated receptor γ coactivator-1α
Pim-1	The regulation protein serine/threonine protein kinases Pim-a
PNM	Paranuclear mitochondria
POLG	Polymerase γ
POLRMT	Mitochondrial RNA polymerase
PPAR	Peroxisome proliferator-activated receptor
PVM	Paravascular mitochondria
ROS	Reactive oxygen species
SIRT	Sirtuins
T2D	Type II diabetes

E.-K. Gidlund (✉)
Department of Physiology and Pharmacology, Karolinska Institutet, Solna, Sweden
e-mail: eva-karin.gidlund@ki.se

P. Kokkinos, P. Narayan (eds.), *Cardiorespiratory Fitness in Cardiometabolic Diseases*,
https://doi.org/10.1007/978-3-030-04816-7_3

TCA	Citrate acid cycle or tricarboxylic acid cycle
TFAM	Mitochondrial transcription factor A
TFB1M/TFB2M	Mitochondrial transcription factor B1/mitochondrial transcription factor B2
TIM	Translocase of the inner membrane
TOM	Translocase of the outer membrane
VO_2 peak	Peak maximal oxygen consumption

Introduction

One of the world's most important intracellular relationships started over billion years ago when free-living aerobic bacteria (prokaryotes) managed to survive an endocytotic engulfment by eukaryotic cells and a successful symbiosis was established. This is known as the endosymbiotic theory which led to one of the most enduring concepts in biology [1]. In 1905, this relationship was recognized and elucidated further by the Russian biologist Constantin Mereschkowsky who postulated a model of intracellular union of two different kinds of cells [2]. However, in the early 1900s, Mereschkowsky did not recognize mitochondria as a product of endosymbiosis, although this symbiotic relationship seems to have formed the organelle that we now know as the mitochondrion. The formation of the mitochondrion made the evolution of more complex multicellular organisms possible [3].

This symbiosis occurred around the same time as oxygen levels in the earth's atmosphere began to rise [4, 5]. This provided a survival benefit for the eukaryotic cell since an oxygen-dependent, highly efficient metabolic system became available [3]. This oxygen-dependent system in the mitochondria is essential for the formation of adenosine triphosphate (ATP) by oxidative phosphorylation. Without the fusion of the eukaryotic cell and these bacteria, all living animals would have been dependent on anaerobic glycolysis for ATP production. In addition, the mitochondria are abundantly present and vital for animal cells, involved in lipid and amino acid metabolism, and play important roles in various cellular processes such as cell proliferation, apoptosis, and cell differentiation [6].

Although mammalian mitochondria have kept some bacterial features, it is estimated that only a small percentage of the mitochondrial proteome of the modern human mitochondria (approximately 10–20%) are derived from the original endosymbiont [7]. However, a number of questions regarding the endosymbiotic theory and formation of modern mitochondria remain unanswered or poorly understood [7, 8].

From a human perspective, the origin of our modern mitochondria has been suggested to come from Africa and is termed the "mitochondrial Eve" [9]. However, this mapping of the origin of our modern mitochondrial DNA (mtDNA) has been extensively discussed and disputed [10]. Moreover, during evolution, different haplogroups of different mitochondria arose through specific mtDNA mutations that have formed different classes of mtDNA pools [11]. Several studies have reported strong evidence of increased disease prevalence and risk as well as certain protective features regarding cardiovascular diseases (CVD) and stroke among different haplogroups [12–14]. Despite different single-nucleotide polymorphism mutations leading to the different mitochondrial haplogroups, physical activity is a major factor that modulates the overall function of mitochondria.

The Magical Mitochondria

Mitochondria are organelles surrounded by two membranes, an outer and an inner membrane, which confine two aqueous compartments, the matrix and the intermembrane space (IMS). Tubular invaginations of the inner mitochondrial membrane form the cristae, which harbor the enzyme complexes of the electron transport chain (ETC) also known as the oxidative phosphorylation system (OXPHOS), which provides the cell with energy in the form of ATP. Other metabolic systems such as the tricarboxylic acid (TCA) cycle and the ®-oxidation, involved in glucose and fatty acid breakdown, can be found within the matrix of the mitochondria [15]. Since the mitochondria are the main source of ATP within the cell, they are commonly referred to as the "powerhouse" of the cell. Mitochondria are present in all tissues in the human body except the red blood cells [16]. Highly metabolic tissues such as the heart, skeletal muscles, and the liver are typically mitochondrially dense tissues [17].

Even though mitochondria are enclosed within a membrane and defined as an organelle, they should not be considered as a single entities, rather a network of interconnected membranes making up a tubular dynamic reticulum within the cell [18, 19]. Fusion and fission dynamics are constantly ongoing events which lead to branching of the reticulum of tubules [19].

Mitochondria are unique organelles since they contain their own circular DNA, and this mtDNA is inherited in a non-Mendelian manner. It is widely accepted that mtDNA is inherited solely from the mitochondria of the oocyte from which the animal develops. This makes it maternally inherited even though a "spillover" of mitochondria from the sperm can occasionally be found [6]. However, sperm mitochondria are lost early in the embryogenesis and therefore do not contribute to the mitochondrial pool [20]. The human mitochondrial genome contains a compact circular, double-stranded molecule of 16,569 base pairs with no known introns and very few non-coding nucleotides. Traditionally, the human mtDNA contains 37 genes coding for 2 ribosomal ribonucleic acids (rRNAs), 22 transfer ribonucleic acids (tRNAs), and 13 polypeptides [15, 20]. The small size of the mtDNA limits its coding capacity and is thought only to account for a small fraction of the organelle's proteome. The 13 well-known proteins encoded by mammalian mtDNA are all components of the ETC. Different versions of the endosymbiotic theory have argued whether there was a massive transfer of genes from the endosymbiont into the nuclear genome during the evolution of the mitochondrion. Almost all of the genes encoding the proteins of modern mitochondria are found in the nuclear genomes of their host cells [21]. Hence, the mitochondrial genomic apparatus does not single-handedly control the organelle's proteome, and the remaining ~77 subunits involved in the ETC are encoded by nuclear genes, as are all proteins required for the transcription, translation, modification, and assembly of the 13 mtDNA proteins [22]. However, this view has recently been challenged, and previously unknown features of mitochondrial gene expression, function, and regulation have been suggested which indicate that the mitochondrial transcriptome and proteome are far more complex than first thought [23, 24]. Technics such as proteomics have estimated the mitochondrial proteome to consist of at least 1000–1500 different proteins, corresponding to 1080 genes [21, 25].

Nuclear genome insertions of mitochondrial origin known as NUMTs have also been identified [26, 27]. In 1967 the first report of DNA fragments with homology to the mitochondrial genome was published [28]. Later, nuclear mitochondrial pseudogenes arose as a concept. A possible explanation for these integrations of mtDNA is incorporation into the nuclear genome during the repair of chromosomal breaks by nonhomologous recombination. Such a hypothesis, of a possible incorporation of mtDNA, is supported by the mtDNA fragments found in the nucleus [29, 30]. There are over 500 NUMTs in the human genome [30, 31]. Although most NUMTs are considered pseudogenes, bioinformatics-based evidence suggests that at least some of the nuclear sequences might be functional genes [32].

The symbiosis between the mitochondrion and the eukaryotic cell created the need for a communication system, to coordinate mitochondrial protein synthesis during biogenesis and to communicate possible mitochondrial malfunctions. Communication from the mitochondria to the nucleus is referred to as retrograde signaling, and communication from the nucleus to the mitochondria is known as antegrade signaling [33]. The mitochondria have traditionally been perceived as a end-function organelle that receive cellular signals and regulate processes such as energy conversion and apoptosis in response to these signals. However, in recent years it has become evident that cellular homeostasis requires a constant and active flow of information between the mitochondria and the nucleus [34]. The research has mainly been focused on a limited number of retrograde signaling molecules and signaling pathways such as sirtuins (SIRT), cytochrome C, reactive oxygen species (ROS), calcium, iron, nitric oxide, and carbon monoxide [35–37]. It has also been shown, in the inflammation response, that mtDNA by itself can act as a retrograde signal [38, 39]. In addition to subcellular signaling programs, mitochondrial factors can even be released from one cell and exert paracrine or endocrine effects on other cells [40]. Beyond these retrograde signals, recent studies have identified a host of mitochondria-linked factors that influence the cellular and extracellular environments, including mitochondria-derived peptides (MDPs) and mitochondria-localized proteins [34, 41, 42]. The first described MDP was humanin [43], and more recently another small peptide also encoded from the mtDNA called MOTS-c has been discovered [44]. These small peptides are encoded from the 16 s rRNA and the 12 s rRNA regions in the mitochondria, respectively, which makes them a "gene within a gene". Studies have shown that these MDPs seem to have functions outside the mitochondria and might be involved in metabolic regulation and insulin sensitivity and to have cyto-protective effects [34, 43, 45–49]. Which function these MDPs actually have in striated muscle such as cardiac and skeletal muscle and their role in metabolism is not yet fully known. However, a recent study in prediabetic males demonstrated that 12 weeks of resistance exercise increased the levels of humanin protein in skeletal muscle [49]. Further, the resistance trained group also exhibited a significant correlation between the humanin levels in serum and improvements in a 2 h glucose loading test. This study indicates that humanin protein might play a role in the regulation of glucose metabolism in prediabetic males and that it is affected by exercise.

The humanin analog, HNG, has also recently been shown to protect cardiac mitochondria against oxidative stress which causes mitochondrial dysfunction [50]. These features make MDPs interesting targets to study further, especially in situations where mitochondrial dysfunction might occur such as in cardiovascular disease (CVD), chronic kidney disease, and type II diabetes [51–54]. Moreover, in 2013 transcriptional profiling identified over 70 different transcription factors that were actively involved in mitochondrial retrograde signaling. Among those, peroxisome proliferator-activated receptor (PPAR)-© γ coactivator 1 α (PGC-1α) and hypoxia-inducible factor (HIF-1) were presented as some of the main candidates affecting retrograde signaling pathways and mitochondrial function [55].

To summarize, mitochondria are unusual and vital organelles, surrounded by two membranes, and contain their own circular DNA. They form a dynamic network which acts as the powerhouse of the cell. The function and appearance of the mitochondria are highly important for the overall cell and whole body function and health.

Heart Muscle Mitochondria

The cardiac mitochondria are densely packed, and approximately 30–35% of the cardiac muscle tissue volume consists of mitochondria [56]. The arrangement of mitochondria within the cardiac muscle tissue is highly ordered and mostly in long and dense rows parallel to the myofilaments [57]. This mitochondrial network ensures that the large demand of ATP by cardiac myocytes is met and appropriately distributed. Mitochondria synthesize approximately 30 kg of ATP/day to provide energy for the basic cellular metabolism and to assure basic physiological functions of the cardiovascular system [58]. Thus, the permanent contractile activity of the myocardium is supplied 95% by mitochondrial respiration, mostly from fatty acid metabolism, to ensure continuous energy production [25].

Depending on where within the cell the mitochondria are located, they are divided into different subgroups called intermyofibrillar mitochondria and subsarcolemmal mitochondria [59]. However, new technics have recently revealed, in cardiomyocytes and in skeletal myocytes, subgroups of mitochondria could actually be differed in more definite groups and divided into paravascular mitochondria (PVM), paranuclear mitochondria (PNM), fiber parallel mitochondria (FPM), I-band mitochondria (IBM), intrafibrillar mitochondria (IFM) and cross-fiber connection mitochondria (CFCM) [60]. As stated above, the mitochondria should not to be considered as single entities rather as a connected network. These networks, which comprise of many mitochondria, are linked through contact sites called intermitochondrial junctions (IMJs). In cardiac and skeletal muscle tissue, the mitochondrial reticulum is segmented into sub-networks which allows a rapid electrical and physical separation of malfunctioning mitochondria. This separation occurs through detachment of IMJs and retraction of elongated mitochondria into condensed structures [61]. In this way, these subgroups of networks protect and limit the cellular impact of local dysfunction while the dynamic disconnection of damaged mitochondria allows the remaining mitochondria to resume normal function within seconds [61]. Thus, mitochondrial network security is comprised of both proactive and reactive mechanisms in striated muscle cells, especially important for hardworking tissues such as the cardiac muscle.

Mitochondrial Replication, Transcription, and Biogenesis

Replication

The main function of the mitochondria is to act as the powerhouse of the cell, as stated above, providing the cell and the whole organism with sufficient amount of ATP. Important in the process to maintain energy demands and function of the mitochondria, the mtDNA needs to be replicated and transcribed. However, in contrast to the nuclear genome, mitochondria are continuously turned over and replicated independent of the cell cycle [62]. In mammalian cells, the mtDNA is a multicopy genome which allows the cell to generally have 10^3–10^4 copies of mtDNA, with 2–10 genomes per organelle [25].

The mtDNA consists of a circular double-stranded (a heavy-strand (HS) and a light-strand (LS)) genome also containing the noncoding regulatory region known as the displacement loop (D-loop), in which the promoter for transcription of both the HS and the LS is located [63]. Almost the entire heavy strand (HS) is transcribed from the other heavy-strand (HS2) promoter (located in proximity to the D-loop), and the entire LS is transcribed from the LS promoter [1]. The HS promoters (H1 and H2) initiate the transcription of the two mitochondrial rRNA molecules [1, 64]. Two different models of mtDNA replication have been proposed, the strand displacement and the symmetric strand-coupled replication model [65]. Mammalian mtDNA molecules replicate by the strand displacement model, and replication is induced by transcription within the noncoding D-loop. In brief, the replication proceeds clockwise from the origin of replication for the HS called the OH site (also known as OriH) until the origin of the LS replication site (OL) is exposed, allowing LS synthesis to proceed clockwise until the entire molecule is copied.

The replication of mtDNA is highly dependent on nuclear events. Proteins known to be of importance for this process are DNA polymerase γ (POLG), mitochondrial single-stranded DNA-binding protein (mtSSB), and the Twinkle helicase (also known as PEO1). The Twinkle helicase has the ability to unwind short segments of mtDNA and thereby aiding the replication process [66]. Unlike nuclear DNA, which is packaged into nucleosomes, mtDNA molecules are tightly associated with the mitochondrial matrix and form compact structures called nucleoids, composed of mtDNA-protein complexes that include proteins involved in replication and transcription such as mtSSB, DNA POLG, and mitochondrial transcription factor A (TFAM) [67].

When the mitochondrial replisome responsible for replication proceeds clockwise past the D-loop region, two thirds of the growing HS is formed before a point is reached at which a growing LS synthesis can start at the OL circle [1, 68]. As a newly exposed single-stranded template sequence in the HS forms a hairpin to constitute OL, HS replication (into an emerging LS) commences in the opposite direction. Both strands are thus replicated as leading strands (5′→3′ directed) rather than lagging strands [69]. The progeny molecules are released as dissimilar free circles. The new double-stranded mtDNA molecule is formed through the removal of the RNA primers, gap filling, introduction of superhelical turns, and finally closure of the circle [1, 68].

Transcription

Transcription of the mtDNA is, just as replication, a unique process within the mitochondria. Depending on which mtDNA strand is to be the template, transcription occurs from the light-strand promoter (LSP) or the heavy-strand promoter (HSP), in opposite directions around the entire genomic circle. In addition, mitochondrial RNA polymerase (POLRMT) and the transcriptional machinery influence the replication process of mtDNA. POLRMT generates the RNA primers used to initiate leading-strand mtDNA synthesis at the OH site for mtDNA replication [70]. Mitochondrial transcription requires nuclear-encoded protein such as POLRMT with assistance and co-activation of the TFAM, together with either mitochondrial transcription factor B1 (TFB1M) or B2 (TFB2M). The genes encoding TFB1M and TFB2M are ubiquitously expressed with the highest mRNA levels detected in the heart, skeletal muscle, and liver, and both TFB1M and TFB2M can form a heterodimeric complex with POLRMT [71]. However, how the mammalian mitochondrial transcription machinery recognizes promoter sequences is not yet fully understood. POLRMT in complex with TFB1M or TFB2M cannot initiate transcription in the absence of TFAM. One possible role for TFAM might be to introduce specific structural alterations in mtDNA, for example, unwinding of the promoter region, which might facilitate transcription initiation [71, 72]. TFAM has also been shown to be upregulated by the nuclear respiratory factor (NRF-1), which coordinates nuclear-encoded respiratory chain expression with mitochondrial gene transcription and replication. Moreover, mitochondrial transcription termination factors (mTERFs) have also been described as a family of additional regulators displaying multiple roles in the regulation of mitochondrial transcription. One function in which mTERFs act seems to involve binding an upstream enhancer of the two mtDNA strands and thereby promoting mitochondrial-encoded gene transcription [25, 73].

Biogenesis

The dynamic network of mitochondria has a central role in cardiac contractility and function. The plasticity of mitochondrial networks is important for meeting the demands of the tissue, which is done by initiating growth, adaptation of mitochondrial structures, and to change the dynamics of the network organization. This plasticity and the dynamic abilities of the network rely on the formation of new mitochondria (biogenesis) and disposal of damaged and old ones (mitophagy).

To enable mitochondrial biogenesis to occur, the mitochondria are highly dependent on mtDNA replication [74]. Even though mitochondrion has its own DNA, it is highly dependent on the nucleus for its function and nuclear-encoded mitochondrial proteins. The small size of the mtDNA limits its coding capacity and is thought only to account for a small fraction of the organelle's entire proteome. Thus, this requires a spatiotemporal coordination between protein synthesis and import and assembly of nuclear-encoded mitochondrial proteins together with mitochondrial-encoded proteins. This process has to occur jointly with the synthesis of phospholipids and mitochondrial membranes. Furthermore, mitochondrial biogenesis is vastly dependent on the ability of the mitochondria to undergo fission/fusion events.

The dynamics of the mitochondrial network are steered, by these opposing processes (fission and fusion), which together work in concert to maintain the overall morphology of mitochondria. The fission and fusion events need to be in balance since an excess of mitochondrial fission events results in mitochondrial fragmentation, whereas an excess of mitochondrial fusion events leads to hypertubulation. To ensure proper mitochondrial function, nuclear-encoded mitochondrial proteins have to be imported from the nucleus to the mitochondria. Nuclear mRNAs are translated in the cytosol to precursor proteins with mitochondria-targeting sequences. They are then escorted and unfolded by molecular chaperones and finally imported into the mitochondrial matrix via the translocase of the outer membrane (TOM) and the translocase of the inner membrane (TIM) [75]. For details regarding the complex transport machinery, see recent review from Wiedemann and Pfanner [76]. The orchestration of factors controlling the fission and fusion events has been reviewed in details elsewhere; see Iqbal and Hood 2015 [77].

In order to initiate mitochondrial biogenesis, a coordination between mitochondrial and nuclear gene expression must take place. This coordination is controlled by the interplay between specific transcription factors such as the nuclear respiratory factors (NRFs), the peroxisome proliferator-activated receptors (PPARs), the estrogen-related receptors (ERR), as well as PGC-1α. The transcription factor coactivator PGC-1α has long been recognized as "the master of mitochondrial biogenesis" and is known to be an important coactivator of NRF-1. In turn, NRF-1 activates TFAM, TFB1M, and TFB2M and thereby stimulates the cell to increase its mitochondrial copy number [78–80]. Recently, TFAM has also been suggested to play a role in the replication and checkpoint system of the mtDNA [81]. These activation pathways demonstrate that mitochondrial replication and transcription are tightly linked to and of major importance for mitochondrial biogenesis [82]. NRF-1 has also been shown to be responsible for the activation of many nuclear-encoded mitochondrial proteins to be transcribed, including OXPHOS proteins. In cardiac tissue, ERRs have been suggested to act as the main coordinator of a transcriptional program involved in energy fluctuations and transport of ATP over the mitochondrial membranes [83]. PGC-1α levels have been shown to correlate with mitochondrial protein levels in both cardiac and skeletal muscle tissue, somewhat supporting its important role in controlling mitochondrial biogenesis [84, 85]. However, in PGC-1α-deficient mice, mitochondrial volume can still be maintained even though mitochondrial genes are reduced suggesting that additional factors and mechanisms might control mitochondrial biogenesis [86, 87]. However, it is important to note that these kinds of animal models show cardiac dysfunction. Factors contributing to the maintenance of mitochondrial volume might be, for example, the recently discovered isoforms of PGC-1α that are transcribed from an alternative promotor, PGC-1β, or the energy-sensing AMP-activated protein kinase (AMPK), or calcium-/calmodulin-dependent protein kinase (CaMK) [88–90]. It has also been shown that the NAD^+-sensing SIRT1 in coordination with AMPK regulates mitochondrial mass, nutrient oxidation, and ATP production to fit the cells' needs via PGC-1α [91, 92]. It is noteworthy that mice lacking both PGC-1α and PGC-1β die shortly after birth and have small hearts and markedly reduced cardiac function probably due to arrest in mitochondrial biogenesis [93].

To initiate mitochondrial biogenesis, external stimuli together with an intercellular response are necessary. External stimuli such as exercise and oxidative stress have been shown to positively stimulate tissue to increase its mitochondrial copy number and are thereby important for mitochondrial biogenesis [94]. Communication between the outer and the inner environment, and the mitochondria, as well as in between different mitochondria is very important to make sure that the demands of the cell are met. Recently, new imaging technics have allowed the visualization of nanotunnels connecting mitochondria with each other [95]. This mitochondrial tool for communication strengthens the importance of seeing the mitochondrial pool as a network rather than single entities. It has also been suggested that the actual nanotunnel might originate from stalled or incomplete fission of an existing mitochondria [96].

Mitochondrial Medicine

Mitochondrial Disorders

Mitochondrial disorders in humans are a group of genetically heterogeneous disorders usually involving mutations in the mtDNA or the nuclear DNA. In population genetics, the variability introduced into mtDNA sequences by mutations has been used to map human history. In epidemiological studies, the prevalence of mtDNA disease was found to be approximately 1:5000 and heteroplasmic mtDNA mutations 1:200 in newborns [97, 98]. Compared to nuclear DNA genes, mtDNA genes have a very high sequence evolution rate and mutational load because of the continuous replication state and high number of mtDNA copies [99].

Mitochondrial diseases can appear at any age, affect any organ system and, depending on where the gene defect lies, originate from an autosome, X chromosomal or maternal inheritance. Currently, mitochondrial disorders cannot be cured, and available treatments are aimed at relieving symptoms [100]. The outcome of these mitochondrial disorders is somewhat varying depending on the organ or tissue affected and also by individual factors affecting patient's protective and/or risk assessments by the alleles. In mammalian cells the mtDNA-linked disorders and their phenotypic variability may also depend on the fact that a mitochondrion can contain both mutated mtDNA and non-mutated mtDNA copies, which makes the mtDNA pool within a mitochondrion highly heteroplastic [99, 101]. Earlier it was thought that the mtDNA heteroplasmy was a rare event; however, new improved molecular methods analyzing mtDNA have revealed presence of heteroplasmic variance in healthy subjects sequenced, even though the levels found were quite low [102]. However, in the presence of heteroplasmy a minimum critical proportion of mutated mtDNA between 60% and 90% (mutant to wild-type DNA) seems necessary before biochemical defects and tissue dysfunction become apparent which migth lead to disease [103]. Specific mitochondrial-linked mutations affecting the heart have been identified, and mitochondrial diseases have been shown to display cardiomyopathies in a frequency of approximately 20–40% of the disorders [104].

Mitochondrial Dysfunction

Mitochondrial dysfunctions that are not classified as genetic disorders have long been recognized to be involved in a vast majority of different diseases including cardiovascular, metabolic, and neurodegenerative diseases [105]. Comparing identical twins discordant for obesity has revealed significant reduced amount of mtDNA and decreased mitochondrial mass in the obese twin [106]. This strengthens the evidence that the mitochondria are highly involved in metabolically related diseases and affected by environmental factors, nutrition, and physical activity. Dysfunction of the mitochondria that effects the energy metabolism and mitochondrial biogenesis appears also to play an important role in cardiac dysfunction and progression to heart failure. Further, both impairments in mitochondrial biogenesis and mitophagy seem to have a role in heart failure [107]. Also, loss of mtDNA in human heart failure has been attributed not to an alteration in genetic control (such as downregulation of PGC-1α), but rather due to increased oxidative damage to the DNA [108]. Furthermore, mitochondrial content depends on the etiology of heart failure, with mtDNA content being increased in patients with dilated cardiomyopathy, yet unchanged in those from ischemic heart disease [109]. However, this increase in mtDNA was also accompanied by increased mtDNA mutations, deletions, and damage rate, indicating an overall mitochondrial dysfunction. Mitochondria also had a greater percentage of mutations and deletions caused by oxidative damage in the dilated cardiomyopathic hearts compared to ischemic heart diseases. Despite this, heart failure subgroups exhibited lower OXPHOS capacity [109]. Thus, heart failure progression can feature a heterogeneously localized increase in the total numbers of defective mitochondria, interspersed with a gradually diminishing pool of normally functioning mitochondria, struggling to sustain cardiac output [109].

As mentioned above, strong evidence exists that links factors such as environment, nutrition, and physical inactivity in the development of overall mitochondrial dysfunction. Beyond cardiomyopathies and heart diseases, mitochondrial dysfunction has been associated with obesity, type II diabetes (T2D), and other commonly age-related diseases. Obesity, in addition of being a risk factor by itself, also increases the risk for other diseases such as cardiovascular disease, cancer, and diabetes [110].

It has been debated what is actually the cause and what is the consequence when it comes to obesity, T2D, and mitochondrial dysfunction. However, mitochondrial dysfunction, if not the cause, is likely to be a key contributor to both obesity and T2D. Obesity leads to processes like inflammation, which in turn have been linked to an increase in the mitochondrial ROS production, which can cause oxidative stress [111]. This stress has been recognized to trigger mitochondrial changes that might lead to mitochondrial dysfunction. Moreover, excess nutrient intake has also been shown to accelerate ROS production by overwhelming the TCA cycle and the OXPHOS system and also to cause imbalance in the mitochondrial fission and fusion events. This type of excessive eating or nutrient-rich environment has been linked to increased fission events generating fragmented and separated mitochondria [112]. For over a decade, studies in T2D patients have shown convincing evidence of mitochondrial dysfunction, mostly displayed as decreased mitochondrial activity, decreased size of the mitochondria, decreased OXPHOS gene activity, and decreased expression of nuclear-encoded genes important for normal mitochondrial function and biogenesis such as PGC-1α [113–119]. Studies of T2D patients are usually performed in tissues such as skeletal muscle and adipose tissue. Therefore it is highly interestingly that the heart of T2D patients has also shown a decreased number of subsarcolemmal mitochondria which have been linked to cardiomyopathy [120].

Aging and Longevity in Connection to Mitochondria

The function and capacity of mitochondria besides being implicated in metabolic disorders and obesity have also been connected to the aging process and life span. Preserved structure of the mitochondria has been suggested to delay the onset of aging. To preserve the morphology of the mitochondria, the regulation protein serine/threonine protein kinases Pim-a (Pim-1) has an important function. Studies in mice with a Pim-1 deficiency show signs of reduced mitochondrial area in the heart and display premature aging [121, 122]. Also factors such as the phospholipid cardiolipin, which is localized in the inner membrane of the mitochondria, have been connected to the aging process [123, 124]. Studies have also shown that mitochondrial OXPHOS capacity and genes connected to this are decreased both in animal and human hearts with aging [125–127]. Several changes shown in heart mitochondria with aging have also been shown in skeletal muscle along with decreased mitochondrial volume, increased oxidative damage, and reduced OXPHOS capacity [128]. In skeletal muscle of aging subjects (over 80 years old), it has been shown by PCR and Southern blotting that over 70% of the mtDNA have random deletions that might play a role in the aging process [129]. Oxidative stress and increased ROS production have been proposed to play a key role in the aging process. According to this theory, as we age, mitochondria accumulate oxidative damage due to the production of ROS during the generation of ATP. This process in turn causes further mitochondrial dysfunction, as ROS are highly reactive and destroy macromolecules such as proteins, lipids, and DNA [130]. In addition, studies of *Drosophila* and mice have shown that overexpression of antioxidant enzymes, such as catalases or superoxide dismutases, increases the life span of these animals [131, 132]. However, this ROS-mitochondrial theory of aging has been disputed since inhibition of mitochondrial function and thereby increased levels of ROS also have been shown to delay aging and increase the life span [133–136]. It is noteworthy that increased ROS levels in connection to increased life span have only been investigated and confirmed in small animals such as *C. elegans*, *Drosophila*, and mice. These studies suggest that ROS, by acting as a signaling molecule and also as a second messenger, might promote an organism's longevity. By acting as a retrograde signaling molecule, ROS can activate HIF-1, which is a nuclear transcription factor that has been linked to increased life span. Activation of the cellular energy sensor AMPK, which can be activated by increased ROS, has also been linked to increased longevity in *C. elegans* [137, 138]. How AMPK mediates this longevity response is currently unknown, but interestingly, AMPK has been shown to increase mitochondrial biogenesis via the activation of SIRT1 and PGC-1α in mammals [139, 140]. This is also somewhat supported by the fact that antioxidant treatment has been shown to abolish long life span caused by the inhibition of mitochondrial respiration, suggesting a requirement of elevated ROS levels for a long life span [136]. Calorie restriction without causing malnutrition has for decades also been shown to increase the life span both in animals and in humans. One important way in which calorie restriction could have been proposed to increase the life span is by increasing the rate of mitochondrial respiration [141–143]. Interestingly, in humans undergoing intervention with calorie restriction, it has also been shown that the mitochondria consume less oxygen than controls but are still producing the same amount of ATP, which suggests that the mitochondria work more efficiently [144]. Calorie restriction has also been shown to induce gene expression of both nuclear and mitochondrial-encoded genes coupled to mitochondrial respiration and also to increase mitochondrial biogenesis [141, 144–147].

Epigenetic Modifications of the Mitochondria

DNA modifications, called epigenetics, in the mitochondrial genome have been known since 1971. Later, mtDNA methylation was recognized as a process occurring within the mammalian mtDNA [148]. However, new techniques have recently evoked the interest of epigenetic modifications affecting the mitochondria [149]. Epigenetics is defined as a phenotype resulting from changes in either gene expression, chromosome changes through posttranslational modifications, histone modifications, or DNA methylation, all without direct alterations in the DNA sequence [150–152]. The mitochondria and the nucleolus are, as stated earlier in this chapter, highly interconnected, and epigenetic modifications in the nuclei can act upon the mitochondria, as it has been shown that the mitochondrial enzyme DNA polymerase γ is regulated by methylation within exon 2 of the nuclear DNA [153]. This methylation thereby regulates and affects the mitochondrial copy number. The mitochondrial genome can also be modified, in a similar manner as the nuclear DNA, by modification of nucleoid structure-forming components, which will affect the opening of the closed structure and can thereby regulate the mtDNA transcription and replication [15, 154]. Methylation of mtDNA in response to oxidative stress has also been examined. However, other epigenetic features, such as mitochondrial noncoding RNAs, are not yet well understood [150, 151, 154].

A number of reports have been associating DNA modifications within the mitochondrial genome with therapeutic drugs, traits and diseases which has provided a new opportunity not only to understand the role of epigenetics in the mitochondrial genome but also to some extent understand the biological function and regulation of the mitochondrial epigenome [149, 155–158]. How factors such as physical activity might spur epigenetic modifications of the mtDNA is still largely unknown. Therefore, much work is still needed before we fully understand the epigenetic regulation of mitochondria and its connection to genetics, physical adaptations, and disease involvement.

In summary, evidence clearly points to the mitochondria as an important target in both the understanding and the treatment of heart failure and cardiovascular diseases [159]. Even though gene therapy might be in the future to reduce mtDNA mutations and mitochondrial dysfunctions, this type of editing is still largely in its infancy compared to nuclear DNA editing. However, this is shaping up to be an interesting and promising field, but many challenges in methodology still need to be overcome.

Exercise Effect on Mitochondria

Acute physical work or exercise constitutes a disturbance in homeostasis and presents a major challenge for the whole body. Chronic exposure to physical work (exercise) that leads to substantial disturbances in homeostasis provides the stimulus for specific adaptations aimed to overcome the challenge, protect the organism from injury, and maintain homeostasis. Evidence of this is provided by the well-documented muscular, cardiovascular, and metabolic chronic adaptations resulting from chronic exercises, such as improved cardiovascular function, oxidative capacity, and insulin sensitivity. These adaptations not only protect the organism against the task at hand (i.e., long distance running) but also appear to render the system resilient to chronic illness. The aforementioned adaptations are mainly due to enhanced oxygen utilization, greater metabolic efficiency, adaptations of heart and skeletal muscle structures and functions, improved peripheral circulation, increased mitochondrial biogenesis and volume, as well as increased OXPHOS enzymes in the mitochondria [90, 160–164]. In this section, an overview of how exercise-induced adaptation affects the mitochondria and how exercise training enhances physical performance which leads to health benefits, largely through adaptations in skeletal muscles, will be presented.

Interventional Evidence and Mechanisms of Exercise-Induced Changes Coupled to the Mitochondria

Exercise affects all organs in the body. Adaptations to exercise are usually seen and studied in high metabolically active tissues which increase their activity during physical activity, such as skeletal and heart muscles, adipose tissue, and liver, organs that are exceedingly affected by exercise [17]. Mitochondrial adaptation, encompassing coordinated improvements in quantity and quality, is recognized as a key factor in the beneficial outcomes of exercise training.

While the benefits of and adaptations to regular exercise have been known for some time, molecular biologists have more recently uncovered networks of signaling pathways and regulatory molecules that coordinate adaptive responses to exercise. It has been suggested that some of the primary mechanisms behind the exercise response seen in mitochondria are due to molecular mechanism such as the activation of signaling kinases and phosphatases via Ca^{2+}, ROS, or ATP-AMP fluctuations, the induction and/or activation of transcriptional regulatory proteins such as the transcription factors PGC-1α and NRF-1/, the import of newly formed precursor proteins into mitochondria, and the coordinated assembly of both mitochondrial and nuclear gene products into an expanding organelle reticulum. Mitochondria are sensitive and responsive to the changes in energy demands that exercise creates, and since the mitochondria oxidize nutrient substrates to generate ATP, they are primarily responsible for meeting the energy demands of prolonged exercise. In 1967, John Holloszy published the first evidence that exercise training promotes mitochondrial biogenesis in rat skeletal muscle [165]. Since then, mitochondrial biogenesis (described in more detail in the Biogenesis section above) has repeatedly proven to be a key component of improved fitness following exercise. This process is known to be highly coordinated and requires the coordination of multiple cellular events, including transcription of two genomes (nuclear and mitochondrial), the synthesis of lipids and proteins, and the coordinated assembly of multi-subunit protein complexes into a functional respiratory chain, as reviewed elsewhere by Hood [166].

The working skeletal muscle responds to the repeated, episodic bouts of muscle contraction related to exercise by functional adaptations such as improved contractile protein function, improved metabolic regulation, and enhanced intracellular signaling leading to increased transcription of nuclear- and mitochondrial-encoded genes. These in turn alter the protein content and enzymatic activity in the skeletal muscles, mitochondrial function, metabolic regulation, intracellular signaling, and transcriptional responses [167–171]. External and internal stimuli from exercise and muscle contraction give rise to signals that trigger the body and in particular the mitochondria to adapt. There are numerous suggested molecular mechanisms that have been associated with the activation of the intracellular orchestra that leads to more efficient and an increased number of mitochondria. One of the most studied factors leading to mitochondrial biogenesis is the transcription coactivator PGC-1α, which can be seen as the primary regulator of transcription of nuclear-encoded genes coupled to mitochondrial biogenesis [172]. Several animal studies, where the PGC-1α gene has been deleted globally or in a muscle-specific manner, have shown strengthening evidence of the importance of PGC-1α in the exercise adaptive response, since these animals display blunted exercise-induced mitochondrial biogenesis or decreased expression of genes important for mitochondrial biogenesis as well as reduced exercise capacity [173–176]. Interestingly, mice overexpressing PGC-1α in muscle show significantly enhanced mitochondrial protein abundance in otherwise fast-twitch muscle fibers [177]. However, as mentioned earlier, PGC-1α does not act alone. ERR α and NRF-1 are recognized as transcription partners of PGC-1α, and transcription of nuclear mitochondrial genes is dependent on this co-activation [178]. Exercise increases the interaction between PGC-1α and NRF-1, and this interaction leads to the transcription of TFAM, a key mitochondrial transcription factor [179]. Exercise has also been shown to stimulate mitochondrial biogenesis by translocation of PGC-1α in the mitochondria, where it forms a complex with TFAM and thereby initiates transcription from the D-loop region [178, 179]. The external and internal cellular signals that activate PGC-1α upstream can be summarized to mechanical stress and/or energy-related changes. Various types of exercise have been shown to increase levels of calcium, which together with the stress-induced p38 mitogen-activated protein kinase (MAPK) activates PGC-1α activity and expression [89, 180, 181]. As an energy-related stimulus, AMPK is one of the most studied factors in exercise intervention studies. In animal studies, exercise-induced AMPK activation has been linked to an increased PGC-1α protein, and in human skeletal muscle cells, it has been shown that AICAR, an AMPK analog, can activate PGC-1α gene expression [89, 91]. A well-known tumor suppressor gene, p53, has also been linked to exercise-induced mitochondrial biogenesis in skeletal muscle [182]. This link seems to involve the activation and regulation of PGC-1α, and p53 has been shown to directly bind to the PGC-1α promoter and thereby increase PGC-1α expression [183]. The metabolic stress that activates p53 and triggers cell-cycle arrest, ROS clearance, or apoptosis has also been shown to be regulated by direct binding of PGC-1α to p53 [184] (Fig. 3.1).

Furthermore, p53 is activated/phosphorylated by muscle contraction and metabolic stress, leading to translocation of p53 which results in the transcription of metabolic genes [185, 186]. PGC-1α is, in this sense, defining the p53 response to metabolic stress such as exercise and can be seen as a critical switch in determining the p53-mediated cell fate. Further support for a potent role of p53 has been evaluated in knockout mice, in which multiple signaling pathways related to mitochondrial biogenesis, e.g., reduced or delayed p38 MAPK, AMPK, and CaMKII responses to acute exercise, along with impaired induction of PGC-1α mRNA have been seen [185]. Studies have also investigated the mechanisms by which AMPK may regulate mitochondrial biogenesis, and this has been shown to involve both direct phosphorylation and deacetylation (via SIRT1) of PGC-1α [187]. However, as mentioned earlier, there are more than one actor steering the exercise-induced apparatus controlling mitochondrial biogenesis. As an e.g of this complexed regulation, it has been shown that mice lacking PGC-1α or SIRT1 have normal increases in mitochondrial biogenesis as a response to exercise [188, 189]. Interestingly, mice lacking the

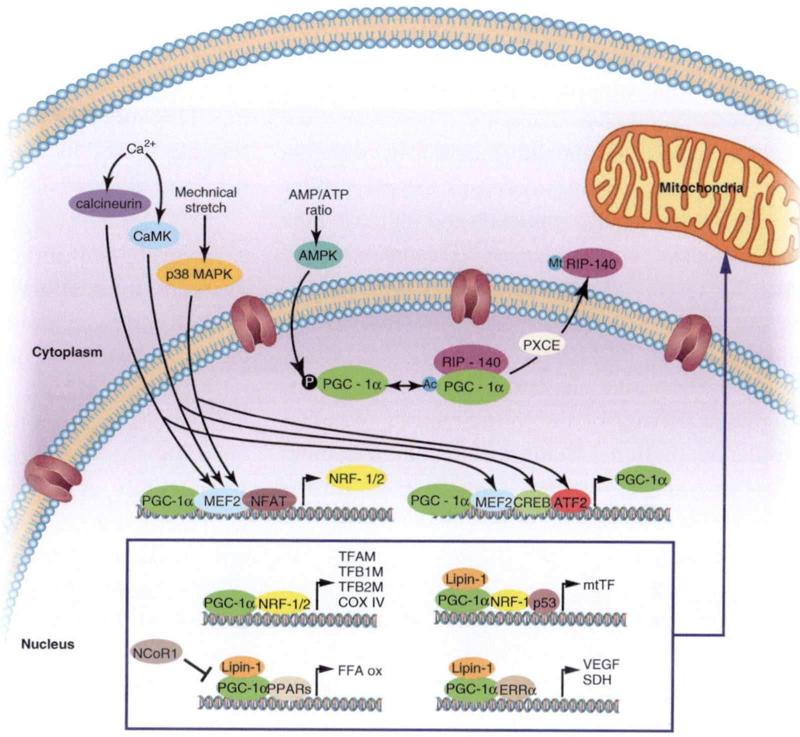

Fig. 3.1 Schematic illustration of a human skeletal muscle cell and its nucleus showing factors involved in exercise-induced adaptations. During and following exercise, stimuli such as mechanical stretch, calcium signaling, and AMP/ATP ratio are affected (displayed in the cytoplasm). Effects of exercise on transcriptional regulation are shown inside the nucleus. The box shows example of nuclear-encoded mitochondrial transcriptions factors that are activated by PGC-1α. (Illustration: Mattias Karlén, copyright Eva-Karin Gidlund)

liver kinase B1 (LKB1), a downstream target of AMPK, do not increase components of the mitochondrial electron transport chain when exposed to exercise training and show reduced exercise capacity [190]. To further understand the complex features that lead to exercise-induced mitochondrial biogenesis, it will be important to establish whether factors other than the AMPK-PGC-1α-SIRT1 pathway are necessary for mediating adaptations to exercise.

Besides PGC-1α, its upstream regulators and mechanical stress or energy-induced signaling pathways that stimulate mitochondrial biogenesis, posttranslational modifications, and translational control systems might also affect the exercise-induced mitochondrial adaptations, as reviewed by Drake et al. [191]. In addition to posttranslational and translational modification, fusion and fission also allow for the dynamic remodeling of mitochondria, which function as a quality control mechanism. However, fusion and fission as exercise-induced events are not well understood. However, after a bout of acute exercise and exercise training, events such as autophagy and mitophagy have been demonstrated to be enhanced, which improves mitochondrial quality [192–194].

Different types of exercise modalities have different effects on the mitochondrial response. Mitochondria appear to adapt and compensate specifically to the type of metabolic stress applied throughout exercise.

Endurance-type training Endurance-type exercise is seen as the primary cause of exercise-induced mitochondrial biogenesis and improved mitochondrial function. Training-induced improvements of mitochondrial volume and mitochondrial enzyme activity were shown in the early 1970s during longitudinal training studies and cross-sectional studies comparing trained and untrained men [195–197]. In light of these findings, later studies of endurance exercise (4–6 weeks) have shown a 30–100% increase in mitochondrial density within the skeletal muscle of healthy humans [198–200]. Over several decades, exercise interventions have also shown increases in total mitochondrial protein amount, enzymes involved in β oxidation, the TCA cycle, and the OXPHOS system [165, 201–203]. Mitochondrial volume is used as a marker of improved oxidative capacity; however two recently published innovative studies have shown that endurance training increases the assemblies of respiratory super-complexes and increased the mitochondrial cristae density. This increase of structures within the mitochondria can be seen as strong indicators of improved and modulated oxidative capacity [204, 205] and imply that important mitochondrial adaptations occur besides the increased density of the mitochondria. Whether similar adaptational changes also adhere to other types of training regimes remains to be further investigated; however, some evidence is discussed below.

Resistance-type training Several studies have shown that resistance exercise in fact can stimulate the signaling cascade that activates mitochondrial biogenesis, although to a relatively lesser degree than endurance exercise and depends on pre-training status and the exercise principles employed [206–208]. Since resistance exercise is much less studied compared to endurance exercise, relatively few studies have investigated the effect of resistance exercise on mitochondrial adaptations and mitochondrial protein synthesis. Interestingly though, available studies indicate that both mitochondrial and myofibrillar protein synthesis increase after a single bout of resistance exercise in healthy untrained individuals. Furthermore, Burd et al. reported in 2012 that a single bout of resistance training increased PGC-1α expression and stimulated mitochondrial protein synthesis [209]. Noteworthy, this result was seen in a fed state where the subjects were given an amino acid supplementation, which has been reported earlier to stimulate mitochondrial protein synthesis [210]. Moreover, 12 weeks of resistance training has been seen in both young and old subjects to increase mitochondrial protein content [211] and increase mitochondrial markers such as citrate synthase (CS) activity and mtDNA copy number [49, 212]. However, utilization of citrate synthase activity as a biomarker is quite equivocal, and apart from increased activity, both decreased [213] and unchanged [207, 214, 215] enzyme activity has been reported after resistance training. This might in part be explained by different training protocols, age, and the pre-training status, as mentioned above.

To evaluate if different training regimes cause different intracellular responses, Coffey et al. studied early signaling responses in skeletal muscle from resistance-only trained and endurance-only trained athletes [206]. After implementing the exercise regimes that the subject was unfamiliar with, the signaling response was examined. Interestingly, AMPK phosphorylation increased in skeletal muscle after cycling in resistance- but not endurance-trained subjects. Conversely, AMPK was elevated after resistance exercise in endurance- but not strength-trained subjects. This pattern also held true when the authors analyzed other factors recognized to be activated by either resistance or endurance training, respectively. The results that the phosphorylation of AMPK increased in cyclists after resistance exercise and in strength-trained athletes after cycling do not support the hypothesis of a selective activation of specific molecular pathways depending on the different exercise types [206]. Rather, this supports the notion that in order to improve performance or elicit a physiological change, the body needs to be stressed and one's workout programs need to vary in order to not reach a progression plateau. Thus, resistance exercise does in fact seem able to stimulate mitochondrial biogenesis although to a lesser degree than endurance training.

High-intensity interval training Apart from the classical endurance- and resistance-type training protocols, high-intensity interval training (HIIT), in particular sprint interval training (SIT), which is characterized by relatively brief, intermittent periods of muscle contraction, often performed with an "all-out" effort (20–30s performed 3–10 times) or at an intensity close to the peak oxygen uptake (VO_2 peak), has been shown to promote mitochondrial adaptations such as biogenesis [216–219]. By comparing different exercise modalities, it has been shown that HIIT seems to have a more beneficial effect on the mitochondrial respiration than initially thought, and this holds true even compared to traditional endurance training [200, 202, 219, 220]. Interestingly, although VO_2 peak improves in response to each exercise modality to a similar extent (approximately 8%), those improvements are primarily attributed to different physiological adaptations. Exercise adaptations seen by HIIT and SIT have primarily been attributed to improvements in skeletal muscle respiratory capacity [202], whereas improvements attendant to more common endurance training have been predominantly determined through hematological adaptations [200]. Even though the energy production during a single sprint is mainly anaerobic, repeated sprints will gradually increase the aerobic contribution favoring a high muscular oxidative capacity important for performance. Interestingly, in untrained subjects SIT exercise seems to induce similar response in mitochondrial biogenesis compared to long-duration cycling (90–120 min at 65% of VO_{2max}) [218].

As mentioned earlier, one of the key controllers of mitochondrial biogenesis is the transcription coactivator PGC-1α. Most studies of acute PGC-1α regulation in humans have used prolonged exercise interventions; however, a surprisingly small dose of very intense interval exercise, equivalent to only 2 min of all-out cycling, has been shown to be sufficient to increase the gene expression of PGC-1α [220]. The energy-sensitive kinase AMPK has been observed to be activated mainly at exercise intensities of about 60% VO_2 peak [221–223]. However, low-intensity exercise at 30–40% of VO_2 peak but performed until exhaustion also activates AMPK in skeletal muscle [222]. A recently published exercise study by Casuso et al. compared high-volume HIIT to sprint interval swimming and found that the sprint-type training resulted in higher muscular stress, but without an increase in systemic oxidation. Interestingly, the high-volume HIIT resulted in a much higher induction of both PGC-1α and AMPK compared to the sprint training [224]. Evidence appears to support that HIIT might act as a stimulus to induce mitochondrial adaptations by stimulating biogenesis and increasing CS activity [225, 226].

Concurrent training Combining endurance and strength training (concurrent training) and the effect on mitochondrial biogenesis have not been well studied. However, if resistance and endurance exercise are performed on separate training sessions, it has been suggested that the mechanism behind improved endurance performance does not seem to be related to changes in mitochondrial content [227, 228]. More recent studies have somewhat challenged this view, by combining resistance and endurance exercise within the same training session. Interestingly, combining aerobic exercise with resistance altered the skeletal muscle transcriptional signature of resistance exercise to initiate important gene programs promoting both myofiber growth and improved oxidative capacity [229].

Also, exercise-induced AMPK activation has been suggested not to interfere with muscle hypertrophy in response to resistance training in men [230]. Further, enhanced CS activity, a marker of mitochondrial biogenesis, has been observed when resistance training was performed immediately after endurance training. Robinson et al. reported recently that both young (18–30 years) and old (65–80 years) individuals had greater activation of mitochondrial markers with 12 weeks of HIIT and combined moderate-intensity aerobic and resistance training but not when performing resistance training alone [211]. Furthermore, in a group of middle-aged men who performed a single bout of endurance (cycling), resistance, and concurrent exercise at different occasions, markers of either oxidative improvements or hypertrophy were analyzed. Interestingly, this study demonstrated that acute concurrent exercise stimulated myofibrillar and mitochondrial protein fractional synthesis rate, protein signaling, and mRNA expression to equivalent number as either cycling or the resistance training alone [231].

A possible explanation for this might be that the molecular signals induced by aerobic/endurance exercises are enhanced when resistance exercise is performed in close proximity and the signals might not interfere as previously thought. Interestingly, in the study by Robinson et al., RNA sequencing of muscle biopsies was performed which revealed a robust increase in mRNA expression of mitochondrial transcripts with HIIT, more so than when subjects performed resistance training or combined aerobic and resistance training [211]. Proteomics data from the same study revealed larger proteomic change in mitochondrial and ribosome proteins when HIIT was performed compared to both resistance and combined aerobic and resistance training. Furthermore, epigenetic analysis revealed a relatively small change (<10%) of DNA promoter methylation and low overlap between transcriptional and proteomic changes [211].

In conclusion, all types of stress on the body will elicit intracellular responses and adaptation. This means that all modes of physical activity have the potential to stimulate the organism and mitochondria to adapt according to external and internal demands. Since the mitochondrion is the powerhouse of the cell and controls aerobic metabolism, it will benefit from aerobic exercise and training. Endurance-type training is therefore a powerful way to stimulate mitochondrial exercise adaptations. However, HIIT seems to effectively improve cardio-metabolic heath in a similar way as endurance and also stimulates mitochondrial biogenesis and oxidative capacity. Lastly, resistance training and concurrent training might also affect the mitochondria by inducing mitochondrial biogenesis, but to a lesser degree than both endurance and HIIT.

Clinical and Public Health Relevance

From an overall health and clinical perspective, it is highly important to have well-functioning mitochondria and to be physically active. However, is it possible to induce mitochondrial biogenesis or improve mitochondrial function by pharmacological treatment? This is a really interesting question and undergoing increasing scrutiny. An increased understanding of the molecular mechanisms that leads to exercise-induced muscle remodeling has spurred development of exercise-mimicking drugs, and activators of AMPK, PPARδ (nuclear receptor activated by PGC-1α), SIRT1, as well as ERRγ have been developed; for details see the review by Fan W and Evans [232]. Other exercise-mimicking drugs, e.g., agonists that activate beta-2-adrenergic receptors such as AICAR, clenbuterol, and formoterol, have also been studied in attempts to induce mitochondrial biogenesis [233]. Apart from these agonists, G-protein-coupled receptors (GPCRs) have gained an increased interest. GPCRs' ligands represent numerous clinically approved receptor agonists, which makes them attractive targets for the identification of therapeutics that induce mitochondrial biogenesis [234, 235]. Besides pharmacological products, some natural products have also been linked to mitochondrial biogenesis and improved mitochondrial function which include resveratrol, epicatechin, curcumin, and some phytoestrogens [236]. These natural/nutritional products have mostly been studied in animal models and cell systems. The most examined product, resveratrol, has shown some promising results and proven to activate the SIRT1-AMPK pathway leading to mitochondrial biogenesis in both in vitro and in vivo studies [236]. Moreover, more therapeutic targets will definitely be developed. Furthermore, recent clinical trials in patients with diagnosed heart failure and decreased ejection fraction have shown promising results from infusion of elamipretide, which is a previously known peptide that targets mitochondrial dysfunction [237].

For decades, researchers and the industry have searched for the "exercise pill": however, to this day no such pills exist that have the potential to replace all the physiological changes and the beneficial effects that exercise brings to the performers. A recent study in mice declared that treatment of PPARδ agonist delayed the exhaustion of running by inducing a glucose-saving shift, and this was said to be a highly potent exercise pill. Nevertheless, even mice that did not exercise but were given the drug displayed a somewhat similar energy shift; however, to get the full exercise-mimicking effect, mice still needed to perform exercise [238].

From a health and a clinical perspective, mitochondrial diseases are also a highlighted research field of interest. In 2017, Zhang et al. earned a lot of attention by publishing a report that described the first birth of a healthy boy after mitochondrial replacement therapy (MRT) by spindle transfer to prevent transmission of mitochondrial disease from mother to child [239]. In this way, three parents gave rise to this child. The child's mother had the mitochondrial mutation that causes Leigh syndrome, and she had the mitochondrial haplogroup I; the donor of the mtDNA had no known mitochondrial mutations and was a mitochondrial haplogroup L2c. According to the authors, the child, who was 7 months old at the time of reporting, was healthy. The mutation load varies in a newborn baby's tissues, and high levels of heteroplasmy are a key issue in MRT, since it can lead to manifestation of disease. An adult human has been estimated to have a total number of 3.72×10^{13} cells with approximately 1×10^{16} cell divisions [240]. Therefore, a slight advantage of cell survival or proliferation with mutant mtDNA can dramatically increase the final level of heteroplasmy. Thus, accordingly to Zhang and colleagues, a trend of the shift in mtDNA heteroplasmy is much more important than the actual heteroplasmy level in the blastocyst in determining the final level of mtDNA mutation in a baby [239]. So, the question of whether mutation load increases with increasing age, and if that will affect the child, is one that cannot be answered definitively at this point. If MRT is the future in mtDNA-linked diseases, it still needs further research.

Besides mtDNA mutations and replacement therapies, the mitochondrial genome and epigenome, as well as the mitochondrial-derived peptides, might be more important than previously thought and highly relevant to achieving health and preventing diseases. But, how and to what degree exercises affect these mitochondrial-encoded genes and the mitochondrial genome and epigenetics are still unknown.

Finally, from a clinical and a public health perspective, as reviewed in different aspects and chapters throughout this book, a healthy weight, regular physical activity and a good nutritional status are key features that affect a person's well-being and health and also one's mitochondria.

Conclusion and Future Directions

In order to maintain health, it has been shown repeatedly that the human body needs a certain amount of physical activity. This need of physical activity is tightly coupled to the activation of gene programs that evolved during the time when we were required to be much more physically active than today. For many years, researchers have focused intensely on trying to understand the mechanisms behind training adaptation such as improved metabolic and mitochondrial function. This has, in part, been done by studying how genes respond to training and lifestyle interventions. Despite substantial progress, significant knowledge gaps remain, even though strong evidence points toward the positive effect of exercise on mitochondria and a connection between mitochondrial function and decreased risk for disease development. The mechanisms of exercise and how it affects all the cells in the body and especially the mitochondria will most certainly continue to be of great scientific and public interest in the future.

The magic of the mitochondria is not fully understood, and the unique structure and functional characteristics of this organelle have raised the ideas of mitochondrial specific drugs. Moreover, retrograde signaling molecules like mitochondrial-derived peptides might have more biological functions than shown previously. These peptides, released from the mitochondria, have already been linked to protective effects in some diseases such as Alzheimer's disease and cancer. If these mitochondrially encoded peptides also have protective effects in cardiovascular diseases needs further assessment. However, we know that exercise increases the size, number, and amount of mitochondria and increases the copy number of the mtDNA, which might be of importance in producing more of these cyto- and neuroprotective peptides.

Furthermore, presence of impaired mitochondrial function and reduced number of mitochondria is usually classified as mitochondrial dysfunction, which is commonly seen in obese individuals and patients with metabolic disorders. Luckily, exercise and regular physical activity seem to have a protective, preventive, and a somewhat therapeutic role in mitochondrial dysfunction. If this is also the case in inherited mitochondrial diseases, it is still under enquiry. However, numerous studies have shown that transcription factors and coactivators such as the exercise-sensitive PGC-1α are highly important for maintaining a good metabolic and mitochondrial function. PGC-1α has also been implicated in novel angiogenic pathways, which may strengthen the notion that exercise-induced activation of PGC-1α might be important for the treatment of, e.g., ischemic heart diseases. Collectively, further developments in the area of mitochondrial medicine and exercise medicine will be very important from a health and disease management perspective.

References

1. Stewart JB, Chinnery PF. The dynamics of mitochondrial DNA heteroplasmy: implications for human health and disease. Nat Rev Genet. 2015;16(9):530–42.
2. Martin W, Kowallik K. Annotated English translation of Mereschkowsky's 1905 paper 'Über Natur und Ursprung der Chromatophoren imPflanzenreiche'. Eur J Phycol. 1999;34(3):287–95.
3. Gray MW, Burger G, Lang BF. Mitochondrial evolution. Science. 1999;283(5407):1476–81.
4. Farquhar J, Bao H, Thiemens M. Atmospheric influence of earth's earliest sulfur cycle. Science. Proc Am Assoc Adv Sci. 2000;289(5480):756–8.
5. Karlberg EOL, Andersson SGE. Mitochondrial gene history and mRNA localization: is there a correlation? Nat Rev Genet. 2003;4(5):391–7.
6. Sato M, Sato K. Maternal inheritance of mitochondrial DNA by diverse mechanisms to eliminate paternal mitochondrial DNA. Biochim Biophys Acta. 2013;1833(8):1979–84.
7. Gray MW. Mosaic nature of the mitochondrial proteome: Implications for the origin and evolution of mitochondria. Proc Natl Acad Sci U S A. 2015;112(33):10133–8.
8. Martin W, Hoffmeister M, Rotte C, Henze K. An overview of endosymbiotic models for the origins of eukaryotes, their ATP-producing organelles (mitochondria and hydrogenosomes), and their heterotrophic lifestyle. Biol Chem. 2001;382(11):1521–39.
9. Cann RL, Stoneking M, Wilson AC. Mitochondrial DNA and human evolution. Nature. 1987;325(6099):31–6.
10. Ankel-Simons F, Cummins JM. Misconceptions about mitochondria and mammalian fertilization: implications for theories on human evolution. Proc Natl Acad Sci U S A. 1996;93(24):13859–63.
11. Endicott P, Ho SYW, Metspalu M, Stringer C. Evaluating the mitochondrial timescale of human evolution. Trends Ecol Evol. 2009;24(9):515–21.
12. Kofler B, Mueller EE, Eder W, Stanger O, Maier R, Weger M, et al. Mitochondrial DNA haplogroup T is associated with coronary artery disease and diabetic retinopathy: a case control study. BMC Med Genet. 2009;10:35.
13. Fernández-Caggiano M, Barallobre-Barreiro J, Rego-Pérez I, Crespo-Leiro MG, Paniagua MJ, Grillé Z, et al. Mitochondrial haplogroups H and J: risk and protective factors for ischemic cardiomyopathy. PLoS One. 2012;7(8):e44128.
14. Kenney MC, Chwa M, Atilano SR, Falatoonzadeh P, Ramirez C, Malik D, et al. Molecular and bioenergetic differences between cells with African versus European inherited mitochondrial DNA haplogroups: implications for population susceptibility to diseases. Biochim Biophys Acta. 2014;1842(2):208–19.
15. Falkenberg M, Larsson N-G, Gustafsson CM. DNA replication and transcription in mammalian mitochondria. Annu Rev Biochem. 2007;76:679–99.
16. Kisch B. Are there mitochondria in red blood cells? Exp Med Surg. 1961;19:278–80.
17. Veltri KL, Espiritu M, Singh G. Distinct genomic copy number in mitochondria of different mammalian organs. J Cell Physiol. Wiley Subscription Services, Inc., A Wiley Company; 1990;143(1):160–4.
18. Kirkwood SP, Munn EA, Brooks GA. Mitochondrial reticulum in limb skeletal muscle. Am J Phys. 1986;251(3 Pt 1):C395–402.
19. Sukhorukov VM, Dikov D, Reichert AS, Meyer-Hermann M. Emergence of the mitochondrial reticulum from fission and fusion dynamics. PLoS Comput Biol. Public Library of Science; 2012;8(10):e1002745.
20. Taanman JW. The mitochondrial genome: structure, transcription, translation and replication. Biochim Biophys Acta. 1999;1410(2):103–23.
21. Karlberg O, Canbäck B, Kurland CG, Andersson SG. The dual origin of the yeast mitochondrial proteome. Yeast. 2000;17(3):170–87.
22. Calvo SE, Mootha VK. The mitochondrial proteome and human disease. Annu Rev Genomics Hum Genet. 2010;11(1):25–44.
23. Hashimoto Y, Ito Y, Niikura T, Shao Z, Hata M, Oyama F, et al. Mechanisms of neuroprotection by

a novel rescue factor humanin from Swedish mutant amyloid precursor protein. Biochem Biophys Res Commun. 2001;283(2):460–8.
24. Mercer TR, Neph S, Dinger ME, Crawford J, Smith MA, Shearwood A-MJ, et al. The human mitochondrial transcriptome. Cell. 2011;146(4):645–58.
25. Rimbaud S, Garnier A, Ventura-Clapier R. Mitochondrial biogenesis in cardiac pathophysiology. Pharmacol Rep. 2009;61(1):131–8.
26. Bensasson D, Zhang D-X, Hartl DL, Hewitt GM. Mitochondrial pseudogenes: evolution's misplaced witnesses. Trends Ecol Evol. Elsevier. 2001;16(6):314–21.
27. Ramos A, Barbena E, Mateiu L, del Mar GM, Mairal Q, Lima M, et al. Nuclear insertions of mitochondrial origin: database updating and usefulness in cancer studies. Mitochondrion. 2011;11(6):946–53.
28. du HG B, Riley FL. Hybridization between the nuclear and kinetoplast DNA's of Leishmania enriettii and between nuclear and mitochondrial DNA's of mouse liver. Proc Natl Acad Sci. 1967;57(3):790–7.
29. Bensasson D. Mitochondrial pseudogenes: evolution's misplaced witnesses. Trends Ecol Evol. 2001;16(6):314–21.
30. Mishmar D, Ruiz-Pesini E, Brandon M, Wallace DC. Mitochondrial DNA-like sequences in the nucleus (NUMTs): insights into our African origins and the mechanism of foreign DNA integration. Hum Mutat. 2004;23(2):125–33.
31. Richly E, Leister D. NUMTs in sequenced eukaryotic genomes. Mol Biol Evol. 2004;21(6):1081–4.
32. Bodzioch M, Lapicka-Bodzioch K, Zapala B, Kamysz W, Kiec-Wilk B, Dembinska-Kiec A. Evidence for potential functionality of nuclearly-encoded humanin isoforms. Genomics. 2009;94(4):247–56.
33. da Cunha FM, Torelli NQ, Kowaltowski AJ. Mitochondrial retrograde signaling: triggers, pathways, and outcomes. Oxidative Med Cell Longev. 2015;2015:482582.
34. Lee C, Yen K, Cohen P. Humanin: a harbinger of mitochondrial-derived peptides? Trends Endocrinol Metab. 2013;24(5):222–8.
35. Verdin E, Hirschey MD, Finley LWS, Haigis MC. Sirtuin regulation of mitochondria: energy production, apoptosis, and signaling. Trends Biochem Sci. 2010;35(12):669–75.
36. Ganta VC, Alexander JS. Focus on carbon monoxide: a modulator of neutrophil oxidants and elastase spatial localization? Am J Physiol Heart Circ Physiol. 2009;297(3):H902–4.
37. Ichikawa Y, Bayeva M, Ghanefar M, Potini V, Sun L, Mutharasan RK, et al. Disruption of ATP-binding cassette B8 in mice leads to cardiomyopathy through a decrease in mitochondrial iron export. Proc Natl Acad Sci USA. National Acad Sciences. 2012;109(11):4152–7.
38. Nakahira K, Haspel JA, Rathinam VAK, Lee S-J, Dolinay T, Lam HC, et al. Autophagy proteins regulate innate immune responses by inhibiting the release of mitochondrial DNA mediated by the NALP3 inflammasome. Nat Immunol. 2011;12(3):222–30.
39. Saki M, Prakash A. DNA damage related crosstalk between the nucleus and mitochondria. Free Radic Biol Med. 2017;107:216–27.
40. Zhang Q, Itagaki K, Hauser CJ. Mitochondrial DNA is released by shock and activates neutrophils via p38 map kinase. Shock. 2010;34(1):55–9.
41. Battersby BJ, Richter U. Why translation counts for mitochondria – retrograde signalling links mitochondrial protein synthesis to mitochondrial biogenesis and cell proliferation. J Cell Sci. 2013;126(19):4331–8.
42. Kadlec AO, Beyer AM, Ait-Aissa K, Gutterman DD. Mitochondrial signaling in the vascular endothelium: beyond reactive oxygen species. Basic Res Cardiol. Springer Berlin Heidelberg; 2016;111(3):26.
43. Hashimoto Y, Niikura T, Tajima H, Yasukawa T, Sudo H, Ito Y, et al. A rescue factor abolishing neuronal cell death by a wide spectrum of familial Alzheimer's disease genes and Abeta. Proc Natl Acad Sci U S A. 2001;98(11):6336–41.
44. Lee C, Zeng J, Drew BG, Sallam T, Martin-Montalvo A, Wan J, et al. The mitochondrial-derived peptide MOTS-c promotes metabolic homeostasis and reduces obesity and insulin resistance. Cell Metab. 2015;21(3):443–54.
45. Muzumdar RH, Huffman DM, Atzmon G, Buettner C, Cobb LJ, Fishman S, et al. Humanin: a novel central regulator of peripheral insulin action. PLoS One. 2009;4(7):e6334.
46. Yen K, Lee C, Mehta H, Cohen P. The emerging role of the mitochondrial-derived peptide humanin in stress resistance. J Mol Endocrinol. 2013;50(1):R11–9.
47. Fuku N, Pareja-Galeano H, Zempo H, Alis R, Arai Y, Lucia A, et al. The mitochondrial-derived peptide MOTS-c: a player in exceptional longevity? Aging Cell. 2015;14(6):921–3.
48. Gong Z, Tas E, Muzumdar R. Humanin and age-related diseases: a new link? Front Endocrinol (Lausanne). 2014;5:210.
49. Gidlund E-K, Walden von F, Venojärvi M, Risérus U, Heinonen OJ, Norrbom J, et al. Humanin skeletal muscle protein levels increase after resistance training in men with impaired glucose metabolism. Physiol Rep. 2016;4(23):e13063.
50. Thummasorn S, Shinlapawittayatorn K, Khamseekaew J, Jaiwongkam T, Chattipakorn SC, Chattipakorn N. Humanin directly protects cardiac mitochondria against dysfunction initiated by oxidative stress by decreasing complex I activity. Mitochondrion. 2018;38:31–40.
51. Ma ZA, Zhao Z, Turk J. Mitochondrial dysfunction and β-cell failure in type 2 diabetes mellitus. Exp Diabetes Res. 2012;2012:703538.
52. Marzetti E, Csiszar A, Dutta D, Balagopal G, Calvani R, Leeuwenburgh C. Role of mitochondrial dysfunction and altered autophagy in cardiovascular aging and disease: from mechanisms to

therapeutics. Am J Physiol Heart Circ Physiol. 2013;305(4):H459–76.
53. Gamboa JL, Billings FT, Bojanowski MT, Gilliam LA, Yu C, Roshanravan B, et al. Mitochondrial dysfunction and oxidative stress in patients with chronic kidney disease. Physiol Rep. 2016;4(9):e12780.
54. Galvan DL, Green NH, Danesh FR. The hallmarks of mitochondrial dysfunction in chronic kidney disease. Kidney Int. 2017;92(5):1051–7.
55. Chae S, Ahn BY, Byun K, Cho YM, Yu M-H, Lee B, et al. A systems approach for decoding mitochondrial retrograde signaling pathways. Sci Signal. American Association for the Advancement of Science. 2013;6(264):rs4.
56. Page E, McCallister LP. Quantitative electron microscopic description of heart muscle cells. Application to normal, hypertrophied and thyroxin-stimulated hearts. Am J Cardiol. 1973;31(2):172–81.
57. Covian R, Balaban RS. Cardiac mitochondrial matrix and respiratory complex protein phosphorylation. Am J Physiol Heart Circ Physiol. 2012;303(8):H940–66.
58. Ferrari R, Censi S, Mastrorilli F, Boraso A. Prognostic benefits of heart rate reduction in cardiovascular disease. Eur Heart J Suppl. 2003;5:G10–4.
59. Palmer JW, Tandler B, Hoppel CL. Biochemical properties of subsarcolemmal and interfibrillar mitochondria isolated from rat cardiac muscle. J Biol Chem. 1977;252(23):8731–9.
60. Glancy B, Hartnell LM, Malide D, Yu Z-X, Combs CA, Connelly PS, et al. Mitochondrial reticulum for cellular energy distribution in muscle. Nature. 2015;523(7562):617–20.
61. Glancy B, Hartnell LM, Combs CA, Fenmou A, Sun J, Murphy E, et al. Power grid protection of the muscle mitochondrial reticulum. Cell Rep. 2017;19(3):487–96.
62. Bogenhagen D, Clayton DA. Mouse L cell mitochondrial DNA molecules are selected randomly for replication throughout the cell cycle. Cell. 1977;11(4):719–27.
63. Montoya J, Christianson T, Levens D, Rabinowitz M, Attardi G. Identification of initiation sites for heavy-strand and light-strand transcription in human mitochondrial DNA. Proc Natl Acad Sci USA. National Academy of Sciences. 1982;79(23):7195–9.
64. Clayton DA. Vertebrate mitochondrial DNA-a circle of surprises. Exp Cell Res. 2000;255(1):4–9.
65. Shadel GS, Clayton DA. Mitochondrial DNA maintenance in vertebrates. Annu Rev Biochem. 1997;66(1):409–35.
66. Wanrooij S, Falkenberg M. The human mitochondrial replication fork in health and disease. Biochim Biophys Acta. 2010;1797(8):1378–88.
67. Spelbrink JN. Functional organization of mammalian mitochondrial DNA in nucleoids: history, recent developments, and future challenges. IUBMB Life. 2010;62(1):19–32.
68. Clayton DA. Transcription and replication of mitochondrial DNA. Hum Reprod. 2000;15(suppl 2):11–7.
69. Abdul Aziz, Mohamed Yusoff, Farizan Ahmad, Zamzuri Idris, Hasnan Jaafar and Jafri Malin Abdullah. Understanding mitochondrial DNA in brain tumorigenesis. In: Molecular considerations and evolving surgical management issues in the treatment of patients with a brain tumor: InTech,United Kingdome; 2015. https://www.intechopen.com/books/molecular-considerations-and-evolving-surgical-management-issues-in-thetreatment-of-patients-with-a-brain-tumor.
70. FustE JM, Wanrooij S, Jemt E, Granycome CE, Cluett TJ, Shi Y, et al. Mitochondrial RNA polymerase is needed for activation of the origin of light-strand DNA replication. Mol Cell. Elsevier. 2010;37(1):67–78.
71. Asin-Cayuela J, Gustafsson CM. Mitochondrial transcription and its regulation in mammalian cells. Trends Biochem Sci. 2007;32(3):111–7.
72. Sologub M, Litonin D, Anikin M, Mustaev A, Temiakov D. TFB2 is a transient component of the catalytic site of the human mitochondrial RNA polymerase. Cell. 2009;139(5):934–44.
73. Roberti M, Polosa PL, Bruni F, Manzari C, Deceglie S, Gadaleta MN, et al. The MTERF family proteins: mitochondrial transcription regulators and beyond. Biochim Biophys Acta. 2009;1787(5):303–11.
74. Medeiros DM. Assessing mitochondria biogenesis. Methods. 2008;46(4):288–94.
75. Hood DA, Joseph A-M. Mitochondrial assembly: protein import. Proc Nutr Soc. 2004;63(2):293–300.
76. Wiedemann N, Pfanner N. Mitochondrial machineries for protein import and assembly. Annu Rev Biochem. 2017;86:685–714.
77. Iqbal S, Hood DA. The role of mitochondrial fusion and fission in skeletal muscle function and dysfunction. Front Biosci. 2015;20:157–72.
78. Fisher RP, Lisowsky T, Parisi MA, Clayton DA. DNA wrapping and bending by a mitochondrial high mobility group-like transcriptional activator protein. J Biol Chem. 1992;267(5):3358–67.
79. Falkenberg M, Gaspari M, Rantanen A, Trifunovic A, Larsson N-G, Gustafsson CM. Mitochondrial transcription factors B1 and B2 activate transcription of human mtDNA. Nat Genet. 2002;31(3):289–94.
80. Scarpulla RC. Metabolic control of mitochondrial biogenesis through the PGC-1 family regulatory network. Biochim Biophys Acta. 2011;1813(7):1269–78.
81. Lyonnais S, Tarrés-Soler A, Rubio-Cosials A, Cuppari A, Brito R, Jaumot J, et al. The human mitochondrial transcription factor A is a versatile G-quadruplex binding protein. Sci Rep. 2017;7:43992.
82. Holt IJ, Reyes A. Human mitochondrial DNA replication. Cold Spring Harb Perspect Biol. 2012;1:4(12).
83. Dufour CR, Wilson BJ, Huss JM, Kelly DP, Alaynick WA, Downes M, et al. Genome-wide orchestration of cardiac functions by the orphan nuclear receptors ERRalpha and gamma. Cell Metab. 2007;5(5):345–56.
84. Lehman JJ, Barger PM, Kovacs A, Saffitz JE, Medeiros DM, Kelly DP. Peroxisome proliferator-activated receptor gamma coactivator-1 promotes cardiac mito-

chondrial biogenesis. J Clin Invest. American Society for Clinical Investigation. 2000;106(7):847–56.
85. Garnier A, Fortin D, Deloménie C, Momken I, Veksler V, Ventura-Clapier R. Depressed mitochondrial transcription factors and oxidative capacity in rat failing cardiac and skeletal muscles. J Physiol. 2003;551(Pt 2):491–501.
86. Leone TC, Lehman JJ, Finck BN, Schaeffer PJ, Wende AR, Boudina S, et al. PGC-1alpha deficiency causes multi-system energy metabolic derangements: muscle dysfunction, abnormal weight control and hepatic steatosis. PLoS Biol. 2005;3(4):e101.
87. Arany Z, He H, Lin J, Hoyer K, Handschin C, Toka O, et al. Transcriptional coactivator PGC-1 alpha controls the energy state and contractile function of cardiac muscle. Cell Metab. 2005;1(4):259–71.
88. Chinsomboon J, Ruas J, Gupta RK, Thom R, Shoag J, Rowe GC, et al. The transcriptional coactivator PGC-1alpha mediates exercise-induced angiogenesis in skeletal muscle. Proc Natl Acad Sci U S A. 2009;106(50):21401–6.
89. Norrbom J, Sällstedt EK, Fischer H, Sundberg CJ, Rundqvist H, Gustafsson T. Alternative splice variant PGC-1 -b is strongly induced by exercise in human skeletal muscle. AJP: Endocrinol Metab. 2011;301(6):E1092–8.
90. Perry CGR, Hawley JA. Molecular basis of exercise-induced skeletal muscle mitochondrial biogenesis: historical advances, current knowledge, and future challenges. Cold Spring Harb Perspect Med. 2018;8(9):a029686.
91. Jäger S, Handschin C, St-Pierre J, Spiegelman BM. AMP-activated protein kinase (AMPK) action in skeletal muscle via direct phosphorylation of PGC-1alpha. Proc Natl Acad Sci USA. National Acad Sciences. 2007;104(29):12017–22.
92. Jeninga EH, Schoonjans K, Auwerx J. Reversible acetylation of PGC-1: connecting energy sensors and effectors to guarantee metabolic flexibility. Oncogene. 2010;29(33):4617–24.
93. Lai L, Leone TC, Zechner C, Schaeffer PJ, Kelly SM, Flanagan DP, et al. Transcriptional coactivators PGC-1alpha and PGC-lbeta control overlapping programs required for perinatal maturation of the heart. Genes & Development Cold Spring Harbor Lab. 2008;22(14):1948–61.
94. Hoppeler H, Fluck M. Plasticity of skeletal muscle mitochondria: structure and function. Med Sci Sports Exerc. 2003;35(1):95–104.
95. Vincent AE, Turnbull DM, Eisner V, Hajnóczky G, Picard M. Mitochondrial Nanotunnels. Trends Cell Biol. 2017;27(11):787–99.
96. Zhang L, Trushin S, Christensen TA, Bachmeier BV, Gateno B, Schroeder A, et al. Altered brain energetics induces mitochondrial fission arrest in Alzheimer's disease. Sci Rep. Nature Publishing Group. 2016;6(1):18725.
97. Elliott HR, Samuels DC, Eden JA, Relton CL, Chinnery PF. Pathogenic mitochondrial DNA mutations are common in the general population. Am J Hum Genet. 2008;83(2):254–60.
98. Gorman GS, Schaefer AM, Ng Y, Gomez N, Blakely EL, Alston CL, et al. Prevalence of nuclear and mitochondrial DNA mutations related to adult mitochondrial disease. Ann Neurol. 2015;77(5):753–9.
99. Wallace DC, Chalkia D. Mitochondrial DNA genetics and the heteroplasmy conundrum in evolution and disease. Cold Spring Harb Perspect Biol. 2013;5(11):a021220.
100. Suomalainen A. Therapy for mitochondrial disorders: little proof, high research activity, some promise. Semin Fetal Neonatal Med. 2011;16(4):236–40.
101. Holt IJ, Harding AE, Morgan-Hughes JA. Deletions of muscle mitochondrial DNA in patients with mitochondrial myopathies. Nature. 1988;331(6158):717–9.
102. Payne BAI, Wilson IJ, Yu-Wai-Man P, Coxhead J, Deehan D, Horvath R, et al. Universal heteroplasmy of human mitochondrial DNA. Hum Mol Genet. 2013;22(2):384–90.
103. Tuppen HAL, Blakely EL, Turnbull DM, Taylor RW. Mitochondrial DNA mutations and human disease. Biochim Biophys Acta. 2010;1797(2):113–28.
104. Brunel-Guitton C, Levtova A, Sasarman F. Mitochondrial Diseases and Cardiomyopathies. Can J Cardiol. 2015;31(11):1360–76.
105. Nunnari J, Suomalainen A. Mitochondria: in sickness and in health. Cell. 2012;148(6):1145–59.
106. Pietiläinen KH, Naukkarinen J, Rissanen A, Saharinen J, Ellonen P, Keränen H, et al. Global transcript profiles of fat in monozygotic twins discordant for BMI: pathways behind acquired obesity. Groop LC, editor. PLoS Med. Public Library of Science; 2008;5(3):e51.
107. Verdejo HE, del Campo A, Troncoso R, Gutierrez T, Toro B, Quiroga C, et al. Mitochondria, myocardial remodeling, and cardiovascular disease. Curr Hypertens Rep. 2012;14(6):532–9.
108. Karamanlidis G, Nascimben L, Couper GS, Shekar PS, del Monte F, Tian R. Defective DNA replication impairs mitochondrial biogenesis in human failing hearts. Circ Res. American Heart Association Inc. 2010;106(9):1541–8.
109. Ahuja P, Wanagat J, Wang Z, Wang Y, Liem DA, Ping P, et al. Divergent mitochondrial biogenesis responses in human cardiomyopathy. Circulation. American Heart Association Inc. 2013;127(19):1957–67.
110. Knight JA. Diseases and disorders associated with excess body weight. Ann Clin Lab Sci. 2011;41(2):107–21.
111. Matsuda M, Shimomura I. Increased oxidative stress in obesity: Implications for metabolic syndrome, diabetes, hypertension, dyslipidemia, atherosclerosis, and cancer. Obes Res Clin Pract. 2013;7(5):e330–41.
112. Putti R, Sica R, Migliaccio V, Lionetti L. Diet impact on mitochondrial bioenergetics and dynamics. Front Physiol. 2015;6:109.
113. Vondra K, Rath R, Bass A, Slabochová Z, Teisinger J, Vitek V. Enzyme activities in quadriceps femoris

muscle of obese diabetic male patients. Diabetologia. 1977;13(5):527–9.
114. Kelley DE, Goodpaster B, Wing RR, Simoneau JA. Skeletal muscle fatty acid metabolism in association with insulin resistance, obesity, and weight loss. Am J Phys. 1999;277(6 Pt 1):E1130–41.
115. Simoneau JA, Veerkamp JH, Turcotte LP, Kelley DE. Markers of capacity to utilize fatty acids in human skeletal muscle: relation to insulin resistance and obesity and effects of weight loss. FASEB J. 1999;13(14):2051–60.
116. Kelley DE, He J, Menshikova EV, Ritov VB. Dysfunction of mitochondria in human skeletal muscle in type 2 diabetes. Diabetes. 2002;51(10):2944–50.
117. Mootha VK, Lindgren CM, Eriksson K-F, Subramanian A, Sihag S, Lehar J, et al. PGC-1alpha-responsive genes involved in oxidative phosphorylation are coordinately downregulated in human diabetes. Nat Genet. 2003;34(3):267–73.
118. Petersen KF, Dufour S, Befroy D, Garcia R, Shulman GI. Impaired mitochondrial activity in the insulin-resistant offspring of patients with type 2 diabetes. N Engl J Med. 2004;350(7):664–71.
119. Sreekumar R, Nair KS. Skeletal muscle mitochondrial dysfunction & diabetes. Indian J Med Res. 2007;125(3):399–410.
120. Croston TL, Thapa D, Holden AA, Tveter KJ, Lewis SE, Shepherd DL, et al. Functional deficiencies of subsarcolemmal mitochondria in the type 2 diabetic human heart. Am J Physiol Heart Circ Physiol. 2014;307(1):H54–65.
121. Mohsin S, Khan M, Nguyen J, Alkatib M, Siddiqi S, Hariharan N, et al. Rejuvenation of human cardiac progenitor cells with Pim-1 kinase. Circ Res. American Heart Association Inc. 2013;113(10):1169–79.
122. Din S, Konstandin MH, Johnson B, Emathinger J, Völkers M, Toko H, et al. Metabolic dysfunction consistent with premature aging results from deletion of Pim kinases. Circ Res. American Heart Association Inc. 2014;115(3):376–87.
123. Petrosillo G, Matera M, Moro N, Ruggiero FM, Paradies G. Mitochondrial complex I dysfunction in rat heart with aging: critical role of reactive oxygen species and cardiolipin. Free Radic Biol Med. 2009;46(1):88–94.
124. Paradies G, Paradies V, De Benedictis V, Ruggiero FM, Petrosillo G. Functional role of cardiolipin in mitochondrial bioenergetics. Biochim Biophys Acta. 2014;1837(4):408–17.
125. Preston CC, Oberlin AS, Holmuhamedov EL, Gupta A, Sagar S, Syed RHK, et al. Aging-induced alterations in gene transcripts and functional activity of mitochondrial oxidative phosphorylation complexes in the heart. Mech Ageing Dev. 2008;129(6):304–12.
126. Niemann B, Chen Y, Teschner M, Li L, Silber R-E, Rohrbach S. Obesity induces signs of premature cardiac aging in younger patients: the role of mitochondria. J Am Coll Cardiol. 2011;57(5):577–85.
127. Niemann B, Pan R, Teschner M, Boening A, Silber R-E, Rohrbach S. Age and obesity-associated changes in the expression and activation of components of the AMPK signaling pathway in human right atrial tissue. Exp Gerontol. 2013;48(1):55–63.
128. Peterson CM, Johannsen DL, Ravussin E. Skeletal muscle mitochondria and aging: a review. J Aging Res. 2012;2012:1–20.
129. Chabi B, de Camaret BM, Chevrollier A, Boisgard S, Stepien G. Random mtDNA deletions and functional consequence in aged human skeletal muscle. Biochem Biophys Res Commun. 2005;332(2):542–9.
130. Hwang AB, Jeong D-E, Lee S-J. Mitochondria and organismal longevity. Curr Genomics. 2012;13(7):519–32.
131. Sun J, Folk D, Bradley TJ, Tower J. Induced overexpression of mitochondrial Mn-superoxide dismutase extends the life span of adult Drosophila melanogaster. Genetics. Genetics Society of America. 2002;161(2):661–72.
132. Schriner SE, Linford NJ, Martin GM, Treuting P, Ogburn CE, Emond M, et al. Extension of murine life span by overexpression of catalase targeted to mitochondria. Science. American Association for the Advancement of Science. 2005;308(5730):1909–11.
133. Dell'Agnello C, Leo S, Agostino A, Szabadkai G, Tiveron C, Zulian A, et al. Increased longevity and refractoriness to Ca2 -dependent neurodegeneration in Surf1 knockout mice. Hum Mol Genet. 2007;16(4):431–44.
134. Copeland JM, Cho J, Lo T, Hur JH, Bahadorani S, Arabyan T, et al. Extension of Drosophila life span by RNAi of the mitochondrial respiratory chain. Curr Biol. 2009;19(19):1591–8.
135. Lee S-J, Hwang AB, Kenyon C. Inhibition of respiration extends C. elegans life span via reactive oxygen species that increase HIF-1 activity. Curr Biol. 2010;20(23):2131–6.
136. Yang W, Hekimi S. A mitochondrial superoxide signal triggers increased longevity in Caenorhabditis elegans. PLoS Biol. 2010;8(12):e1000556.
137. Onken B, Driscoll M. Metformin induces a dietary restriction-like state and the oxidative stress response to extend C. elegans Healthspan via AMPK, LKB1, and SKN-1. PLoS One. 2010;5(1):e8758.
138. Hwang AB, Ryu E-A, Artan M, Chang H-W, Kabir MH, Nam H-J, et al. Feedback regulation via AMPK and HIF-1 mediates ROS-dependent longevity in Caenorhabditis elegans. Proc Natl Acad Sci U S A. 2014;111(42):E4458–67.
139. Reznick RM, Shulman GI. The role of AMP-activated protein kinase in mitochondrial biogenesis. J Physiol. 2006;574(Pt 1):33–9.
140. Hardie DG. AMP-activated protein kinase: an energy sensor that regulates all aspects of cell function. Genes Dev. 2011;25(18):1895–908.
141. Fontana L, Meyer TE, Klein S, Holloszy JO. Long-term calorie restriction is highly effective in reducing the risk for atherosclerosis in humans. Proc

Natl Acad Sci USA. National Acad Sciences. 2004;101(17):6659–63.
142. Heilbronn LK, De Jonge L, Frisard MI, DeLany JP, Larson-Meyer DE, Rood J, et al. Effect of 6-month calorie restriction on biomarkers of longevity, metabolic adaptation, and oxidative stress in overweight individuals. JAMA. 2006;295(13):1539.
143. Fernström M, Bakkman L, Loogna P, Rooyackers O, Svensson M, Jakobsson T, et al. Improved muscle mitochondrial capacity following gastric bypass surgery in obese subjects. OBES SURG. Springer US. 2016;26(7):1391–7.
144. López-Lluch G, Hunt N, Jones B, Zhu M, Jamieson H, Hilmer S, et al. Calorie restriction induces mitochondrial biogenesis and bioenergetic efficiency. Proc Natl Acad Sci USA. National Acad Sciences. 2006;103(6):1768–73.
145. Faulks SC, Turner N, Else PL, Hulbert AJ. Calorie restriction in mice: effects on body composition, daily activity, metabolic rate, mitochondrial reactive oxygen species production, and membrane fatty acid composition. J Gerontol A Biol Sci Med Sci. 2006;61(8):781–94.
146. Civitarese AE, Carling S, Heilbronn LK, Hulver MH, Ukropcova B, Deutsch WA, et al. Calorie restriction increases muscle mitochondrial biogenesis in healthy humans. PLoS Med. Public Library of Science. 2007;4(3):e76.
147. Finley LWS, Lee J, Souza A, Desquiret-Dumas V, Bullock K, Rowe GC, et al. Skeletal muscle transcriptional coactivator PGC-1α mediates mitochondrial, but not metabolic, changes during calorie restriction. Proc Natl Acad Sci USA. National Acad Sciences. 2012;109(8):2931–6.
148. Manev H, Dzitoyeva S. Progress in mitochondrial epigenetics. Biomol Concepts. 2013;4(4):381–9.
149. Iacobazzi V, Castegna A, Infantino V, Andria G. Mitochondrial DNA methylation as a next-generation biomarker and diagnostic tool. Mol Genet Metab. 2013;110(1–2):25–34.
150. Chinnery PF, Elliott HR, Hudson G, Samuels DC, Relton CL. Epigenetics, epidemiology and mitochondrial DNA diseases. Int J Epidemiol. 2012;41(1):177–87.
151. Lambertini L, Byun H-M. Mitochondrial epigenetics and environmental exposure. Curr Environ Health Rep. Springer International Publishing. 2016;3(3):214–24.
152. Hernández-Aguilera A, Fernández-Arroyo S, Cuyàs E, Luciano-Mateo F, Cabre N, Camps J, et al. Epigenetics and nutrition-related epidemics of metabolic diseases: Current perspectives and challenges. Food Chem Toxicol. 2016;96:191–204.
153. Kelly RDW, Mahmud A, McKenzie M, Trounce IA, St John JC. Mitochondrial DNA copy number is regulated in a tissue specific manner by DNA methylation of the nuclear-encoded DNA polymerase gamma A. Nucleic Acids Res. 2012;40(20):10124–38.
154. Stimpfel M, Jancar N, Virant-Klun I. New challenge: mitochondrial epigenetics? Stem Cell Rev. Springer US. 2017;4(2):13–4.
155. Sadakierska-Chudy A, Frankowska M, Filip M. Mitoepigenetics and drug addiction. Pharmacol Ther. 2014;144(2):226–33.
156. Sitarz KS, Elliott HR, Karaman BS, Relton C, Chinnery PF, Horvath R. Valproic acid triggers increased mitochondrial biogenesis in POLG-deficient fibroblasts. Mol Genet Metab. 2014;112(1):57–63.
157. Menga A, Palmieri EM, Cianciulli A, Infantino V, Mazzone M, Scilimati A, et al. SLC25A26overexpression impairs cell function via mtDNA hypermethylation and rewiring of methyl metabolism. FEBS J. 2017;284(6):967–84.
158. Matilainen O, Quirós PM, Auwerx J. Mitochondria and epigenetics – crosstalk in homeostasis and stress. Trends Cell Biol. 2017;27(6):453–63.
159. Brown DA, Perry JB, Allen ME, Sabbah HN, Stauffer BL, Shaikh SR, et al. Expert consensus document: mitochondrial function as a therapeutic target in heart failure. Nat Rev Cardiol. 2017;14(4):238–50.
160. Holloszy JO, Booth FW. Biochemical adaptations to endurance exercise in muscle. Annu Rev Physiol. 1976;38:273–91.
161. Booth FW, Roberts CK. Linking performance and chronic disease risk: indices of physical performance are surrogates for health. Br J Sports Med. 2008;42(12):950–2.
162. Chimen M, Kennedy A, Nirantharakumar K, Pang TT, Andrews R, Narendran P. What are the health benefits of physical activity in type 1 diabetes mellitus? A literature review. Diabetologia. 2012;55(3):542–51.
163. Russell AP, Foletta VC, Snow RJ, Wadley GD. Skeletal muscle mitochondria: a major player in exercise, health and disease. Biochim Biophys Acta. 2014;1840(4):1276–84.
164. Roh J, Rhee J, Chaudhari V, Rosenzweig A. The role of exercise in cardiac aging: from physiology to molecular mechanisms. Circ Res. American Heart Association Inc. 2016;118(2):279–95.
165. Holloszy JO. Biochemical adaptations in muscle. Effects of exercise on mitochondrial oxygen uptake and respiratory enzyme activity in skeletal muscle. J Biol Chem. 1967;242(9):2278–82.
166. Hood DA. Invited review: contractile activity-induced mitochondrial biogenesis in skeletal muscle. J Appl Physiol. 2001;90(3):1137–57.
167. Green HJ, Helyar R, Ball-Burnett M, Kowalchuk N, Symon S, Farrance B. Metabolic adaptations to training precede changes in muscle mitochondrial capacity. J Appl Physiol. 1992;72(2):484–91.
168. Adams GR, Hather BM, Baldwin KM, Dudley GA. Skeletal muscle myosin heavy chain composition and resistance training. J Appl Physiol. 1993;74(2):911–5.
169. Spina RJ, Chi MM, Hopkins MG, Nemeth PM, Lowry OH, Holloszy JO. Mitochondrial enzymes increase in muscle in response to 7-10 days of cycle exercise. J Appl Physiol. 1996;80(6):2250–4.

170. Pilegaard H, Saltin B, Neufer PD. Exercise induces transient transcriptional activation of the PGC-1alpha gene in human skeletal muscle. J Physiol. 2003;546(Pt 3):851–8.
171. Benziane B, Burton TJ, Scanlan B, Galuska D, Canny BJ, Chibalin AV, et al. Divergent cell signaling after short-term intensified endurance training in human skeletal muscle. Am J Physiol Endocrinol Metab. 2008;295(6):E1427–38.
172. Vega RB, Huss JM, Kelly DP. The coactivator PGC-1 cooperates with peroxisome proliferator-activated receptor α in transcriptional control of nuclear genes encoding mitochondrial fatty acid oxidation enzymes. Mol Cell Biol. American Society for Microbiology. 2000;20(5):1868–76.
173. Handschin C, Chin S, Li P, Liu F, Maratos-Flier E, Lebrasseur NK, et al. Skeletal muscle fiber-type switching, exercise intolerance, and myopathy in PGC-1α muscle-specific knock-out animals. J Biol Chem. American Society for Biochemistry and Molecular Biology. 2007;282(41):30014–21.
174. Geng T, Li P, Okutsu M, Yin X, Kwek J, Zhang M, et al. PGC-1 plays a functional role in exercise-induced mitochondrial biogenesis and angiogenesis but not fiber-type transformation in mouse skeletal muscle. AJP: Cell Physiology. 2009;298(3):C572–9.
175. Leick L, Lyngby SS, Wojtasewski JF, Pilegaard H. PGC-1α is required for training-induced prevention of age-associated decline in mitochondrial enzymes in mouse skeletal muscle. Exp Gerontol. 2010;45(5):336–42.
176. Zechner C, Lai L, Zechner JF, Geng T, Yan Z, Rumsey JW, et al. Total skeletal muscle PGC-1 deficiency uncouples mitochondrial derangements from fiber type determination and insulin sensitivity. Cell Metab. 2010;12(6):633–42.
177. Lin J, Wu H, Tarr PT, Zhang C-Y, Wu Z, Boss O, et al. Transcriptional co-activator PGC-1α drives the formation of slow-twitch muscle fibres. Nature. 2002;418(6899):797–801.
178. Safdar A, Little JP, Stokl AJ, Hettinga BP, Akhtar M, Tarnopolsky MA. Exercise increases mitochondrial PGC-1alpha content and promotes nuclear-mitochondrial cross-talk to coordinate mitochondrial biogenesis. J Biol Chem. 2011;286(12):10605–17.
179. Wu Z, Puigserver P, Andersson U, Zhang C, Adelmant G, Mootha V, et al. Mechanisms controlling mitochondrial biogenesis and respiration through the thermogenic coactivator PGC-1. Cell. 1999;98(1):115–24.
180. Akimoto T, Pohnert SC, Li P, Zhang M, Gumbs C, Rosenberg PB, et al. Exercise stimulates Pgc-1alpha transcription in skeletal muscle through activation of the p38 MAPK pathway. J Biol Chem [Internet]. 2005;280(20):19587–93. Available from: http://eutils.ncbi.nlm.nih.gov/entrez/eutils/elink.fcgi?dbfrom=pubmed&id=15767263&retmode=ref&cmd=prlinks
181. Zhang Y, Uguccioni G, Ljubicic V, Irrcher I, Iqbal S, Singh K, et al. Multiple signaling pathways regulate contractile activity-mediated PGC-1α gene expression and activity in skeletal muscle cells. Physiol Rep. 2014;1:2(5).
182. Park J-Y, Wang P-Y, Matsumoto T, Sung HJ, Ma W, Choi JW, et al. p53 improves aerobic exercise capacity and augments skeletal muscle mitochondrial DNA content. Circ Res. 2009;105(7):705. –12–11pfollowing712.
183. Aquilano K, Baldelli S, Pagliei B, Cannata SM, Rotilio G, Ciriolo MR. p53 orchestrates the PGC-1α-mediated antioxidant response upon mild redox and metabolic imbalance. Antioxid Redox Signal. 2013;18(4):386–99.
184. Sen N, Satija YK, Das S. PGC-1α, a key modulator of p53, promotes cell survival upon metabolic stress. Mol Cell. Elsevier. 2011;44(4):621–34.
185. Saleem A, Carter HN, Hood DA. p53 is necessary for the adaptive changes in cellular milieu subsequent to an acute bout of endurance exercise. AJP: Cell Physiology. 2013;306(3):C241–9.
186. Saleem A, Hood DA. Acute exercise induces tumour suppressor protein p53 translocation to the mitochondria and promotes a p53-Tfam-mitochondrial DNA complex in skeletal muscle. J Physiol. 2013;591(Pt 14):3625–36.
187. Cantó C, Auwerx J. PGC-1α, SIRT1 and AMPK, an energy sensing network that controls energy expenditure. Curr Opin Lipidol. 2009;20(2):98–105.
188. Adhihetty PJ, Uguccioni G, Leick L, Hidalgo J, Pilegaard H, Hood DA. The role of PGC-1 on mitochondrial function and apoptotic susceptibility in muscle. AJP: Cell Physiology. 2009;297(1):C217–25.
189. Philp A, Chen A, Lan D, Meyer GA, Murphy AN, Knapp AE, et al. Sirtuin 1 (SIRT1) deacetylase activity is not required for mitochondrial biogenesis or peroxisome proliferator activated receptor- coactivator-1 (PGC-1) deacetylation following endurance exercise. J Biol Chem. 2011;286(35):30561–70.
190. Tanner CB, Madsen SR, Hallowell DM, Goring DMJ, Moore TM, Hardman SE, et al. Mitochondrial and performance adaptations to exercise training in mice lacking skeletal muscle LKB1. AJP: Endocrinol Metab. 2013;305(8):E1018–29.
191. Drake JC, Wilson RJ, Yan Z. Molecular mechanisms for mitochondrial adaptation to exercise training in skeletal muscle. FASEB J. 2016;30(1):13–22.
192. Twig G, Hyde B, Shirihai OS. Mitochondrial fusion, fission and autophagy as a quality control axis: the bioenergetic view. Biochim Biophys Acta. 2008;1777(9):1092–7.
193. Lira VA, Okutsu M, Zhang M, Greene NP, Laker RC, Breen DS, et al. Autophagy is required for exercise training-induced skeletal muscle adaptation and improvement of physical performance. FASEB J. 2013;27(10):4184–93.
194. Pagano AF, Py G, Berna H, Candau RB, Sanchez AMJ. Autophagy and protein turnover signaling in slow-twitch muscle during exercise. Med Sci Sports Exerc. 2014;46(7):1314–25.
195. Varnauskas E, Bjorntorp P, Fahlen M, Prerovsky I, Stenberg J. Effects of physical training on exercise

blood flow and enzymatic activity in skeletal muscle. Cardiovasc Res. 1970;4(4):418–22.
196. Hoppeler H, Lüthi P, Claassen H, Weibel ER, Howald H. The ultrastructure of the normal human skeletal muscle. Pflugers Arch. Springer-Verlag. 1973;344(3):217–32.
197. Booth FW, Narahara KA. Vastus lateralis cytochrome oxidase activity and its relationship to maximal oxygen consumption in man. Pflugers Arch. Springer-Verlag. 1974;349(4):319–24.
198. Hoppeler H, Howald H, Conley K, Lindstedt SL, Claassen H, Vock P, et al. Endurance training in humans: aerobic capacity and structure of skeletal muscle. J Appl Physiol. 1985;59(2):320–7.
199. Hood DA, Uguccioni G, Vainshtein A, D'souza D. Mechanisms of exercise-induced mitochondrial biogenesis in skeletal muscle: implications for health and disease. Compr Physiol. 2011;1(3):1119–34.
200. Montero D, Cathomen A, Jacobs RA, Flück D, de Leur J, Keiser S, et al. Haematological rather than skeletal muscle adaptations contribute to the increase in peak oxygen uptake induced by moderate endurance training. J Physiol. 2015;593(20):4677–88.
201. Baldwin KM, Klinkerfuss GH, Terjung RL, Molé PA, Holloszy JO. Respiratory capacity of white, red, and intermediate muscle: adaptative response to exercise. Am J Phys. 1972;222(2):373–8.
202. Jacobs RA, Fluck D, Bonne TC, Burgi S, Christensen PM, Toigo M, et al. Improvements in exercise performance with high-intensity interval training coincide with an increase in skeletal muscle mitochondrial content and function. J Appl Physiol. 2013;115(6):785–93.
203. Scalzo RL, Peltonen GL, Binns SE, Shankaran M, Giordano GR, Hartley DA, et al. Greater muscle protein synthesis and mitochondrial biogenesis in males compared with females during sprint interval training. FASEB J. 2014;28(6):2705–14.
204. Nielsen J, Gejl KD, Hey-Mogensen M, Holmberg H-C, Suetta C, Krustrup P, et al. Plasticity in mitochondrial cristae density allows metabolic capacity modulation in human skeletal muscle. J Physiol. 2017;595(9):2839–47.
205. Greggio C, Jha P, Kulkarni SS, Lagarrigue S, Broskey NT, Boutant M, et al. Enhanced respiratory chain supercomplex formation in response to exercise in human skeletal muscle. Cell Metab. 2017;25(2):301–11.
206. Coffey VG, Zhong Z, Shield A, Canny BJ, Chibalin AV, Zierath JR, et al. Early signaling responses to divergent exercise stimuli in skeletal muscle from well-trained humans. FASEB J. 2006;20(1):190–2.
207. Wilkinson SB, Phillips SM, Atherton PJ, Patel R, Yarasheski KE, Tarnopolsky MA, et al. Differential effects of resistance and endurance exercise in the fed state on signalling molecule phosphorylation and protein synthesis in human muscle. J Physiol. 2008;586(15):3701–17.
208. Vissing K, McGee SL, Farup J, Kjølhede T, Vendelbo MH, Jessen N. Differentiated mTOR but not AMPK signaling after strength vs endurance exercise in training-accustomed individuals. Scand J Med Sci Sports. 2013;23(3):355–66.
209. Burd NA, Andrews RJ, West DWD, Little JP, Cochran AJR, Hector AJ, et al. Muscle time under tension during resistance exercise stimulates differential muscle protein sub-fractional synthetic responses in men. J Physiol. 2012;590(2):351–62.
210. Bohé J, Low A, Wolfe RR, Rennie MJ. Human muscle protein synthesis is modulated by extracellular, not intramuscular amino acid availability: a dose-response study. J Physiol. 2003;552(Pt 1):315–24.
211. Robinson MM, Dasari S, Konopka AR, Johnson ML, Manjunatha S, Esponda RR, et al. Enhanced protein translation underlies improved metabolic and physical adaptations to different exercise training modes in young and old humans. Cell Metab. 2017;25(3):581–92.
212. Tang JE, Hartman JW, Phillips SM. Increased muscle oxidative potential following resistance training induced fibre hypertrophy in young men. Appl Physiol Nutr Metab. 2006;31(5):495–501.
213. Kon M, Ohiwa N, Honda A, Matsubayashi T, Ikeda T, Akimoto T, et al. Effects of systemic hypoxia on human muscular adaptations to resistance exercise training. Physiol Rep. 2014;1:2(6).
214. Wang N, Hikida RS, Staron RS, Simoneau JA. Muscle fiber types of women after resistance training–quantitative ultrastructure and enzyme activity. Pflugers Arch. 1993;424(5–6):494–502.
215. Porter C, Reidy PT, Bhattarai N, Sidossis LS, Rasmussen BB. Resistance exercise training alters mitochondrial function in human skeletal muscle. Med Sci Sports Exerc. 2015;47(9):1922–31.
216. MacDougall JD, Hicks AL, MacDonald JR, McKelvie RS, Green HJ, Smith KM. Muscle enzymatic adaptations to sprint interval training. Medicine &amp Science in Sports &amp Exercise. 1996;28(Supplement):21.
217. Barnett C, Carey M, Proietto J, Cerin E, Febbraio MA, Jenkins D. Muscle metabolism during sprint exercise in man: influence of sprint training. J Sci Med Sport. 2004;7(3):314–22.
218. Gibala MJ, Little JP, Van Essen M, Wilkin GP, Burgomaster KA, Safdar A, et al. Short-term sprint interval versus traditional endurance training: similar initial adaptations in human skeletal muscle and exercise performance. J Physiol. 2006;575(Pt 3):901–11.
219. Burgomaster KA, Howarth KR, Phillips SM, Rakobowchuk M, Macdonald MJ, McGee SL, et al. Similar metabolic adaptations during exercise after low volume sprint interval and traditional endurance training in humans. J Physiol. 2008;586(1):151–60.
220. Gibala MJ, McGee SL, Garnham AP, Howlett KF, Snow RJ, Hargreaves M. Brief intense interval exercise activates AMPK and p38 MAPK signaling and increases the expression of PGC-1 in human skeletal muscle. J Appl Physiol. 2009;106(3):929–34.
221. Wojtaszewski JFP, Nielsen P, Hansen BF, Richter EA, Kiens B. Isoform-specific and exercise

intensity-dependent activation of 5′-AMP-activated protein kinase in human skeletal muscle. J Physiol. 2000;528(1):221–6.
222. Wojtaszewski JFP, Mourtzakis M, Hillig T, Saltin B, Pilegaard H. Dissociation of AMPK activity and ACCβ phosphorylation in human muscle during prolonged exercise. Biochem Biophys Res Commun. 2002;298(3):309–16.
223. Chen Z-P, Stephens TJ, Murthy S, Canny BJ, Hargreaves M, Witters LA, et al. Effect of exercise intensity on skeletal muscle AMPK signaling in humans. Diabetes. 2003;52(9):2205–12.
224. Casuso RA, Plaza-Díaz J, Ruiz-Ojeda FJ, Aragón-Vela J, Robles-Sanchez C, Nordsborg NB, et al. High-intensity high-volume swimming induces more robust signaling through PGC-1α and AMPK activation than sprint interval swimming in m. triceps brachii. PLoS One. 2017;12(10):e0185494.
225. Gibala M. Molecular responses to high-intensity interval exercise. Appl Physiol Nutr Metab. 2009;34(3):428–32.
226. Hood MS, Little JP, Tarnopolsky MA, Myslik F, Gibala MJ. Low-volume interval training improves muscle oxidative capacity in sedentary adults. Med Sci Sports Exerc. 2011;43(10):1849–56.
227. Hickson RC, Dvorak BA, Gorostiaga EM, Kurowski TT, Foster C. Potential for strength and endurance training to amplify endurance performance. J Appl Physiol. 1988;65(5):2285–90.
228. Bell GJ, Syrotuik D, Martin TP, Burnham R, Quinney HA. Effect of concurrent strength and endurance training on skeletal muscle properties and hormone concentrations in humans. Eur J Appl Physiol. Springer-Verlag. 2000;81(5):418–27.
229. Lundberg TR, Fernandez-Gonzalo R, Tesch PA, Rullman E, Gustafsson T. Aerobic exercise augments muscle transcriptome profile of resistance exercise. AJP: Regulatory, Integrative and Comparative Physiology. 2016:ajpregu.00035.2016.
230. Lundberg TR, Fernandez-Gonzalo R, Tesch PA. Exercise-induced AMPK activation does not interfere with muscle hypertrophy in response to resistance training in men. J Appl Physiol. 2014;116(6):611–20.
231. Donges CE, Burd NA, Duffield R, Smith GC, West DWD, Short MJ, et al. Concurrent resistance and aerobic exercise stimulates both myofibrillar and mitochondrial protein synthesis in sedentary middle-aged men. J Appl Physiol. 2012;112(12):1992–2001.
232. Fan W, Evans RM. Exercise mimetics: impact on health and performance. Cell Metab. 2017;25(2):242–7.
233. Zamora M, Pardo R, Villena JA. Pharmacological induction of mitochondrial biogenesis as a therapeutic strategy for the treatment of type 2 diabetes. Biochem Pharmacol. 2015;98(1):16–28.
234. Overington JP, Al-Lazikani B, Hopkins AL. How many drug targets are there? Nat Rev Drug Discov. Nat Publ Group. 2006;5(12):993–6.
235. Pang J, Xu X, Getman MR, Shi X, Belmonte SL, Michaloski H, et al. G protein coupled receptor kinase 2 interacting protein 1 (GIT1) is a novel regulator of mitochondrial biogenesis in heart. J Mol Cell Cardiol. 2011;51(5):769–76.
236. Cameron RB, Beeson CC, Schnellmann RG. Development of therapeutics that induce mitochondrial biogenesis for the treatment of acute and chronic degenerative diseases. J Med Chem. 2016;59(23):10411–34.
237. Daubert MA, Yow E, Dunn G, Marchev S, Barnhart H, Douglas PS, et al. Novel mitochondria-targeting peptide in heart failure treatment. Circ Heart Fail. 2017;10(12):e004389.
238. Fan W, Waizenegger W, Lin CS, Sorrentino V, He M-X, Wall CE, et al. PPARδ promotes running endurance by preserving glucose. Cell Metab. 2017;25(5):1186–93. e4.
239. Zhang J, Liu H, Luo S, Lu Z, Chávez-Badiola A, Liu Z, et al. Live birth derived from oocyte spindle transfer to prevent mitochondrial disease. Reprod Biomed Online. 2017;34(4):361–8.
240. Bianconi E, Piovesan A, Facchin F, Beraudi A, Casadei R, Frabetti F, et al. An estimation of the number of cells in the human body. Ann Hum Biol. 2013;40(6):463–71.

Effect of Exercise on Adult Stem Cells

4

Nabanita Kundu, Cleyton C. Domingues, and Sabyasachi Sen

Abbreviations

ADMA	Asymmetric dimethylarginine
ALPL	Alkaline phosphatase, liver/bone/kidney
BAT	Brown adipose tissue
BMP	Bone morphogenic protein
C/EBPα	CCAAT/enhancer-binding protein α
CAD	Coronary artery disease
CDC	Centers for Disease Control and Prevention
CVD	Cardiovascular disease
Drp-1	Dynamin-related protein-1
EPCs	Endothelial progenitor cells
INS	Insulin
ION	Idiopathic osteonecrosis
MFN1 and 2	Mitofusins 1 and 2
MSCs	Mesenchymal stem cells
NIDDK	National Institute of Diabetes and Digestive and Kidney Diseases
NO	Nitric oxide
PGC1α	Peroxisome proliferator-activated receptor gamma coactivator 1-alpha
POMC	Proopiomelanocortin
PPARγ-2	Peroxisome proliferator-activated receptor gamma-2
ROS	Reactive oxygen species
RUNX2	Runt-related transcription factor 2
SDF-1	Stromal cell-derived factor 1
SDF1alpha	Stromal cell-derived alpha protein
T2DM	Type 2 diabetes mellitus
UCP-1	Uncoupling protein 1
VEGF	Vascular endothelial growth factor
WAT	White adipose tissue

Introduction

Over the past decades, obesity, diabetes, hypertension, stroke, and coronary artery diseases (CAD) have been rising dangerously worldwide and have reached epidemic proportions. According to the National Institute of Diabetes and Digestive and Kidney Diseases (NIDDK), NIH-USA, more than two in every three adults are overweight or obese, and more than one in three adults are obese [1]. The World Health Organization has estimated that 422 billion people are suffering from diabetes [2]. Moreover, Centers for Disease Control and Prevention (CDC) has also reported that 1 out of 3 adults suffers from hypertension, 1 out of every 20 deaths is due to stroke, and 1 out of every 4 deaths

N. Kundu · C. C. Domingues · S. Sen (✉)
Department of Medicine, George Washington University, Washington, DC, USA
e-mail: ssen1@gwu.edu

P. Kokkinos, P. Narayan (eds.), *Cardiorespiratory Fitness in Cardiometabolic Diseases*,
https://doi.org/10.1007/978-3-030-04816-7_4

is due to CAD in the USA [3–5]. According to CDC, 84 million Americans also have prediabetes [6], a condition associated with increased risk of type 2 diabetes and cardiovascular disease (CVD) which includes hypertension, CAD, and stroke. In addition, increased mortality rates associated with these health conditions are associated with a large economic burden. Indeed, CDC estimates that the annual medical cost for obesity and its complications in the USA was annually \$147 billion in 2008 [7]. The American Diabetes Association reported that it costs \$245 billion to treat diabetes and related complications in the USA [8]. Approximately \$46 billion was used to treat hypertension in 2015, \$34 billion for stroke, and \$200 billion for heart disease in 2016, according to CDC reports [3–5].

Finding effective ways to prevent cardiometabolic diseases reported above has been a challenge, particularly in countries where the western-style diet and sedentary behavior are prevalent. Strong evidence suggests that regularly performed exercise attenuates the development of obesity, diabetes, and CVD [9]. Additionally, according to CDC, physical exercise not only reduces risk of developing type 2 diabetes and CVD but also helps reduce body weight in addition to lowering the risk of developing certain cancers [10]. Moreover, exercise strengthens bones and muscles and improves mental health, and daily activity prevents falls, by improving balance. In combination with reduced calorie intake, exercise increases life expectancy irrespective of age, ethnicity, body habitus, and body mass [11].

In addition to the traditional clinical parameters used to evaluate the effects of exercise on human health, studying the impact of exercise on adult stem cells may offer a novel insight into the mechanism(s) modulating the impact of exercise on health outcomes. This may also help us understand the mechanism of the positive effects of exercise.

Adult Stem Cells Are Influenced by Exercise

Stem cells are nonspecialized cells which can differentiate into some or all of the major specialized cell types of tissues or organs. Predominantly, there are two types of stem cells: embryonic and somatic/adult stem cells. While the role of stem cells on embryonic development has remained the main focus in regenerative medicine for years, the interest in adult stem cells and the role they play in disease and health are more recent.

Adult stem cells are found in different tissues including the bone marrow, peripheral blood, blood vessels, skeletal muscle, adipose tissue, brain, and many other tissues by forming niche for specific and multitasking work. For endothelial progenitor cells (EPCs) and mesenchymal stem cells (MSCs), the bone marrow is the main reservoir. MSCs can also be found in other tissues (i.e., adipose tissue) besides the bone marrow [12]. Predominantly, adult stem cells such as EPCs and MSCs are responsible for daily tissue or cell maintenance, remodeling, regeneration of multiple tissues, and especially replenishing cells dying from apoptosis [13]. Often, adult stem cells respond to tissue-specific signals, such as stromal cell-derived factor 1-alpha (SDF1alpha), by migrating to injured areas that need regeneration. Exercise can therefore play an important role in the function and fate of these adult stem cells by altering extracellular matrix composition, reducing inflammation, and promoting their migratory capacity [14].

Obesity, diabetes, dyslipidemia, and hyperglycemia all play an important role in causation of cardiometabolic diseases. They also appear to play a role in mitochondrial fragmentation and dysfunction (Fig. 4.1) [15, 16]. Based on effects of exercise on mitochondrial fission, it could play an important role in mitochondrial repair and biogenesis and cellular respiration. It was reported that both endurance and resistance training increase peroxisome proliferator-activated receptor gamma coactivator 1-alpha (PGC1α) which lead to more mitochondrial fusion followed by mitochondrial biogenesis [17]. However, it has also been reported that mitochondrial function could be improved by increasing electron transport chain function and mitochondrial dynamics without increasing mitochondrial biogenesis [18]. Exercise training decreases activation of the mitochondrial fission protein dynamin-related protein-1 (DRP-1) in insulin-resistant human skeletal

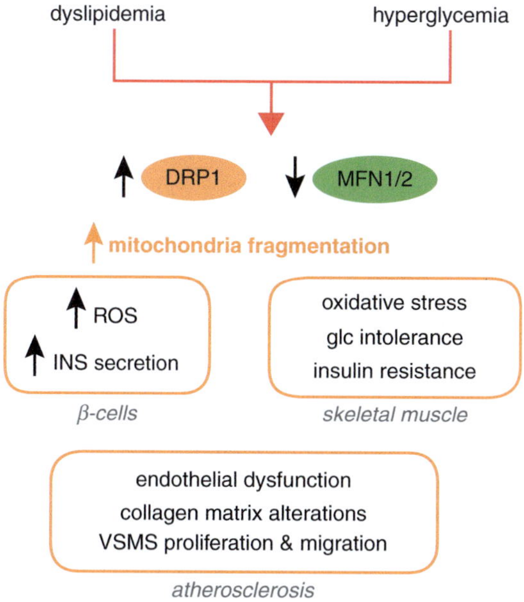

Fig. 4.1 Mitochondrial shape alterations in T2 diabetes: mitochondrial fragmentation or fission and impaired mitochondrial trafficking are hallmarks of T2DM. These changes in mitochondrial dynamics lead to pathological responses in β cells, skeletal muscle, adipocytes, and vessels. Exercise can reduce mitochondrial fission and can be used as a hallmark for exercise effectiveness

muscle [19]. Cumulatively, exercise enhances mitochondrial function which affects a stem cell more than a mature cell by improving the stem cell function [20].

Effect of Exercise on Endothelial Progenitor Cells (EPCs) and Mesenchymal Stromal Cells (MSCs)

Effects on EPCs

Human EPCs are circulating cells, available in the peripheral blood, bone marrow, and umbilical cord. Most commonly, EPCs are defined by cell surface markers such as CD34+ or CD34+/kinase-insert-domain-containing receptor (KDR)+ or CD34+/KDR+/CD133+ [21]. EPCs play an important role in angiogenesis and neovascularization, predominantly, by incorporation into the endothelium or by its paracrine properties that favor de novo vessel formation [22]. Both type 1 diabetes mellitus and T2DM often lead to the vascular damage and vaso-occlusive disease. In this regard, EPCs play a vital role in repair and regeneration of blood vessels. Metabolic disorders like diabetes, either type 1 or 2, dramatically decrease EPC numbers and impair their function. Therefore, EPCs play a key role for diabetes and CVD treatment outcome measures. Physical activity increases the production and numbers of circulating EPCs [23]. This improvement in the number of EPCs could be explained based on an anti-apoptotic effect that is partially dependent on nitric oxide (NO) [24, 25]. Similarly, in at least one study, exercise has been shown to reduce phosphatidylinositol 3-kinase (PI3-kinase)-mediated apoptosis which depends on NO [26]. Prostaglandin E1-mediated upregulation of EPC is also linked to the improvement of EPC function and increased angiogenesis [27]. The findings of another study suggest that improvement in EPC numbers may be related to and preceded by an increase in plasma vascular endothelial growth factor (VEGF). In patients with CAD, exercise-induced transient myocardial ischemia, which provides the stimulus for increases in EPC concentrations via a VEGF-dependent mechanism, helped improve organ function by improving tissue perfusion [28]. Additionally, patients with chronic heart failure show increased EPC counts by increasing not only plasma VEGF but also stromal cell-derived factor 1 (SDF-1) levels post exercise [29].

Age is also a major factor reducing EPC numbers, with the number of CD34+/KDR+EPC being twice as high in young population compared to older group at resting state. Studies have demonstrated that exercise increases the number of EPCs in middle age and older persons [30, 31]. Interestingly, the number of EPCs following exercise was elevated irrespective of age group [31].

In addition to the increased concentrations of EPCs, evidence suggests that exercise improves the function of these cells [32, 33]. Sen et al. (2015) showed that a home exercise program improves $CD34^+$ cell function by increasing migration of EPCs in the presence of the chemotactic factor SDF-1α. These results indicate that regularly performed exercise leads to enhanced vasculoneogenesis within a relatively short time [32]. It has also been reported that exercise substantially influences SDF-1α concentrations [33]. In addition, atherosclerotic plaque regression has been demonstrated in response to exercise [34]. Other studies have reported that supervised exercise training boosts the circulating EPC counts and reduces asymmetric dimethylarginine (ADMA) levels leading to an increased angiogenesis, improvement of endothelial function, and decreased atherosclerosis. Collectively, the aforementioned findings suggest that exercise-induced cell mobilization and reduction of ADMA may serve as a physiological repair mechanism for atherosclerosis [35–37].

Exercise training normalized the EPC levels and function in SHR that were exercise trained (SHR-T) which was accompanied by an increase in VEGF and NO levels. In addition, oxidative stress levels were normalized in SHR-T. Similar results were found in the number and function of bone marrow EPC. Exercise training repaired the peripheral capillary rarefaction in hypertension by a signaling pathway VEGF/endothelial nitric oxide synthase (eNOS)-dependent in SHR-T. Moreover, improvement in EPC was significantly related to angiogenesis [38].

Our data and discussion show that CD34+ cells can act as a robust biomarker in metabolic diseases such as obesity, prediabetes, and type 2 diabetes [21, 32]. Exercise repairs the impairment of EPCs in hypertension, which could be associated with peripheral revascularization, suggesting a mechanism for its potential therapeutic application in vascular diseases. In spontaneously hypertensive rats, exercise normalized the EPC levels and functions, impaired by hypertension. Moreover, improvement in EPC was significantly related to angiogenesis, suggesting that exercise may promote neovascularization, and a potential mechanism for the exercise-related therapeutic applications in vascular diseases [38]. In an interesting review, Wahl et al. [39] proposed that exercise promotes mechanical stress in the tissue and vasculature. This mechanical force directly or indirectly regulates EPC's fate. Collectively, exercise promotes release of growth factors and other molecules such as interleukin-6 (IL-6) and NO which facilitate EPC production from the bone marrow and their differentiation. Therefore, exercise may stimulate migration of CD34+ cells and homing to the hypoxic tissue, thereby improving angiogenesis and vasculogenesis [39].

Expectedly, the exercise-related favorable effects of EPCs are modulated by exercise intensity, duration, and volume. A direct relationship has been shown between exercise duration and the number of circulating EPCs [28]. Moderate- and high-intensity exercise of 30 min has been shown to increase circulating EPC number. However, this increase is not observed when exercise time is reduced to 10 min [40]. This finding suggests that exercise duration plays a significant role on EPC number and possibly function. Moreover, a maximal bout of exercise stimulates a significant shift of CD34+ cells toward CD34+/KDR+ cells or in other words improves maturity of an undecided progenitor cell toward an endothelial lineage cell [41].

Effects on MSC

Mesenchymal stromal cells (MSCs) are multipotent cells which can differentiate into osteoblasts, adipocytes, and chondrocytes. As mentioned above, MSCs can be obtained from different sources: umbilical cord blood, bone marrow, adipose tissue, pancreatic islet, fetal liver, and lung [42–45]. Often, MSCs are defined by specific markers such as CD44, CD73, CD90, and CD105 but not CD31, CD34, and CD45 [46].

Exercise can have an impact on MSCs, and it may facilitate MSC migration by increasing IL-6 and recruiting stem cell in the site of injury [47]. Additionally, MSC secretome is responsible for hematopoietic stem and progenitor cell (HSPC) mobilization and proliferation, and exercise induces homing of HSPCs to extramedullary sites [48]. Several studies support improvement of MSC transplantation following exercise training. In two animal studies, treadmill exercise increased the therapeutic effects of MSC transplantation in traumatic brain injury (TBI) in a rat model [49]. In a similar study, exercise increased the efficiency of MSC transplantation in cerebral ischemic rats by reducing apoptosis [50].

In human studies, the use of stromal vascular fraction cells (a well-known mixed cell population enriched in MSCs) combined with exercise helps improve pain in patients with knee osteoarthritis [51]. Interestingly, exercise also facilitates MSC transplantation in idiopathic osteonecrosis (ION) of the femoral head by increasing vascularization in the bone graft [52].

Exercise plays a vital role in differentiation of multipotent MSCs such as promoting bone differentiation. Li et al. indicated that mechanical force increases osteoblast differentiation by increasing runt-related transcription factor (RUNX2) and is responsible for reduction of adipogenic peroxisome proliferator-activated receptor gamma-2 (PPARγ-2) and CCAAT/enhancer-binding protein α (C/EBPα), indicating a reduction of adipogenesis [53]. Curiously, the effect of exercise on osteogenesis has been observed for bone marrow-derived MSCs, but not for adipose-derived MSCs [54]. However, bone differentiation markers such as RUNX2; alkaline phosphatase, liver/bone/kidney (ALPL); and osteocalcin were significantly upregulated in a MSC-containing stromal fraction from a veteran population subjected to exercise indicating osteogenic differentiation [54]. Cook and Genever postulated how signaling pathways can orchestrate MSC differentiation and showed that both bone morphogenic protein (BMP) and wingless-type MMTV integration site (WNT) signaling pathways play an important role in MSC differentiation. WNT signaling promotes osteoblast differentiation by upregulating RUNX2 and inhibiting PPARγ. On the other hand, BMP activates osteogenic differentiation by activating RUNX2 (Fig. 4.1) [55].

Exercise can also increase the number of bone marrow-derived MSCs [56]. Furthermore, elevated activity of alkaline phosphatase and increased levels of osteopontin and osteocalcin were noted in mice subjected to exercises indicating an improvement of musculoskeletal function [56]. In addition to the effect of exercises on MSC osteogenic differentiation, it has been shown that exercise can improve cartilage repair when followed by MSC transplantation [57].

Another important fact about the effect of exercise on MSCs can be extrapolated from data obtained in white adipose tissue (WAT) that undergoes a browning process. These cells, which have been called beige/brite cells, express uncoupling protein 1 (UCP-1) and therefore have thermogenic capacity similarly to a brown adipose tissue (BAT). However, they differ from WAT once they have multilocular morphology and also express unique gene markers (i.e., Tbx1) which are not expressed in both WAT and BAT [58]. Thus, WAT browning process contributes to increased energy expenditure and helps prevent/treat obesity. The WAT process can occur via proopiomelanocortin (POMC) neurons which are subjected to insulin and leptin actions. Nevertheless, in obesity condition, a hypothalamic inflammation process is established, and it impairs insulin and leptin signaling in this tissue, thus preventing WAT browning. An alternative way to reduce this inflammation in the hypothalamus and increase POMC neurons' gene expression is by practicing physical exercises [[59] and references therein]. Another mechanism to activate the WAT browning process is via irisin. It has been proposed that physical exercises increase the level of this hormone which promotes a higher utilization of the energy reserve in the cells and thermogenesis by increasing UCP-1 expression in WAT. In contrast, irisin levels are reduced in people with obesity and T2DM [[59] and references therein]. Therefore, POMC neurons and irisin activities seem to be crucial as mediators of the physical exercise and control of energy homeostasis.

Although MSCs can be differentiated in both white and brown adipocytes, these cells have different precursors. While Myf5+ precursor is induced to transform into brown pre-adipocyte and then into mature brown adipocyte, white pre-adipocyte and mature white adipocyte are originated from Myf5- precursor [60]. However, it remains unclear whether physical exercise would play a role on MSC (Myf5- precursor) differentiation via POMC or irisin as described above for white adipocytes.

Conclusion

Although relatively limited, information strongly supports a pleotropic, favorable effect of exercise on adult progenitor/stem cells MSC and EPCs as cellular markers of cardiovascular health [61] and exercise physiology [32]. In addition, it appears that these changes occur relatively quickly (within weeks of exercise) and at exercise intensities that most middle-aged and older individuals can tolerate. This potentially has significant clinical and public health implication. Exercise can be implemented to large populations as a preventive and therapeutic modality for a number of chronic diseases. These two, EPC and MSC, may also provide promising cellular biomarkers to easily evaluate exercise efficacy for different populations and different disease entities.

References

1. NIDDK, NIH, Overweight and obesity statistics, 2014. https://www.niddk.nih.gov/health-information/health-statistics/overweight-obesity.
2. World Health Organization. Fact sheet. Diabetes. 2017. http://www.who.int/mediacentre/factsheets/fs312/en/.
3. Center for Disease Control and Prevention. High blood pressure facts. 2016. https://www.cdc.gov/dhdsp/data_statistics/fact_sheets/fs_bloodpressure.htm.
4. Center for Disease Control and Prevention. Stroke fact sheet. 2017. https://www.cdc.gov/stroke/facts.htm.
5. Center for Disease Control and Prevention. Heart disease fact. 2017. https://www.cdc.gov/heartdisease/facts.htm.
6. Center for Disease Control and Prevention. National diabetes statistics report. 2017. https://www.cdc.gov/diabetes/data/statistics/statistics-report.html.
7. Center for Disease Control and Prevention. Adult obesity facts. 2017. https://www.cdc.gov/obesity/data/adult.html.
8. American Diabetes Association. Economic costs of diabetes in the U.S. in 2012. Diabetes Care. 2013;36(4):1033–46.
9. Kokkinos P. Physical activity, health benefits, and mortality risk. ISRN Cardiol. 2012;2012:718789.
10. Center for Disease Control and Prevention. Physical activity and health. 2015. https://www.cdc.gov/physicalactivity/basics/pa-health/index.htm.
11. Moore SC, Patel AV, Matthews CE, Berrington de Gonzalez A, Park Y, Katki HA, et al. Leisure time physical activity of moderate to vigorous intensity and mortality: a large pooled cohort analysis. PLoS Med. 2012;9(11):e1001335.
12. Hass R, Kasper C, Böhm S, Jacobs R. Different populations and sources of human mesenchymal stem cells (MSC): A comparison of adult and neonatal tissue-derived MSC. Cell Commun Signal. 2011;9:12.
13. Yoder MC. Human endothelial progenitor cells. Cold Spring Harb Perspect Med. 2012;2(7):a006692.
14. Van Craenenbroeck EM, Conraads VM. Endothelial progenitor cells in vascular health: focus on lifestyle. Microvasc Res. 2010;79(3):184–92.
15. Pernas L, Scorrano L. Mito-morphosis: mitochondrial fusion, fission, and cristae remodeling as key mediators of cellular function. Annu Rev Physiol. 2016;78:505–31.
16. Schrepfer E, Scorrano L. Mitofusins, from mitochondria to metabolism. Mol Cell. 2016;61(5):683–94.
17. Yan Z, Lira VA, Greene NP. Exercise training-induced regulation of mitochondrial quality. Exerc Sport Sci Rev. 2012 Jul;40(3):159–64.
18. Gusdon AM, Callio J, Distefano G, O'Doherty RM, Goodpaster BH, Coen PM, et al. Exercise increases mitochondrial complex I activity and DRP1 expression in the brains of aged mice. Exp Gerontol. 2017;90:1–13.
19. Fealy CE, Mulya A, Lai N, Kirwan JP. Exercise training decreases activation of the mitochondrial fission protein dynamin-related protein-1 in insulin-resistant human skeletal muscle. J Appl Physiol. 2014;117(3):239–45.
20. Hsu YC, Wu YT, Yu TH, Wei YH. Mitochondria in mesenchymal stem cell biology and cell therapy: from cellular differentiation to mitochondrial transfer. Semin Cell Dev Biol. 2016;52:119–31.
21. Kundu N, Domingues CC, Chou C, Ahmadi N, Houston S, Jerry DJ, Sen S. J Am Heart Assoc. 2017;6(4). pii: e005146. https://doi.org/10.1161/JAHA.116.005146. PMID: 28365567.
22. Boppart MD, Lisio M, Witkowski S. Exercise and stem cells. Prog Mol Biol Transl Sci. 2015;135:423–56.
23. Laufs U, Werner N, Link A, Endres M, Wassmann S, Jürgens K, et al. Physical training increases endothelial progenitor cells, inhibits neointima formation, and enhances angiogenesis. Circulation. 2004;109(2):220–6.
24. Steiner S, Niessner A, Ziegler S, Richter B, Seidinger D, Pleiner J, et al. Endurance training increases the number of endothelial progenitor cells in patients with cardiovascular risk and coronary artery disease. Atherosclerosis. 2005;181(2):305–10.
25. Jenkins NT, Witkowski S, Spangenburg EE, Hagberg JM. Effects of acute and chronic endurance exercise on intracellular nitric oxide in putative endothelial progenitor cells: role of NAPDH oxidase. Am J Physiol Heart Circ Physiol. 2009;297(5):H1798–805.

26. Zhang KR, Liu HT, Zhang HF, Zhang QJ, Li QX, Yu QJ, et al. Long-term aerobic exercise protects the heart against ischemia/reperfusion injury via PI3 kinase-dependent and Akt-mediated mechanism. Apoptosis. 2007;12(9):1579–88.
27. Gensch C, Clever Y, Werner C, Hanhoun M, Böhm M, Laufs U. Regulation of endothelial progenitor cells by prostaglandin E1 via inhibition of apoptosis. J Mol Cell Cardiol. 2007;42(3):670–7.
28. Adams V, Lenk K, Linke A, Lenz D, Erbs S, Sandri M, et al. Increase of circulating endothelial progenitor cells in patients with coronary artery disease after exercise-induced ischemia. Arterioscler Thromb Vasc Biol. 2004;24(4):684–90.
29. Sarto P, Balducci E, Balconi G, Fiordaliso F, Merlo L, Tuzzato G, et al. Effects of exercise training on endothelial progenitor cells in patients with chronic heart failure. J Card Fail. 2007;13(9):701–8.
30. Hoetzer GL, Van Guilder GP, Irmiger HM, Keith RS, Stauffer BL, DeSouza CA. Aging, exercise, and endothelial progenitor cell clonogenic and migratory capacity in men. J Appl Physiol (1985). 2007;102(3):847–52.
31. Thijssen DH, Vos JB, Verseyden C, van Zonneveld AJ, Smits P, Sweep FC, et al. Haematopoietic stem cells and endothelial progenitor cells in healthy men: effect of aging and training. Aging Cell. 2006;5(6):495–503.
32. Sen S, Witkowski S, Lagoy A, Islam AM. A six-week home exercise program improves endothelial function and $CD34^+$ circulating progenitor cells in patients with pre-diabetes. Journal of Endocrinology and Metabolism. 2015;5(1–2):163–71.
33. Van Craenenbroeck EM, Bruyndonckx L, Van Berckelaer C, Hoymans VY, Vrints CJ, Conraads VM. The effect of acute exercise on endothelial progenitor cells is attenuated in chronic heart failure. Eur J Appl Physiol. 2011;111(9):2375–9.
34. Ajijola OA, Dong C, Herderick EE, Ma Q, Goldschmidt-Clermont PJ, Yan Z. Voluntary running suppresses proinflammatory cytokines and bone marrow endothelial progenitor cell levels in apolipoprotein-E-deficient mice. Antioxid Redox Signal. 2009;11(1):15–23.
35. Schlager O, Giurgea A, Schuhfried O, Seidinger D, Hammer A, Gröger M, et al. Exercise training increases endothelial progenitor cells and decreases asymmetric dimethylarginine in peripheral arterial disease: a randomized controlled trial. Atherosclerosis. 2011;217(1):240–8.
36. Van Craenenbroeck EM, Beckers PJ, Possemiers NM, Wuyts K, Frederix G, Hoymans VY, et al. Exercise acutely reverses dysfunction of circulating angiogenic cells in chronic heart failure. Eur Heart J. 2010;31(15):1924–34.
37. Rehman J, Li J, Parvathaneni L, Karlsson G, Panchal VR, Temm CJ, et al. Exercise acutely increases circulating endothelial progenitor cells and monocyte–/macrophage-derived angiogenic cells. J Am Coll Cardiol. 2004;43(12):2314–8.
38. Fernandes T, Nakamuta JS, Magalhães FC, Roque FR, Lavini-Ramos C, Schettert IT, et al. Exercise training restores the endothelial progenitor cells number and function in hypertension: implications for angiogenesis. J Hypertens. 2012;30(11):2133–43.
39. Wahl P, Brixius K, Bloch W. Exercise-induced stem cell activation and its implication for cardiovascular and skeletal muscle regeneration. Minim Invasive Ther Allied Technol. 2008;17(2):91–9.
40. Laufs U, Urhausen A, Werner N, Scharhag J, Heitz A, Kissner G, et al. Running exercise of different duration and intensity: effect on endothelial progenitor cells in healthy subjects. Eur J Cardiovasc Prev Rehabil. 2005;12(4):407–14.
41. Van Craenenbroeck EM, Vrints CJ, Haine SE, Vermeulen K, Goovaerts I, Van Tendeloo VF, et al. A maximal exercise bout increases the number of circulating CD34+/KDR+ endothelial progenitor cells in healthy subjects. Relation with lipid profile. J Appl Physiol (1985). 2008;104(4):1006–13.
42. Sen S, Domingues CC, Rouphael C, Chou C, Kim C, Yadava N. Genetic modification of human mesenchymal stem cells helps to reduce adiposity and improve glucose tolerance in an obese diabetic mouse model. Stem Cell Res Ther. 2015;6:242. PMID: 26652025
43. Zanini C, Bruno S, Mandili G, Baci D, Cerutti F, Cenacchi G, et al. Differentiation of mesenchymal stem cells derived from pancreatic islets and bone marrow into islet-like cell phenotype. PLoS One. 2011;6(12):e28175.
44. Stagg J, Galipeau J. Mechanisms of immune modulation by mesenchymal stromal cells and clinical translation. Curr Mol Med. 2013;13(5):856–67.
45. Dominici M, Le Blanc K, Mueller I, Slaper-Cortenbach I, Marini F, Krause D, et al. Minimal criteria for defining multipotent mesenchymal stromal cells. The International Society for Cellular Therapy position statement. Cytotherapy. 2006;8(4):315–7.
46. Schmidt A, Bierwirth S, Weber S, Platen P, Schinköthe T, Bloch W. Short intensive exercise increases the migratory activity of mesenchymal stem cells. Br J Sports Med. 2009;43(3):195–8.
47. Emmons R, Niemiro GM, Owolabi O, De Lisio M. Acute exercise mobilizes hematopoietic stem and progenitor cells and alters the mesenchymal stromal cell secretome. J Appl Physiol. 2016;120(6):624–32.
48. Shin MS, Park HK, Kim TW, Ji ES, Lee JM, Choi HS, et al. Neuroprotective effects of bone marrow stromal cell transplantation in combination with treadmill exercise following traumatic brain injury. Int Neurourol J. 2016;20(Suppl 1):S49–56.
49. Zhang YX, Yuan MZ, Cheng L, Lin LZ, Du HW, Chen RH, et al. Treadmill exercise enhances therapeutic potency of transplanted bone mesenchymal stem cells in cerebral ischemic rats via anti-apoptotic effects. BMC Neurosci. 2015;16:56. Arch Phys Med Rehabil 2015; 96(3):532–9.
50. Gibbs N, Diamond R, Sekyere EO, Thomas WD. Management of knee osteoarthritis by combined stromal vascular fraction cell therapy, platelet-rich plasma, and musculoskeletal exercises: a case series. J Pain Res. 2015;8:799–806.

51. Aoyama T, Fujita Y, Madoba K, Nankaku M, Yamada M, Tomita M, et al. Rehabilitation program after mesenchymal stromal cell transplantation augmented by vascularized bone grafts for idiopathic osteonecrosis of the femoral head: a preliminary study. Arch Phys Med Rehabil. 2015;96(3):532–9.
52. Li R, Liang L, Dou Y, Huang Z, Mo H, Wang Y, et al. Mechanical strain regulates osteogenic and adipogenic differentiation of bone marrow mesenchymal stem cells. Biomed Res Int. 2015;2015:873251.
53. Liu SY, He YB, Deng SY, Zhu WT, Xu SY, Ni GX. Exercise affects biological characteristics of mesenchymal stromal cells derived from bone marrow and adipose tissue. Int Orthop. 2017;41(6):1199–209.
54. Kundu N, Domingues CC, Paal E, Kokkinos P, Nylen E, Sen S. Effect of aerobic and resistance exercise training on fat derived mesenchymal stromal cells (MSCs) in subjects with prediabetes. Mol Ther. 2017;25(5):115. ASGCT Conference Abstract.
55. Cook D, Genever P. Regulation of mesenchymal stem cell differentiation. Adv Exp Med Biol. 2013;786:213–29.
56. Marędziak M, Śmieszek A, Chrząstek K, Basinska K, Marycz K. Physical activity increases the total number of bone-marrow-derived mesenchymal stem cells, enhances their osteogenic potential, and inhibits their Adipogenic properties. Stem Cells Int. 2015;2015:379093.
57. Yamaguchi S, Aoyama T, Ito A, Nagai M, Iijima H, Tajino J, et al. The effect of exercise on the early stages of mesenchymal stromal cell-induced cartilage repair in a rat osteochondral defect model. PLoS One. 2016;11(3):e0151580.
58. Stanford KI, Middelbeek RJW, Goodyear LJ. Exercise effects on white adipose tissue: Beiging and metabolic adaptations. Diabetes. 2015;64:2361–8.
59. Rodrigues KCC, Pereira RM, Campos TDP, Moura RF, Silva ASR, Cintra DE, et al. The role of physical exercise to improve the browning of white adipose tissue via POMC neurons. Front Cell Neurosci. 2018;12:88.
60. Park A, Kim WK, Bae KH. Distinction of white, beige and brown adipocytes derived from mesenchymal stem cells. World J Stem Cell. 2014;6(1):33–42.
61. Dore FJ, Domingues CC, Ahmadi N, Kundu N, Kropotova Y, Houston S, Rouphael C, Mammadova A, Witkin L, Khiyami A, Amdur RL, Sen S. The synergistic effects of saxagliptin and metformin on CD34+ endothelial progenitor cells in early type 2 diabetes patients: a randomized clinical trial. Cardiovasc Diabetol. 2018;17:65.

Exercise Metabolism in Health and Disease

5

Anastassios Philippou, Costas Chryssanthopoulos, Maria Maridaki, George Dimitriadis, and Michael Koutsilieris

Abbreviations

1-RM	One-repetition maximum
Acetyl-CoA	Acetyl coenzyme A
ADP	Adenosine diphosphate
AMP	Adenosine monophosphate
AMPK	AMP-activated protein kinase
AT	Anaerobic threshold
ATP	Adenosine triphosphate
ATPase	Adenosine triphosphatase
BCAA	Branched-chain amino acids
BCOADH	Branched-chain 2-oxoacid dehydrogenase
CK	Creatine kinase
CPK	Creatine phosphokinase
Cr	Creatine
$FADH_2$	Flavin adenine dinucleotide
FAT/CD 36	Fatty acid translocase
FATP	Fatty acid transport protein
FFA	Free fatty acids
FT	Free testosterone
G-6-P	Glucose-6-phosphate
GH	Growth hormone
GLUT4	Glucose transporter type 4
GSDV	Glycogen storage disease type V
HbA1c	(Glycated) hemoglobin A1c
HDL-C	High-density lipoprotein cholesterol
HGP	Hepatic glucose output
HIF-1	Hypoxia-inducible factor-1
HIIT	High-intensity interval training
HSL	Hormone-sensitive lipase
IGF-1	Insulin-like growth factor-1
IL	Interleukin
IMP	Inosine monophosphate
LDH	Lactate dehydrogenase
LDL-C	Low-density lipoprotein cholesterol
LDM	Low-density microsomes
LT	Lactate threshold
MCT1	Monocarboxylate transporter 1
mPTP	Mitochondrial permeability transition pore
MTGL	Muscle triacylglycerol lipase
NAD	Nicotinamide adenine dinucleotide
NADH	Reduced form of NAD
NH_4^+	Ammonium
NO	Nitric oxide

A. Philippou · C. Chryssanthopoulos
M. Koutsilieris (✉)
Department of Physiology, Medical School, National and Kapodistrian University of Athens, Athens, Greece
e-mail: mkoutsil@med.uoa.gr

M. Maridaki
Department of Sports Medicine & Biology of Physical Activity, Faculty of Physical Education and Sport Science, National and Kapodistrian University of Athens, Athens, Greece

G. Dimitriadis
Second Department of Internal Medicine-Research Institute and Diabetes Center, "Attikon" University Hospital, Medical School, National and Kapodistrian University of Athens, Athens, Greece

P. Kokkinos, P. Narayan (eds.), *Cardiorespiratory Fitness in Cardiometabolic Diseases*, https://doi.org/10.1007/978-3-030-04816-7_5

PCr	Phosphocreatine
PDH	Pyruvate dehydrogenase complex
PFK	Phosphofructokinase
PGC-1α	Peroxisome proliferator-activated receptor gamma coactivator 1-alpha
PHOS	Glycogen phosphorylase
RER	Respiratory exchange ratio
ROS	Reactive oxygen species
SHBG	Sex hormone-binding globulin
SIRTs	Sirtuins
SNARE	Soluble *N*-ethylmaleimide-sensitive factor attachment protein receptors
T1D	Diabetes mellitus type 1
T2D	Diabetes mellitus type 2
TCA	Tricarboxylic acid cycle
TGs	Triglycerides
VCO_2	Volume of carbon dioxide expired
V_E	Volume of air inspired or expired
VLDL-C	Very low-density lipoprotein cholesterol
VO_2	Volume of oxygen uptake
VO_2max	Maximal oxygen uptake

Exercise Metabolism: An Overview

In vertebrates, movement is accomplished by the contraction of skeletal muscles attached to bones via tendons. The compound adenosine triphosphate (ATP), considered the energy currency of the human body, provides the energy requirements of the working muscles. The chemical energy incorporated into the ATP is released as ATP is hydrolyzed by adenosine triphosphatase (ATPase), providing the energy for the thin myofilaments of actin to slide on the thick myofilaments of myosin. During the initial 7–10 s of maximum or near maximum physical effort, the ATP requirements are met almost exclusively by the energy compound phosphocreatine (PCr) stored within the muscles. As ATP is degraded to adenosine diphosphate (ADP), the phosphate from the stored PCr binds to ADP and ATP is formed. As activity continues beyond approximately 10 s, the limited supplies of PCr are exhausted, and the intensity of the activity (or exercise) begins to decline. However, this allows the necessary time for the glycolytic pathways to maximize their capacity to form ATP and become the predominant supplier of energy for the working muscles for the next few minutes.

Anaerobic metabolism occurs in the cytosol. The formation of ATP via the glycolytic pathways (anaerobically) involves the degradation of glycogen and glucose to pyruvate and lactate (Fig. 5.1). Muscle glucose and glycogen primarily serve the energy needs of the host muscle. Glucose entering the myocytes is phosphorylated by the enzyme hexokinase to form glucose-6-phosphate (G-6-P). This is an irreversible step as the muscle lacks the enzyme glucokinase (found in the liver) responsible for dephosphorylation of G-6-P and the exit of glucose from the cell into the bloodstream. Thus, muscle glycogen can be degraded to glucose as needed by the host muscle but cannot exit the muscle cells (enter the bloodstream) to serve the energy needs of other organs.

Aerobic metabolism takes place in the mitochondrion. ATP is formed either from pyruvate entering the mitochondrion or acetyl coenzyme A (Acetyl-CoA) formed from blood-borne or intramuscular fatty acids through β-oxidation (Fig. 5.1). Aerobic metabolism is a much more efficient process, and the amount of ATP formed is much higher than the ATP formed anaerobically.

Proteins in the form of amino acids may also support ATP resynthesis via aerobic metabolism. However, the contribution of amino acid oxidation to total energy demand is almost negligible during high-intensity exercise, whereas during prolonged exercise, it accounts for about 3–6% of the total ATP resynthesis [1, 2]. Nevertheless, amino acid oxidation may contribute more to total energy expenditure especially when body carbohydrate levels are low [3].

ATP concentrations are maintained fairly constant, even during maximal exercise intensity as energy substrates such as PCr and muscle glyco-

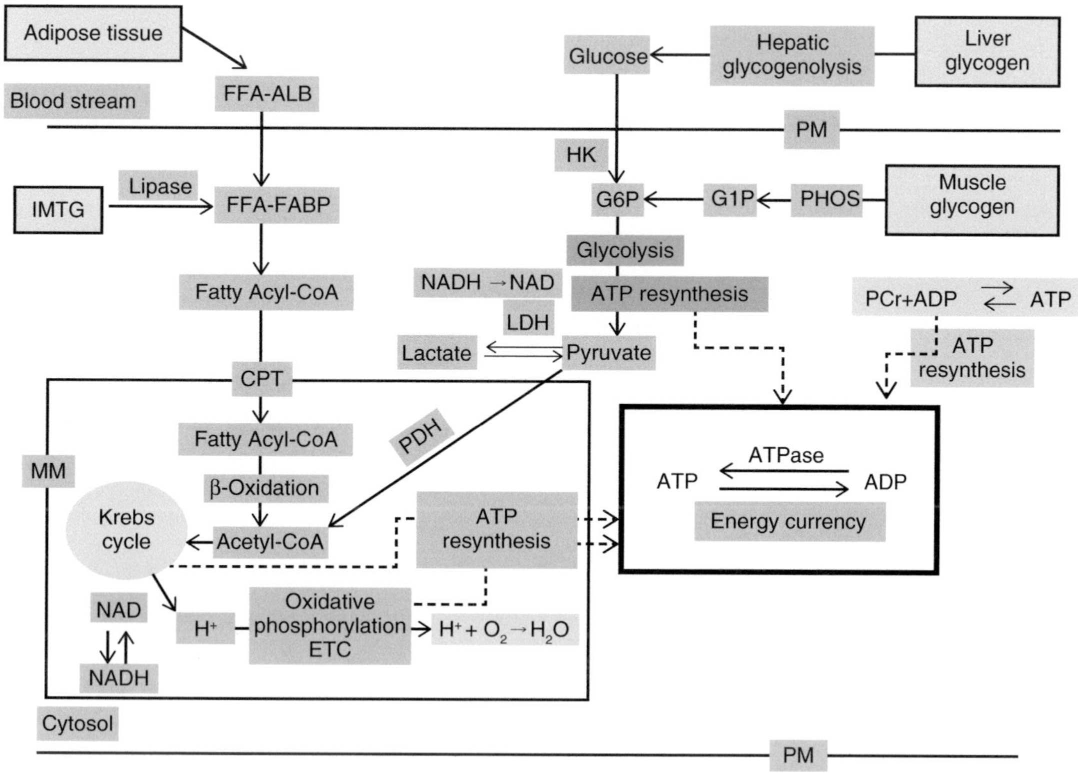

Fig. 5.1 A simplified overview of energy production in skeletal muscle. Acetyl-CoA acetyl-coenzyme A, acyl-CoA acyl-coenzyme A, ADT adenosine diphosphate, ATP adenosine triphosphate, ATPase adenosine triphosphatase, CPT carnitine palmitoyltransferase, ETC electron transport chain, FFA-ALB free fatty acids-albumin, FFA-FABP free fatty acid-fatty acid binding protein, G1P glucose-1phosphate, G6P glucose-6-phosphate, HK hexokinase, IMTG intramuscular triglycerides, LDH lactate dehydrogenase, MM mitochondrial membrane, NAD nicotinamide adenine dinucleotide, NADH nicotinamide adenine dinucleotide reduced form, PCr phosphocreatine, PDH pyruvate dehydrogenase, PHOS phosphorylase, PM plasma membrane

gen replenish the ATP utilized for the task at hand. Substrate use for ATP formation is modulated by the exercise intensity. At very high exercise intensities, PCr contribution to ATP regeneration is high. During a 30-s all-out effort of cycling or running, postexercise PCr were reduced by about 75–80%, and ATP levels by less than 30% [4, 5]. In endurance type of exercise to volitional fatigue, muscle glycogen was reduced by more than 80%, whereas ATP by only 6% [6]. Muscle fiber heterogeneity also plays a considerable role in substrate use for ATP formation and utilization [7].

The aforementioned metabolic pathways do not function independently, but in an integrative manner, where the main factor determining the relative contribution of aerobic and anaerobic metabolism is exercise intensity. If we consider a person starting exercise at a low intensity equivalent to 5 $Km.h^{-1}$, and this intensity requires a volume of oxygen uptake (VO_2) of 14 $ml.kg^{-1}.min^{-1}$, this oxygen demand is about fourfold higher than the resting of VO_2 that is about 3.5 $ml.kg^{-1}.min^{-1}$. The amount of energy for this initial stage of exercise is also supported by anaerobic metabolism, since aerobic metabolism is slow and cannot meet instantaneously the VO_2 required (Fig. 5.2). The amount of oxygen not provided, that is, illustrated in Fig. 5.2 above the VO_2 line, is referred to as oxygen deficit. If the individual continues exercise to volitional fatigue in a graded exercise intensity fashion, where intensity is increased every 3 min, a maximal oxygen uptake (VO_2max) level will be reached (Fig. 5.3).

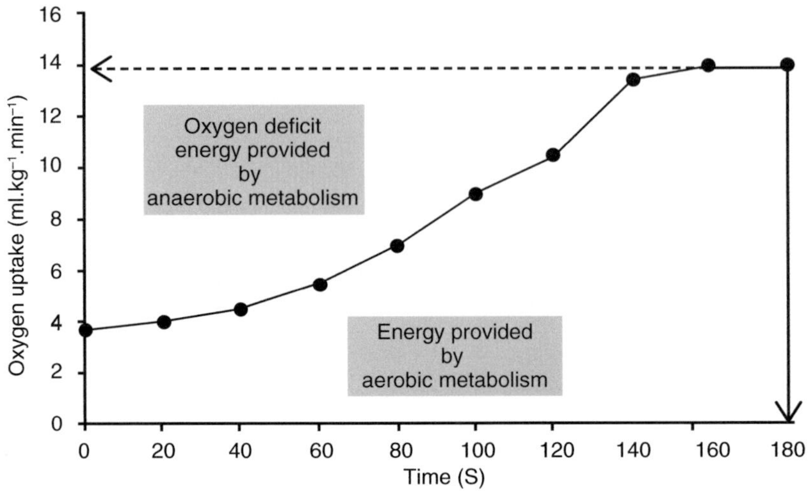

Fig. 5.2 Initial stage of a hypothetical grated exercise test of a healthy individual on a treadmill

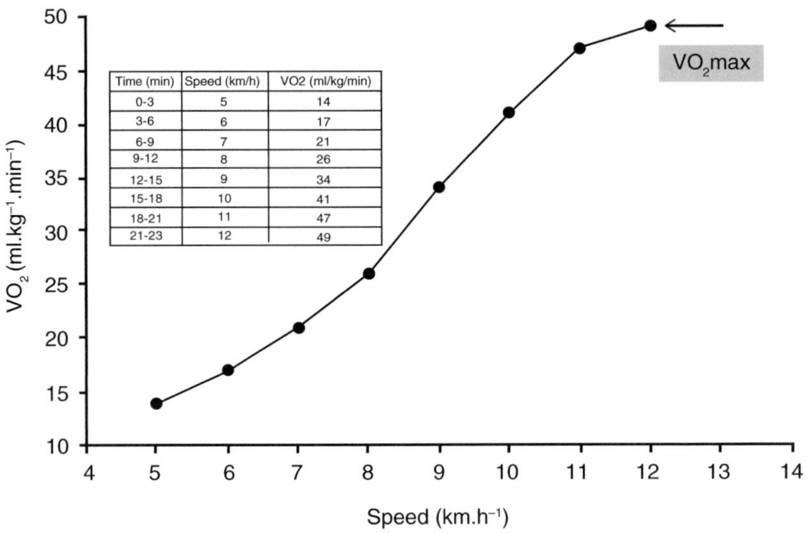

Fig. 5.3 Hypothetical grated exercise test to volitional fatigue of a healthy individual on a treadmill

The energy demand exercising above the VO_2max level is mainly supported by anaerobic metabolism (Fig. 5.4).

Muscle Fiber Types

Skeletal muscles are comprised by different fiber types that possess distinct morphological, histochemical, biochemical, or physiological characteristics [8]. In fact, based on myosin heavy chain gene expression, muscle fibers have an almost continuous spectrum of ATP usage and muscle contraction speeds [9, 10].

In humans, skeletal muscle fibers are broadly classified as type I (slow twitch) and type II (fast twitch). Type II fibers are further classified into three major subtypes (types IIa, IIb, and IIX) [11]. Type I fibers are, aerobically oriented fibers, designed for long-duration exercise. They have an extended capillary network and numerous mitochondria and produce a low level of force. On the other spectrum, type IIb and IIX fibers are fast twitch, have a larger diameter than type I, and therefore can produce more force. They are designed for higher exercise intensities, with their energy demands met predominantly by the glycolytic pathways, but they fatigue fast. Finally,

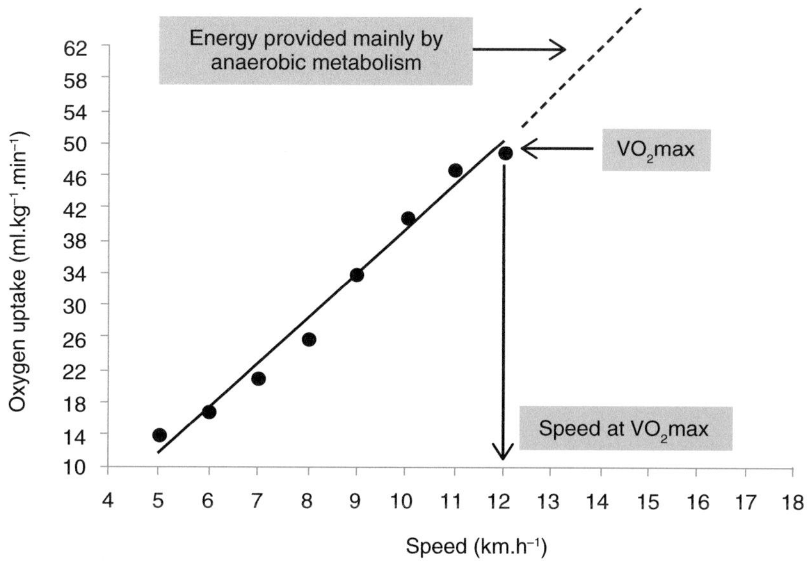

Fig. 5.4 When exercise intensity exceeds that at which VO_2max is achieved, the energy needs are met mainly by anaerobic metabolism

type IIa fibers are considered intermediate fibers, having characteristics of both type I and II [12]. The recruitment of the different fiber types is mainly dictated by the exercise intensity and the level of force developed by the muscle. For exercise intensities up to 40% of VO_2max, type I fibers are the predominant fibers recruited. As the intensity increases, progressively more type IIa fibers are recruited. For intensities >75% VO_2max, type IIa and especially IIb fibers are recruited, as intensities approach > 90% VO_2max [13]. Whether fibers can be altered as a result of chronic and specific exercise training has been scrutinized for years. The consensus is that fibers are likely to be altered to accommodate the demand imposed by the type of work. Thus, the glycolytic capacity of aerobically oriented fibers (type I) can be enhanced if these fibers are exposed to anaerobic work and vice versa [14].

In medicine, fiber typing may be important for certain fibers are prone to disease genetic myopathies, while others seem to be resistant. Some of these diseases include Duchenne muscle dystrophy, myotonic dystrophy, facioscapulohumeral muscular dystrophy, Pompe disease, and certain myosinopathies. In addition, metabolic and chronic disorders such as obesity, type 2 diabetes, heart failure, chronic obstructive pulmonary disease, or aging-related sarcopenia affect certain fiber types, while other fiber types seem to be resistant [15] (Table 5.1). The capacity of the muscle to alter the characteristics of its fibers may provide beneficial effects in the prevention and treatment of these diseases [10, 15].

Energy Substrates

ATP

Skeletal muscles store a relatively small amount of ATP which can support muscle contractions for only a few seconds. No differences in ATP concentration in different fiber types of human skeletal muscle have been observed [4, 16, 17]. A decline in muscle ATP concentrations is associated with muscle fatigue. Muscle fatigue is a protective mechanism designed to prevent ATP decline to levels associated with muscle rigor or serious muscle damage [18, 19].

Phosphocreatine (PCr)

Skeletal muscle PCr reserves are about three times higher than ATP levels. Its function is to replenish ATP via rephosphorylation of ADP. PCr stores are higher in type II compared to type I fibers [17, 20, 21]. Furthermore, PCr content may be increased by dietary manipulation and in

Table 5.1 Muscle disorders and morphological and functional changes of affected fiber types

Morphological/functional change	Fiber type affected	Muscle disorder
Atrophy-degeneration	Type IIx	Duchenne muscular dystrophy
	Type I	Myotonic dystrophy type 1 Myosinopathies Muscle inactivity (injury, bed rest)
	Type II Type IIa	Myosinopathies Pompe disease (mouse model) Aging/sarcopenia
Fiber type shift	Type II → type I	Facioscapulohumeral muscular dystrophy Congenital fiber type disproportion Heart failure (diaphragm) Chronic obstructive pulmonary disease (diaphragm)
	Type I → type IIx	Obesity Type 2 diabetes Muscle inactivity (injury, bed rest)
	Type I→ type II	Heart failure (limb muscles) Chronic obstructive pulmonary disease (limb muscles)
Reduced force generation	Type I	Myotonic dystrophy type 1
	Type II	Facioscapulohumeral muscular dystrophy

Modified from Ref. [15]

particular creatine supplementation and exercise [22]. The outcome varies among individuals and seems to be affected by factors such as dietary habits (vegetarians vs. omnivorous) or age (children vs. elderly) [23].

Glycogen

Glycogen is the main form of carbohydrates used for muscular work. It is also the most advantageous energy fuel in terms of ATP resynthesis since glycogen degradation is accomplished both aerobically and anaerobically. Glycogen is a polymerized form of glucose stored mainly in muscle and liver tissue. Its structure is in branch form in a treelike formation. This arrangement provides an advantage to enzymes phosphorylase and transferase to rapidly reach the various terminal sides of glycogen formation and speed up glycogen breakdown, making glycolysis a very fast metabolic pathway. Similarly, the many end points of the treelike formation provide multiple sites to the glycogen synthase for glucose unit addition through the process of glycogenesis. Ultimately, glycogen, this important substrate, can be degraded and resynthesized quickly [24].

About 75% of glycogen is stored between myofibrils as inter-myofibrillar glycogen, while the rest of the total glycogen pool is situated in the myofibrils and beneath the sarcolemma (intra-myofibrillar and sub-sarcolemmal glycogen, respectively) [25, 26]. In healthy individuals, muscle glycogen concentration varies depending on the tissue, the preceding physical activity, the person's recent diet, fitness status, fiber type, and possibly gender [26–28]. The liver tissue can accommodate approximately 85 kg wet weight^{-1}, or approximately 100 g of glycogen for the average liver weighing 1.2 kg [24]. In recent years, the use of ^{13}C magnetic resonance spectroscopy studies has shown that liver glycogen content does not differ between trained and untrained individuals and declines significantly during submaximal endurance exercise of about 60–70% VO_2max [27, 29, 30]. Conversely, muscle glycogen levels are usually 20–66% higher in endurance trained compared with untrained individuals. This may be attributable to increased insulin sensitivity observed with exercise training [27]. Furthermore, muscle glycogen is higher in type II fiber types compared to type I [4, 6, 16, 31]. Muscle glycogen stored can be increased by manipulation in diet and exercise, the so-called carbohydrate loading strategy or supercompensation, often used by endurance athletes to improve performance [28]. Whether this supercompensation response differs between males and females still remains controversial [2, 32, 33].

Finally, the existence of several types of glycogen storage diseases caused by various enzyme deficiencies [34], although rare, produces metabolic abnormalities in the liver, muscle, and brain and is associated with abnormal glucose and fat metabolism.

Lipids

Lipids are stored mainly in the adipose tissue and muscle in the form of triacylglycerols. There is considerable variation among individuals in terms of total body fat stores that can exceed 50% of the total body weight in severely obese. In general, females have a higher body fat content than males, and sportsmen usually have lower body fat levels than inactive individuals, although there is also a great variability in fat weight among athletes [35].

Intramuscular triglycerides are stored in the form of lipid droplets close to the mitochondria. Their amount varies between muscle groups and between fiber types, with type I to have a higher content as reported in muscle biopsy and magnetic resonance spectroscopy studies [36, 37]. The quantification of intramuscular triglycerides and their contribution to energy metabolism is problematic due to the fact that these fat reserves are not as nicely distributed in the muscle as glycogen [38]. However, studies combining immunofluorescence microscopy, stable isotope, and muscle biopsy techniques have demonstrated that muscle triglycerides are important energy contributors during prolonged exercise (≥3 h) of low to moderate (approximately ≤60% VO_2max) intensity [39].

Metabolic Pathways

As mentioned previously the energy source for muscular work is ATP. For work to continue, a constant supply of ATP is needed. This is accomplished via the anaerobic and aerobic pathways.

Anaerobic Metabolism During Exercise

The ATP-PCr System

During the hydrolysis of ATP by myofibrillar ATPase, ADP, hydrogen ions, and inorganic phosphate are formed as well as 30.5 kj of free energy per mole of ATP [40]:

$$\begin{aligned} \mathrm{ATP} + \mathrm{H_2O} &\leftrightarrow \mathrm{ADP} + \mathrm{Pi} \\ &+ \mathrm{H^+} - 30.5\,\mathrm{kj}(\mathrm{kilojoules}) \end{aligned} \quad (5.1)$$

This energy release provides the "driving or power stroke" by which the myosin attachment at a 90° angle to the binding sites on actin to change to a 45° angle resulting in the shortening in the muscle [41]. For the detachment of myosin from actin to take place, ATP is also required to bind to myosin. So, ATP is regenerated by the conversion of ADP and inorganic phosphate, so that ATP is again available to myosin. The majority of the energy spent (about 70–75%) in the contracting muscle is used by the myosin ATPase activity, with the remaining amount to be used by enzymes involved in Na^+, K^+, and Ca^{2+} ATPase [42].

The amount of energy stored in the form of ATP is limited (about 25 $mmol.kg^{-1}dw$) and, if not resynthesized, can only provide energy for approximately 3–5 s of sprinting or about 15 s of aerobic exercise [42]. One way of the anaerobic ATP provision is accomplished via the breakdown of PCr, a reaction catalyzed by creatine phosphokinase (CPK) or creatine kinase (CK), leading to the formation of ATP and creatine (Cr):

$$\mathrm{PCr} + \mathrm{ADP} + \mathrm{H^+} \leftrightarrow \mathrm{ATP} + \mathrm{Cr} \quad (5.2)$$

During maximal efforts lasting more than 10 s, ATP stores decline in the exercising muscle, while ADP and adenosine monophosphate (AMP) are formed. This allows the formation of some ATP by a reaction (5.3) catalyzed by adenylate kinase [42]:

$$2\mathrm{ADP} \leftrightarrow \mathrm{ATP} + \mathrm{AMP} \quad (5.3)$$

The produced AMP is quickly broken down by the enzyme AMP deaminase to inosine monophosphate (IMP) and ammonium (NH_4^+):

$$AMP + H^+ \rightarrow IMP + NH_4^+ \quad (5.4)$$

Since NH_4^+ is toxic, it is transported in the liver through blood circulation and converted to urea. The formation of IMP is important in maintaining ADP and AMP at low levels in the muscle cell sustaining in this way enough free energy from ATP breakdown to support muscle contraction [19].

The above three reactions (5.2, 5.3, and 5.4) formulate the "ATP-PCr system" [43], "the phosphagen system" [19], or "anaerobic alactic system" since no oxygen or lactate formation is involved [44]. As highlighted earlier, the importance of this system is that energy can be provided at a very high rate almost instantaneously, something that cannot be accomplished by glycolysis or aerobic metabolism. This system has played a crucial role in our survival, as immediate action is required in many instances to avoid injury. Activities that require high levels of muscle power (weightlifting, shot put, hammer and discus throw, jumping, etc.) are also supported by the phosphagen system.

Glycolysis

ATP generated via glycolysis involves ten chemical reactions with lactate as the end product formed by pyruvate, a reaction catalyzed by lactate dehydrogenase (LDH). The net result for the muscle is the formation of 2ATP molecules when G-6-P is derived from glucose and three molecules when the initial substrate is glycogen. This pathway can be summarized as follows:

$$\begin{aligned} &\text{Glycogen} + 3\text{ADP} + 3\text{Pi} \rightarrow 3\text{ATP} \\ &\quad + 2\text{Lactate} + 2\text{H}^+ \end{aligned} \quad (5.5)$$

A central reaction in glycolytic pathway is considered the transformation of 3-phosphogly ceraldehyde to 1,3-diphosphoglycerate by glyceraldehyde phosphate dehydrogenase, where nicotinamide adenine dinucleotide (NAD^+) is reduced to NADH [40]. The ratio of NAD/NADH, the so-called redox (reduction-oxidation) status of the muscle, plays a significant role as substrate in electron transport chain and oxidative phosphorylation since for every pair of electrons transported by NADH to the electron transport chain, three molecules of ATP are generated. Furthermore, NAD and NADH have the role of activators or inhibitors in muscle metabolism [42].

Although not as fast as ATP-PCr system, glycolysis can also regenerate ATP very quickly and is activated within the very first second of muscle contraction by various factors such as Ca^{2+}, ADP, AMP, IMP, fructose-6-phosphate, Pi, and Mg^{2+} in an allosteric fashion [44]. It can support sporting activities that require high level of ATP resynthesis for several seconds such as sprinting during various games like soccer, basketball, football, handball, and several others. Furthermore, glycolysis provides the extra energy needed when intensity exceeds that of VO_2max (Fig.5.4) or when oxygen is not available. In addition, both the phosphagen system and glycolysis support ATP regeneration at the initiation of exercise (Fig. 5.1) as well as when exercise intensity changes to a higher intensity level, allowing the necessary time for the aerobic pathways to match the ATP demands (Fig. 5.3).

Regulation of Anaerobic Pathways

The regulation of anaerobic pathways is mainly achieved by activation or inhibition of the enzymes catalyzing the various reactions. With the initiation of muscle contractions, the accompanied increase in Ca^{2+}stimulates myofibrillar ATPase. This stimulation moves ATP hydrolysis reaction (5.1) to the right, resulting in a decrease in ATP concentrations and a subsequent elevation of ADP and Pi. These changes produce a mass-action effect stimulating CPK to displace reaction (5.2) to the right replacing the previously hydrolyzed ATP but "spending" PCr stores [45]. It should be noted that as mentioned earlier, although ATP concentrations do not massively change even in maximal fatiguing exercise, small changes of this molecule have a larger impact on the concentrations of ADP and AMP which together with ATP formulate the total adenylate pool [46].

The enzyme phosphofructokinase (PFK) responsible for the conversion of fructose-6-phosphate to fructose-1,6-diphosphate is regarded as the key enzyme in the control of glycolysis [46]. In activities like sprinting, the increase in the rate of glycolysis exceeds 1000-fold compared to resting rate [40]. Increased cellular levels of inorganic phosphate (5.1), as a result of ATP hydrolysis, as well as AMP by adenylate kinase (5.3), enhance PFK activity. On the other hand, when ATP demand is not high and ATP levels rise, PFK activity is reduced. A high rate of glycolysis will also result in an increased H^+ accumulation (5.5) that will lower muscle pH inhibiting in this way PFK. This is considered a protective mechanism, designed to prevent further lactate formation leading to extreme acidosis [46]. ATP activity is also inhibited by increased citrate concentrations, an intermediate of Krebs cycle, indicating that when ATP is regenerated by aerobic metabolism there is no need for high rates of ATP formation through glycolysis.

In muscle glycogenolysis, the main control is exerted by glycogen phosphorylase (PHOS) that degrades glycogen to G1P (Fig. 5.1). This enzyme has two forms: PHOS *a*, the more active, and PHOS *b*, the less active which are interconvertible by phosphatase and kinase enzymes. When the muscle is at rest, most of PHOS is in its less active *b* form [40]. Activators of PHOS from *b* to *a* form are ADP, AMP, IMP, Pi, Ca^{2+}, and adrenaline, whereas inhibitors are H^+, G6P, and ATP [44, 47, 48]. Also, the availability of substrates in the form of exogenous oral carbohydrates, blood-borne fatty acids, or muscle glycogen itself may influence the rate of muscle glycogenolysis [6, 31, 49–52].

Lactate Metabolism

Lactate is the end product of glycolysis formed after pyruvate is reduced to lactate by LDH according to the following chemical reaction:

$$\text{Pyruvate} + \text{NADH} + \text{H}^+ \leftrightarrow \text{Lactate} + \text{NAD}^+$$

Often the term lactic acid is used instead of lactate and vice versa. Lactic acid, when formed, is unstable within the physiological muscle and blood pH range and immediately more than 99% of lactic acid releases a proton and dissociates into lactate anions and protons (H+) [53]. Therefore, since lactate is measured, this term will be used in this chapter. In biochemical terms, the above reaction is important because lactate regenerates NAD in the cytosol that is necessary in the glyceraldehyde phosphate dehydrogenase which in turn converts 3-phosphoglyceraldehyde to 1,3-diphosphoglycerate. In this way the glycolytic flux and redox status of the muscle (NAD/NADH) are maintained; otherwise, glycolysis would slow down resulting in a reduced glycolytic rate of ATP resynthesis. This becomes very important not so much during high-intensity exercise, where PCr stores are significantly reduced within seconds and consequently the muscle relies more on glycolysis, but in endurance events such as marathon running. Fast marathoners rely mainly on carbohydrate oxidation during exercise; however, this requires a high rate of glycogenolysis and simultaneously the ability to remove and metabolize lactate for energy [54, 55].

Two misconceptions exist regarding lactate. First, lactate is associated with metabolic acidosis and fatigue. However, the lactate molecule itself is not responsible for acidosis. In reality, the production of lactate coincides with the formation of H^+ that reduces pH-inhibiting key enzymes of glycolysis such as PFK [56]. In fact, to some extent, lactate contributes to proton buffering since in the LDH reaction (conversion of pyruvate to lactate), two electrons and one proton from NADH and another proton from solution are used [19].

Second, especially in the past, lactate was considered a waste product of glycolysis due to hypoxia and was associated with fatigue especially during high-intensity exercise [57]. Also, postexercise lactate metabolism was linked to the oxygen depth, the phenomenon of elevated oxygen uptake during the postexercise period [58]. However, since the 1970s, the multidimensional metabolic role of lactate was realized gradually [53, 57]. The application of muscle biopsy; arteriovenous, magnetic resonance spectroscopy; and tracer techniques enabled researchers to focus not simply on lactate accumulation during or after exercise but on lactate formation (appearance), removal, and transport between and within various tissues such as the muscle, liver, heart, and brain [59–61]. For example aerobically trained individuals demonstrate a delayed blood lactate accumulation during progressive exercise compared to anaerobic or untrained people, as indicated by the higher anaerobic threshold they possess [62], suggesting that lactate formation and removal can be modulated by exercise training. This is discussed later on in this chapter.

Currently, the general consensus is that lactate formation is not due to hypoxic conditions of the working muscles since an increased lactate production and accumulation also occurs under aerobic conditions [53, 57].

The concept that lactate produced by the working muscles is taken up and metabolized by other tissues was introduced in the mid-1980s by George A. Brooks and was termed lactate shuttle, although today is known as cell-to-cell lactate shuttle [63]. He reported that about 75% of the lactate during submaximal exercise is removed and oxidized and only about 20% is converted to glucose. Lactate continues to be oxidized during the recovery period, but significant amounts are used for glycogen repletion through gluconeogenesis in the muscle and liver. However, these tissues do not replace their glycogen via this mechanism unless feeding is provided, with the exception of the heart that supercompensates its glycogen stores even during fasting [63]. The cell-to-cell shuttle has been proposed not only for the muscle but other tissues like the brain, heart, and liver.

Lactate can also be transported to oxidative (type I) fibers within the exercising muscle, to inactive oxidative fibers, and used as energy source. It can also exit the working muscle and be transported to less active muscle groups or to inactive glycolytic (type II) muscle fibers where it is either oxidized or converted to glycogen and stored [53, 57]. The liver can also oxidize or convert lactate to glucose, where this newly formed glucose can be either returned to exercising muscle through the Cori cycle pathway or stored as liver glycogen. Also, lactate in the systemic circulation can be directly oxidized in heart and brain tissue. Regarding the brain, astrocytes take-up blood glucose and convert it to lactate that in turn is transported to nearby neurons where it can be oxidized to regenerate ATP in the mitochondria [53, 57]. Therefore, taking into account all these possible pathways, lactate today is considered as a metabolic intermediate that connects glycolytic with oxidative metabolism [54].

In medicine, lactate metabolism has recently being incorporated in the study of cancer metabolism and treatment [64]. On the basis of Warburg effect, where in the presence of oxygen, cancer cells rely on glycolysis for energy production accompanied by high rates of lactate formation, it has been suggested that a treatment approach would have been to neglect glucose to cancer cells and provide as alternative fuel lactate, the so-called lactate-protected hypoglycemia treatment [65]. Although this idea is attractive, cancer metabolism is far more complicated with a diverse collection of normal and cancer cells whose metabolism is different in an in vitro environment compared to poorly understood tumor microenvironment [53, 64]. Nevertheless, it seems that as our understanding on lactate metabolism increases, this molecule will have the potential to offer more in health and disease in the future.

Lactate Threshold: How Is It Affected by Fitness?

In 1964 Wasserman and McIlroy introduced the term "anaerobic threshold" (AT) when attempting to define (without assessing blood lactate) the exercise intensity where energy production shifted from a mainly aerobic metabolism to that combining both anaerobic and aerobic patterns [66].

When VO_2max is directly assessed, ventilatory rates (V_E; volume of air inspired or expired per minute), volume of carbon dioxide expired (VCO_2), VCO_2/VO_2 ratio referred as the respiratory exchange ratio (RER or simply R), and the ventilatory equivalent for oxygen (VO_2/V_E) are also assessed. As the workload increases, a point is reached where these values increase disproportionally to exercise intensity [67]. This reflects the point at which the increasing metabolic demands due to the increased workload can no longer be met mainly by aerobic metabolism. Consequently, an increase in the relative contribution to energy needs is met by anaerobic metabolism and especially by glycolysis. This point has been coined as the "anaerobic or ventilator threshold."

This exercise level is also marked by an increase in lactate concentration accompanied by an increase in H^+ which is eventually transported out of the muscle in the circulation and blood pH is reduced. Thus, this threshold can also be detected using blood lactate measurements and is therefore referred to as lactate threshold (LT). An example of such determination is presented in Fig. 5.5. Because the AT and LT do not always coincide and, at times, the term onset of blood lactate accumulation (OBLA) has been introduced, in this case, the LT is defined as the exercise intensity at which a lactate accumulation of 4 mmol.l^{-1} is observed [68]. As illustrated in Fig. 5.5, this blood lactate level occurs at 9 km·h^{-1}. Below this workload, lactate remains fairly constant despite an increase in exercise intensity and an expected increase in glycolysis (Fig. 5.5). This indicates that lactate formed below workload of 9 km.h^{-1} is metabolized by the working muscle (via the cell-to-cell shuttles discussed above), and therefore lactate concentrations do not rise until the 9 km.h^{-1} workload is exceeded.

Since the original study by Wasserman and McIlroy in 1964, much criticism and debate has taken place, mainly regarding the link between what is observed and the actual changes occurring within the exercising muscle. This is due to methodological constraints and the difficulty in measuring intracellular partial pressure of oxygen during incremental exercise [56]. However, LT and AT still remain valuable functional parameters for doctors and sports scientists [69–71].

Can the Lactate Threshold Be Altered?

The LA is determined by mainly two factors: genetics and the level of physical fitness. Since there is little one can do with our genetic makeup, AT can only be altered by physical activity. The change in AT occurs in two ways. First, regularly performed aerobic activities lead to an increased VO_2max. The increase in VO_2max dictates that O_2 consumption at a given submaximal workload will be lower postexercise training compared to pre-training. As an example, let us assume that VO_2max prior to exercise training was 40 ml^{-1}.kg^{-1}.min^{-1} and following training increased to 50 ml^{-1}.kg-^{1}.min^{-1}. If we assume that LT occurs at approximately 50% of VO_2max, the AT for this individual prior to exercise training will occur at 20 ml^{-1}.kg^{-1}.min^{-1} and at 25 ml^{-1}.kg^{-1}.min^{-1} after training. Thus, following exercise training, the workload necessary to shift the working muscle from predominantly aerobic to anaerobic metabolism is increased.

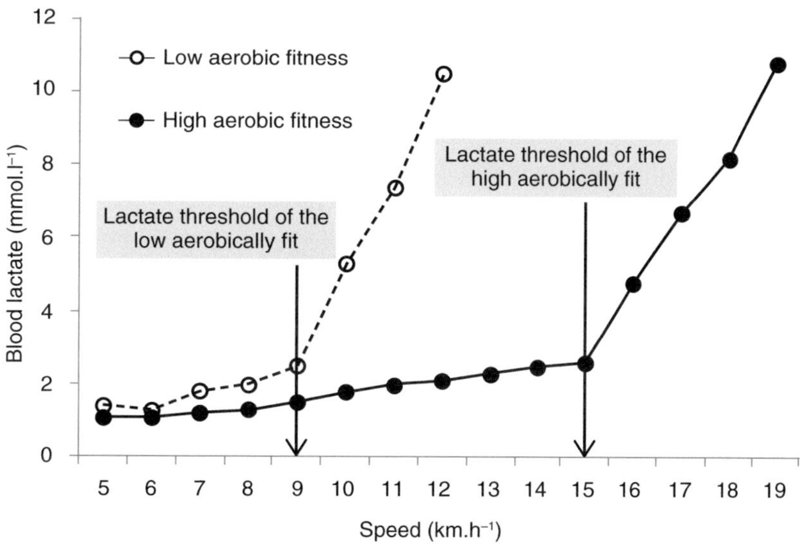

Fig. 5.5 A hypothetical lactate threshold during grated exercise test to volitional fatigue for low and high aerobically trained individuals

The second way AT is altered is via the increased efficiency of the aerobic pathways resulting from training. In other words, the metabolic alterations in aerobic enzymes such as succinate dehydrogenase, malate dehydrogenase, citrate synthase, a higher number and size of mitochondria, improved capillary network, and a high percentage of type I muscle fibers [68, 69, 72, 73] render the aerobically trained muscle capable of exercising at higher exercise intensities and accumulating even less blood lactate [74]. Thus, the AT of highly trained individuals occurs at about 75% and not at 50% as is the case with sedentary individuals. This is illustrated in Fig. 5.5 where an individual with low aerobic fitness may have a LT at 9 $km^{-1} \cdot h^{-1}$, while for someone with high aerobic fitness, LT can occur at 15 $Km^{-1} \cdot h^{-1}$.

Aerobic Metabolism During Exercise

Aerobic metabolism involves more complex energy systems than anaerobic metabolism, since all three major macronutrients, carbohydrates, fats, and proteins, contribute to the production of ATP. All aerobic chemical reactions take place in the mitochondria, situated mostly near the myofibrils, but may also be scattered in the sarcoplasm. A common molecule of all macronutrients is acetyl-Coa, although some other metabolites from fat or protein origin may "join" the oxidative phosphorylation process at glycolysis or Krebs cycle pathways.

The main characteristic of this system is that it can provide a much higher amount of ATP to the working muscle and for fats this may be almost unlimited, but its major disadvantage is that this energy is given at a substantially lower rate compared to anaerobic metabolism. For example, the net ATP yield of PCr system is 1 ATP, and glucose/glycogen 2–3 ATP. In contrast, the complete aerobic oxidation of glucose/glycogen yields 38–39 ATP, and a fatty acid like palmitate per mol 129 ATP. The maximum rates of ATP resynthesis by the aforementioned systems are approximately 2.25, 1.10, and 0.25–0.70 $ATP \cdot kg^{-1}$ $ww.s^{-1}$, for PCr, glycolysis, and Krebs cycle, respectively [40, 75].

Carbohydrate Metabolism

Blood-borne glucose and muscle glycogen are the carbohydrate substrates converted to pyruvate and then enter mitochondria as acetyl-CoA (Fig. 5.1). This reaction is catalyzed by the pyruvate dehydrogenase complex (PDH), situated in the inner mitochondrial membrane. PDH consists of three enzymes: pyruvate dehydrogenase, dihydrolipoamide acetyltransferase, and dihydrolipoamide reductase [40]. This chemical reaction is important since acetyl-CoA is the main substrate for the Krebs cycle. Once acetyl-CoA is formed, it cannot be converted back to pyruvate. Therefore, PDH is controlled by hormones and various effectors allosterically [40].

The Krebs cycle, also known as tricarboxylic acid cycle (TCA) or citric acid cycle, consists of a series of reactions that begins with the combination of oxaloacetate and acetyl-CoA to form citrate. These reactions are summarized as follows [40]:

$$\text{Acetyl-CoA} + 3H_2 0 \rightarrow 2CO_2 + 4[2H] + \text{CoASH}(\text{Coenzyme A})$$

Each cycle generates four pairs of hydrogen atoms ([2H]) which are carried to the electron transport chain by NADH and flavin adenine dinucleotide ($FADH_2$). Through the aerobic process of oxidative phosphorylation, the complete oxidation of acetyl-CoA yields 12 ATP molecules per cycle. A complete oxidation of glucose yields a total of 38 ATP, and glycogen yields 39 ATP. This is 19 and 13 times higher, respectively, compared to 2 and 3 ATP generated anaerobically.

Regulation of Hepatic Glucose Production

Liver plays a dominant role in blood homeostasis during exercise by releasing glucose into the bloodstream; otherwise, exercise would have been impossible to be carried out [76]. Splanchnic glucose increases almost linearly to exercise intensities up to 60% VO_2max and exponentially above this level, despite a gradual decrease in blood flow to the hepatosplanchnic area due to blood redistribution favoring the exercising muscles [77]. This exponential increase of blood glucose at higher exercise intensities shows that hepatic glucose production (HGP) and glucose uptake by the muscle do not match, indicating that regulation of HGP during exercise may not be via a feedback mechanism (i.e., blood glucose concentration) [77]. This mismatch suggests that hormonal and neural factors may affect to at least some extent HGP during exercise. In a study using somatostatin to modulate glucagon and insulin, during exercise at low intensity (40% VO_2max) for 2 h, the absence of glucagon totally abolished HGP, while in the absence of insulin, there was a threefold increase in HGP compared to rest [78]. There is evidence to suggest that these two hormones and especially glucagon may be more important in maintaining blood homeostasis late into a long-duration exercise rather than at the beginning [79].

The fact that epinephrine stimulates glycogen degradation during exercise led to the assumption that epinephrine stimulates HGP during exercise [76]. However, collective findings from human and animal studies show that when sympathoadrenergic activity is reduced, splanchnic glucose production is not impaired [77]. This leads to the conclusion that in addition to glucagon, insulin, or epinephrine, other mechanisms may be involved in the regulation of HGP during exercise [76, 77].

Regulation of Muscle Glucose Uptake

Glucose diffuses from capillaries to the muscle membrane through interstitial fluid by facilitated diffusion and is converted to G-6-P by hexokinase. Thus, blood supply, transport, and phosphorylation inside the muscle cell are potential sites of regulation of glucose uptake by the exercising muscle [80]. Simply, glucose uptake increases with increasing exercise intensity and duration to support the continuous energy demands of exercising muscle [81–83]. In the classical studies by Ahlborg and co-workers, when blood glucose gradually declined to about 2.5–3 $mmol.l^{-1}$ over 3.5–4 h of cycling, muscle glucose uptake was also reduced [81, 82]. On the other hand, when exogenous carbohydrate was provided during cycling, hypoglycemia was prevented and glucose uptake was maintained [84, 85]. These finding support that blood glucose concentration is an important factor for muscle glucose uptake during exercise.

The diffusion of glucose into the muscle cell is facilitated by the insulin-mediated translocation of GLUT-4 transporters from intracellular storage depots to the sarcolemma and transverse tubules. It is also well accepted that exercise has an insulin-like effect, translocating GLUT-4 to the surface of the cell through different molecular mechanisms and independent from insulin [80, 86]. Various factors identified as potential activators of GLUT-4 include Ca^{2+}, AMP-activated protein kinase (AMPK), reactive oxygen species (ROS), nitric oxide (NO), soluble *N*-ethylmaleimide-sensitive factor attachment protein receptors (SNARE), and GTPases especially RabGTPase proteins (members of the Ras small GTPases superfamily) [86–89]. Furthermore, epinephrine seems to reduce glucose uptake possibly due to stimulation of muscle glycogenolysis, resulting in an elevated G-6-P concentration. In turn hexokinase, the enzyme responsible for glucose phosphorylation, is inhibited [90]. Finally, lowering muscle glycogen content by 60 min single-legged cycling 16 h before a subsequent two-legged exercise bout increased muscle glucose uptake by threefold in the exercising leg (lower glycogen leg) compared to the control leg, suggesting that muscle glycogen levels may influence muscle glucose uptake [91].

Cross Talk Between Skeletal Muscle and Liver Metabolism in Exercise

During muscle contractions, skeletal muscle releases cytokines referred to as myokines [92]. In fact, the muscle is considered an endocrine organ that releases various myokines such as interleukin (IL) IL-6, IL-8, IL-15, brain-derived neurotrophic factor, leukemia inhibitory factor, fibroblast growth factor 21, and follistatin-like 1 [93]. In particular, muscle-derived IL-6, among other actions, may act in a hormonelike fashion increasing HGP and lipolysis in adipose tissue [94, 95]. In a study involving cycling at 40% VO_2max for 2 h with high and low IL-6 infusion rates, the use of stable $6,6^2H_2$ isotopes demonstrated higher rates of appearance and disappearance of blood glucose when the IL-6 infusion rates were high. This supports the view that IL-6 influences glucose homeostasis during exercise [95]. Furthermore, muscle-derived IL-6 has been observed to stimulate liver CXL-1 chemokine expression, a small cytokine that is involved in the processes of angiogenesis, inflammation, and wound healing, in exercising mice [96]. Thus, it is theorized that the exercising muscle communicates with distant organs such as the liver, adipose tissue, and brain by the release of myokines. This muscle-to-organ cross talk may play a significant role in the prevention of metabolic-related diseases such as obesity, diabetes, and cancer [93, 97].

Fat Metabolism

Acetyl-CoA is also generated from fat metabolism. Fats in the form of triacylglycerols are degraded to fatty acids and glycerol by a hormone-sensitive lipase through the process of lipolysis. Once in the circulation, glycerol is either taken by the liver to form triacylglycerols, converted to glucose through gluconeogenesis, or converted to dihydroxyacetone phosphate and enters glycolysis.

Fatty acids in the circulation are bound to albumin, whereas fatty acids in the muscle are also bound to binding proteins (Fig. 5.1). When fatty acids enter the muscle cells, they are converted to fatty acyl-CoA, which, in turn with the aid of carnitine, crosses the mitochondrial matrix. This is catalyzed by carnitine acyltransferase, also named carnitine palmitoyltransferase. This enzyme exists in two forms, one bound to the outer mitochondrial membrane (carnitine acyltransferase I) producing acyl carnitine and the other on the inner mitochondrial membrane that reverses the previous reaction producing acyl-CoA and carnitine [46]. Inside the mitochondrion, fatty acyl-CoA gradually loses two carbons to form acetyl-CoA, which enters Krebs cycle following the same pathway pyruvate follows (Fig. 5.1). Fatty acids yield more ATP depending on the number of their carbon atoms. For example, a 16-atom fatty acid will generate a net yield of 130 ATP molecules. Due to the complexity of mobilization, transport, and b-oxidation processes, however, the rate of ATP resynthesis by fatty acids is the slowest among all the fuels available [75].

Regulation of Muscle Fat Metabolism

The potential sites for regulation in skeletal muscle fat metabolism are (a) lipolysis of the adipose tissue and the delivery of fatty acids to the muscle, (b) movement of fatty acids across sarcolemma, (c) control of these molecules through the mitochondrial membrane, and (d) regulation of triacylglycerol lipase activity [98].

The hormone-sensitive lipase (HSL) responsible for lipolysis is activated by catecholamines which through β-adrenergic receptors activate lipolytic cascade and HSL is phosphorylated [99]. When participants cycled for 30 min at three different exercise intensities, 25%, 65%, and 85% VO_2max, fatty acid uptake, and oxidation decreased with the highest exercise intensity [100]. The investigators concluded that this was the outcome of reduced blood flow to the adipose tissue. However, in a subsequent study where fatty acid concentration was maintained high at exercise levels of 85% VO_2max, the uptake and oxidation of fatty acids increased, but was still lower than the levels achieved when exercising at 65% VO_2max. This suggests that intramuscular factors may be responsible for the rate of fat oxidation at higher exercise intensities [101].

Regarding the movement of fatty acids across muscle membrane during exercise, three fatty acid transport proteins, fatty acid binding protein in plasma membrane ($FABP_{pm}$), the fatty acid translocase (FAT/CD36), and fatty acid transport protein (FATP) have attracted considerable attention [102, 103]. In particular, evidence supports that FAT/CD36 is translocated from intracellular space to the muscle membrane during muscle contraction, and this coincides with increased fatty acid transport to the muscle [98]. Furthermore, more recent observations suggest that FAT/CD36 translocation is activated by insulin. This transporter is also present in the subcellular and intra-myofibrillar mitochondria, and its mitochondrial content is correlated with mitochondrial fatty acid oxidation, indicating that it is involved in regulating fatty acid oxidation in human skeletal muscle [103–105]. Another potential regulatory factor in fat oxidation is the muscle triacylglycerol lipase (MTGL). Methodological constraints have not allowed MTGL to be studied thoroughly. However, it seems that it is activated during aerobic exercise and contributes to energy supply by the degradation of muscle triacylglycerols which play an important role in providing fatty acids for oxidation during exercise [39, 98, 103].

Proteins as an Energy Source During Exercise

As mentioned earlier the protein contribution to ATP resynthesis is minimum. The muscle has the capacity to oxidize seven amino acids (alanine, asparagines, aspartate, glutamate, isoleucine, leucine, and valine), with some evidence suggesting that lysine may also be oxidized [106]. However, during exercise the main amino acids oxidized are isoleucine, leucine, and valine, the so-called branched-chain amino acids (BCAA). This is indicated by isotope tracer studies, a large muscle uptake of BCAA, and specific enzyme activation [107]. The BCAA are first transaminated to their keto acid analogues by branched-chain aminotransferase, and the formulated keto acids are oxidized by a mitochondrial branched-chain 2-oxoacid dehydrogenase enzyme (BCOADH) [106]. The BCOADH is considered to be the rate-limiting enzyme for BCAA oxidation and exists in active dephosphorylated form and less active phosphorylated form [106, 107]. This enzyme is activated during endurance exercise in human muscle [108–110]. This activation seems to be related to the glycogen status in the muscle, since when glycogen stores are low BCOADH is activated more, whereas when glycogen stores are high, the enzyme is not activated [110, 111]. This is linked to the observation that based on sweat urea N measurements low carbohydrate stores elevate protein degradation during exercise [112]. However, the contribution of BCAA to total energy expenditure during endurance activities is calculated to be only about 3–6% [1, 2]. Nevertheless, there is the view that amino acids may interact with TCA during prolonged exercise. As exercise progresses and glycogen stores become depleted, an increase in leucine oxidation may lead to a carbon drain on the TCA cycle, reduce its flux, and lead to fatigue [3, 111]. However, this mechanism may not be quantitatively important by others since changes in TCA cycle intermediates may be unrelated to oxidative energy provision in skeletal muscle [113].

Finally, in resistance exercise there is an increased protein turnover in the postexercise period that remains negative (i.e., protein breakdown >protein resynthesis) if the exercising individual remains in postabsorptive condition [107, 114].

Factors Determining Substrate Preference During Exercise

Substrate preference for ATP resynthesis in healthy individuals is dependent on four main factors, exercise intensity, duration, fitness status, and diet, while gender and environmental factors may also influence substrate utilization. The contribution of PCr is mainly at exercise intensities exceeding 100% VO_2max or when exercise intensity increases abruptly (Figs. 5.3 and 5.4). Therefore, the main fuels used are carbohydrates and fats, while proteins contribute approximately <5–6% to the total energy turnover [1, 2].

Possibly the strongest factor dictating the relative contribution of fats and carbohydrates is exercise intensity. At low exercise intensity levels of about 25% VO_2max plasma fatty acids are the main contributors. As intensity increases, the contribution of fats decreases proportionally, with a marked decrease observed at exercise intensities above 80% of VO_2max, while the contribution of muscle glycogen and plasma glucose increases proportionally [100, 115]. However, fat oxidation in absolute amounts (i.e., g/min) increases up to exercise intensities of 40–65% VO_2max [115, 116]. It seems that an increased glycolytic flux may inhibit fatty acids from entering the mitochondria, leading to diminished lipid oxidation [117, 118]. However, since all the aforementioned studies were based on indirect calorimetry, there is the concern that at high exercise intensities, fat oxidation might have been underestimated due to metabolic perturbations [119].

Another major factor that alters substrate preference is the duration of exercise. In general, at fixed exercise intensity, fat oxidation increases, while carbohydrate contribution decreases as exercise progresses. At low to moderate exercise intensities (about 25–60% VO_2max), fats gradually become the main fuels for energy especially when activity lasts for hours. For example, in one of the classical studies by Ahlborg and coworkers, they reported that during 4 h of exercise at approximately 30% of VO_2max the relative contribution of free fatty acid rose progressively to 62% of the total energy requirements after 40 min of exercise. The contribution of glucose fell from 40% during the initial exercise of 40 min to 30% between 90 and 240 min [81].

Similarly, in another study, plasma fatty acids provided more than 80% of total energy expenditure during 2 h of cycling at 25% VO_2max [100]. Finally, Edwards and colleagues reported that a runner exercising for 6 hours, about 84% of the energy requirements are derived from fats [120]. The increased free fatty acid (FFA) oxidation over time is associated with a progressive decrease in glycogen stores lending support to the concept that carbohydrate availability may play a role in the regulation of fat oxidation during exercise [117].

It is also well documented that aerobic fitness status and diet influence substrate use. This occurs as a result of metabolic adaptations occurring at peripheral fat tissues and within the muscle cells enabling the trained muscle to oxidize relatively more fat and less carbohydrate [121–123]. This is of particular importance for the endurance athlete since the limiting factor in performance is glycogen stores. Shifting the balance to utilizing more fat than glycogen for a given task (marathon run) delays glycogen depletion and, therefore, delays fatigue [56].

The effect of diet on substrate use was demonstrated almost a century ago when Krogh and Lindhard showed that after a high-fat low-carbohydrate diet RER values were lower from baseline, indicating higher oxidation of FFA [124]. More recent studies confirmed this early finding and reported that a high-carbohydrate diet reduces fat oxidation, whereas a diet rich in fat produces the opposite result [125]. Similarly, carbohydrate oxidation increased during exercise after a carbohydrate load 3–4 h prior to exercise compared to an overnight fast [126–128]. It takes at least 6 h at the postabsorptive state before exercise metabolic responses are similar to a fast of 8–12 h [129].

Finally, environmental conditions may play a role in substrate use especially when these conditions divert from a thermoneutral environment. In general, when exercise is performed in the heat, there is an increase in muscle glycogenolysis and liver glucose output, reduced fat utilization, and also an enhanced and no increase in muscle glucose uptake, leading to an elevation in blood glucose concentration. These responses seem to be related to high muscle temperature and a sympathoadrenal response [130].

Sex-Related Differences in Substrate Preference During Exercise

It is well established that sex-related metabolic and hormonal differences in exercise exist and should be considered [131, 132]. Males rely to a greater extent on carbohydrate oxidation, while females rely more on lipid oxidation displaying a lower RER during exercise. Indeed, at any given relative exercise intensity, women oxidize less carbohydrate and more fat than men [133, 134]. However, other studies reported no gender differences in the substrate preference [115, 135]. The rationale for the possible increased fat oxidation by females may be that estrogen promotes fat oxidation, as indicated when estrogen supplementation is administered in males [136]. Female hormones or the relatively greater proportion of type I fibers in women compared to men may explain the differences between the patterns of energy substrate utilization in men and women [132, 137]. In addition, elevated levels of GH in women, both at rest and at peak response to exercise, could also contribute to the sex-related differences in substrate use [132]. Furthermore, variations in ovarian hormone levels throughout the menstrual cycle may alter exercise metabolism in women [138].

Specifically, the female sex hormone, estrogen, is a factor that in both sexes affects energy substrate selection during exercise; however, it does not appear to be the sole determinant for substrate selection in females [139]. Estrogen, specifically 17β-estradiol, decreases carbohydrate oxidation and promotes lipid oxidation during prolonged, moderate-intensity exercise [140–142]. Moreover, during the luteal phase compared to the follicular phase of the menstrual cycle, higher levels of circulating estrogen and thus a higher relative rate of fat oxidation as well as a higher estradiol response to an acute bout of exercise have been observed [132, 143, 144]. In addition, a greater reliance on lipids as a fuel source was found in females compared to males during prolonged, moderate-intensity exercise, indicated by a lower RER in women. Moreover, women in the follicular phase had higher glycogen use as well as glucose appearance and disappearance rates than women in the luteal phase [141]. Interestingly, during the follicular phase of the menstrual cycle, women exhibit an increase in circulating estradiol after an acute bout of aerobic or resistance exercise, in contrast with men, although circulating levels of estrogen do not differ significantly between women and men [143, 145, 146]. Moreover, there is evidence supporting that overall fat oxidation may not be different between sexes, but the type of fat may differ with females to use more myocellular triacylglycerols [147, 148]. The issue becomes more complex due to the anti-estrogenic action of progesterone and other confounding variables such as exercise intensity and nutritional status that may obscure any estrogen's possible effect [138].

Cardiac Metabolism During Exercise

Myocardial metabolism is a complex network of highly regulated metabolic pathways and an integral part of the function of the heart, both as consumer and provider of energy, matching cardiac energy demand and supply with precision [149]. Cardiac metabolism in health and disease has been studied extensively in vitro, in animal models and in humans under resting conditions [150–153]. However, few studies in vivo have been conducted in healthy humans during exercise. This is due to technical and practical difficulties as well as to the invasive nature of these procedures, where the methods commonly used are catheterization of aorta and coronary sinus and use of radioactive and nonradioactive isotopes [154].

Metabolism of Energy Substrate in Heart During Exercise

The basic principles of cellular metabolism in various tissues apply also to cardiac muscle cells, with some quantitative differences. The cardiac muscle is designed to function aerobically, as it is endowed by an abundance of blood supply. Under resting conditions, most of the energy requirements of the heart are derived from fatty acids.

During exercise, cardiac output may increase more than sevenfold exceeding 40 $l \cdot min^{-1}$ in elite endurance athletes [11]. Therefore, the heart muscle requires large amounts of energy and is the largest energy consumer relative to its weight in the body [155]. Since the ATP content of the heart muscle is low (5 $\mu mol \cdot g^{-1}$ww), ATP homeostasis must be maintained for myocardium to function properly [151]. To support ATP resynthesis, the myocardium uses a variety of substrates such as fatty acids, glucose, lactate, pyruvate, ketones, and amino acids [155]. However, the main substrates that have been directly studied and seem to contribute during exercise to the oxygen extraction ratio of the myocardium are free fatty acids, glucose, and lactate [156–162]. During exercise, the preferred fuel for the cardiac muscle is lactate released form the exercising muscle followed by FFA. However, under ischemic conditions (i.e., coronary artery obstruction), the heart is forced to switch to anaerobic glycolysis for its energy needs. This situation is not sustainable, and if blood supply is not restored within minutes, the heart suffers irreparable damage. The relation between energy supply, mechanical function, and intracellular pH of the myocardium, both in healthy and diseased conditions, has been fundamental to cardiology.

Glucose

Glucose utilization for the myocardium occurs especially under hypoxic conditions, resulting in lactate formation [159, 162]. Multiple functions in myocardium are also mediated by glucose and its metabolites, and failure to control the levels of intracellular glucose metabolites has been implicated in the generation of ROS, as well as the development of insulin resistance. Moreover, excessive accumulation of glucose metabolites has been associated with various myocardial pathologies [149].

Free Fatty Acids

Long-chain free fatty acids are the myocardium's predominant fuel for respiration [163]. The pathway of long-chain FFA metabolism (oxidation) is initiated with their liberation from triglycerides (TGs) and ends with the entry of acetyl-CoA into the Krebs cycle. Acetyl-CoA is committed to oxidation by the system of β-oxidation, inside the mitochondria [164]. The rate of oxidation of FFA in the myocardium is somehow related to the activity of Krebs cycle and the rate of oxidative phosphorylation, and changes in flux through pathways of fatty acid metabolism reflect changes in substrate provision to the myocardium [149].

Ketone Bodies

Concentrations of ketone bodies in the plasma can dramatically rise during exercise, and their uptake, which is concentration-dependent, is a key feature in myocardial metabolism. The ketone bodies have access to the Krebs cycle in the heart [165]; however, the rate of oxidation is not sufficient to meet the energy demands of the myocardium [166, 167]. Interestingly, pyruvate carboxylation accounts for at least 3–6% of Krebs cycle flux in the heart [149].

Amino Acids

An integral part of energy metabolism in the heart is also amino acids, and one of the main functions of transaminases in myocardium under physiologic conditions is the supply of carbon skeletons for the Krebs cycle [168]. In addition, alanine is also an end product of anaerobic glucose metabolism, like lactate, and it is easily transphosphorylated to ATP, while this reaction results in anaerobic energy production independently of lactate formation [149].

As in skeletal muscle and other tissues, most of the metabolic energy is used to form ATP in the mitochondria, and this ATP acts as the conveyer of energy for cardiac muscle contraction and other cellular functions, such as ion movements and intracellular protein turnover. As in any other bodily organ, it is impossible to separate metabolism from function in the heart. The heart converts substrates and oxygen to contractile function and heat, and there is positive correlation between the work output, the rate of ATP turnover, the rate of oxygen consumption, and the rate of substrate input and utilization. However, it is certain that for a given physiologic environment, the myocardium oxidizes the most efficient substrate [149].

Preferred Substrate for Energy Needs of the Heart During Exercise

Metabolism of oxidizable substrates for energy supply fuels ATP production in the mitochondria for the contractile function of the myocardium. About 2/3 of the energy from the hydrolyzed ATP is used in contractile machinery with the remaining to support ion pumps such as Ca^{2+}, Na^{+}, and K^{+}. The main driving force of energy metabolism in cardiac muscle is the rate of energy turnover and not its stored ATP [149, 169–171].

The intermediary metabolism of energy substrates supports the contractile function of the myocardium, and the bulk of the energy for this function is derived from oxidative phosphorylation of ADP. Indeed, in well-oxygenated healthy myocardium, ATP resynthesis is accomplished almost exclusively (>98%) by oxidative phosphorylation in the mitochondria, and only a small fraction (<2%) is derived from glycolysis [172]. Interestingly, the myocardium has the capability of maintaining and controlling, even during high-intensity exercise, the same levels of high-energy phosphate compounds (PCr and ATP) as well as their ratio observed at rest, suggesting that the intracellular-free ADP concentration, differently from skeletal muscle, does not function as a primary system to control cardiac muscle during exercise [173, 174]. Indeed, using ^{31}P NMR technology in vivo it was observed that even a threefold increase in myocardial oxygen did not alter cytosolic ATP, ADP, and Pi concentrations [175].

In particular, the total lactate dehydrogenase (LDH) and phosphofructokinase (PFK) activity is high, and, therefore, cardiac muscle should have the ability to release significant energy via anaerobic glycolysis [176, 177]. However, the myocardium also has a high aerobic capacity, and, therefore, both at rest and during maximal exercise, myocardial energy demands are met mostly by aerobic metabolism without detectable contribution of anaerobic glycolysis, even during maximal exercise [178, 179]. Notably, in a healthy heart the coronary circulation has the capacity to supply the myocardium with blood and oxygen without the need of anaerobic myocardial metabolism [176]. Indeed, aerobic metabolism is predominant in myocardium and the predominant fuel for energy supply is FFA. Glucose is not a preferred substrate by the cardiac muscle, and when it is limitedly used, myocardium first oxidizes glycogen, followed by the aerobic, again, breakdown of glucose and lactate, without the need of anaerobic metabolism. Interestingly, during high-intensity exercise, when blood levels of lactate rise, the healthy preferred substrate for the myocardium is lactate, which replaces all other energy-providing substrates as heart's fuel for respiration [149, 180–183].

Molecular Mechanisms of Exercise-Induced Metabolic Adaptations in Cardiac Muscle

Exercise-induced physiologic cardiac adaptations include mitochondrial biogenesis, ultimately leading to enhanced fatty acid and glucose metabolism. Consequently, metabolic homeostasis is preserved [179]. Metabolite profiling before and after exercise showed a subset of metabolites that regulate glucose and lipid metabolism[184], suggesting that metabolites and other molecules regulate various physiological processes, possibly including the myocardium response to exercise [185].

Moreover, sirtuins (SIRTs), a family of NAD-dependent deacetylases, regulate a variety of functions in the cells, including growth, metabolism, apoptosis, and aging [186]. SIRT1 and SIRT3 are the most studied in the cardiac tissue and both are upregulated by exercise. SIRT1 has pro-growth and pro-survival functions in cardiac muscle cells [187], while SIRT3 is a mitochondrial sirtuin [188] and protects the heart against oxidative stress. It has also been reported that it may modulate the opening of the mitochondrial permeability transition pore (mPTP) [189, 190]. Additionally, it regulates cardiac metabolism via activation of 5' AMP-activated protein kinase (AMPK) and peroxisome proliferator-activated receptor gamma coactivator 1-alpha (PGC-1α), both of which inhibit maladaptive remodeling of myocardium [189].

Furthermore, exercise upregulates PGC-1α, as potent mediator of oxidative phosphorylation and mitochondrial biogenesis. PGC-1α-deficiency results in inability of the myocardium to meet energy demands, indicating the importance of energy and metabolic homeostasis in myocardial health [179]. PGC-1α has also been shown to regulate a pathway of angiogenesis which is independent of the hypoxia-inducible factor-1 (HIF-1), therefore providing a mechanism for coordinately regulating blood supply and mitochondrial function in the exercising myocardium [185, 191].

Future Considerations of Cardiac Metabolism

Both in physiological and pathological conditions, the cardiac muscle has enormous energy demands, and myocardial metabolic dysregulation is a noticeable feature of cardiovascular disease [185]. The importance of energy substrate metabolism in the myocardium is increasingly appreciated in heart disease, diabetes, and cancer. Changes in the physiologic environment of the heart directly result in alterations of its metabolic fluxes, suggesting that an integral part of cardiac adaptation to its environment is metabolic signals, while metabolic remodeling both triggers and sustains structural and functional remodeling of the heart [192]. Notably, pathological cardiac remodeling has been associated with a switch from the fatty acid utilization, which is the primary energy substrate for the adult heart, to glucose metabolism, as it happens in ischemic conditions. Since aerobic exercise training has been shown to promote not only efficient fatty acid and glucose handling but also mitochondrial biogenesis in the heart [179], aerobic exercise benefits in myocardial metabolic dysregulation should be further characterized and utilized, as they cannot be fully reproduced by any novel and improved, exercise-mimicking treatment for heart disease [185].

Exercise-Induced Chronic Metabolic Adaptations

Regularly performed exercises of adequate intensity, duration, and volume lead to chronic adaptations. These adaptations are specific to the exercise mode, encompass both morphological and function changes, and include all systems involved in the physical task. The ultimate outcome is improved functional capacity of the individual resulting in an improved oxidative capacity of the working muscle [26, 193–197]. A major metabolic change due to endurance training is the exercise-induced mitochondrial biogenesis resulting in a higher mitochondrial content, volume, and oxidative capacity [198].

This process involves multiple molecular events ultimately resulting in improved functional capacity of the individual [198, 199] and significant health implications, as these adaptations attenuate the aged-induced sarcopenia and apoptosis that can lead to pathological conditions such as autoimmune and neurodegenerative diseases [199].

The increase in the number, volume, and oxidative capacity of mitochondria is accompanied by increased mitochondrial enzyme concentration and activity and increases in capillary density [197, 200, 201]. Collectively, these adaptations increase the capacity of the muscle to oxidize fats and carbohydrates more efficiently, sparing in this way the limited body glycogen stores [56]. This is significant for athletes engaged in long-duration activities (marathon run), where one of the limiting factors of performance is glycogen depletion leading to fatigue.

Significant reduction in the rate of muscle glycogenolysis with endurance training has been reported in several studies [200, 202–204]. However, others dispute these findings, as change in the rate of muscle glycogenolysis is not accompanied by a higher activation of phosphorylase, indicating that other factors such as ADP, AMP, and Pi may have an influence [203]. Furthermore, studies using isotopes have reported a reduced rate of liver glycogenolysis as indicated by the lower rate of glucose appearance in the systemic circulation [204–206]. Conflicting results have also been reported regarding gluconeogenesis [205, 207]. Muscle glucose uptake is also reduced as a result of training at pre-training exercise intensity of 60% VO_2max [206, 208, 209]. However, at higher pre-training exercise intensities (80–100% VO_2max), post training muscle glucose uptake is increased [210].

Studies have shown clearly that fat oxidation is enhanced with aerobic training [206–209]. However, it is difficult to clearly distinguish fat oxidation from blood-borne fatty acids with that from intramuscular stores. Methodological constraints in arterial-venous difference and tracer procedures have resulted in conflicting results regarding the extent to which blood-borne fatty acid oxidation is elevated [211]. It is not clear if there are exercise-related improvements in intramuscular triglycerides oxidation. Accurate assessments are hampered by the variability of biopsy samples as well as the potential that some of the fatty acids from circulation may not be oxidized in the muscle but replace intramuscular fat stores [211]. However, it is the discrepancy between total fat oxidized by indirect calorimetry and that from tracer data which suggests that intramuscular fatty acids are oxidized to a greater extent after training [211, 212].

Another clear training response is the lower lactate concentrations after aerobic training. This reflects an enhanced metabolic clearance rate as judged by the rate of lactate disappearance at any given concentration [59, 213, 214]. The precise mechanism(s) facilitating lactate clearance is not understood. However, several concepts are proposed including (1) enhanced mitochondrial oxidative capacity, (2) an increase in the expression of monocarboxylate transporter 1 (MCT1) which facilitates lactate uptake by mitochondria, and (3) alteration of LDH activity to its H-LDH isoenzyme that favors lactate oxidation to pyruvate [215].

Hormonal Regulation of Exercise Metabolism

Hormones are sensitive to exercise-induced stress and play various roles in muscle metabolism during exercise or even in the regenerative and adaptive mechanisms following exercise-induced muscle damage [44, 137, 216].

Specifically, hormones regulate in part the release of energy from carbohydrate and lipid stores during exercise, the synthesis of glycogen and TGs following meals, and the resynthesis of muscle protein. Within the context of energy storage and energy production during exercise, the role of catecholamines, insulin, glucagon, and cortisol in the metabolic regulation of carbohydrate and lipid metabolism will be considered, along with the mechanisms that elicit the metabolic responses. Moreover, as exercise is accompanied by changes in catabolic and anabolic hormones, as well as muscle protein synthesis, the roles of growth hormone (GH), testosterone, and estrogen will also be described.

The increased energy demands during exercise are modulated by the synergistical work of pancreatic hormones, insulin and glucagon, resulting in elevated blood glucose [137, 217, 218]. Specifically, during exercise, insulin and the contractile activity of the exercising muscles act synergistically, but through independent mechanisms, to facilitate translocation of glucose transporter type 4 (GLUT4) receptors to the cell membrane and increase glucose uptake of the exercising muscles [137, 219, 220]. Although glucose transporters on plasma membranes are activated by both insulin and exercise independently [221–226], insulin inhibits the transcriptional biosynthesis of GLUT4, and, thus, it leads to a marked reduction of the GLUT4 pool of the low-density microsomes (LDM), where GLUT4 is stored. However, exercise not only increases the GLUT4 translocation from LDM compartment to the plasma membrane but also increases the biosynthesis of GLUT4, thus leading to only a small decrease of GLUT4 pool in LDM [221, 227–229]. Interestingly, in fat cells only insulin, and not exercise, accelerates the GLUT4 translocation velocity from LDM to the plasma membrane [221, 230].

Long-term muscular activity during prolonged moderate exercise results in greater insulin sensitivity, and, thus, blood insulin levels decrease [231–233]. Thus, during an ultra-long distance running, a rise of insulin antagonists, i.e., cortisol, glucagon, and GH, has been observed in the early stages of ultra-long running, which was inversely proportional to the intake of carbohydrates [234]. During endurance exercise, there are a number of potential sites of control which can regulate the interaction of substrate (carbohydrate and lipid) metabolism. These include availability of intra- and extra-muscular substrates which are controlled by diet and the action of key hormones, such as insulin and the catecholamines, the abundance of proteins such as GLUT4, and the activity of key enzymes involved in the regulation of metabolic pathways. Thus, interestingly, within the context of interactions between hormonal actions and metabolic regulation, insulin, apart from acting to lower blood glucose, it may also stimulate glycolysis by inducing increased synthesis of key glycolytic enzymes [44].

In addition to insulin and glucagon, blood glucose during exercise is also modulated by cortisol and epinephrine. Exercise-induced stress results in the release of both these hormones, and both mediate the maintenance of blood glucose levels.

Specifically, epinephrine, a stress hormone secreted by the adrenal medulla, stimulates glycogen phosphorylase activity in the liver and muscle, thereby increasing glucose availability for the exercising muscles. Cortisol, also a stress hormone, is secreted from the adrenal gland and promotes muscle protein breakdown, thus making certain glucogenic amino acids available for gluconeogenesis (after 20–30 min or more) and ultimately resulting in increased blood glucose levels [137].

In summary, exercise facilitates an increase in circulating cortisol, catecholamines, glucagon, and GH and a suppression of insulin release. Consequently, these hormones synergistically increase glycolysis, glycogenolysis both in the muscle and liver, lipolysis in muscle and adipose tissue, gluconeogenesis in the liver, and protein degradation in the muscle and liver. Ultimately, this leads to an increase in substrate availability to meet the increased energy demands of the working muscles.

In addition to the effects of the hormones on energy availability during exercise, it is also important to appreciate that hormones regulate the recovery process following exercise. This includes not only resynthesis of muscle glycogen stores ready for the next training session but also promotion of protein synthesis in the muscle. For instance, increased release of GH in response to exercise may have an anabolic effect or improve postexercise recovery time [44].

Hormonal Responses in High-Intensity Anaerobic Exercise and in Prolonged Aerobic Exercise

Repeated high-intensity (near maximal or supramaximal) exercise bouts of activity lasting only seconds to a few minutes, interspersed with exercise of low to moderate intensity (active recovery) or complete inactivity, have become popular recently. The major sources of energy during such activities are derived from anaerobic processes. On the other hand, aerobic processes provide the energy sources of physical activity that is performed for durations from a few minutes to hours and causes an increased heart rate and respiratory volume to meet the oxygen requirements of the exercising muscles [44, 235, 236].

A growing interest has been developed regarding the metabolic characteristics and adaptations of high-intensity exercise training [237]. In this context, the acute hormonal and metabolic responses to high-intensity anaerobic exercise have received particular interest. More specifically, high metabolic stimuli, such as high levels of lactate, changes in the acid base status, and large decreases in pH, which are induced by high-intensity interval training (HIIT), elicit certain hormonal responses that may be different from the traditional anaerobic work and appear to result even in aerobic adaptations [238–240]. Metabolic disturbances appear to play a key role in causing acute hormonal responses and long-term adaptations to HIIT, and it has been speculated that the acute metabolic disturbances and the consequent hormonal increases after HIIT may play a positive role in optimizing training adaptations and eliciting health benefits. The hormonal responses to HIIT indicate their involvement in adaptation mechanisms potentially as part of a regulatory network to support a normal adaptation process to HIIT. However, the influence of the duration of intervals and recovery, the different exercise intensities, and the work/rest ratio on the acute hormonal responses to HIIT and particularly on its long-term adaptations should be further investigated and optimized [237]. Moreover, it remains to be elucidated if these responses and adaptations have significant health implications, such as the improvement of some cardiometabolic risk factors reported in special populations [241].

Exercise represents a powerful stimulus for the sympathoadrenergic system, which is important for the metabolic adaptation to exercise [217, 242, 243]. Specifically, during exercise the stimulation and the subsequent increase in plasma catecholamines depend on the duration of exercise (total work), workload, and the muscle mass recruited, as well as on the emotional stress, however, not on the power output pattern, in both continuous and interval exercise training. Particularly during high-intensity exercise, the sympathoadrenergic system and catecholamines affect the substrate mobilization, while particularly noradrenaline is a potent stimulator of muscle glycolysis [137]. Moreover, although the concentration of blood glucose strongly influences the extent of the insulin secretion, however, insulin release is inhibited by stimulation of adrenoceptors on pancreatic beta-cells, as it occurs during exhaustive exercise due to the increased levels of catecholamines. Increases in catecholamine concentrations are higher in intense anaerobic exercise than prolonged aerobic exercise in both young and adults [137, 244, 245]. The adrenergic inhibition of the insulin secretion by the exercise-induced elevated catecholamine levels supports the substrate supply during exercise; glycogenolysis and lipolysis are inhibited by insulin, while, in contrast, catecholamines that oppose the action of insulin stimulate these processes [137]. Thus, the inhibition of insulin release results in reduced glycogenesis in liver and muscle and intensifies glycogen mobilization in muscle and the glycogenolytic and gluconeogenetic glucose output from the liver [217]. In addition, within the context of hormonal-induced substrate mobilization, repeated bouts of high-intensity sprints have been shown to result in increased blood levels of glucagon, with no effect of sex on those changes [246]. Nevertheless, exercise training-induced changes in hormone concentrations such as norepinephrine, insulin, and glucagon are unable to explain all of the effects that occur between liver glucose production and muscle glucose uptake during exercise, and it has been proposed that, possibly, the actual rate of muscle glucose uptake acts as a feedback signal to regulate glucose output from the liver [44, 209].

Growth hormone possesses both anabolic and catabolic actions. It stimulates cellular uptake of amino acids and their incorporation into various proteins, including those of the muscle. It also acts as a repartitioning agent fostering fat metabolism via mobilization of TGs. In adults, GH levels increase during exercise; however, its secretion is pulsatile in nature, and, thus, it is difficult to interpret its peak values during exercise [106, 137, 247, 248]. There is evidence that GH responses are much higher in HIIT compared to high-volume aerobic training and that the increase in blood GH levels is in part a consequence of the decreased blood pH following HIIT [240].

It is important to mention that, when examining GH response to exercise, insulin-like growth factor-1 (IGF-1) should be taken into consideration. IGF-1 is a hormone that mediates many actions of GH, and the GH-IGF-1 axis, among other primary actions, has been suggested to mediate many of the anabolic effects associated with resistance, anaerobic, and aerobic exercise [249, 250]. Specifically, during exercise IGF-1 levels appear to be independent of GH responses, while there has been an inconsistency of findings regarding the IGF-1 response to exercise, with studies reporting a decrease, increase, or no change in blood IGF-1 [251, 252]. Most studies reported significant increases in IGF-1 after high-intensity exercise stimuli, while IGF-1 response to exercise appears to depend on type, intensity, and duration of exercise. Particularly regarding IGF-1 and glucose response, it is not clear to what extent endogenously produced IGF-1 contributes to glucose homeostasis, although there is evidence that exogenous IGF-1 can lower blood glucose [132].

Serum levels of hormones such as GH, IGF-1, testosterone, estradiol, dehydroepiandrosterone, and cortisol have been found to be similarly increased in response to an acute bout of moderate endurance exercise in adult females of a wide range of age, indicating that increasing age does not necessarily inhibit the hormonal response to a bout of aerobic exercise in women [145]. In addition, the effect of exercise training on the hormonal responses of GH, IGF-1, testosterone, free testosterone (FT), and sex hormone-binding globulin (SHBG) to a sub-maximum aerobic exercise bout was investigated in older men before and after 4 months of resistance or moderate aerobic training. Aerobic training or leg-only resistance training did not change the resting hormonal concentration of older men. There was an increase in testosterone and FT concentration immediately after both sub-maximum aerobic exercise and resistance exercise bout, which was higher after the 4-month resistance training but not after the aerobic training. In contrast, GH/IGF-1 response to sub-maximum aerobic exercise bout appeared to be blunted regardless of training status [253].

Gender Differences in Hormonal Responses in Anaerobic and Aerobic Exercise

Significantly higher GH responses in men compared to women after aerobic, anaerobic, or resistance exercise have been reported [132]. Moreover, females and males show a different pattern of GH release in the circulation during exercise, which peaks sooner and return to baseline more quickly in women, while men exhibit a more prolonged response. There are also noticeable sex-related differences in GH levels at rest, and subsequently higher peaks of GH during exercise in women. These differences in GH response have been attributed to a lack of testosterone response to exercise in women. Testosterone is a steroid hormone with anabolic potential on a number of tissues, including muscle and, hence, can impact muscle growth and exercise performance. Indeed, data suggest that this hormone may affect both anaerobic and aerobic performance [254, 255], with greater increases in FT being reported after HIIT than endurance exercise [256]. Women exhibit little or no increase in circulating testosterone in response to exercise [132, 257], and, hence, GH may compensate for the anabolic requirements triggered by acute exercise. In addition, the higher resting basal level of GH in women compared to men is dependent on the phase of the menstrual cycle, when estrogen levels affect accordingly circulating GH levels (reviewed in [132]). The sex-associated differences in GH response to exercise can affect the control of blood glucose in both sexes; increases in GH stimulate lipolysis and lipid oxidation while suppressing glucose oxidation and, consequently, increasing blood glucose levels [257]. Thus, higher levels of GH at rest in women, due to higher levels of estrogen, may preserve blood glucose levels to a greater extent in women compared with men [132, 257].

Nevertheless, the majority of studies investigating the GH/IGF-1 axis responses to exercise reported a similar relative increase in both sexes during and after exercise longer than 10 min [132, 257–259], while slight decreases in IGF-1 responses to ultra-endurance exercise were revealed, again similarly occurring in both sexes [132, 260]. Acute bouts of HIIT have been shown to lead or not to significant differences in IGF-1 responses in male compared to females, while the increase in IGF-1 in response to HIIT does not appear to be depended on the phase of the menstrual cycle of the female subjects [132, 250].

Moreover, it was showed that long-duration, low-intensity, or moderate aerobic exercise bouts produced significantly lower epinephrine and norepinephrine levels in women than in men, while there is a sex-related difference in sensitivity of lipolytic activity to catecholamines during exercise. Catecholamines increase lipolysis during exercise, and despite their lower levels in women compared to men, there has been evidence for elevated levels of lipolysis in women during exercise, implying a greater sensitivity to the lipolytic action of the catecholamines in females. Thus, during exercise-induced elevation of epinephrine, women have relatively greater fat oxidation and lipolysis than men [132, 259]. In addition, blood glucagon increases in both sexes following prolonged submaximal exercise, with the majority of studies reporting a lower glucagon response to moderate exercise in females compared to males [132, 259, 261].

Exercise Metabolism: Clinical Implications

Diabetes Mellitus (Type 1 and 2)

Diabetes mellitus refers to a group of metabolic disorders which are characterized by chronically increased circulating glucose levels (hyperglycemia). There are two main forms of diabetes, type 1 (T1D) and type 2 (T2D). T1D usually begins in youth, also known as juvenile-onset diabetes, whereas T2D usually begins in adulthood, and thus it is referred to as adult-onset diabetes [262].

Hyperglycemia is a common feature of both forms of diabetes; however, the cause is different. In T1D an autoimmune destruction of the beta-cells in the pancreas that produce insulin results in no insulin production in most patients (a minority of T1D patients has some remaining β-cell function). These patients require exogenous insulin, and for this reason, this type of diabetes mellitus is also known as insulin-dependent. Its etiology remains unknown; however, environmental factors, genetic disposition, and autoimmune reactions have been implicated [263]. Exogenous insulin use has been greatly contributed to the prevention of hyperglycemia and management of T1D. Exercise has also been shown to be effective in the management of hyperglycemia by improving glucose uptake form of the exercising muscles [137, 219, 221–226, 264].

T2D, accounting for up to 95% of all cases, is characterized by insulin resistance, in which the response to insulin in the muscle, liver, and fat cells is inadequate. However, endogenous production of insulin in many instances is also impaired. T2D, also known as non-insulin-dependent diabetes mellitus, as exogenous administration of insulin may not be necessary, and insulin resistance can be managed using diet and exercise to enhance insulin sensitivity [262]. Since insulin is required for muscle cells, liver cells, and adipocytes to take up and store glucose [262, 265], insulin resistance and insulin deficiency lead to hyperglycemia. Hyperglycemia is associated with blood vessel wall and nerve damage, eventually leading to various complications and premature mortality, usually from cardiovascular disease [266–271]. Moreover, increased physical activity and enhanced cardiorespiratory fitness are well accepted as an effective approach to attenuate and even prevent the development of T2D in individuals with prediabetes [266, 269, 272].

Diabetes Mellitus and Exercise

The improved glucose uptake by exercise, due to increased GLUT4 density in plasma membrane, has therapeutic consequences for both T1D and T2D. Specifically, both acute exercise and especially chronic exercise training lead to an insulin-independent increase in glucose uptake by GLUT4. This partially compensates for the absence of the insulin-stimulated glucose uptake in T1D. In T2D, characterized by insulin receptor and post-receptor defects and insulin resistance, acute and chronic exercise not only improves GLUT4 function but also enhances B-cell function and improvement of insulin sensitivity [217, 273, 274].

It is not clear whether there are sex-related differences in insulin sensitivity in response to exercise, since some studies have reported that women show a greater improvement of insulin sensitivity in response to acute bouts of submaximal exercise, while, conversely, others have shown that men and women exhibit a similar improvement of insulin sensitivity [132]. Furthermore, the phase of the menstrual cycle may also affect insulin sensitivity during exercise in women, as a significant decrease in insulin sensitivity was found during the luteal phase compared to the follicular phase (reviewed in [132]).

Type 1 Diabetes Mellitus and Exercise

The findings on the specific effects of exercise training on the glycemic control of patients with T1D are conflicting. Some reported no improvement in glycosylated hemoglobin (HbA1c) concentrations with physical training, whereas an inverse association between physical activity levels and HbA1c in T1D patients has been reported in a comprehensive review [263]. Moreover, the Position Statement of the American Diabetes Association for physical activity/exercise and diabetes [275] states that regular physical activity/exercise has an important role in the treatment of T1D and related benefits, including improved long-term weight and glycemic control, insulin sensitivity, lipid profile, and endothelial function, as well as fitness level and overall well-being [263, 264, 275–279].

Individuals with T1D who take up exercise have specific needs, as both exercise and insulin therapy play a key role in glycemic control. Since exercise enhances glucose uptake, exogenous insulin administration (injection) and carbohydrate ingestion must be coordinated with exercise. Specifically, when to exercise in relations to the meal and/or insulin injection, how hard (intensity), and how long (duration) are important consideration to maintain glycemic control [276]. Failure to appropriately coordinate blood glucose, dietary needs, and exogenous insulin administration prior, during, or following exercise can lead to unfavorable health outcomes [280, 281].

In particular, the increased release of counter-regulatory hormones to provide with energy for exercise of longer duration increases the risk of hypoglycemia particularly after endurance exercise. This risk persists for up to 15 h after the completion of exercise. It has been reported that overnight hypoglycemia is common in children with T1D after exercise, underlining the importance of blood glucose management in these patients when exercise is performed afternoon [262].

Various exercise strategies, including a single, all-out 10-s sprint before or after a bout of prolonged, moderate aerobic exercise, have been developed for the prevention of postexercise hypoglycemia in individuals with T1D. Indeed, there is evidence that high-intensity exercise has a stronger impact on glycemic control than moderate exercise. The risk of hypoglycemia is also lower with HIIT compared with moderate-intensity continuous training, as HIIT stimulates glucose production in the liver more than moderate-intensity exercise. Thus, athletes with T1D must be instructed so as to avoid exercise-induced hypoglycemia, by monitoring blood glucose and adjusting insulin and diet [263, 282].

Overall, although balancing exercise and food intake and adjusting insulin dosage are a challenge individualized for the T1D athlete in order to prevent either hyperglycemia or hypoglycemia, it is attainable, and physical activity/exercise recommendations should be adapted to the specific needs of each individual with T1D. Exercise training must be regular and in accordance with insulin treatment and adjustment, as well as with dietary regulation [263, 275, 276, 278, 280, 281, 283]. Both aerobic exercise and strength training of moderate-intensity exercise are advisable, as well as their combination, for at least 30 min daily. Exercise training has been recommended to be of approximately the same intensity and, if possible, at the same time of day [263]. Moreover, while exercise is safe and beneficial for individuals with T1D and avoiding exercise carries greater risks than being active, however, in order to reduce the risk of some complications, precautions must be taken. Thus, it has been suggested that physical activity should be postponed when blood glucose levels are higher than 14 mmol/L accompanied by ketonuria, or higher than 17 mmol/L without ketonuria, until this condition has been corrected. The same applies to blood glucose levels lower than 7 mmol/L [263].

Type 2 Diabetes Mellitus and Exercise

T2D is a progressive disease in which insulin resistance leads to poor glycemic control (hyperglycemia), and since this condition is not due to the lack of insulin, the body continues to secrete more insulin in response to the hyperglycemic state, resulting in hyperinsulinemia [262, 276]. There is a large body of evidence that physical exercise reduces the risk of developing T2D, while, also, exercise is one of the three cornerstones in the treatment of T2D along with healthy diet and medication [262, 263, 276, 277]. Specifically, many studies have indicated that regular physical activity plays a key role in controlling blood glucose in patients with T2D. In particular, a meta-analysis revealed that exercise lowers postprandial glucose but not fasting glucose in T2D, and this is important because, unlike medications, exercise is effective in reducing postprandial glycemic excursions just within a few days [263, 284]. Moreover, exercise improves glucose tolerance, insulin sensitivity, and HbA1c, while muscle contraction triggers glucose transport by insulin-independent mechanisms [262]. Indeed, physical exercise leads to an increase in insulin sensitivity and, consequently, in glucose uptake in insulin-sensitive tissues, however, with a lower consumption of insulin. Thus, the aforementioned long-term effect of exercise on glycemic levels can be expected [263]. A detailed coverage of the topic is provided by the Position Statement of the American Diabetes Association for physical activity/exercise and diabetes, briefly discussed below [275], and the American College of Sports Medicine (ACSM) and the American

Diabetes Association Joint Position Statement for Exercise and T2D [285].

Observational and intervention studies, randomized controlled trials, and meta-analyses of controlled clinical trials concerning the effects of physical activity on T2D have shown health benefits of regular physical activity/exercise for the treatment of T2D. In particular, it has been revealed that aerobic exercise training significantly reduces HbA1c levels in individuals with T2D, while strength training also increases insulin-mediated glucose uptake in skeletal muscle and significantly decreases HbA1c in patients with T2D. Interestingly, no differences have been reported between aerobic training and resistance training regarding the effect on HbA1c changes [263, 286]. Specifically, progressive resistance training was found to be effective in improving insulin sensitivity in both children and adults. Indeed, strengthening skeletal muscle is strongly associated with improved glycemic control, since approximately 85% of glucose uptake takes place directly in skeletal muscle [276, 287]. In addition, HIIT improves glycemic control and induces cardiometabolic adaptations similar to those of moderate aerobic exercise in prediabetes and T2D, while it provides greater benefits to functional capacity in patients with T2D [263, 286, 288]. On the other hand, a clear advantage of various activities of moderate-intensity exercise lasting for 20–60 min per day to HIIT exercise for diabetes prevention was not identified [286]. Nevertheless, structured exercise training consisted of aerobic exercise, resistance training, or their combination was revealed by a meta-analysis to be associated with HbA1c reduction in patients with T2D. Interestingly, a combination of resistance training and aerobic training is probably the optimal form of exercise for patients with T2D. Furthermore, structured exercise training of more than 150 min/week has been associated with greater HbA1c improvements compared with that of 150 min or less/week [263, 289].

Overall, the Position Statement of the American Diabetes Association (2016) provides a clinically oriented review and evidence-based recommendations about physical activity and exercise in people with diabetes. Briefly, exercise improves blood glucose control in T2D, contributes to weight loss, improves well-being, and reduces cardiovascular risk factors. Moreover, regular exercise may prevent or delay the development of T2D and also has considerable health benefits for people with T1D. Blood glucose management through exercise includes various challenges related to diabetes type, activity type, and presence of diabetes-related complications [275]. In view of the optimum exercise prescription for reducing the risk of T2D, initially 150 min per week of moderate-intensity physical activity and building up to 200–300 min per week was proven effective in improving insulin sensitivity and, thus, can help in preventing T2D. More specifically, exercise recommendations include low- to moderate-intensity exercise (40–70% of maximum oxygen uptake) performed on at least three non-consecutive days each week, starting with 10–15 min and progressing up to 60 min per session over time [262]. The mode of exercise may depend on personal preference and include a variety of activities, comprised of aerobic and resistance exercises. More studies are needed to establish specific guidelines regarding the independent and synergistic effects of quantity and intensity of the various types of exercise [263, 285]. Although the health benefits of physical activity/exercise outweigh the risks, exercise should be postponed in T2D patients when blood glucose levels are >17 mmol/L or <7 mmol/L, until they have been corrected [263].

An important determinant of T2D risk is obesity, and although obesity and physical inactivity are both independent predictors of T2D risk, the power of this association is much greater for obesity compared with physical inactivity [262]. Indeed, obesity plays a pivotal role in the pathogenesis of insulin resistance in skeletal muscle; nevertheless, exercise represents one of the most effective interventions for reversing insulin resistance in skeletal muscle of obese patients at high risk for T2D [290]. Due to the strong association between physical activity, obesity, and T2D, there is currently great interest in these areas, as these conditions are related in part to a general decline in physical activity, while several new hormones discovered have enhanced understanding the mechanisms underlying diabetes and obesity [262]. Severe metabolic dysregulation in diabetes and obesity can reduce the benefit from exercise; however, the intact response of key metabolic regulators in exercising muscle of diabetic patients indicates the effectiveness of exercise to treat these diseases [291].

Dyslipidemia-Hyperlipidemia

Hyperlipidemia or dyslipidemia is a group of disorders of lipid and lipoprotein metabolism characterized by increased circulating levels of certain forms of cholesterol and TGs. Isolated hypercholesterolemia and combined dyslipidemia are the most common types of dyslipidemia, occurring as a result of excessive fat intake and leading to increased risk of atherosclerosis [263, 292]. Regular exercise favorably modulates blood lipid profile and is considered as one of the mechanisms responsible at least in part, for the protective effects of exercise against the development of vascular diseases [280]. Moreover, epidemiological and cross-sectional observational studies indicate that physical activity prevents the development of hyperlipidemia [293–295].

Specifically, a systematic review assessing the effect of supervised exercise interventions on lipid profiles in patients with T2D concluded that exercise is effective in lowering low-density lipoprotein cholesterol (LDL-C) and elevating high-density lipoprotein cholesterol (HDL-C) levels in diabetic patients [263, 296]. There is also evidence supporting that a large volume of exercise training resulted in a beneficial effect on the blood lipid profile independently of weight loss [297]. Collectively, it is concluded that regular physical activity reduces TG and increases HDL-C levels in the blood [298, 299]. The amount of exercise required for favorable changes in the lipoprotein-lipid profile is approximately 7 miles or more per week. A dose-response relationship between miles run per week, HDL-C, and other lipoprotein-lipid levels was noted with most changes occurring when running 7–14 miles per week at mild to moderate intensities [300]. These findings are confirmed by an interventional study demonstrating that high-volume exercise had a more favorable impact on lipoprotein-lipid metabolism than exercise intensity [301].

Studies have also shown that exercise has favorable effects on postprandial lipid profile. Non-fasting TG levels were reduced significantly following exercise training in individuals with metabolic syndrome [302]. Moreover, a single exercise session appears to be as effective in lowering non-fasting TG as continuous aerobic exercise, with effects lasting till the following day [252, 303]. Similarly, short-term (4 days) aerobic exercise had effects on postprandial TG, LDL-C, and VLDL-C, but no changes in HDL-C were noted [304].

Collectively, the current literature suggests that aerobic exercise has a favorable effect on lipoprotein-lipid metabolism. An exercise intensity, duration, and volume threshold as well as an interaction between the exercise components (intensity, duration, frequency) appear to exist beyond which favorable changes can occur in a dose-response pattern [305, 306].

McArdle Disease

McArdle disease, also known as glycogen storage disease type V (GSDV) or myophosphorylase deficiency, is an inherited metabolic disorder characterized by the inability of skeletal muscle to degrade glycogen. Patients with McArdle disease are deficient in muscle glycogen phosphorylase [307–309]. Myophosphorylase is the only isoform of glycogen phosphorylase expressed in skeletal muscle only. Hence, McArdle disease is considered a relatively benign myopathy, as it affects only skeletal muscle in contrast with other metabolic disorders where, apart from muscle, other tissues and organs are also affected [310, 311].

The enzyme myophosphorylase is involved in muscle glycogen degradation to glucose-1-phosphate. Consequently, muscle phosphorylase deficiency renders the muscle incapable to mobilize and utilize muscle glycogen during an aerobic metabolism [312, 313]. Since glycolysis is blocked upstream, muscles can still take up and utilize blood glucose [311]; hence, glycolysis in skeletal muscles of McArdle disease patients is not totally impaired. However, the substantially limited pyruvate formation generated from the limited glycolytic activity [314] leads to abnormally low substrate influx through the Krebs cycle and reduced rates of acetyl-CoA formation, thereby inhibiting the Krebs cycle oxidative phosphorylation [307, 311]. Consequently, VO_2max is approximately 40% lower than normal controls. This leads to a disproportionate elevation in exercise heart rate and ventilation rate which reduced blood flow to the exercising muscles, partial ischemia, and exacerbated symptoms [307, 311]. Muscle stiffness, fatigue, myalgia, and weakness, induced by exercise and relieved by rest, are also typical symptoms in these patients. If these symptoms are ignored and exercise is continued, painful cramping and contracture of the exercising muscles occurs, followed by myoglobinuria [307] and, in some cases, muscle damage or rhabdomyolysis [311, 314].

Free fatty acids are the primary energy substrate that is utilized by skeletal muscle, through oxidative phosphorylation, in the resting state as well as during low-intensity aerobic activity. Although acetyl-CoA is generated from free fatty acid metabolism, the capacity of the McArdle disease patients to utilize FFA without exercise training is limited [307, 313, 314]. Disorders that alter energy provision to the muscle, irrespective of whether they affect lipid or carbohydrate metabolism, essentially result in chronic muscle weakness or, most frequently in McArdle disease, exercise intolerance. Exercise intolerance is characterized by acute crises of muscle pain, stiffness, and undue fatigue, accompanied by muscle contractures, especially at the beginning of exercise, which are attenuated with exercise cessation; however, these crises can result in muscle damage or rhabdomyolysis [311, 314]. McArdle disease patients are likely to adapt a sedentary lifestyle exposing these patients to secondary health risks such as obesity, T2D, and cardiovascular disease [311, 315, 316].

Exercise Intervention Studies in McArdle's Disease

The exercise-related health benefits for McArdle disease patients were first documented in patients who followed a supervised aerobic cycling exercise program at moderate intensity, for 45 min/session, three times per week for 8 weeks. The aerobic exercise training resulted in attenuated exercise intolerance compared to baseline [311, 317]. A similar exercise training program resulted in increased peak work capacity, VO_2 peak, cardiac output, and some key mitochondrial enzymes compared to baseline [318]. Favorable training effects were also reported in nine patients who followed a walking or cycling exercise training program including five sessions per week for 32 weeks at duration and intensities similar to the abovementioned studies. VO_2 peak and other variables of exercise capacity were found to be increased with training along with a reduction in serum CK levels [319], indicating that chronic muscle activity may counterbalance muscle wasting and damage. Overall, aerobic exercise interventions are proven to be safe and efficacious for McArdle disease patients [311, 320]. Significant improvement in work capacity without any serious complication for McArdle disease patients were also reported in a similar study, with exercise-related beneficial effects attributed to improved blood flow and mitochondrial metabolism [321].

The effects of resistance exercise have also been evaluated in an adolescent male patient and in seven adult McArdle patients of both sexes [322, 323]. A 15-year-old patient followed a 6-week, light- to moderate-intensity exercise program (two sessions/week, at 65–70% of his one-repetition maximum; 1-RM). After the intervention, his 1-RM power performance improved without any myoglobinuria episodes reported, while, interestingly, he became virtually asymptomatic in terms of exercise limitation [322]. In adult patients, 16-week light to moderate resistance exercise training consisting of two sessions per week, followed by an 8-week detraining period, resulted in a significant beneficial effect on total lean mass, without any major contraindication reported and non-exhibited fixed muscle weakness or limitations in the daily life activities [323].

In conclusion, regular aerobically oriented physical activity or structured exercise programs of moderate intensity are safe and can attenuate the severity of McArdle disease for these patients [307, 319, 320, 324]. Carbohydrate ingestion prior to exercise is currently the only useful therapy for this disease [313, 314, 320]. This approach appears to improve exercise tolerance to submaximal and maximum workloads and help prevent exercise-induced muscle damage and reduce the threat of renal failure [325, 326]. Some evidence also supports that low to moderate resistance exercises are safe and efficacious for McArdle disease patients. However, HIIT and other forms of high resistance exercises should be avoided.

Conclusions

The paramount importance of the human organism is to maintain metabolic homeostasis. On this basis, ATP levels in skeletal and heart muscle are maintained fairly constant through continuous resynthesis of ATP via anaerobic and aerobic metabolism. The main factor dictating the dominant metabolic pathway and the type of substrate used is exercise intensity, whereas exercise duration, fitness status, gender, diet, and environmental temperature play a secondary role in exercise metabolism. Metabolic pathways do not function independently, but synergistically, by interactions with the exercising muscles and distant organs such as the liver, heart, and brain. Hormones, secreted by cells of the endocrine system, regulate activity of cells in other parts of the body. They are sensitive to exercise-induced stress and modulate metabolism during exercise, not only in skeletal muscle but also in various other organs. Several clinical implications for health benefits of special populations rely on exercise metabolism alterations.

References

1. Phillips SM, Atkinson SA, Tarnopolsky MA, MacDougall JD. Gender differences in leucine kinetics and nitrogen balance in endurance athletes. J Appl Physiol (1985). 1993;75:2134–41.
2. Tarnopolsky MA, Atkinson SA, Phillips SM, MacDougall JD. Carbohydrate loading and metabolism during exercise in men and women. J Appl Physiol (1985). 1995;78:1360–8.
3. Wagenmakers AJ. Muscle amino acid metabolism at rest and during exercise: Role in human physiology and metabolism. Exerc Sport Sci Rev. 1998;26:287–314.
4. Greenhaff PL, Nevill ME, Soderlund K, Bodin K, Boobis LH, Williams C, et al. The metabolic responses of human type i and ii muscle fibres during maximal treadmill sprinting. J Physiol. 1994;478(Pt 1):149–55.
5. Bogdanis GC, Nevill ME, Boobis LH, Lakomy HK, Nevill AM. Recovery of power output and muscle metabolites following 30 s of maximal sprint cycling in man. J Physiol. 1995;482(Pt 2):467–80.
6. Tsintzas OK, Williams C, Boobis L, Greenhaff P. Carbohydrate ingestion and single muscle fiber glycogen metabolism during prolonged running in men. J Appl Physiol (1985). 1996;81:801–9.
7. Sargeant AJ. Structural and functional determinants of human muscle power. Exp Physiol. 2007;92:323–31.
8. Scott W, Stevens J, Binder-Macleod SA. Human skeletal muscle fiber type classifications. Phys Ther. 2001;81:1810–6.
9. Pette D, Staron RS. Myosin isoforms, muscle fiber types, and transitions. Microsc Res Tech. 2000;50:500–9.
10. Schiaffino S, Reggiani C. Fiber types in mammalian skeletal muscles. Physiol Rev. 2011;91:1447–531.
11. Astrand P-O, Rodahl K, Dahl HA, Stromme B. Textbook of work physiology. Physiological bases of exercise. Champaign: Human Kinetics; 2003.
12. Zierath JR, Hawley JA. Skeletal muscle fiber type: Influence on contractile and metabolic properties. PLoS Biol. 2004;2:e348.
13. Sale DG. Influence of exercise and training on motor unit activation. Exerc Sport Sci Rev. 1987;15:95–151.
14. Pette D. The adaptive potential of skeletal muscle fibers. Can J Appl Physiol. 2002;27:423–48.
15. Talbot J, Maves L. Skeletal muscle fiber type: using insights from muscle developmental biology to dissect targets for susceptibility and resistance to muscle disease. Wiley Interdiscip Rev Dev Biol. 2016;5:518–34.
16. Greenhaff PL, Soderlund K, Ren JM, Hultman E. Energy metabolism in single human muscle fibres during intermittent contraction with occluded circulation. J Physiol. 1993;460:443–53.
17. Gray SR, Soderlund K, Ferguson RA. ATP and phosphocreatine utilization in single human muscle fibres during the development of maximal power output at elevated muscle temperatures. J Sports Sci. 2008;26:701–7.
18. Kent-Braun JA, Fitts RH, Christie A. Skeletal muscle fatigue. Compr Physiol. 2012;2:997–1044.
19. Baker JS, McCormick MC, Robergs RA. Interaction among skeletal muscle metabolic energy systems during intense exercise. J Nutr Metab. 2010;2010:905612.

20. Tesch PA, Thorsson A, Fujitsuka N. Creatine phosphate in fiber types of skeletal muscle before and after exhaustive exercise. J Appl Physiol (1985). 1989;66:1756–9.
21. Sahlin K, Soderlund K, Tonkonogi M, Hirakoba K. Phosphocreatine content in single fibers of human muscle after sustained submaximal exercise. Am J Physiol. 1997;273:C172–8.
22. Harris RC, Soderlund K, Hultman E. Elevation of creatine in resting and exercised muscle of normal subjects by creatine supplementation. Clin Sci (Lond). 1992;83:367–74.
23. Solis MY, Artioli GG, Otaduy MCG, Leite CDC, Arruda W, Veiga RR, et al. Effect of age, diet, and tissue type on PCr response to creatine supplementation. J Appl Physiol (1985). 2017;123:407–14.
24. Gollnick PD. Energy metabolism and prolonged exercise. In: Lamb DR, Murray M, editors. Perspectives in exercise science and sports medicine, volume 1:prolonged exercise. Indianapolis: Benchmark Press; 1988. p. 1–42.
25. Gejl KD, Ortenblad N, Andersson E, Plomgaard P, Holmberg HC, Nielsen J. Local depletion of glycogen with supramaximal exercise in human skeletal muscle fibres. J Physiol. 2017;595:2809–21.
26. Hearris MA, Hammond KM, Fell JM, Morton JP. Regulation of muscle glycogen metabolism during exercise: implications for endurance performance and training adaptations. Nutrients. 2018;10:1–21.
27. Gonzalez JT, Fuchs CJ, Betts JA, van Loon LJ. Liver glycogen metabolism during and after prolonged endurance-type exercise. Am J Physiol Endocrinol Metab. 2016;311:E543–53.
28. Hawley JA, Schabort EJ, Noakes TD, Dennis SC. Carbohydrate-loading and exercise performance. An update. Sports Med. 1997;24:73–81.
29. Stevenson EJ, Thelwall PE, Thomas K, Smith F, Brand-Miller J, Trenell MI. Dietary glycemic index influences lipid oxidation but not muscle or liver glycogen oxidation during exercise. Am J Physiol Endocrinol Metab. 2009;296:E1140–7.
30. Gonzalez JT, Fuchs CJ, Smith FE, Thelwall PE, Taylor R, Stevenson EJ, Trenell MI, Cermak NM, van Loon LJ. Ingestion of glucose or sucrose prevents liver but not muscle glycogen depletion during prolonged endurance-type exercise in trained cyclists. Am J Physiol Endocrinol Metab. 2015;309:E1032–9.
31. Tsintzas OK, Williams C, Boobis L, Greenhaff P. Carbohydrate ingestion and glycogen utilization in different muscle fibre types in man. J Physiol. 1995;489(Pt 1):243–50.
32. Tarnopolsky MA, Zawada C, Richmond LB, Carter S, Shearer J, Graham T, et al. Gender differences in carbohydrate loading are related to energy intake. J Appl Physiol (1985). 2001;91:225–30.
33. Walker JL, Heigenhauser GJ, Hultman E, Spriet LL. Dietary carbohydrate, muscle glycogen content, and endurance performance in well-trained women. J Appl Physiol (1985). 2000;88:2151–8.
34. Shin YS. Glycogen storage disease: Clinical, biochemical, and molecular heterogeneity. Semin Pediatr Neurol. 2006;13:115–20.
35. Fleck SJ. Body composition of elite American athletes. Am J Sports Med. 1983;11:398–403.
36. Essen B, Jansson E, Henriksson J, Taylor AW, Saltin B. Metabolic characteristics of fibre types in human skeletal muscle. Acta Physiol Scand. 1975;95:153–65.
37. Watt MJ, Heigenhauser GJ, Spriet LL. Intramuscular triacylglycerol utilization in human skeletal muscle during exercise: Is there a controversy? J Appl Physiol (1985). 2002;93:1185–95.
38. Wendling PS, Peters SJ, Heigenhauser GJ, Spriet LL. Variability of triacylglycerol content in human skeletal muscle biopsy samples. J Appl Physiol (1985). 1996;81:1150–5.
39. Stellingwerff T, Boon H, Jonkers RA, Senden JM, Spriet LL, Koopman R, et al. Significant intramyocellular lipid use during prolonged cycling in endurance-trained males as assessed by three different methodologies. Am J Physiol Endocrinol Metab. 2007;292:E1715–23.
40. Newsholme EA, Leech AR. Biochemistry for the medical sciences. Chichester: Wiley; 1983.
41. Metzeger JM. Mechanism of chemomechanical coupling in skeletal muscle during work. In: Lamb DR, Gisolfi CV, editors. Energy metabolism in exercise and sport, vol. 5. Dubuque: Brown & Benchmark; 1992. p. 1–51.
42. Spriet LL. Anaerobic metabolism during exercise. In: Hargreaves M, Spriet L, editors. Exercise metabolism. Champaign: Human Kinetics; 2006. p. 7–27.
43. Kenney LW, Wilmore JH, Costill DL. Physiology of sport and exercise. 5th ed. Champaign: Human Kinetics, Champaign, IL; 2012.
44. MacLaren D, Morton J. Biochemistry for sport and exercise metabolism. Champaign: Wiley-Blackwell; 2011.
45. Sahlin K. Metabolic factors in fatigue. In: Hargreaves M, Spriet L, editors. Exercise metabolism. Champaign: Human Kinetics; 2006. p. 163–86.
46. Berg JM, Tymoczko JL, Stryer L. Biochemistry. 5th ed. New York: W.H. Freeman and Company; 2002.
47. Chasiotis D. The regulation of glycogen phosphorylase and glycogen breakdown in human skeletal muscle. Acta Physiol Scand Suppl. 1983;518:1–68.
48. Rush JW, Spriet LL. Skeletal muscle glycogen phosphorylase a kinetics: Effects of adenine nucleotides and caffeine. J Appl Physiol (1985). 2001;91:2071–8.
49. Costill DL, Coyle E, Dalsky G, Evans W, Fink W, Hoopes D. Effects of elevated plasma FFA and insulin on muscle glycogen usage during exercise. J Appl Physiol Respir Environ Exerc Physiol. 1977;43:695–9.
50. Dyck DJ, Peters SJ, Wendling PS, Chesley A, Hultman E, Spriet LL. Regulation of muscle glycogen phosphorylase activity during intense aerobic cycling with elevated FFA. Am J Phys. 1996;270:E116–25.

51. Hargreaves M, McConell G, Proietto J. Influence of muscle glycogen on glycogenolysis and glucose uptake during exercise in humans. J Appl Physiol (1985). 1995;78:288–92.
52. Howlett KF, Spriet LL, Hargreaves M. Carbohydrate metabolism during exercise in females: effect of reduced fat availability. Metabolism. 2001;50:481–7.
53. Ferguson BS, Rogatzki MJ, Goodwin ML, Kane DA, Rightmire Z, Gladden LB. Lactate metabolism: historical context, prior misinterpretations, and current understanding. Eur J Appl Physiol. 2018;118:691–728.
54. Brooks GA. Lactate: link between glycolytic and oxidative metabolism. Sports Med. 2007;37:341–3.
55. O'Brien MJ, Viguie CA, Mazzeo RS, Brooks GA. Carbohydrate dependence during marathon running. Med Sci Sports Exerc. 1993;25:1009–17.
56. Robergs RA, Roberts SO. Exercise physiology. Exercise, performance, and clinical applications. Boston: WCB, McGraw-Hill; 1997.
57. Gladden LB. Lactate metabolism: a new paradigm for the third millennium. J Physiol. 2004;558:5–30.
58. Margaria R, Edwards RHT, Dill DB. The possible mechanisms of contracting and paying the oxygen debt and the role of lactic acid in muscular contraction. Am J Physiol. 1933;106:689–715.
59. Bergman BC, Wolfel EE, Butterfield GE, Lopaschuk GD, Casazza GA, Horning MA, et al. Active muscle and whole body lactate kinetics after endurance training in men. J Appl Physiol (1985). 1999;87:1684–96.
60. Nielsen HB, Clemmesen JO, Skak C, Ott P, Secher NH. Attenuated hepatosplanchnic uptake of lactate during intense exercise in humans. J Appl Physiol (1985). 2002;92:1677–83.
61. Mangia S, Garreffa G, Bianciardi M, Giove F, Di Salle F, Maraviglia B. The aerobic brain: lactate decrease at the onset of neural activity. Neuroscience. 2003;118:7–10.
62. Green JM, Hornsby JH, Pritchett RC, Pritchett K. Lactate threshold comparison in anaerobic vs. aerobic athletes and untrained participants. Int J Exerc Sci. 2014;7:329–38.
63. Brooks GA. The lactate shuttle during exercise and recovery. Med Sci Sports Exerc. 1986;18:360–8.
64. Goodwin ML, Gladden LB, Nijsten MW, Jones KB. Lactate and cancer: revisiting the warburg effect in an era of lactate shuttling. Front Nutr. 2014;1:27.
65. Nijsten MW, van Dam GM. Hypothesis: using the warburg effect against cancer by reducing glucose and providing lactate. Med Hypotheses. 2009;73:48–51.
66. Wasserman K, McIlroy MB. Detecting the threshold of anaerobic metabolism in cardiac patients during exercise. Am J Cardiol. 1964;14:844–52.
67. Yoshida T, Nagata A, Muro M, Takeuchi N, Suda Y. The validity of anaerobic threshold determination by a douglas bag method compared with arterial blood lactate concentration. Eur J Appl Physiol Occup Physiol. 1981;46:423–30.
68. Sjodin B, Jacobs I, Svedenhag J. Changes in onset of blood lactate accumulation (obla) and muscle enzymes after training at obla. Eur J Appl Physiol Occup Physiol. 1982;49:45–57.
69. Coyle EF. Integration of the physiological factors determining endurance performance ability. Exerc Sport Sci Rev. 1995;23:25–63.
70. Ghosh AK. Anaerobic threshold: its concept and role in endurance sport. Malays J Med Sci. 2004;11:24–36.
71. Agostoni P, Corra U, Cattadori G, Veglia F, Battaia E, La Gioia R, et al. Prognostic value of indeterminable anaerobic threshold in heart failure. Circ Heart Fail. 2013;6:977–87.
72. Rusko H, Rahkila P, Karvinen E. Anaerobic threshold, skeletal muscle enzymes and fiber composition in young female cross-country skiers. Acta Physiol Scand. 1980;108:263–8.
73. Bassett DR Jr, Howley ET. Limiting factors for maximum oxygen uptake and determinants of endurance performance. Med Sci Sports Exerc. 2000;32:70–84.
74. Kenney LWW, Costill JH, D.L. Physiology of sport and exercise. 5th ed. Champaign: Human Kinetics; 2012.
75. Jeukendrup AE, Gleeson M. Sports nutrition. An introduction to energy production and performance. 1st ed. Champaign: Human Kinetics; 2004.
76. Trefts E, Williams AS, Wasserman DH. Exercise and the regulation of hepatic metabolism. Prog Mol Biol Transl Sci. 2015;135:203–25.
77. Kjaer M. Hepatic metabolism during exercise. In: Hargreaves M, Spriet L, editors. Exercise metabolism. Champaign: Human Kinetics; 2006. p. 45–70.
78. Lavoie C, Ducros F, Bourque J, Langelier H, Chiasson JL. Glucose metabolism during exercise in man: the role of insulin and glucagon in the regulation of hepatic glucose production and gluconeogenesis. Can J Physiol Pharmacol. 1997;75:26–35.
79. Tuttle KR, Marker JC, Dalsky GP, Schwartz NS, Shah SD, Clutter WE, et al. Glucagon, not insulin, may play a secondary role in defense against hypoglycemia during exercise. Am J Physiol. 1988;254:E713–9.
80. Rose AJ, Richter EA. Skeletal muscle glucose uptake during exercise: how is it regulated? Physiology (Bethesda). 2005;20:260–70.
81. Ahlborg G, Felig P, Hagenfeldt L, Hendler R, Wahren J. Substrate turnover during prolonged exercise in man. Splanchnic and leg metabolism of glucose, free fatty acids, and amino acids. J Clin Invest. 1974;53:1080–90.
82. Ahlborg G, Felig P. Lactate and glucose exchange across the forearm, legs, and splanchnic bed during and after prolonged leg exercise. J Clin Invest. 1982;69:45–54.
83. Katz A, Broberg S, Sahlin K, Wahren J. Leg glucose uptake during maximal dynamic exercise in humans. Am J Physiol. 1986;251:E65–70.
84. Jeukendrup AE, Raben A, Gijsen A, Stegen JH, Brouns F, Saris WH, et al. Glucose kinetics during

prolonged exercise in highly trained human subjects: effect of glucose ingestion. J Physiol. 1999;515(Pt 2):579–89.

85. Angus DJ, Febbraio MA, Hargreaves M. Plasma glucose kinetics during prolonged exercise in trained humans when fed carbohydrate. Am J Physiol Endocrinol Metab. 2002;283:E573–7.
86. Richter EA, Hargreaves M. Exercise, GLUT4, and skeletal muscle glucose uptake. Physiol Rev. 2013;93:993–1017.
87. Merry TL, McConell GK. Skeletal muscle glucose uptake during exercise: a focus on reactive oxygen species and nitric oxide signaling. IUBMB Life. 2009;61:479–84.
88. Richter EA, Ruderman NB. AMPK and the biochemistry of exercise: implications for human health and disease. Biochem J. 2009;418:261–75.
89. Katz A. Role of reactive oxygen species in regulation of glucose transport in skeletal muscle during exercise. J Physiol. 2016;594:2787–94.
90. Watt MJ, Howlett KF, Febbraio MA, Spriet LL, Hargreaves M. Adrenaline increases skeletal muscle glycogenolysis, pyruvate dehydrogenase activation and carbohydrate oxidation during moderate exercise in humans. J Physiol. 2001;534:269–78.
91. Steensberg A, van Hall G, Keller C, Osada T, Schjerling P, Pedersen BK, et al. Muscle glycogen content and glucose uptake during exercise in humans: Influence of prior exercise and dietary manipulation. J Physiol. 2002;541:273–81.
92. Pedersen BK, Akerstrom TC, Nielsen AR, Fischer CP. Role of myokines in exercise and metabolism. J Appl Physiol (1985). 2007;103:1093–8.
93. Pedersen L, Hojman P. Muscle-to-organ cross talk mediated by myokines. Adipocyte. 2012;1:164–7.
94. Pedersen BK, Febbraio MA. Muscle as an endocrine organ: focus on muscle-derived interleukin-6. Physiol Rev. 2008;88:1379–406.
95. Febbraio MA, Hiscock N, Sacchetti M, Fischer CP, Pedersen BK. Interleukin-6 is a novel factor mediating glucose homeostasis during skeletal muscle contraction. Diabetes. 2004;53:1643–8.
96. Pedersen L, Pilegaard H, Hansen J, Brandt C, Adser H, Hidalgo J, et al. Exercise-induced liver chemokine CXCL-1 expression is linked to muscle-derived interleukin-6 expression. J Physiol. 2011;589:1409–20.
97. Pedersen BK, Febbraio M. Muscle-derived interleukin-6--a possible link between skeletal muscle, adipose tissue, liver, and brain. Brain Behav Immun. 2005;19:371–6.
98. Spriet LL. Regulation of skeletal muscle fat oxidation during exercise in humans. Med Sci Sports Exerc. 2002;34:1477–84.
99. Horowitz JF. Adipose tissue lipid mobilization during exercise. In: Hargreaves M, Spriet L, editors. Exercise metabolism. Champaign: Human Kinetics; 2006. p. 89–104.
100. Romijn JA, Coyle EF, Sidossis LS, Gastaldelli A, Horowitz JF, Endert E, et al. Regulation of endogenous fat and carbohydrate metabolism in relation to exercise intensity and duration. Am J Physiol. 1993;265:E380–91.
101. Romijn JA, Coyle EF, Sidossis LS, Zhang XJ, Wolfe RR. Relationship between fatty acid delivery and fatty acid oxidation during strenuous exercise. J Appl Physiol (1985). 1995;79:1939–45.
102. Luiken JJ, Glatz JF, Bonen A. Fatty acid transport proteins facilitate fatty acid uptake in skeletal muscle. Can J Appl Physiol. 2000;25:333–52.
103. Hargreaves M, Spriet LL. Exercise metabolism: fuels for the fire. Cold Spring Harb Perspect Med. 2018;8(8):1–15.
104. Holloway GP, Luiken JJ, Glatz JF, Spriet LL, Bonen A. Contribution of FAT/CD36 to the regulation of skeletal muscle fatty acid oxidation: an overview. Acta Physiol (Oxf). 2008;194:293–309.
105. Holloway GP, Bonen A, Spriet LL. Regulation of skeletal muscle mitochondrial fatty acid metabolism in lean and obese individuals. Am J Clin Nutr. 2009;89:455S–62S.
106. Tarnopolsky MA. Protein metabolism in strength and endurance activities. In: Lamb DR, Murray R, editors. The metabolic bases of performance in exercise and sport. Carmel: Cooper Publishing Group; 1999. p. 125–63.
107. Gibala MJ. Effect of exercise on skeletal muscle protein and amino acid metabolism in humans. In: Hargreaves M, Spriet L, editors. Exercise metabolism. Champaign: Human Kinetics; 2006. p. 137–61.
108. Wagenmakers AJ, Brookes JH, Coakley JH, Reilly T, Edwards RH. Exercise-induced activation of the branched-chain 2-oxo acid dehydrogenase in human muscle. Eur J Appl Physiol Occup Physiol. 1989;59:159–67.
109. Rush JW, MacLean DA, Hultman E, Graham TE. Exercise causes branched-chain oxoacid dehydrogenase dephosphorylation but not AMP deaminase binding. J Appl Physiol (1985). 1995;78:2193–200.
110. van Hall G, MacLean DA, Saltin B, Wagenmakers AJ. Mechanisms of activation of muscle branched-chain alpha-keto acid dehydrogenase during exercise in man. J Physiol. 1996;494(Pt 3):899–905.
111. Wagenmakers AJ, Beckers EJ, Brouns F, Kuipers H, Soeters PB, van der Vusse GJ, et al. Carbohydrate supplementation, glycogen depletion, and amino acid metabolism during exercise. Am J Physiol. 1991;260:E883–90.
112. Lemon PW, Mullin JP. Effect of initial muscle glycogen levels on protein catabolism during exercise. J Appl Physiol Respir Environ Exerc Physiol. 1980;48:624–9.
113. Gibala MJ. Regulation of skeletal muscle amino acid metabolism during exercise. Int J Sport Nutr Exerc Metab. 2001;11:87–108.
114. Phillips SM, Tipton KD, Aarsland A, Wolf SE, Wolfe RR. Mixed muscle protein synthesis and breakdown after resistance exercise in humans. Am J Physiol. 1997;273:E99–107.

115. Romijn JA, Coyle EF, Sidossis LS, Rosenblatt J, Wolfe RR. Substrate metabolism during different exercise intensities in endurance-trained women. J Appl Physiol (1985). 2000;88:1707–14.
116. Achten J, Gleeson M, Jeukendrup AE. Determination of the exercise intensity that elicits maximal fat oxidation. Med Sci Sports Exerc. 2002;34:92–7.
117. Coyle EF, Jeukendrup AE, Wagenmakers AJ, Saris WH. Fatty acid oxidation is directly regulated by carbohydrate metabolism during exercise. Am J Physiol. 1997;273:E268–75.
118. Sidossis LS, Gastaldelli A, Klein S, Wolfe RR. Regulation of plasma fatty acid oxidation during low- and high-intensity exercise. Am J Physiol. 1997;272:E1065–70.
119. Bergman BC, Brooks GA. Respiratory gas-exchange ratios during graded exercise in fed and fasted trained and untrained men. J Appl Physiol (1985). 1999;86:479–87.
120. Edwards HT, Margaria R, Dill DB. Metabolic rate, blood sugar and utilization of carbohydrate. Am J Physiol. 1934;108:203–9.
121. Martin WH. Effect of endurance training on fatty acid metabolism during whole body exercise. Med Sci Sports Exerc. 1997;29:635–9.
122. Kiens B. Effect of endurance training on fatty acid metabolism: Local adaptations. Med Sci Sports Exerc. 1997;29:640–5.
123. Nicklas BJ. Effects of endurance exercise on adipose tissue metabolism. Exerc Sport Sci Rev. 1997;25:77–103.
124. Krogh AL, J. The relative value of fat and carbohydrate as sources of muscular energy. Biochem J. 1920;14:290–363.
125. Jeukendrup AE. Periodized nutrition for athletes. Sports Med. 2017;47:51–63.
126. Wright DA, Sherman WM, Dernbach AR. Carbohydrate feedings before, during, or in combination improve cycling endurance performance. J Appl Physiol (1985). 1991;71:1082–8.
127. Chryssanthopoulos C, Williams C. Pre-exercise carbohydrate meal and endurance running capacity when carbohydrates are ingested during exercise. Int J Sports Med. 1997;18:543–8.
128. Chryssanthopoulos C, Williams C, Nowitz A, Kotsiopoulou C, Vleck V. The effect of a high carbohydrate meal on endurance running capacity. Int J Sport Nutr Exerc Metab. 2002;12:157–71.
129. Montain SJ, Hopper MK, Coggan AR, Coyle EF. Exercise metabolism at different time intervals after a meal. J Appl Physiol (1985). 1991;70: 882–8.
130. Febbraio MA. Temperature, muscle metabolism and performance. In: Lamb DR, Murray R, editors. The metabolic basis of performance in exercise and sport. Traverse City: Cooper Publishing Group; 1999. p. 315–53.
131. Devries MC. Sex-based differences in endurance exercise muscle metabolism: impact on exercise and nutritional strategies to optimize health and performance in women. Exp Physiol. 2016;101:243–9.
132. Brockman NK, Yardley JE. Sex-related differences in fuel utilization and hormonal response to exercise: implications for individuals with type 1 diabetes. Appl Physiol Nutr Metab. 2018;43(6):541–52.
133. Tarnopolsky LJ, MacDougall JD, Atkinson SA, Tarnopolsky MA, Sutton JR. Gender differences in substrate for endurance exercise. J Appl Physiol (1985). 1990;68:302–8.
134. Horton TJ, Pagliassotti MJ, Hobbs K, Hill JO. Fuel metabolism in men and women during and after long-duration exercise. J Appl Physiol (1985). 1998;85:1823–32.
135. Marliss EB, Kreisman SH, Manzon A, Halter JB, Vranic M, Nessim SJ. Gender differences in glucoregulatory responses to intense exercise. J Appl Physiol (1985). 2000;88:457–66.
136. Hamadeh MJ, Devries MC, Tarnopolsky MA. Estrogen supplementation reduces whole body leucine and carbohydrate oxidation and increases lipid oxidation in men during endurance exercise. J Clin Endocrinol Metab. 2005;90:3592–9.
137. Boisseau N, Delamarche P. Metabolic and hormonal responses to exercise in children and adolescents. Sports Med. 2000;30:405–22.
138. Oosthuyse T, Bosch AN. The effect of the menstrual cycle on exercise metabolism: implications for exercise performance in eumenorrhoeic women. Sports Med. 2010;40:207–27.
139. Numao S, Hayashi Y, Katayama Y, Matsuo T, Tanaka K. Sex differences in substrate oxidation during aerobic exercise in obese men and postmenopausal obese women. Metabolism. 2009;58:1312–9.
140. Devries MC, Hamadeh MJ, Graham TE, Tarnopolsky MA. 17beta-estradiol supplementation decreases glucose rate of appearance and disappearance with no effect on glycogen utilization during moderate intensity exercise in men. J Clin Endocrinol Metab. 2005;90:6218–25.
141. Devries MC, Hamadeh MJ, Phillips SM, Tarnopolsky MA. Menstrual cycle phase and sex influence muscle glycogen utilization and glucose turnover during moderate-intensity endurance exercise. Am J Physiol Regul Integr Comp Physiol. 2006;291:R1120–8.
142. Isacco L, Duche P, Boisseau N. Influence of hormonal status on substrate utilization at rest and during exercise in the female population. Sports Med. 2012;42:327–42.
143. Kraemer RR, Heleniak RJ, Tryniecki JL, Kraemer GR, Okazaki NJ, Castracane VD. Follicular and luteal phase hormonal responses to low-volume resistive exercise. Med Sci Sports Exerc. 1995;27:809–17.
144. Riddell MC, Partington SL, Stupka N, Armstrong D, Rennie C, Tarnopolsky MA. Substrate utilization during exercise performed with and without glucose ingestion in female and male endurance trained athletes. Int J Sport Nutr Exerc Metab. 2003;13:407–21.
145. Copeland JL, Consitt LA, Tremblay MS. Hormonal responses to endurance and resistance exercise in females aged 19-69 years. J Gerontol A Biol Sci Med Sci. 2002;57:B158–65.

146. Fragala MS, Kraemer WJ, Denegar CR, Maresh CM, Mastro AM, Volek JS. Neuroendocrine-immune interactions and responses to exercise. Sports Med. 2011;41:621–39.
147. Roepstorff C, Steffensen CH, Madsen M, Stallknecht B, Kanstrup IL, Richter EA, et al. Gender differences in substrate utilization during submaximal exercise in endurance-trained subjects. Am J Physiol Endocrinol Metab. 2002;282:E435–47.
148. Steffensen CH, Roepstorff C, Madsen M, Kiens B. Myocellular triacylglycerol breakdown in females but not in males during exercise. Am J Physiol Endocrinol Metab. 2002;282:E634–42.
149. Taegtmeyer H. Cardiomyocyte metabolism: all is in flux. Muscle Fundamental Biol Mech Dis. 2012;1:187–202.
150. Abdel-aleem S, Lowe JE, editors. Cardiac metabolism in health and disease. Dordrecht: Springer Science+Business Media, B.V; 1998.
151. Stanley WC, Recchia FA, Lopaschuk GD. Myocardial substrate metabolism in the normal and failing heart. Physiol Rev. 2005;85:1093–129.
152. Lopaschuk GD, Dhalla NS, editors. Cardiac energy metabolism in health and disease. New York: Springer; 2014.
153. Schwarzer M, Doenst T, editors. The scientist's guide to cardiac metabolism. Amsterdam: Academic; 2016.
154. Taegtmeyer H, Young ME, Lopaschuk GD, Abel ED, Brunengraber H, Darley-Usmar V, et al. American Heart Association Council on Basic Cardiovascular Sciences. Assessing cardiac metabolism: a scientific statement from the American heart association. Circ Res. 2016;118:1659–701.
155. Lopaschuk GD, Kelly DP. Signalling in cardiac metabolism. Cardiovasc Res. 2008;79:205–7.
156. Keul J. Myocardial metabolism in athletes. In: Pernow B, Saltin B, editors. Muscle metabolism during exercise. New York/London: Plenum Press; 1971.
157. Kaijser L, Lassers BW, Wahlqvist ML, Carlson LA. Myocardial lipid and carbohydrate metabolism in fasting men during prolonged exercise. J Appl Physiol. 1972;32:847–58.
158. Lassers BW, Wahlqvist ML, Kaijser L, Carlson LA. Effect of nicotinic acid on myocardial metabolism in man at rest and during exercise. J Appl Physiol. 1972;33:72–80.
159. Gertz EW, Wisneski JA, Stanley WC, Neese RA. Myocardial substrate utilization during exercise in humans. Dual carbon-labeled carbohydrate isotope experiments. J Clin Invest. 1988;82:2017–25.
160. Stanley WC. Myocardial lactate metabolism during exercise. Med Sci Sports Exerc. 1991;23:920–4.
161. Kaijser L, Berglund B. Myocardial lactate extraction and release at rest and during heavy exercise in healthy men. Acta Physiol Scand. 1992;144:39–45.
162. Kemppainen J, Fujimoto T, Kalliokoski KK, Viljanen T, Nuutila P, Knuuti J. Myocardial and skeletal muscle glucose uptake during exercise in humans. J Physiol. 2002;542:403–12.
163. Bing RJ. The metabolism of the heart. Trans Am Coll Cardiol. 1955;5:8–14.
164. Bremer J, Wojtczak AB. Factors controlling the rate of fatty acid -oxidation in rat liver mitochondria. Biochim Biophys Acta. 1972;280:515–30.
165. Williamson JR, Krebs HA. Acetoacetate as fuel of respiration in the perfused rat heart. Biochem J. 1961;80:540–7.
166. Zimmerman AN, Meijler FL, Hulsmann WC. The inhibitory effect of acetoacetate on myocardial contraction. Lancet. 1962;2:757–8.
167. Taegtmeyer H, Hems R, Krebs HA. Utilization of energy-providing substrates in the isolated working rat heart. Biochem J. 1980;186:701–11.
168. Krebs HA. Some aspects of the regulation of fuel supply in omnivorous animals. Adv Enzyme Regul. 1972;10:397–420.
169. Balaban RS. Cardiac energy metabolism homeostasis: Role of cytosolic calcium. J Mol Cell Cardiol. 2002;34:1259–71.
170. Balaban RS, Kantor HL, Katz LA, Briggs RW. Relation between work and phosphate metabolite in the in vivo paced mammalian heart. Science. 1986;232:1121–3.
171. Kupriyanov VV, Lakomkin VL, Kapelko VI, Steinschneider A, Ruuge EK, Saks VA. Dissociation of adenosine triphosphate levels and contractile function in isovolumic hearts perfused with 2-deoxyglucose. J Mol Cell Cardiol. 1987;19:729–40.
172. Stanley WC, Chandler MP. Energy metabolism in the normal and failing heart: potential for therapeutic interventions. Heart Fail Rev. 2002;7:115–30.
173. Gollnick PD. Metabolic regulation in skeletal muscle: influence of endurance training as exerted by mitochondrial protein concentration. Acta Physiol Scand Suppl. 1986;556:53–66.
174. Kuno S, Ogawa T, Katsuta S, Itai Y. In vivo human myocardial metabolism during aerobic exercise by phosphorus-31 nuclear magnetic resonance spectroscopy. Eur J Appl Physiol Occup Physiol. 1994;69:488–91.
175. Balaban RS, Heineman FW. Control of mitochondrial respiration in the heart in vivo. Mol Cell Biochem. 1989;89:191–7.
176. Grubbstrom J, Berglund B, Kaijser L. Myocardial blood flow and lactate metabolism at rest and during exercise with reduced arterial oxygen content. Acta Physiol Scand. 1991;142:467–74.
177. Jansson E, Sylven C. Activities of key enzymes in the energy metabolism of human myocardial and skeletal muscle. Clin Physiol. 1986;6:465–71.
178. Conway MA, Bristow JD, Blackledge MJ, Rajagopalan B, Radda GK. Cardiac metabolism during exercise in healthy volunteers measured by 31P magnetic resonance spectroscopy. Br Heart J. 1991;65:25–30.
179. Arany Z, He H, Lin J, Hoyer K, Handschin C, Toka O, et al. Transcriptional coactivator pgc-1 alpha controls the energy state and contractile function of cardiac muscle. Cell Metab. 2005;1:259–71.

180. Goodwin GW, Taegtmeyer H. Improved energy homeostasis of the heart in the metabolic state of exercise. Am J Physiol Heart Circ Physiol. 2000;279:H1490–501.
181. Goodwin GW, Taylor CS, Taegtmeyer H. Regulation of energy metabolism of the heart during acute increase in heart work. J Biol Chem. 1998;273:29530–9.
182. Goodwin GW, Ahmad F, Doenst T, Taegtmeyer H. Energy provision from glycogen, glucose, and fatty acids on adrenergic stimulation of isolated working rat hearts. Am J Physiol. 1998;274:H1239–47.
183. Chatham JC. Lactate – the forgotten fuel! J Physiol. 2002;542:333.
184. Lewis GD, Farrell L, Wood MJ, Martinovic M, Arany Z, Rowe GC, et al. Metabolic signatures of exercise in human plasma. Sci Transl Med. 2010;542:33ra37.
185. Mann N, Rosenzweig A. Can exercise teach us how to treat heart disease? Circulation. 2012;126:2625–35.
186. Finkel T, Deng CX, Mostoslavsky R. Recent progress in the biology and physiology of sirtuins. Nature. 2009;460:587–91.
187. Ferrara N, Rinaldi B, Corbi G, Conti V, Stiuso P, Boccuti S, et al. Exercise training promotes SIRT1 activity in aged rats. Rejuvenation Res. 2008;11:139–50.
188. Pillai VB, Sundaresan NR, Jeevanandam V, Gupta MP. Mitochondrial SIRT3 and heart disease. Cardiovasc Res. 2010;88:250–6.
189. Sundaresan NR, Gupta M, Kim G, Rajamohan SB, Isbatan A, Gupta MP. SIRT3 blocks the cardiac hypertrophic response by augmenting Foxo3a-dependent antioxidant defense mechanisms in mice. J Clin Invest. 2009;119:2758–71.
190. Hafner AV, Dai J, Gomes AP, Xiao CY, Palmeira CM, Rosenzweig A, et al. Regulation of the mPTP by SIRT3-mediated deacetylation of CypD at lysine 166 suppresses age-related cardiac hypertrophy. Aging (Albany NY). 2010;2:914–23.
191. Arany Z, Foo SY, Ma Y, Ruas JL, Bommi-Reddy A, Girnun G, et al. HIF-independent regulation of VEGF and angiogenesis by the transcriptional coactivator PGC-1alpha. Nature. 2008;451:1008–12.
192. Young ME, McNulty P, Taegtmeyer H. Adaptation and maladaptation of the heart in diabetes: Part ii: potential mechanisms. Circulation. 2002;105:1861–70.
193. Hellsten Y, Nyberg M. Cardiovascular adaptations to exercise training. Compr Physiol. 2015;6:1–32.
194. McKenzie DC. Respiratory physiology: adaptations to high-level exercise. Br J Sports Med. 2012;46:381–4.
195. Gabriel DA, Kamen G, Frost G. Neural adaptations to resistive exercise: mechanisms and recommendations for training practices. Sports Med. 2006;36:133–49.
196. Hedayatpour N, Falla D. Physiological and neural adaptations to eccentric exercise: mechanisms and considerations for training. Biomed Res Int. 2015;2015:193741.
197. Holloszy JO, Coyle EF. Adaptations of skeletal muscle to endurance exercise and their metabolic consequences. J Appl Physiol Respir Environ Exerc Physiol. 1984;56:831–8.
198. Lundby C, Jacobs RA. Adaptations of skeletal muscle mitochondria to exercise training. Exp Physiol. 2016;101:17–22.
199. Hood DA, Uguccioni G, Vainshtein A, D'Souza D. Mechanisms of exercise-induced mitochondrial biogenesis in skeletal muscle: implications for health and disease. Compr Physiol. 2011;1: 1119–34.
200. Kiens B, Essen-Gustavsson B, Christensen NJ, Saltin B. Skeletal muscle substrate utilization during submaximal exercise in man: effect of endurance training. J Physiol. 1993;469:459–78.
201. Laughlin MH, Roseguini B. Mechanisms for exercise training-induced increases in skeletal muscle blood flow capacity: differences with interval sprint training versus aerobic endurance training. J Physiol Pharmacol. 2008;59(Suppl 7):71–88.
202. Green HJ, Jones S, Ball-Burnett ME, Smith D, Livesey J, Farrance BW. Early muscular and metabolic adaptations to prolonged exercise training in humans. J Appl Physiol (1985). 1991;70:2032–8.
203. Chesley A, Heigenhauser GJ, Spriet LL. Regulation of muscle glycogen phosphorylase activity following short-term endurance training. Am J Physiol. 1996;270:E328–35.
204. Phillips SM, Green HJ, Tarnopolsky MA, Heigenhauser GJ, Grant SM. Progressive effect of endurance training on metabolic adaptations in working skeletal muscle. Am J Physiol. 1996;270:E265–72.
205. Coggan AR, Swanson SC, Mendenhall LA, Habash DL, Kien CL. Effect of endurance training on hepatic glycogenolysis and gluconeogenesis during prolonged exercise in men. Am J Physiol. 1995;268:E375–83.
206. Mendenhall LA, Swanson SC, Habash DL, Coggan AR. Ten days of exercise training reduces glucose production and utilization during moderate-intensity exercise. Am J Physiol. 1994;266:E136–43.
207. Bergman BC, Horning MA, Casazza GA, Wolfel EE, Butterfield GE, Brooks GA. Endurance training increases gluconeogenesis during rest and exercise in men. Am J Physiol Endocrinol Metab. 2000;278:E244–51.
208. Coggan AR, Kohrt WM, Spina RJ, Bier DM, Holloszy JO. Endurance training decreases plasma glucose turnover and oxidation during moderate-intensity exercise in men. J Appl Physiol (1985). 1990;68:990–6.
209. Phillips SM, Green HJ, Tarnopolsky MA, Heigenhauser GF, Hill RE, Grant SM. Effects of training duration on substrate turnover and oxidation during exercise. J Appl Physiol (1985). 1996;81:2182–91.
210. Kristiansen S, Gade J, Wojtaszewski JF, Kiens B, Richter EA. Glucose uptake is increased in trained

vs. Untrained muscle during heavy exercise. J Appl Physiol (1985). 2000;89:1151–8.
211. Phillips SM. Endurance training-induced adaptations in substrate turnover and oxidation. In: Hargreaves M, Spriet L, editors. Exercise metabolism. Champaign: Human Kinetics; 2006. p. 187–213.
212. Purdom T, Kravitz L, Dokladny K, Mermier C. Understanding the factors that effect maximal fat oxidation. J Int Soc Sports Nutr. 2018;15:3.
213. MacRae HS, Dennis SC, Bosch AN, Noakes TD. Effects of training on lactate production and removal during progressive exercise in humans. J Appl Physiol (1985). 1992;72:1649–56.
214. Messonnier LA, Emhoff CA, Fattor JA, Horning MA, Carlson TJ, Brooks GA. Lactate kinetics at the lactate threshold in trained and untrained men. J Appl Physiol (1985). 2013;114:1593–602.
215. Dubouchaud H, Butterfield GE, Wolfel EE, Bergman BC, Brooks GA. Endurance training, expression, and physiology of LDH, MCT1, and MCT4 in human skeletal muscle. Am J Physiol Endocrinol Metab. 2000;278:E571–9.
216. Philippou A, Maridaki M, Tenta R, Koutsilieris M. Hormonal responses following eccentric exercise in humans. Hormones (Athens). 2017;16:405–13.
217. Weicker H, Strobel G. Endocrine regulation of metabolism during exercise. In: Steinacker JM, Ward SA, editors. The physiology and pathophysiology of exercise tolerance. New York: Springer Science & Business Media; 1996.
218. Benardot D, editor. Advanced sports nutrition. 2nd ed. Champaign: Human Kinetics; 2012.
219. Nesher R, Karl IE, Kipnis DM. Dissociation of effects of insulin and contraction on glucose transport in rat epitrochlearis muscle. Am J Physiol. 1985;249:C226–32.
220. Etgen GJ Jr, Memon AR, Thompson GA Jr, Ivy JL. Insulin- and contraction-stimulated translocation of GTP-binding proteins and GLUT4 protein in skeletal muscle. J Biol Chem. 1993;268:20164–9.
221. Farrell PA. Exercise effects on regulation of energy metabolism by pancreatic and gut hormones. Perspectives in Exerc Science and Sports Med Energy Supply in Exercise and Sport. 1992;5:383–434.
222. Ploug T, Galbo H, Richter EA. Increased muscle glucose uptake during contractions: no need for insulin. Am J Physiol. 1984;247:E726–31.
223. Ploug T, Galbo H, Ohkuwa T, Tranum-Jensen J, Vinten J. Kinetics of glucose transport in rat skeletal muscle membrane vesicles: effects of insulin and contractions. Am J Physiol. 1992;262:E700–11.
224. Hamada T, Arias EB, Cartee GD. Increased submaximal insulin-stimulated glucose uptake in mouse skeletal muscle after treadmill exercise. J Appl Physiol (1985). 2006;101:1368–76.
225. Richter EA, Ploug T, Galbo H. Increased muscle glucose uptake after exercise. No need for insulin during exercise. Diabetes. 1985;34:1041–8.
226. Slentz CA, Gulve EA, Rodnick KJ, Henriksen EJ, Youn JH, Holloszy JO. Glucose transporters and maximal transport are increased in endurance-trained rat soleus. J Appl Physiol (1985). 1992;73:486–92.
227. Flores-Riveros JR, Kaestner KH, Thompson KS, Lane MD. Cyclic AMP-induced transcriptional repression of the insulin-responsive glucose transporter (GLUT4) gene: identification of a promoter region required for down-regulation of transcription. Biochem Biophys Res Commun. 1993;194:1148–54.
228. Goodyear LJ, Hirshman MF, Valyou PM, Horton ES. Glucose transporter number, function, and subcellular distribution in rat skeletal muscle after exercise training. Diabetes. 1992;41:1091–9.
229. Neufer PD, Shinebarger MH, Dohm GL. Effect of training and detraining on skeletal muscle glucose transporter (GLUT4) content in rats. Can J Physiol Pharmacol. 1992;70:1286–90.
230. Kono T, Robinson FW, Blevins TL, Ezaki O. Evidence that translocation of the glucose transport activity is the major mechanism of insulin action on glucose transport in fat cells. J Biol Chem. 1982;257:10942–7.
231. Goodyear LJ, Kahn BB. Exercise, glucose transport, and insulin sensitivity. Annu Rev Med. 1998;49:235–61.
232. Wallberg-Henriksson H. Exercise and diabetes mellitus. Exerc Sport Sci Rev. 1992;20:339–68.
233. Richter EA, Galbo H, Sonne B, Holst JJ, Christensen NJ. Adrenal medullary control of muscular and hepatic glycogenolysis and of pancreatic hormonal secretion in exercising rats. Acta Physiol Scand. 1980;108:235–42.
234. Raschka C, Schuhmann R, Plath M, Parzeller M. Changes of hormone values during an ultra long distance run. In: Steinacker JM, Ward SA, editors. The physiology and pathophysiology of exercise tolerance. New York: Springer Science & Business Media; 1996.
235. American College of Sports Medicine. ACSM's guidelines for exercise testing and prescription. 10th ed. Philadelphia: Lippincott Williams & Wilkins; 2016.
236. American College of Sports Medicine. ACSM's guidelines for exercise testing and prescription. 5th ed. Philadelphia: Lippincott Williams & Wilkins; 1995.
237. Wahl P. Hormonal and metabolic responses to high intensity interval training. J Sports Med Doping Stud. 2013;3:1–2.
238. Wahl P, Zinner C, Achtzehn S, Bloch W, Mester J. Effect of high- and low-intensity exercise and metabolic acidosis on levels of GH, IGF-I, IGFBP-3 and cortisol. Growth Hormon IGF Res. 2010;20:380–5.
239. Gibala MJ, Little JP, van Essen M, Wilkin GP, Burgomaster KA, Safdar A, et al. Short-term sprint interval versus traditional endurance training: similar initial adaptations in human skeletal muscle and exercise performance. J Physiol. 2006;575:901–11.
240. Gordon SE, Kraemer WJ, Vos NH, Lynch JM, Knuttgen HG. Effect of acid-base balance on the growth hormone response to acute high-

intensity cycle exercise. J Appl Physiol (1985). 1994;76:821–9.
241. Batacan RB Jr, Duncan MJ, Dalbo VJ, Tucker PS, Fenning AS. Effects of high-intensity interval training on cardiometabolic health: a systematic review and meta-analysis of intervention studies. Br J Sports Med. 2017;51:494–503.
242. Strobel G, Friedmann B, Jost J, Bartsch P. Plasma and platelet catecholamine and catecholamine sulfate response to various exercise tests. Am J Physiol. 1994;267:E537–43.
243. Cryer PE. Physiology and pathophysiology of the human sympathoadrenal neuroendocrine system. N Engl J Med. 1980;303:436–44.
244. Kindermann W, Schnabel A, Schmitt WM, Biro G, Cassens J, Weber F. Catecholamines, growth hormone, cortisol, insulin, and sex hormones in anaerobic and aerobic exercise. Eur J Appl Physiol Occup Physiol. 1982;49:389–99.
245. Pullinen T, Mero A, MacDonald E, Pakarinen A, Komi PV. Plasma catecholamine and serum testosterone responses to four units of resistance exercise in young and adult male athletes. Eur J Appl Physiol Occup Physiol. 1998;77:413–20.
246. Justice TD, Hammer GL, Davey RJ, Paramalingam N, Guelfi KJ, Lewis L, et al. Effect of antecedent moderate-intensity exercise on the glycemia-increasing effect of a 30-sec maximal sprint: a sex comparison. Physiol Rep. 2015;3:1–10.
247. Vierck J, O'Reilly B, Hossner K, Antonio J, Byrne K, Bucci L, Dodson M. Satellite cell regulation following myotrauma caused by resistance exercise. Cell Biol Int. 2000;24:263–72.
248. Galbo H. Endocrine factors in endurance. In: Shepard RJ, Astrand PO, editors. Endurance in sport. Oxford: Blackwell Scientific Publications; 1992.
249. Philippou A, Maridaki M, Pneumaticos S, Koutsilieris M. The complexity of the IGF1 gene splicing, posttranslational modification and bioactivity. Mol Med. 2014;20:202–14.
250. Eliakim A, Nemet D, Most G, Rakover N, Pantanowitz M, Meckel Y. Effect of gender on the GH-IGF-I response to anaerobic exercise in young adults. J Strength Cond Res. 2014;28:3411–5.
251. Philippou A, Papageorgiou E, Bogdanis G, Halapas A, Sourla A, Maridaki M, et al. Expression of IGF-1 isoforms after exercise-induced muscle damage in humans: characterization of the MGF E peptide actions in vitro. In Vivo. 2009;23:567–75.
252. Gatti R, De Palo EF, Antonelli G, Spinella P. IGF-I/IGFBP system: metabolism outline and physical exercise. J Endocrinol Investig. 2012;35:699–707.
253. Lovell DI, Cuneo R, Wallace J, McLellan C. The hormonal response of older men to sub-maximum aerobic exercise: the effect of training and detraining. Steroids. 2012;77:413–8.
254. Hartgens F, Kuipers H. Effects of androgenic-anabolic steroids in athletes. Sports Med. 2004;34:513–54.
255. Tamaki T, Uchiyama S, Uchiyama Y, Akatsuka A, Roy RR, Edgerton VR. Anabolic steroids increase exercise tolerance. Am J Physiol Endocrinol Metab. 2001;280:E973–81.
256. Hackney AC, Hosick KP, Myer A, Rubin DA, Battaglini CL. Testosterone responses to intensive interval versus steady-state endurance exercise. J Endocrinol Invest. 2012;35:947–50.
257. Kraemer WJ, Gordon SE, Fleck SJ, Marchitelli LJ, Mello R, Dziados JE, et al. Endogenous anabolic hormonal and growth factor responses to heavy resistance exercise in males and females. Int J Sports Med. 1991;12:228–35.
258. Pullinen T, Mero A, Huttunen P, Pakarinen A, Komi PV. Resistance exercise-induced hormonal responses in men, women, and pubescent boys. Med Sci Sports Exerc. 2002;34:806–13.
259. Davis SN, Galassetti P, Wasserman DH, Tate D. Effects of gender on neuroendocrine and metabolic counterregulatory responses to exercise in normal man. J Clin Endocrinol Metab. 2000;85:224–30.
260. Berg U, Enqvist JK, Mattsson CM, Carlsson-Skwirut C, Sundberg CJ, Ekblom B, et al. Lack of sex differences in the IGF-IGBP response to ultra endurance exercise. Scand J Med Sci Sports. 2008;18:706–14.
261. Horton TJ, Grunwald GK, Lavely J, Donahoo WT. Glucose kinetics differ between women and men, during and after exercise. J Appl Physiol (1985). 2006;100:1883–94.
262. Buckley J. Endocrine factors in endurance. In: Maclaren D, Spurway N, editors. Exercise physiology in special populations. Advances in sport and exercise science. Livingstone: Churchill; 2008.
263. Pedersen BK, Saltin B. Exercise as medicine – evidence for prescribing exercise as therapy in 26 different chronic diseases. Scand J Med Sci Sports. 2015;25(Suppl 3):1–72.
264. Yardley JE, Hay J, Abou-Setta AM, Marks SD, McGavock J. A systematic review and meta-analysis of exercise interventions in adults with type 1 diabetes. Diabetes Res Clin Pract. 2014;106:393–400.
265. Krentz AJ, Bailey CJ. Type 2 diabetes in practice. London: Royal Society of Medicine Press; 2001.
266. Kokkinos P, Faselis C, Narayan P, Myers J, Nylen E, Sui X, Zhang J, Lavie CJ. Cardiorespiratory fitness and incidence of type 2 diabetes in united states veterans on statin therapy. Am J Med. 2017;130:1192–8.
267. Kokkinos P. Physical activity, health benefits, and mortality risk. ISRN Cardiol. 2012;2012:718789.
268. Lavie CJ, De Schutter A, Parto P, Jahangir E, Kokkinos P, Ortega FB, et al. Obesity and prevalence of cardiovascular diseases and prognosis-the obesity paradox updated. Prog Cardiovasc Dis. 2016;58:537–47.
269. Nylen ES, Gandhi SM, Kheirbek R, Kokkinos P. Enhanced fitness and renal function in type 2 diabetes. Diabet Med. 2015;32:1342–5.

270. Kokkinos P, Sheriff H, Kheirbek R. Physical inactivity and mortality risk. Cardiol Res Pract. 2010;2011:924945.
271. Goff DC Jr, Lloyd-Jones DM, Bennett G, Coady S, D'Agostino RB, Gibbons R, et al. 2013 ACC/AHA Guideline on the Assessment of Cardiovascular Risk: a report of the American College of Cardiology/American Heart Association Task Force on Practice Guidelines. Circulation. 2013;129:S49–73.
272. Nylen E, Ni D, Myersb J, Manchin C, Plunkett M, Kokkinos P. Cardiorespiratory fitness impact on all-cause mortality in prediabetic veterans. J Endocrinol Metab. 2015;5:215–9.
273. Dela F, von Linstow ME, Mikines KJ, Galbo H. Physical training may enhance beta-cell function in type 2 diabetes. Am J Physiol Endocrinol Metab. 2004;287:E1024–31.
274. Hawley JA. Exercise as a therapeutic intervention for the prevention and treatment of insulin resistance. Diabetes Metab Res Rev. 2004;20:383–93.
275. Colberg SR, Sigal RJ, Yardley JE, Riddell MC, Dunstan DW, Dempsey PC, et al. Physical activity/exercise and diabetes: a position statement of the american diabetes association. Diabetes Care. 2016;39:2065–79.
276. Kerksick CM, Fox E. Sports nutrition needs for child and adolescent athletes. Boca Raton: CRC Press; 2016.
277. Reyes LM, Davenport MH. Exercise as a therapeutic intervention to optimize fetal weight. Pharmacol Res. 2018;132:160–7.
278. Gallen IW. Exercise for people with type 1 diabetes. Med Sport Sci. 2014;60:141–53.
279. Moser O, Yardley JE, Bracken RM. Interstitial glucose and physical exercise in type 1 diabetes: integrative physiology, technology, and the gap in-between. Nutrients. 2018;10:1–15.
280. MacDonald MJ. Postexercise late-onset hypoglycemia in insulin-dependent diabetic patients. Diabetes Care. 1987;10:584–8.
281. Gallen IW, Hume C, Lumb A. Fuelling the athlete with type 1 diabetes. Diabetes Obes Metab. 2011;13:130–6.
282. Guelfi KJ, Jones TW, Fournier PA. New insights into managing the risk of hypoglycaemia associated with intermittent high-intensity exercise in individuals with type 1 diabetes mellitus: implications for existing guidelines. Sports Med. 2007;37:937–46.
283. Yardley JE, Sigal RJ. Exercise strategies for hypoglycemia prevention in individuals with type 1 diabetes. Diabetes Spectr. 2015;28:32–8.
284. MacLeod SF, Terada T, Chahal BS, Boule NG. Exercise lowers postprandial glucose but not fasting glucose in type 2 diabetes: a meta-analysis of studies using continuous glucose monitoring. Diabetes Metab Res Rev. 2013;29:593–603.
285. Colberg SR, Albright AL, Blissmer BJ, Braun B, Chasan-Taber L, Fernhall B, et al. Exercise and type 2 diabetes: American college of sports medicine and the american diabetes association: joint position statement. Exercise and type 2 diabetes. Med Sci Sports Exerc. 2010;42:2282–303.
286. De Nardi AT, Tolves T, Lenzi TL, Signori LU, Silva A. High-intensity interval training versus continuous training on physiological and metabolic variables in prediabetes and type 2 diabetes: a meta-analysis. Diabetes Res Clin Pract. 2018;137:149–59.
287. Lee S, Kim Y. Effects of exercise alone on insulin sensitivity and glucose tolerance in obese youth. Diabetes Metab J. 2013;37:225–32.
288. Church TS, Blair SN, Cocreham S, Johannsen N, Johnson W, Kramer K, Mikus CR, Myers V, Nauta M, Rodarte RQ, Sparks L, Thompson A, et al. Effects of aerobic and resistance training on hemoglobin A1c levels in patients with type 2 diabetes: a randomized controlled trial. JAMA. 2010;304:2253–62.
289. Umpierre D, Ribeiro PA, Kramer CK, Leitao CB, Zucatti AT, Azevedo MJ, et al. Physical activity advice only or structured exercise training and association with HbA1c levels in type 2 diabetes: a systematic review and meta-analysis. JAMA. 2011;305:1790–9.
290. Kwak HB. Exercise and obesity-induced insulin resistance in skeletal muscle. Integr Med Res. 2013;2:131–8.
291. Plomgaard P, Weigert C. Do diabetes and obesity affect the metabolic response to exercise? Curr Opin Clin Nutr Metab Care. 2017;20:294–9.
292. Kopin L, Lowenstein C. Dyslipidemia. Ann Intern Med. 2017;167:ITC81–96.
293. Leon AS, Sanchez OA. Response of blood lipids to exercise training alone or combined with dietary intervention. Med Sci Sports Exerc. 2001;33:S502–15; discussion S528–509
294. Breneman CB, Polinski K, Sarzynski MA, Lavie CJ, Kokkinos PF, Ahmed A, et al. The impact of cardiorespiratory fitness levels on the risk of developing atherogenic dyslipidemia. Am J Med. 2016;129:1060–6.
295. Sui X, Sarzynski MA, Lee DC, Kokkinos PF. Impact of changes in cardiorespiratory fitness on hypertension, dyslipidemia and survival: An overview of the epidemiological evidence. Prog Cardiovasc Dis. 2017;60:56–66.
296. Hayashino Y, Jackson JL, Fukumori N, Nakamura F, Fukuhara S. Effects of supervised exercise on lipid profiles and blood pressure control in people with type 2 diabetes mellitus: a meta-analysis of randomized controlled trials. Diabetes Res Clin Pract. 2012;98:349–60.
297. Mann S, Beedie C, Jimenez A. Differential effects of aerobic exercise, resistance training and combined exercise modalities on cholesterol and the lipid profile: review, synthesis and recommendations. Sports Med. 2014;44:211–21.
298. Kodama S, Tanaka S, Saito K, Shu M, Sone Y, Onitake F, Suzuki E, Shimano H, Yamamoto S, Kondo K, Ohashi Y, Yamada N, Sone H. Effect of aerobic exercise training on serum levels of high-density lipoprotein cholesterol: a meta-analysis. Arch Intern Med. 2007;167:999–1008.

299. Pronk NP. Short term effects of exercise on plasma lipids and lipoproteins in humans. Sports Med. 1993;16:431–48.
300. Kokkinos PF, Holland JC, Narayan P, Colleran JA, Dotson CO, Papademetriou V. Miles run per week and high-density lipoprotein cholesterol levels in healthy, middle-aged men. A dose-response relationship. Arch Intern Med. 1995;155:415–20.
301. Kraus WE, Houmard JA, Duscha BD, Knetzger KJ, Wharton MB, McCartney JS, et al. Effects of the amount and intensity of exercise on plasma lipoproteins. N Engl J Med. 2002;347:1483–92.
302. Mestek ML, Plaisance EP, Ratcliff LA, Taylor JK, Wee SO, Grandjean PW. Aerobic exercise and postprandial lipemia in men with the metabolic syndrome. Med Sci Sports Exerc. 2008;40:2105–11.
303. Pafili ZK, Bogdanis GC, Tsetsonis NV, Maridaki M. Postprandial lipemia 16 and 40 hours after low-volume eccentric resistance exercise. Med Sci Sports Exerc. 2009;41:375–82.
304. Sabaka P, Kruzliak P, Balaz D, Komornikova A, Celovska D, Cammarota G, et al. Effect of short term aerobic exercise on fasting and postprandial lipoprotein subfractions in healthy sedentary men. Lipids Health Dis. 2015;14:151.
305. Kokkinos PF, Narayan P, Colleran J, Fletcher RD, Lakshman R, Papademetriou V. Effects of moderate intensity exercise on serum lipids in African-American men with severe systemic hypertension. Am J Cardiol. 1998;81:732–5.
306. Durstine JL, Grandjean PW, Cox CA, Thompson PD. Lipids, lipoproteins, and exercise. J Cardiopulm Rehabil. 2002;22:385–98.
307. Quinlivan R, Buckley J, James M, Twist A, Ball S, Duno M, et al. McArdle disease: a clinical review. J Neurol Neurosurg Psychiatry. 2010;81:1182–8.
308. Mc AB. Myopathy due to a defect in muscle glycogen breakdown. Clin Sci. 1951;10:13–35.
309. Nogales-Gadea G, Santalla A, Ballester-Lopez A, Arenas J, Martin MA, Godfrey R, et al. Exercise and preexercise nutrition as treatment for McArdle disease. Med Sci Sports Exerc. 2015;48:673–9.
310. Delaney NF, Sharma R, Tadvalkar L, Clish CB, Haller RG, Mootha VK. Metabolic profiles of exercise in patients with McArdle disease or mitochondrial myopathy. Proc Natl Acad Sci USA. 2017;114:8402–7.
311. Nogales-Gadea G, Godfrey R, Santalla A, Coll-Canti J, Pintos-Morell G, Pinos T, et al. Genes and exercise intolerance: Insights from McArdle disease. Physiol Genomics. 2016;48:93–100.
312. Kaczor JJ, Robertshaw HA, Tarnopolsky MA. Higher oxidative stress in skeletal muscle of McArdle disease patients. Mol Genet Metab Rep. 2017;12:69–75.
313. Quinlivan R, Martinuzzi A, Schoser B. Pharmacological and nutritional treatment for McArdle disease (glycogen storage disease type v). Cochrane Database Syst Rev. 2014;11:CD003458.
314. Santalla A, Nogales-Gadea G, Ortenblad N, Brull A, de Luna N, Pinos T, et al. McArdle disease: a unique study model in sports medicine. Sports Med. 2014;44:1531–44.
315. Nogales-Gadea G, Consuegra-Garcia I, Rubio JC, Arenas J, Cuadros M, Camara Y, et al. A transcriptomic approach to search for novel phenotypic regulators in McArdle disease. PLoS One. 2012;7:e31718.
316. Munguia-Izquierdo D, Santalla A, Lucia A. Cardiorespiratory fitness, physical activity, and quality of life in patients with McArdle disease. Med Sci Sports Exerc. 2015;47:799–808.
317. Ollivier K, Hogrel JY, Gomez-Merino D, Romero NB, Laforet P, Eymard B, et al. Exercise tolerance and daily life in McArdle's disease. Muscle Nerve. 2005;31:637–41.
318. Andersen ST, Haller RG, Vissing J. Effect of oral sucrose shortly before exercise on work capacity in McArdle disease. Arch Neurol. 2008;65:786–9.
319. Mate-Munoz JL, Moran M, Perez M, Chamorro-Vina C, Gomez-Gallego F, Santiago C, et al. Favorable responses to acute and chronic exercisein McArdle patients. Clin J Sport Med. 2007;17:297–303.
320. Quinlivan R, Vissing J, Hilton-Jones D, Buckley J. Physical training for McArdle disease. Cochrane Database Syst Rev. 2011;12:CD007931.
321. Haller RG, Wyrick P, Taivassalo T, Vissing J. Aerobic conditioning: an effective therapy in McArdle's disease. Ann Neurol. 2006;59:922–8.
322. Garcia-Benitez S, Fleck SJ, Naclerio F, Martin MA, Lucia A. Resistance (weight lifting) training in an adolescent with McArdle disease. J Child Neurol. 2013;28:805–8.
323. Santalla A, Munguia-Izquierdo D, Brea-Alejo L, Pagola-Aldazabal I, Diez-Bermejo J, Fleck SJ, et al. Feasibility of resistance training in adult McArdle patients: clinical outcomes and muscle strength and mass benefits. Front Aging Neurosci. 2014;6:334.
324. Garber CE, Blissmer B, Deschenes MR, Franklin BA, Lamonte MJ, Lee IM, et al. American College of Sports Medicine Position Stand. Quantity and quality of exercise for developing and maintaining cardiorespiratory, musculoskeletal, and neuromotor fitness in apparently healthy adults: guidance for prescribing exercise. Med Sci Sports Exerc. 2011;43:1334–59.
325. Andersen ST, Vissing J. Carbohydrate- and protein-rich diets in McArdle disease: effects on exercise capacity. J Neurol Neurosurg Psychiatry. 2008;79:1359–63.
326. Reason SL, Westman EC, Godfrey R, Maguire E. Can a low-carbohydrate diet improve exercise tolerance in McArdle disease? J Rare Disord Diagn Ther. 2017;3:1–5.

Exercise and the Endothelium

6

Joshua C. Tremblay and Kyra E. Pyke

Introduction

The vascular endothelium is a single layer of cells that lines the luminal surface of blood vessels. Endothelial cell signaling is involved in determining vascular tone, structure, and permeability as well as thrombosis and thus plays a key role in determining vascular health [1, 2]. Endothelial cells respond to both chemical and mechanical stimuli, and given their position in the vascular lumen, they are constantly exposed to changing hemodynamic forces. Changes in blood flow alter the frictional force (shear stress) of the blood against the vessel wall. Shear stress is sensed via several endothelial membrane structures resulting in biochemical signaling. This conversion of the frictional force of the flowing blood into a biochemical response is called shear stress transduction [3–5]. Chronically, the magnitude and pattern of shear stress to which the endothelium is exposed play a key role in determining its function and structure [6, 7].

Regular exercise reduces cardiovascular disease risk, and the multifaceted mechanisms of this beneficial effect likely include improvements in endothelial function, mediated at least in part by exercise-induced elevations in shear stress [8]. Exercise causes large changes in arterial shear stress which vary depending on the nature of the exercise (e.g., modality, intensity) and the location in the arterial tree [9, 10]. Although chronic exercise alters many variables that could influence endothelial function (e.g., blood pressure [11], blood lipid levels [12]), the repeated exposure to increases in shear stress during exercise appears to be critical to exercise-induced adaptations in endothelial function [13, 14]. This includes stimulating alterations in endothelial gene expression which result in a more vasoprotective or "atherosclerosis-inhibiting" (antiatherogenic) cell phenotype [15]. In the first part of this chapter, we will review the role of endothelial function in the development of atherosclerosis, describe the methods used to quantify endothelial function in humans, and review the association between metrics of endothelial function and cardiovascular event risk. The remainder of the chapter will focus on reviewing the evidence regarding the impact of exercise training on endothelial function in a range of populations and the mechanisms underlying the beneficial effects.

Endothelial Function and Atherosclerosis

Atherosclerosis is an inflammatory disease wherein modified lipid molecules, macrophages, and smooth muscle cells accumulate in the vascular wall

J. C. Tremblay · K. E. Pyke (✉)
Queen's University, School of Kinesiology and Health Studies, Kingston, ON, Canada
e-mail: pykek@queensu.ca

P. Kokkinos, P. Narayan (eds.), *Cardiorespiratory Fitness in Cardiometabolic Diseases*,
https://doi.org/10.1007/978-3-030-04816-7_6

between the endothelium and the smooth muscle cell layer forming plaques that may eventually restrict blood flow through the vessel lumen [1]. The pathogenesis of atherosclerosis is complex and has been reviewed in detail elsewhere [16, 17]. It involves the adhesion of monocytes (a type of leukocyte) to the endothelium followed by their infiltration and differentiation to macrophages. Macrophages envelop oxidized low-density lipoprotein cholesterol in the vessel wall forming foam cells which aggregate to form fatty streaks, the first stage of atherosclerotic lesions. Lesions grow larger and more complex as smooth muscle cell proliferation contributes to the plaque and a fibrous cap forms. The primary clinical manifestations of atherosclerosis include myocardial infarction and stroke. These events occur most often as a result of plaque rupture, initiating the formation of a thrombus (blood clot), which can rapidly limit blood flow by occluding the lumen [18, 19]. The endothelium is a critically positioned barrier that circulating factors must adhere to or infiltrate to participate in plaque formation [1].

The role of endothelial dysfunction in the initiation and pathogenesis of atherosclerosis is well established and has been recently reviewed [17]. Depending on their environment, endothelial cells can exert a pro- or antiatherogenic influence, and the magnitude and pattern of shear stress exposure are critical determinants of which phenotype is expressed [1, 17]. When exposed to laminar flow and a high mean shear stress, the endothelium exhibits an antiatherogenic phenotype (Fig. 6.1). This includes (but is not limited to) increased expression of the enzyme endothelial nitric oxide synthase (eNOS) and in turn increased bioavailability of the vasodilator nitric oxide (NO) [15, 20]. In addition to causing vasorelaxation, NO inhibits vascular smooth muscle cell proliferation and thrombus formation, thus inhibiting atherosclerotic lesion progression and complication [21]. In contrast, low mean shear

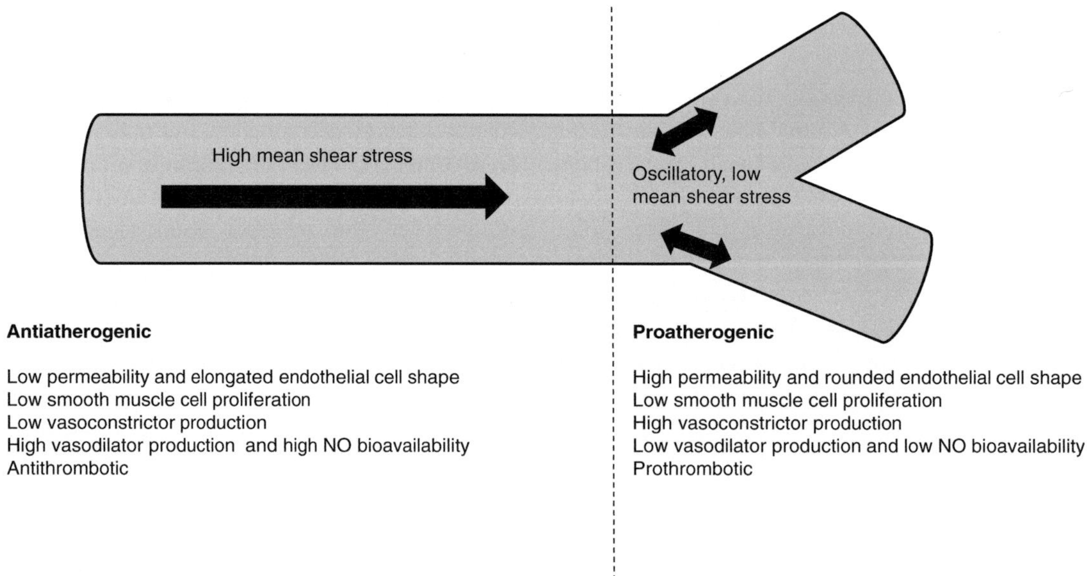

Fig. 6.1 Impact of local shear stress on endothelial cell phenotype. Chronic shear stress exposure has an important impact on endothelial cell function and structure. High levels of shear stress promote an endothelial cell phenotype that inhibits the initiation/progression of atherosclerosis in a number of ways (antiatherogenic). In contrast when mean shear stress is low, which can be accompanied by a disturbed pattern of reversing forward and back flow (oscillatory shear stress), this results in an endothelial phenotype that increases vulnerability to atherosclerotic lesions (proatherogenic). The importance of shear stress magnitude/pattern in determining vulnerability to atherosclerosis is demonstrated in vivo by the localization of lesions to arterial branch points where mean shear stress is low [24]. NO nitric oxide – important vasodilator released from the endothelium in response to shear stress. (Adapted from Cahill and Redmond [1])

stress, which can occur when there is alternating forward and back flow (termed oscillatory shear stress), promotes a proatherogenic endothelial cell phenotype. This includes endothelial gene expression and a cell morphology that encourages atherosclerotic progression [1, 6, 15] (Fig. 6.1). For example, when cultured endothelial cells are seeded onto tubes exposed to oscillatory shear stress via a pump system, this decreases eNOS expression and increases expression of the vasoconstrictor endothelin-1 [22], which also stimulates smooth muscle cell proliferation [23]. The clearest in vivo evidence of the importance of shear stress to atherosclerosis progression is the observation of localization of atherosclerotic lesions to arterial branch points where flow is disturbed (non-laminar) and mean shear stress is low [24, 25].

In summary, endothelial dysfunction precedes and plays a role in the pathogenesis of atherosclerosis. Endothelial dysfunction is characterized by an endothelial phenotype that encourages thrombosis and smooth muscle cell proliferation with lowered vasodilator production and increased vasoconstrictor formation. The pattern and magnitude of chronic shear stress exposure are critical determinants of endothelial cell phenotype and thus vulnerability to atherosclerotic lesions; a high level of laminar shear stress is antiatherogenic, while an oscillatory, low mean level of shear stress is proatherogenic.

Endothelial Function Assessment in Humans

There are several ways to assess endothelial function in humans, and some approaches measure circulating factors that reflect endothelial repair processes, damage to the endothelial cells, or endothelial clotting function (e.g., endothelial cell progenitor cells, endothelial microparticles, or von Willebrand factor). The most common techniques stimulate endothelial-dependent dilation such that the magnitude of dilation reflects endothelial function (more dilation = better endothelial function). However, influencing vascular tone is only one of the many functions of the endothelium, and testing endothelial-dependent dilation alone likely does not provide a fully comprehensive representation of all "endothelial functions." Nevertheless, endothelial-dependent dilation and the other roles of the endothelium are not mutually exclusive; for example, NO is a key vasodilator produced by the endothelium, and its bioavailability is important to the endothelium's role in inhibition of thrombosis and smooth muscle cell proliferation [21]. Given the pervasive use of assessments that interrogate endothelium-dependent vasodilation, this chapter will focus on these approaches. In this section the methods used to assess microvascular and conduit artery endothelial function in both the coronary and limb circulations will be reviewed. Importantly, microvascular and conduit artery endothelial functions are not always well correlated suggesting that they can change independently and/or along a distinct time course [26].

Microvascular

The microvasculature refers to the arterioles (also known as resistance vessels) and capillaries. However in this chapter, the use of the term will refer to arteriolar function only. Changes in arteriolar smooth muscle tone result in large changes in arteriolar diameter and therefore the resistance to flow (decrease in diameter = increase in resistance). Thus the tone of arterioles controls perfusion to the downstream tissue by altering resistance. The gold standard methodology for the assessment of microvascular endothelial function involves estimating endothelial-dependent dilation in response to arterial infusion of acetylcholine (Ach). When acetylcholine binds to muscarinic receptors on the endothelium, this stimulates the production of vasodilators, predominantly NO, resulting in vasodilation [27–29]. The change in local blood flow following infusion is used as the index of microvascular endothelial function and NO bioavailability [30]. This is because the increase in blood flow reflects decreased vascular resistance due to endothelial-dependent, NO-mediated vasodilation in the whole microvascular bed downstream from the infusion site. Rather than blood flow, changes in calculated vascular resistance or vascular conductance (the inverse of resistance; reflects degree of vasodilation in the vascular bed) can also be reported as the index of endothelial function.

Coronary artery microvascular endothelial function is involved in myocardial perfusion and therefore is clinically relevant [31, 32]. However, coronary function can only be invasively assessed via arterial catheterization (Fig. 6.2a) [30, 32]. This limits its feasibility outside of coronary artery disease patients. Fortunately, microvascular endothelial function can be assessed more noninvasively in the limbs. To assess forearm microvascular endothelial function, Ach is infused into the brachial or radial artery, and forearm blood flow is assessed via venous occlusion plethysmography or duplex ultrasound [33] (Fig. 6.2b). The increase in forearm blood flow (FBF_{Ach}) reflects the degree of receptor-mediated endothelial-dependent microvascular dilation and therefore endothelial function [33]. Skin microvascular endothelial function can be assessed with transdermal application of Ach via iontophoresis or microdialysis infusion of Ach [34]. The reactive hyperemia (peak blood flow) or conductance following limb occlusion is also reported as a fully noninvasive index of microvascular function; however, it is less specific to endothelial function per se than Ach-induced dilation (i.e., it may also reflect endothelial-independent mechanisms of dilation) [35]. Similarly, peripheral arterial tonometry during reactive hyperemia provides an index of microvascular function, although changes in the

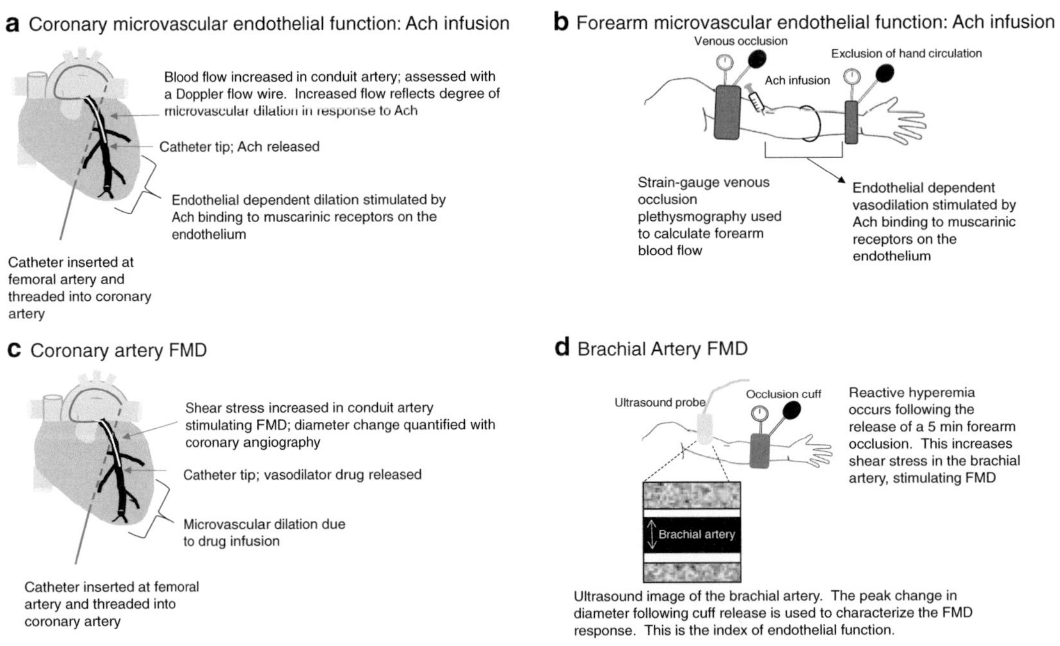

Fig. 6.2 Schematic representation of endothelial function assessment techniques. (**a**) Invasive assessment of coronary endothelial-dependent microvascular vasodilation stimulated by infusion of Ach into the coronary microvascular circulation. The increase in coronary artery blood flow reflects the magnitude of microvascular dilation and provides the index of endothelial function. (**b**) Less invasive assessment of forearm endothelial-dependent microvascular vasodilation stimulated by Ach infusion via a catheter inserted into the brachial artery. The increase in forearm blood flow measured with brachial artery ultrasound (not pictured) or strain-gauge venous occlusion plethysmography reflects the magnitude of microvascular dilation and provides the index of endothelial function. (**c**) Invasive assessment of coronary conduit artery FMD. Conduit artery diameter is assessed via coronary angiography. A shear stress stimulus is created via the infusion of a vasodilator drug downstream from the site of diameter assessment. The change in conduit artery diameter in response to the shear stress (i.e., the FMD response) is the index of endothelial function. (**d**) Noninvasive assessment of brachial artery FMD. Brachial artery diameter is assessed via ultrasound. A shear stress stimulus is created via the release of a 5 min forearm occlusion (which stimulates forearm microvascular vasodilation; reducing resistance to flow in the forearm). The peak change in brachial artery diameter in response to the shear stress (i.e., the FMD response) is the index of endothelial function. Ach acetylcholine, FMD flow-mediated dilation

pulse wave measured at the finger (which reflect the degree of microvascular dilation), rather than changes in forearm blood flow, are assessed as the index of function [35].

A low blood flow response to Ach could presumably reflect either a low endothelial bioavailability of NO (i.e., endothelial dysfunction) or a failure of the vascular smooth muscle to respond to NO produced by the endothelium. To confirm that low blood flow in response to Ach is indicative of endothelial dysfunction per se, responses to Ach are often tested in conjunction with flow responses to infusion of an exogenous NO donor (e.g., nitroglycerine) [30]. If the increase in blood flow in response to Ach is low and blood flow in response to NO donor infusion is intact, this confirms endothelial dysfunction.

Conduit Artery

Conduit arteries are large, elastic vessels (e.g., the aorta, brachial artery, and femoral artery) that accommodate bulk flow with low resistance. Compared to the arterioles, they are relatively uninvolved in controlling perfusion, although in the aorta, coronary, and lower limb vasculature, they are prone to atherosclerosis which can result in an aneurysm or critical flow limitation (e.g., angina, myocardial infarction, intermittent claudication). Similar to the microvasculature, conduit coronary artery diameter changes in response to Ach infusion. The change in diameter can be directly measured via quantitative angiography and interpreted as an index of endothelial function. Ach results in vasodilation in healthy arteries and a paradoxical conduit artery constriction in coronary artery disease patients [30]. However, shear stress, rather than Ach, is used more frequently to stimulate and assess conduit artery endothelial function. As indicated above, endothelial cells are sensitive to blood flow-associated shear stress, and their acute response to increases in shear stress involves the release of vasodilators. This response is termed flow-mediated dilation, or FMD. The magnitude of FMD in response to experimenter-imposed increases in shear stress provides the primary index of conduit artery endothelial function [36]. Although several vasodilators are released in response to shear stress and may participate in FMD, evidence to date supports that NO typically makes an important contribution [37–39].

Coronary artery FMD can be assessed invasively via catheterization and infusion of drugs to decrease downstream resistance and increase flow and shear stress in a coronary conduit artery [30] (Fig. 6.2c). In 1992 Celermajer and colleagues [40] introduced a technique that allows noninvasive assessment of limb conduit artery FMD. A shear stress stimulus is created with reactive hyperemia following the release of a ~5 min limb occlusion, and ultrasound imaging of the feeding conduit artery permits assessment of the resulting FMD response (Fig. 6.2d). While this remains the most popular assessment technique, induction of sustained increases in shear stress via limb heating or small muscle mass exercise is also gaining popularity as an alternative way to increase shear stress for FMD assessment [41]. FMD can be assessed in the arms and the legs and has been reported in the brachial, radial, superficial femoral, and popliteal arteries. Upper limb FMD has been shown to correlate with coronary artery FMD and is therefore often considered a noninvasive surrogate for coronary artery endothelial function [42, 43] and marker of systemic endothelial function.

As with the microcirculation, administration of endothelial-independent NO donors (e.g., glycerol trinitrite (GTN)) is often done in conjunction with FMD testing. For noninvasive assessment, GTN is administered sublingually, and the conduit artery dilation in response to GTN serves as the index of vascular smooth muscle function [44]. If responses to GTN are intact, this isolates an impaired FMD response to endothelial dysfunction specifically.

Endothelial Function and Cardiovascular Disease Risk

Atherosclerosis leads to cardiovascular events including myocardial infarction, stroke, and angina. If endothelial dysfunction precedes and plays a role in the pathogenesis of atherosclerosis, it follows that endothelial dysfunction should serve as an "early warning system" for cardiovascular

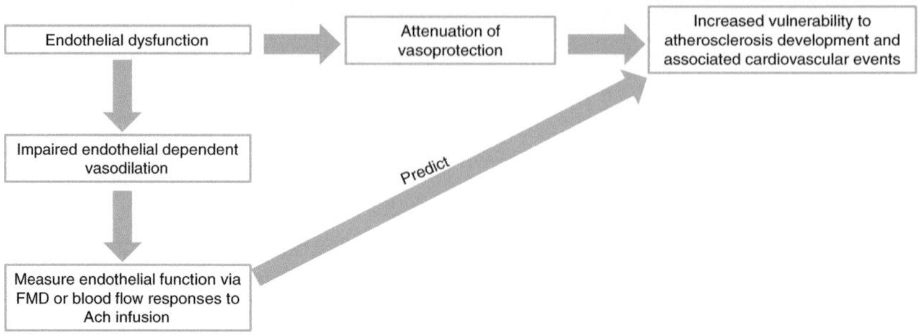

Fig. 6.3 Conceptual model summarizing how endothelial dysfunction assessed in conduit arteries (FMD) or the microvasculature (Ach infusion) provides prognostic information regarding the occurrence of cardiovascular events

disease risk (Fig. 6.3). In this section we review the evidence that endothelial-dependent dilation can predict future cardiovascular events in asymptomatic adults and those with diagnosed cardiovascular disease.

Microvascular

A smaller coronary microvascular vasodilation following Ach infusion has been shown to predict greater cardiovascular event risk in patients undergoing cardiac catheterization [45]. However invasive coronary testing is not widely performed over a range of initial levels of cardiovascular risk. Using less invasive testing of the arm microvasculature, FBF_{Ach} has been shown to predict events in patients with coronary artery disease [46, 47]. As mentioned above, reactive hyperemic flow is used as an index of limb microvascular function and likely involves a combination of endothelial-dependent and endothelial-independent vasodilatory mechanisms. In a study involving ~1500 male firefighters with a low cardiovascular risk burden and no overt cardiovascular disease at study entry, the magnitude of forearm reactive hyperemia in the first cardiac cycle following cuff occlusion was an independent predictor of cardiovascular events [48]. Finally, in a meta-analysis of 6 studies (~1600 participants with cardiovascular disease) using the peripheral arterial tonometry reactive hyperemia technique, a 1SD decrease in the natural log of the reactive hyperemia index was associated with a doubling of cardiovascular event risk, after controlling for traditional cardiovascular risk factors [49]. Taken together, these data suggest that microvascular endothelial function assessed via responses to Ach has prognostic value in patients with cardiovascular disease. Less endothelial-specific indices of microvascular function also appear to have prognostic value in asymptomatic adults and patients with cardiovascular disease.

Conduit Artery

Greater coronary conduit artery paradoxical constriction in response to infusion of Ach has been shown to predict greater cardiovascular event risk in patients undergoing catheterization [45]. However, as with microvascular testing in the coronary circulation, this invasive procedure is not performed in a wide range of populations. Brachial artery FMD is the most commonly used method in clinical research [49], and it is inversely related to the severity of coronary artery disease (larger number of coronary arteries affected = lower FMD [50]). In the absence of diagnosed disease, it has been demonstrated repeatedly that brachial artery FMD is lower in the presence of cardiovascular risk factors [51–53]. Several meta-analyses have identified that lower brachial artery FMD is associated with increased risk of cardiovascular events after adjusting for traditional risk factors [49, 54, 55]. In the most recent meta-analysis, Matsuzawa et al. [49] reported an 8% decrease in risk of a cardiovascular event for every 1% increase in FMD in individuals without cardiovascular disease at study entry. In individuals with diagnosed disease at study entry, the effect was stronger such that there was a 16% decrease in event risk for every 1% increase in FMD. Ras et al. [54] found a similar influence of initial health status. In addition, a smaller study did not identify an association between FMD and events in male firefighters free from overt cardiovascular disease and with a low cardiovascular risk factor burden at study entry [48]. Thus, while FMD appears to provide some prognostic insight in both asymptomatic adults and cardiovascular disease patients, the predictive value of endothelial function for event risk may be more robust in the latter. It is also important to note that despite efforts to standardize the FMD technique, considerable variability in FMD magnitude remains between research groups, such that what characterizes "impaired" FMD in an at-risk group in one study may be equivalent to the mean FMD value in another study's healthy control group [56]. As such, while FMD may provide useful insight regarding vascular health at the group level, there is no clear reference value for FMD suggesting that an individual is "at risk" [57].

Exercise and Endothelial Function

Exercise confers substantial cardiovascular risk reduction, although traditional risk factors cannot exclusively explain the benefits. For instance, in a prospective study of 27,055 women, <60% of physical activity-related reductions in the rate of cardiovascular events were attributed to known and novel risk factors [58]. Enhanced endothelial function may explain, in part, the remaining ~40% risk reduction [59, 60]. Indeed, aerobic training has been shown to improve microvascular and conduit artery endothelial function in clinical populations without altering traditional risk factors [61], providing support for a role of exercise in improving endothelial function through mechanisms independent of traditional risk factor reduction.

In this part of the chapter, we discuss the influence of habitual training for athletic competition on endothelial function, as well as the impact of exercise training interventions on endothelial function in young (i.e., aged 20–35 years), healthy adults and in elderly and clinical populations. While cross-sectional studies permit characterization of the impact of habitual exercise on endothelial function, they may be confounded by other factors that differ between groups (i.e., genetics, diet, sleep) that may contribute to any differences in endothelial function. Longitudinal studies (training studies) provide a greater opportunity to attribute changes in endothelial function to the training itself. However, training studies are often short in duration. After reviewing the training study evidence, we examine the influence of sex and exercise modality (i.e., aerobic versus resistance training, interval versus continuous training) on training-induced adaptations in endothelial function. Lastly, we summarize purported mechanisms whereby exercise training modulates endothelial function, focusing specifically on shear stress and oxidative stress.

Endothelial Function in Athletes

> A man is only as old as his arteries. –Dr. Thomas Sydenham (1624–1689)

Aging is accompanied by a reduction in endothelial function and associated attenuation of vasoprotection (Fig. 6.4) [62]. The rate and onset of dysfunction appear to be modifiable by habitual exercise wherein exercise mitigates and in some instances prevents the so-called vascular aging. The following sections discuss findings from cross-sectional investigations of microvascular and conduit artery endothelial function comparing master athletes to healthy, sedentary older adults.

Microvascular

Endurance-trained elderly individuals have been shown not only to have greater FBF_{Ach} compared to age-matched sedentary peers but also only slightly reduced increases in forearm blood flow compared to younger endurance-trained individuals [63]. By contrast, in sedentary middle-aged and older men, reduced increases in forearm blood flow compared to younger sedentary men have been reported [64]. The benefit of habitual training for competition (primarily endurance training) on microvascular function was recently summarized in a meta-analysis including 14 studies that assessed microvascular function using Ach infusion, post-occlusion reactive hyperemia, or heating-induced increases

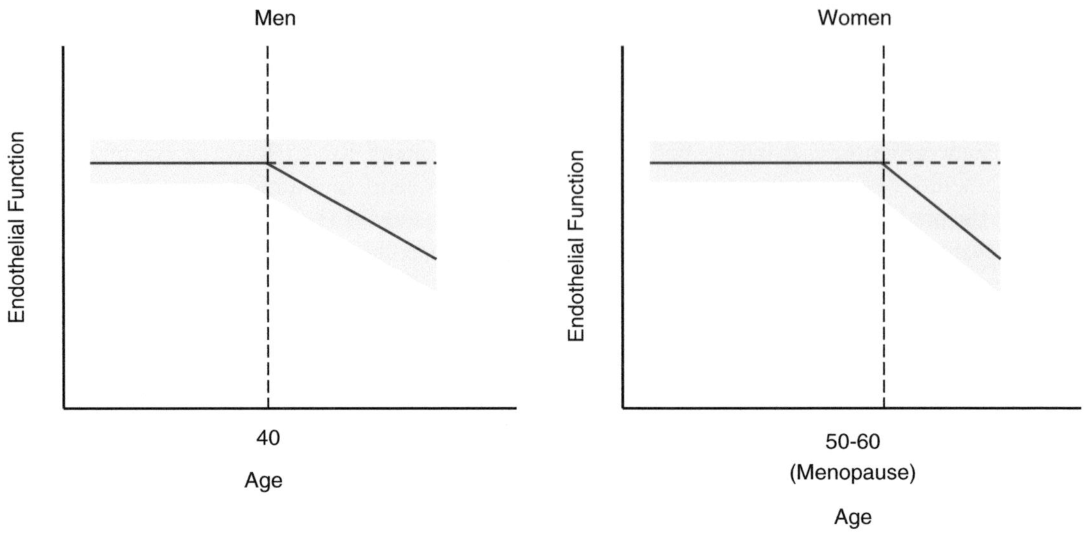

Fig. 6.4 Age-related decline in endothelial function in men and women. The age-related decline may be abrogated by habitual exercise, as depicted by the dotted line. In men, the reduction in endothelial function manifests in middle age (~40 years), while in women the reduction typically appears at the onset of menopause or in the perimenopausal phase in women not taking hormone replacement therapy. (Adapted from Celermajer et al. [62])

in blood flow. After pooling results from the 14 studies, master athletes and young athletes demonstrated enhanced microvascular vasodilatory function compared to age-matched sedentary peers [65]. Furthermore, endothelium-independent vasodilation in response to NO donors was also improved in athletes compared to controls, suggesting that the enhanced vasodilation may be attributed at least in part to the greater vascular smooth muscle response, rather than exclusive improvements in endothelial function.

As a whole, the evidence to date suggests that habitual athletic training has a beneficial effect on microvascular function that includes improvements in endothelial function specifically. It is also important to note that these findings describe the systemic influence of long-term exercise training on microvascular function. In these studies while microvascular function was typically assessed in the forearm, most athletes were endurance runners or cyclists. Thus, the benefits of exercise appear to extend beyond the exercised/trained limb.

Conduit Artery

Flow-mediated dilation begins to decrease in men in their 40s and in women at the onset of menopause (Fig. 6.4) [62]. Similar to microvascular endothelial function, FMD of endurance-trained older men has been shown to resemble that of young men, whereas sedentary aging appears to be accompanied by a lower FMD [66]. Specifically, Eskurza et al. [66] observed an FMD of ~8 ± 2% in young, sedentary men; ~5 ± 1% in old, sedentary men; and ~7 ± 2% in older, endurance-trained men, while endothelium-independent vasodilation was similar between groups. The endurance-trained men had been engaged in vigorous aerobic endurance exercise more than three times a week for more than 2 years. This suggests that exercise can prevent age-associated decreases in conduit artery endothelial function.

The impact of long-term training on conduit artery function was supported by a recent meta-analysis indicating that elderly athletes (>50 years; primarily endurance-trained men) had greater brachial artery FMD and enhanced smooth muscle function compared to sedentary peers [67]. These findings indicate that long-term training can attenuate an age-associated decline in vascular function [67]. Furthermore, these athletes primarily trained the lower limbs, such that improved brachial artery function indicates a systemic effect of the training.

However, similar to the findings in the microvasculature, because both FMD and vascular smooth muscle responses to an NO donor were enhanced in master athletes, whether the improvement in FMD is due to enhanced endothelial function or greater smooth muscle responsiveness is not entirely clear.

In the same conduit artery function meta-analysis, and in contrast to the findings in the microvasculature, neither FMD nor smooth muscle function was augmented in young athletes versus young sedentary adults [67]. The absence of group differences in young adults may relate to structural changes in the conduit arteries of young athletes (discussed in the *Exercise training and endothelial function in young, healthy humans* section). Therefore, cross-sectional evidence comparing athletes to age-matched peers suggests that the benefit of habitual training is more evident in older athletes, perhaps due to the increased risk of endothelial dysfunction with sedentary aging.

Men and postmenopausal women may not experience the same degree of exercise-induced protection against age-associated endothelial dysfunction. Although there is evidence to suggest that endurance-trained postmenopausal women have preserved FMD [68], others report that endurance-trained postmenopausal women exhibit similar FMD to sedentary postmenopausal women [69]. This suggests a potential sex-specific effect of exercise on the preservation of endothelial function; however, the benefit of habitual exercise may persist in women using hormone replacement therapy [70]. Collectively, the evidence suggests that estrogen may play a modulatory role in the exercise-associated preservation of endothelial function in women, as discussed in the *Sex differences in the effects of exercise training on endothelial function* section.

Exercise Training and Endothelial Function in Young, Healthy Adults

Studies examining the influence of exercise training on endothelial function in young, healthy adults typically involve a 4–12-week training intervention. Some studies have provided only pre- and post-training assessments, while others have performed multiple mid-training assessments to provide insight regarding the time course of adaptations. The following sections focus on the influence of aerobic exercise training.

Microvascular

A limited number of studies have investigated the effects of aerobic exercise training on microvascular function. Kingwell et al. [71] did not observe any effect of 4 weeks of cycling training on FBF_{Ach}. However, training increased the influence of NO on basal tone, as reflected by a greater reduction in FBF at rest during infusion of the eNOS inhibiter L-NMMA post-training. Interrogating the skin microvasculature, Wang [72] observed increased cutaneous perfusion in response to iontophoretically applied Ach after 8 weeks of cycling training in young, sedentary men. Shenouda et al. [73] found that peak upper and lower limb reactive hyperemia was unchanged after 6 and 12 weeks of moderate-intensity continuous training and sprint interval training in sedentary men [73]. Similarly, Currie et al. [74] found that the peak change in calf vascular conductance (indicative of microvascular vasodilation during reactive hyperemia) was unaltered after 6 days of endurance exercise training for 2 h per day. Taken together there is some evidence to suggest that microvascular endothelial function may be improved with exercise training in young, healthy humans; however, findings are mixed and may depend on the index used to assess microvascular endothelial function.

Conduit Artery

A summary of studies that have assessed FMD in young, healthy adults before and during/after an exercise training intervention is included in Table 6.1. Generally, FMD of the upper and lower limb improves with exercise training in young healthy humans, although some studies

Table 6.1 The impact of aerobic exercise training on flow-mediated dilation (FMD) in young, healthy adults. Studies that measured FMD mid-training intervention to assess the time course of adaptation are included

Author	Year	N (female)	Age	Length	Pre-training FMD	Mid- or post-training FMD
Brachial artery						
Clarkson et al. [85]	1999	25 (0)	20	10 weeks	2.2 ± 2.4%	3.9 ± 2.5%*
Tinken et al. [75]	2008	13 (0)	22 ± 2	2 weeks	5.9 ± 1.9%	9.1 ± 2.1%*
				4 weeks	5.9 ± 1.9%	8.4 ± 2.3%*
				6 weeks	5.9 ± 1.9%	7.6 ± 1.7%
				8 weeks	5.9 ± 1.9%	6.9 ± 2.4%
Birk et al. [13]	2012	11 (0)	22 ± 2	2 weeks	5.8 ± 4.1%	8.6 ± 3.8%*
				4 weeks	5.8 ± 4.1%	7.4 ± 3.5%
				8 weeks	5.8 ± 4.1%	6.0 ± 2.3%
Spence et al. [131]	2013	9 (0)	27 ± 5	6 months	5.5 ± 4.3%	7.3 ± 3.7%
Scholten et al. [86]	2014	20 (20)	32 ± 4	12 weeks	11.8 ± 3.5%	13.3 ± 3.6%*
Bailey et al. [116]	2016	9 (9)	25 ± 5	8 weeks	6.8%	8.1%*
Shenouda et al. [73]	2017	10 (0)	28 ± 9	6 weeks	9.3 ± 2.9	9.9 ± 3.9%
				12 weeks	9.3 ± 2.9	7.9 ± 2.5%
Popliteal artery						
Rakobowchuk et al. [84]	2008	10 (5)	23 ± 2	6 weeks	4.8%	7%*
Tinken et al. [75]	2008	13 (0)	22 ± 2	2 weeks	6.2 ± 2.6%	9.2 ± 2.0%*
				4 weeks	6.2 ± 2.6%	9.5 ± 2.2%*
				6 weeks	6.2 ± 2.6%	7.8 ± 1.7%*
				8 weeks	6.2 ± 2.6%	6.6 ± 2.2%
Shenouda et al. [73]	2017	10 (0)	28 ± 9	6 weeks	3.8 ± 4.5%	4.3 ± 4.1%
				12 weeks	3.8 ± 4.5%	4.6 ± 3.9
Superficial femoral artery						
Spence et al. [131]	2013	10 (0)	27 ± 5	6 months	4.5 ± 2.0%	6.4 ± 2.2%
Scholten et al. [86]	2014	20 (20)	32 ± 4	12 weeks	8.7 ± 3.2%	10.5 ± 2.8%*

Data are presented as mean ± SD, and significant difference from pre-training ($P < 0.05$) is denoted by *
FMD flow-mediated dilation

have observed that this adaptation is short lived. Several studies have reported a peak improvement in FMD that manifests after 2–4 weeks of aerobic training. Following the peak, FMD begins to return to pre-training levels such that it is no longer elevated from baseline at the sixth week of training in young, healthy men [13, 73, 75]. This pattern of FMD improvement is commonly hypothesized to be an evidence of initial functional changes that are then superseded by a structural adaptation [8, 76, 77].

It is thought that conduit artery structural adaptation in the form of expansive remodeling, wherein lumen diameter increases and wall thickness decreases [78], may serve to normalize shear stress in the face of repeated exercise-induced elevations in blood flow [77]. Shear stress is equal to the viscosity of the blood multiplied by the blood flow velocity divided by the vessel diameter (shear stress = viscosity x velocity ÷ vessel diameter) [79]. Thus, increases in vessel diameter will tend to decrease shear stress. A larger conduit artery diameter, as a result of exercise training, could decrease the stimulus for endothelial improvement during each exercise bout and/or decrease the stimulus for FMD during FMD assessment. Either of these outcomes could contribute to a regression of observed FMD improvements over time with continued training.

In animal studies, exposing an artery to chronically high shear stress causes endothelium-dependent vascular remodeling, leading to a larger arterial diameter [80, 81]. In humans there is both cross-sectional [65, 78, 82] and longitudinal evidence [73, 78, 83] to suggest that exercise training results in conduit artery remodeling to increase diameter. However, this is not always observed [13, 75, 84–86]. Indeed, studies that have observed a regression of brachial artery FMD improvement with continued training have not reported decreases in the stimulus for FMD or clear evidence of brachial artery remodeling [13, 75]. Further research is required to fully understand the interaction between functional and structural conduit artery adaptations and regression of training-induced improvements in FMD in young healthy adults.

Exercise Training and Endothelial Function in Aging and Clinical Populations

Endothelial function is typically impaired in older adults or persons with cardiovascular risk factors and disease compared to young and healthy controls. The following section addresses whether the impaired endothelial function in these populations is improved with exercise training.

Microvascular

DeSouza et al. [64] had sedentary middle-aged and older men perform 30–45 min of brisk walking 3–6 days per week for 3 months and observed a 30% improvement in FBF_{Ach}. After the training, FBF_{Ach} was similar to young adults, suggesting that age-associated endothelial dysfunction is reversible. Exercise training has also been shown to reverse cutaneous microvascular endothelial dysfunction, assessed as the increase in cutaneous vascular conductance in response to acetylcholine microdialysis infusion in sedentary elderly subjects [87]. Similarly, and as recently reviewed by Green et al. in [8], exercise has been shown to improve microvascular endothelial function in individuals with hypertension [88], type 2 diabetes [89], obesity [90], hypercholesterolemia [91], coronary artery disease [92], and heart failure [93]. Hambrecht et al. [30] trained patients with coronary artery disease six times per day for 10 min at 80% of peak heart rate for 4 weeks. After exercise training, the patients demonstrated a 78% increase in coronary artery blood flow during Ach infusion, suggesting a cardioprotective improvement in endothelial function with exercise training. However, findings have not been unanimous, and in some instances, FBF_{Ach} is unchanged after training [94, 95], perhaps reflecting irreversible endothelial dysfunction and/or insufficient training stimuli. Collectively, exercise training appears to improve limb and coronary microvascular endothelial function and potentially reverses the adverse influences of sedentary aging and/or cardiovascular risk factors and disease.

Conduit Artery

Evidence regarding FMD in populations with cardiovascular risk factors or established cardiovascular disease also supports that pre-existing endothelial dysfunction is amenable to improvement with exercise training. A meta-analysis of randomized controlled trials with FMD measured pre- and postexercise training confirmed that aerobic, resistance, and combined exercise training improves conduit artery endothelial function in participants with a wide range of cardiovascular risk factors and diagnosed disease [96]. Unlike young, healthy participants, improvements in FMD in patient groups appear to persist regardless of the duration of exercise training [96, 97]. For instance, patients with hypercholesterolemia, coronary artery disease, chronic heart failure, and type 2 diabetes demonstrated increased FMD following 8 weeks of exercise training [61]. Similarly, prolonged exercise training interventions (24 weeks) have elicited improvements in FMD in heart transplant patients [98], patients with peripheral artery disease [99], and coronary artery disease [100, 101]. Although the effects of exercise training on endothelial function in at-risk populations are promising, the duration of the training interventions performed to date has been relatively short. Longer-duration exercise interventions are required to discern whether improvements in endothelial function confer vasoprotection and decreased risk of events in populations with established risk factors and disease [57].

Sex Differences in the Effects of Exercise Training on Endothelial Function

Estrogen, like exercise, promotes enhanced endothelial function and is vasoprotective [102]. In the context of exercise training, a synergistic or additive effect of exercise and estrogen has been suggested [103]. Although young women demonstrate a lower prevalence of cardiovascular disease compared to men, once women become postmenopausal, the prevalence is similar between the two [104–107]. This corresponds to a reduction in endothelial function postmenopause (Fig. 6.4) [62, 108], suggesting a role of attenuated endothelial vasoprotection. This is supported by evidence that postmenopausal women have 3.4 times greater risk of atherosclerosis compared to similarly aged premenopausal women [109]. Indeed, endothelial function, assessed by FMD, begins to decline in the perimenopausal phase and worsens postmenopause [110]. Microvascular and conduit artery endothelial function improve with estrogen therapy, suggesting an essential role for the loss of estrogen in driving the reduction in endothelial function [111, 112].

Microvascular

In recently postmenopausal women not undertaking hormone replacement therapy (HRT) (<5 years past their final menstrual period), a 12-week high-intensity aerobic exercise training intervention improved leg vascular responses to Ach infusion, suggesting that lower limb microvascular endothelial function is amenable to improvement early postmenopause [113]. In the same cohort, high-intensity exercise training increased eNOS expression in the quadriceps muscle, demonstrating a possible mechanism whereby exercise training can improve endothelial function in recently postmenopausal women [114]. Whether this microvascular endothelial function plasticity persists later in menopause is unclear. Santos-Parker et al. [115] found that both endurance-trained (6 ± 4 years postmenopausal) and sedentary (10 ± 10 years postmenopausal) women not taking HRT displayed blunted FBF_{Ach} compared to premenopausal sedentary women. There is evidence that HRT influences the impact of training on conduit artery endothelial function (see *Conduit artery* section below). Further studies investigating whether exercise training in older postmenopausal women improves microvascular endothelial function, and whether HRT interacts with exercise training, are warranted.

Conduit Artery

There is limited evidence regarding the influence of exercise training on FMD in young women (Table 6.1). Scholten et al. [86] trained 20 women for 12 weeks (cycling) and observed an increase in brachial and superficial femoral FMD. In a shorter-duration training study, Bailey et al. [116] demonstrated an increase in brachial artery FMD after 8 weeks of a cycling intervention. Thus, young healthy women appear to demonstrate improved FMD following aerobic exercise training, although more studies are warranted. The majority of studies investigating the impact of exercise training on endothelial function in postmenopausal women have focused on conduit artery endothelial function. Pierce et al. [69] trained sedentary postmenopausal women and older men 6 days/week for 8 weeks (brisk walking). Older sedentary men, but not postmenopausal women, demonstrated improved FMD post-intervention. In support of these findings, a cross-sectional comparison of endurance-trained postmenopausal women and older men versus sedentary age-matched peers revealed that FMD was similar regardless of training status in postmenopausal women, while older endurance-trained men had superior FMD to sedentary peers [69]. Similarly, 12 weeks of walking/jogging 4 days/week did not improve FMD in a separate cohort of postmenopausal women [117]; neither did 18 weeks of resistance or aerobic training [118], 2 weeks of high-intensity interval training [119], or 12 weeks of aerobic training [117]. Importantly, the women in the aforementioned studies were not undergoing HRT.

Moreau et al. [112] investigated the role of HRT in training-induced adaptations to endothelial function. They performed a placebo-controlled trial administering postmenopausal women HRT (oral or transdermal estradiol) or placebo for 12 weeks. Women continued treatment and underwent a 12-week aerobic exercise training protocol (5–7 days/week, 65–80% max HR). Estradiol treatment alone improved FMD, and the exercise intervention resulted in a further improvement in FMD in the HRT group; however, the placebo group showed no improvement in FMD, even after exercise training. These observations suggest an obligatory role for estradiol in facilitating exercise-induced improvements in FMD in postmenopausal women. The antioxidant effects of estradiol may be relevant to the aerobic exercise-induced improvements in FMD observed in postmenopausal women on HRT. This is supported by the observations of Moreau et al. [112], who found that infusion of the antioxidant ascorbic acid had no effect on FMD in trained postmenopausal women on HRT (suggesting an absence of relevant oxidative stress), while it acutely "rescued" FMD in trained postmenopausal women not on HRT.

Not all studies have found this essential role of HRT. In contrast to the aforementioned findings, studies administering 8, 10, 16, and 24 weeks of moderate-intensity aerobic training have found improved FMD in postmenopausal women not on HRT [68, 121–124]. Further, a cross-sectional investigation showed that endurance-trained postmenopausal women not on HRT demonstrated similar FMD to younger women [68]. Postmenopausal women with additional risk factors, such as obesity, also appear to demonstrate improvement in FMD with exercise training. Swift et al. [125] assigned obese postmenopausal women (~one third taking HRT) to one of three doses of aerobic exercise training for a 6-month period and observed a similar increase in FMD among training groups, suggesting that exercise-associated improvements can occur with a variety of exercise regimens. Similarly, after 10 weeks of moderate-intensity aerobic training, Azadpour et al. [121] observed that obese postmenopausal women had an 86% improvement in FMD [121]. In agreement with these findings, compared to sedentary peers, a larger FMD response has been observed in overweight postmenopausal women who are physically active [126]. The timing of the exercise intervention (i.e., immediately postmenopausal versus late postmenopause [110, 112–114, 123]), the presence of comorbidities [125], and the intensity and duration of exercise training [118, 119, 125] appear to influence whether endothelial function can be improved with training in postmenopausal women. Further research is necessary to identify whether there is an ideal training window in the menopausal transition and to better elucidate the interactive role of estradiol and exercise on endothelial function.

Impact of Exercise Modality on Endothelial Function

Studies investigating the impact of exercise training interventions on endothelial function have adopted heterogeneous exercise programs. The following section touches briefly on the influence of aerobic exercise intensity and aerobic versus resistance training on endothelial function.

Microvascular

The influence of resistance exercise training on microvascular function has been assessed using the peak and the area under the curve of reactive hyperemia. Eight weeks of progressive resistance exercise training improved peak reactive hyperemia in older, but not young women, while the area under the curve increased in both groups [127]. By contrast, in young, healthy men, 6 weeks [128, 129] and 12 weeks [129] of resistance training increased peak and area under the curve of reactive hyperemia. Therefore, resistance training may be an effective exercise modality to improve microvascular function in postmenopausal women and young men, but less so in young healthy women, although there is limited evidence.

To assess the influence of aerobic exercise intensity on microvascular endothelial function, Goto et al. [130] assessed FBF_{Ach} before and after 12 weeks of mild- (25% VO_2 max), moderate- (50% VO_2 max), or high (75% VO_2 max)-intensity aerobic exercise training in young, healthy men. Moderate-, but not mild- nor high-intensity, training improved FBF_{Ach} [130], perhaps due to insufficient stimulus (mild intensity) or an exaggerated increased oxidative stress (high intensity). Whether the exercise intensity differentially influences the effect of exercise training in populations at increased cardiovascular risk merits future investigation.

Conduit Artery

A meta-analysis of randomized controlled trials, which implemented aerobic, resistance, or combined (aerobic and resistance) training (primarily in participants at increased cardiovascular risk), demonstrated that training improved FMD regardless of the exercise modality [96]. Thus, in populations that often present with endothelial dysfunction, FMD appears to be amenable to improvement with both resistance and aerobic training. In one study comparing the effects of 6 months of resistance versus aerobic exercise training in young, healthy men, those in the resistance training group demonstrated an improvement in FMD, while those assigned to 6 months of endurance training did not [131]. In a shorter-duration study, neither 6 nor 12 weeks of resistance training in young men improved FMD [129], suggesting that in young, healthy men, a long duration of resistance exercise training is necessary to improve FMD. These findings also suggest that resistance and aerobic training may result in a different time course of FMD adaptation in young healthy adults (improved FMD present after 6 months of training for the former but not the latter modality), but this awaits confirmation with additional studies.

The intensity of aerobic exercise may also influence the effect of training on FMD. A meta-analysis of randomized trials that investigated high-intensity interval training and moderate-intensity continuous training in populations at increased cardiovascular risk suggested that high-intensity interval training evokes a superior improvement in FMD compared to moderate-intensity continuous training [132]. Furthermore, in their meta-analysis sample comprised primarily of adults with cardiovascular or metabolic disease, Ashor et al. [96] identified a dose-dependent relationship between aerobic exercise training intensity (both relative and absolute) and the improvement in endothelial function (improvements in FMD following resistance training were predicted by exercise frequency rather than intensity). In contrast, in young, healthy adults, sprint interval training has elicited either similar or inferior improvements in FMD compared to moderate-intensity continuous training [73, 84]; one study in young, healthy adults reported that neither heavy nor moderate interval training improved FMD [133]. Therefore, the influence of aerobic exercise intensity appears to differ based on cardiovascular risk or pre-training presence of compromised endothelial function, and those at increased risk may obtain the greatest benefit from high-intensity aerobic training. A summary of studies that have assessed exercise training intervention on postmenopausal women is presented in Table 6.2.

Mechanisms of Exercise-Induced Modulation of Endothelial Function

Recent reviews of the mechanisms responsible for improved vascular function with exercise are available elsewhere [8, 76]. Briefly, the mechanisms discussed include hemodynamic stimuli including circumferential strain and shear stress, as well as changes in autonomic function and oxidative stress. Here, we will address the role of shear stress and oxidative stress in the process of exercise-induced improvements in endothelial function.

Table 6.2 The impact of exercise training on endothelial function in postmenopausal women

Author	Year	*N*	Age	Time postmenopause (years)	HRT	Length	Impact of training on endothelial function
Azadpour et al. [121]	2016	12	58 ± 4	9.9 ± 4.0	N	10 weeks	Moderate intensity aerobic training improved FMD
Akazawa et al. [122]	2012	11	59 ± 5	>2	N	8 weeks	Aerobic exercise improved FMD
Bailey et al. [123]	2016	14	52 ± 4	1–4	N	16 weeks	Moderate intensity aerobic exercise improved FMD
Black et al. [68]	2009	6	57 ± 5	NR	N	24 weeks	Moderate intensity walking and cycling improved FMD
Casey et al. [118]	2007	13	59 ± 5	8.0 ± 5.9	N	18 weeks	Resistance training did not change FMD
		10	60 ± 7	9.5 ± 6.8	N	18 weeks	Treadmill walking did not change FMD
Klonizakis et al. [119]	2014	11	64 ± 7	NR	N	2 weeks	High-intensity interval training did not change FMD
Moreau et al. [112]	2013	10	56 ± 7	8.8 ± 8.0	N	12 weeks	Brisk walking did not change FMD
		15	57 ± 4	8.5 ± 5.6	Oral E2	12 weeks	Brisk walking improved FMD
		11	57 ± 4	6.2 ± 5.1	Transdermal E2	12 weeks	Brisk walking improved FMD
Nyberg et al. [113]	2016	16	54 ± 4	3.1 ± 2	N	12 weeks	High-intensity training increased leg vascular conductance responses to Ach infusion
Nyberg et al. [114]	2017	16	54 ± 4	3.1 ± 2	N	12 weeks	High-intensity training increased leg eNOS protein content
Pierce et al. [69]	2011	15	63 ± 4	9.4 ± 6.6	N	8 weeks	Brisk walking did not change FMD
Swift et al. [125]	2012	68	57 ± 6	NR	32.4%	6 months	4 kcal/kg/week improved FMD
		32	56 ± 6	NR	37.5%	6 months	8 kcal/kg/week improved FMD
		32	56 ± 7	NR	34.4%	6 months	12 kcal/kg/week improved FMD
Swift et al. [117]	2014	8	56 ± 2	NR	N	12 weeks	Aerobic training did not change FMD
		16	57 ± 6	NR	N	12 weeks	Aerobic training did not change FMD
Yoshizawa et al. [124]	2010	10	57 ± 3	NR	N	8 weeks	Aerobic training improved FMD

Data are presented as mean ± SD
E2–17 beta estradiol, *FMD* flow-mediated dilation, *N* no, *NR* not reported

Shear Stress

Exercise increases blood flow and, as a result, the shear stress exerted on the endothelium. Large muscle mass exercise (e.g., cycling) increases shear stress not only in the vessels feeding the metabolically active muscle but also systemically. For example, cycling, walking, and leg kicking all substantially increase shear stress in the brachial artery [134]. Training studies that have prevented the exercise-associated increases in shear stress provide strong evidence for shear stress being essential to improving endothelial function (Fig. 6.5). For example, Tinken et al. [14] performed 8 weeks of bilateral handgrip exercise training, with one arm cuffed to mitigate increases in shear stress. Only the uncuffed arm demonstrated improvements in endothelial function. Similarly, Birk et al. [13] performed 8 weeks of cycle training with one forearm cuffed and the other uncuffed. The uncuffed arm demonstrated improvements in endothelial function, whereas in the cuffed arm (i.e., smaller increase in shear stress), endothelial function did not change. Collectively, the aforementioned studies implicate augmented shear stress as essential to training-induced endothelial adaptation.

To assess whether repeated increases in shear stress without exercise can induce similar endothelial adaptations, researchers have examined the impact of heat therapy/training on FMD. Heating induces a sustained increase in shear stress [135]; thus, if repeated increases in shear stress are responsible for inducing endothelial adaptations, heat therapy would be expected to improve endothelial function. Assessing local adaptations, Naylor et al. [136] performed bilateral forearm heating training for 8 weeks, cuffing one arm to mitigate the increase in shear stress. Similar to exercise, endothelial func-

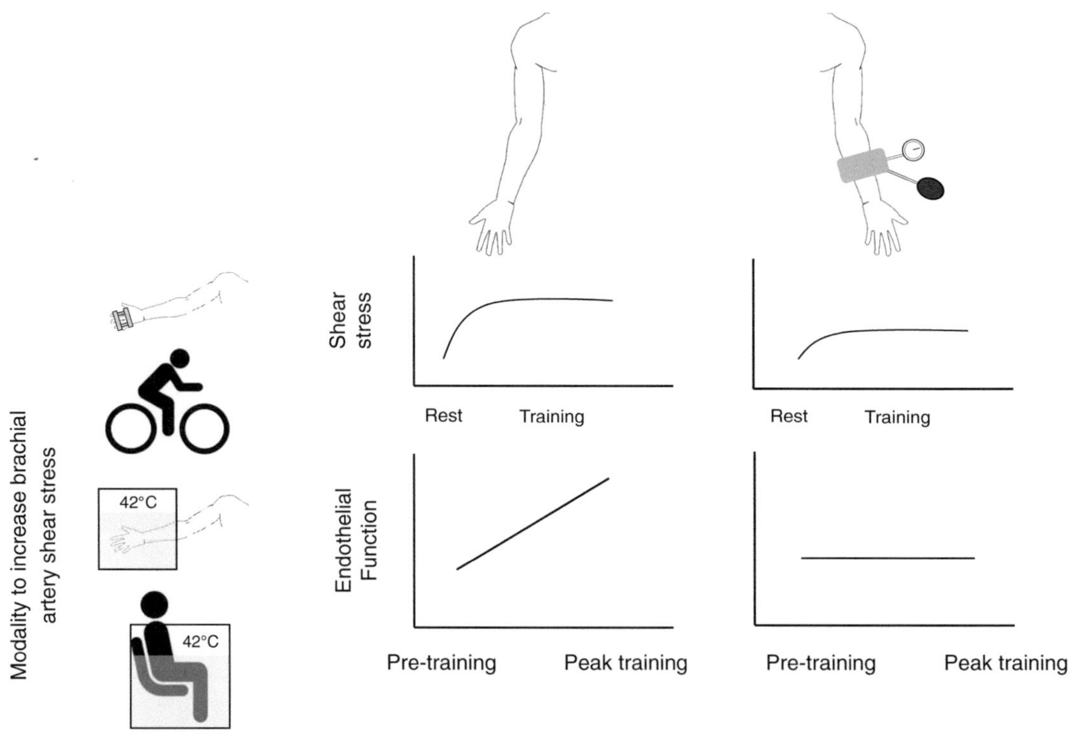

Fig. 6.5 Shear stress mediates the improvement in endothelial function and structure in young, healthy men. Investigations that have implemented a unilateral forearm cuff during training to mitigate the increase in shear stress during handgrip exercise [14], cycling [13], forearm heating [136], and lower body heating [137] have all demonstrated improved endothelial function and structure in the uncuffed arm, but not the cuffed arm. Cuffing the forearm mitigates the increase in shear stress experienced during the training sessions. As a result, flow-mediated dilation improves only in the uncuffed arm (i.e., the one exposure to training-associated increases in shear stress). (Adapted from Green et al. [8])

tion improved after 2 weeks of training in the uncuffed arm, while no changes occurred in the cuffed arm. Carter et al. [137] performed a similar study using leg heating to increase core temperature, and hence brachial artery shear stress, for an 8-week training period. The cuffed arm showed no change in FMD throughout the training period, but the uncuffed arm showed an improvement after 4 weeks. These findings have been corroborated by Brunt et al. [138], who performed 8 weeks (4–5 times/week) of hot tub therapy in young, healthy, sedentary adults. The intervention increased FMD from 5.6% to 10.9%, while also improving reactive hyperemia, indicating a simultaneous improvement in microvascular function. Further, in patients with heart failure, 3 weeks of sauna therapy improved FMD [139]. Collectively, these studies provide evidence that even in the absence of exercise, increases in shear stress facilitate endothelial adaptation.

A primary mechanism whereby shear stress improves endothelial function is via increased expression of eNOS. Two to 3 h of endothelial cell exposure to high shear stress in isolated coronary arterioles elicits an increase in eNOS mRNA expression [140, 141], and the increase in eNOS correlates with the increase in shear stress [142]. In animal models, increased eNOS protein expression has also been observed after 7–10 days of exercise training [143, 144]. An impact of training on eNOS has also been shown after 4 weeks of supervised aerobic exercise training (three times for 10 min each on a rowing and cycle ergometer daily) in patients with coronary artery disease. In internal mammary artery tissue sampled during bypass surgery, patients who had undertaken the exercise training demonstrated increased eNOS protein expression and phosphorylation [92]. Phosphorylation of the enzyme is essential for its production of NO [145, 146]. Collectively, increased eNOS expression and phosphorylation facilitate an improved NO bioavailability and, hence, endothelium-dependent vasodilation. The latter is supported by evidence that training-induced improvements in FMD are abolished after eNOS inhibition. Hornig et al. found that after 4 weeks of daily handgrip exercise training, in patients with chronic heart failure, radial artery FMD increased [147]. Inhibition of eNOS reversed the improvements in FMD, suggesting that the improvement was mediated by enhanced NO bioavailability. Whether improved NO bioavailability post-training directly results in a clinically relevant improvement in vasoprotection and reduced risk of cardiovascular events requires further study.

Oxidative Stress

At low levels reactive oxygen species (ROS) can play an important role in cell signaling [148]. Indeed, there is evidence that ROS, particularly hydrogen peroxide, can play a vasodilatory role and participate in FMD [149–151]. However, oxidative stress, a state characterized by increased ROS and reduced antioxidant defenses, reduces NO bioavailability [152]. ROS, such as superoxide, interact with NO to form peroxynitrite, preventing its vasodilatory actions [153]. Further, ROS can decrease the bioavailability of the essential cofactor for eNOS, which can lead to eNOS uncoupling, a state in which eNOS produces superoxide instead of NO [152]. Improvements in FMD with acute antioxidant administration suggest that oxidative stress is present and is impairing FMD, while a lack of change, or a decrease in FMD with antioxidant administration, suggests that a healthy ROS to antioxidant balance is present in the vasculature [148, 154].

Aging and certain disease states are associated with increased oxidative stress [155, 156] that appears to negatively influence endothelial function. This is supported by observations that acute antioxidant administration improves endothelial function in sedentary older men [63, 66, 157, 158], in estrogen-deficient postmenopausal women [112], and patients with hypertension [159], chronic obstructive pulmonary disease [160], coronary artery disease [161], and type 2 diabetes [162]. In contrast, in young healthy adults, FMD is typically not improved by antioxidant administration [66, 163], suggesting that either oxidative stress is not present or at least that it is not having a deleterious impact on endothelial function [148].

While a single bout of aerobic [164] and resistance [165] exercise increases ROS production, training has an antioxidant effect [166]. Thus, an enhanced antioxidant system with exercise training may play an integral role in improving endothelial function in populations characterized by oxidative stress, although studies directly examining this are limited. However, some evidence that an antioxidant impact of exercise plays a role in exercise-induced improvements in endothelial function is provided by both cross-sectional and intervention studies. Eskurza et al. [66] found that older sedentary men demonstrated improved FMD following antioxidant infusion, while FMD was unchanged in young or endurance-trained older men. In agreement with these observations, Donato et al. [167] found that before training, antioxidant administration improved FMD in sedentary older men, while after 6 weeks of knee-extensor training, this was no longer the case. This suggests that post-training, oxidative stress was no longer having a negative impact on endothelial function.

Conclusions (Summary Fig. 6.6)

Endothelial function plays a critical role in promoting vascular health and protecting against atherosclerosis. Endothelium-dependent vasodilation is considered to be indicative of, at least in part, NO bioavailability, and its assessment in both the microvasculature and conduit artery predicts cardiovascular event risk. In young, healthy populations, exercise training improves endothelial function, although this is sometimes reported as a transient improvement that may coincide with vascular structural remodeling. In the elderly and populations at increased cardiovascular risk, there is ample evidence that exercise training results in sustained improvement in both microvascular and conduit artery endothelial function. The improvements manifest systemically, in that they are not restricted to the exercising limb(s). Studies to date have focused primarily on endurance exercise. However there is evidence that resistance exercise also has a beneficial impact on endothelial function. Exercise-induced improvements in endothelial function appear to be due in part to improvements in NO bioavailability as a result of increased shear stress exposure and increased antioxidant defense/reduced oxidative stress. The magnitude of exercise training-induced improvements in endothelial function may relate to aerobic exercise intensity and resistance exercise session frequency [96]. Collectively, these improvements may afford cardio–/vasoprotection and contribute to exercise-induced reductions in cardiovascular event risk.

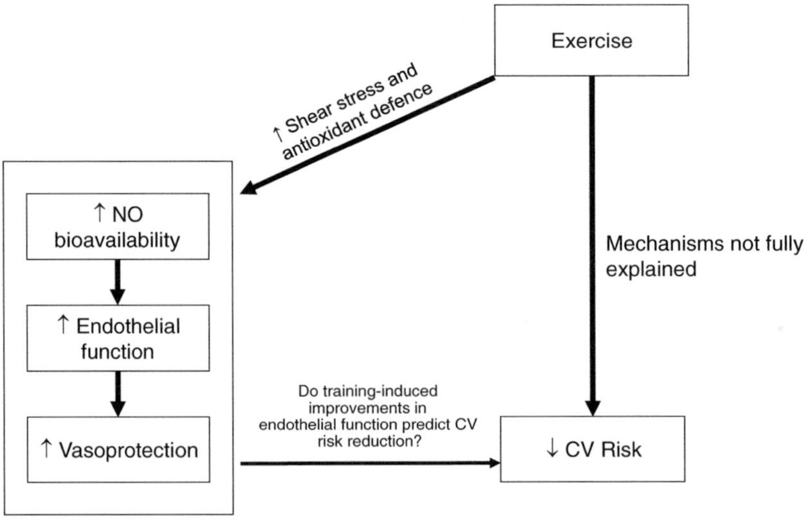

Fig. 6.6 Conceptual model summarizing how exercise could improve endothelial function and how this may translate to reduced cardiovascular event risk

References

1. Cahill PA, Redmond EM. Vascular endothelium - gatekeeper of vessel health. Atherosclerosis. 2016;248:97–109.
2. Gutierrez E, Flammer AJ, Lerman LO, Elizaga J, Lerman A, Fernandez-Aviles F. Endothelial dysfunction over the course of coronary artery disease. Eur Heart J. 2013;34(41):3175–81.
3. Tarbell JM, Pahakis MY. Mechanotransduction and the glycocalyx. J Intern Med. 2006;259(4):339–50.
4. Chatterjee S, Fisher AB. Mechanotransduction in the endothelium: role of membrane proteins and reactive oxygen species in sensing, transduction, and transmission of the signal with altered blood flow. Antioxid Redox Signal. 2014;20(6):899–913.
5. Chien S. Mechanotransduction and endothelial cell homeostasis: the wisdom of the cell. Am J Physiol Heart Circ Physiol. 2007;292(3):H1209–H24.
6. Kadohama T, Akasaka N, Nishimura K, Hoshino Y, Sasajima T, Sumpio BE. p38 Mitogen-activated protein kinase activation in endothelial cell is implicated in cell alignment and elongation induced by fluid shear stress. Endothelium. 2006;13(1):43–50.
7. Cunningham KS, Gotlieb AI. The role of shear stress in the pathogenesis of atherosclerosis. Lab Investig. 2005;85(1):9–23.
8. Green DJ, Hopman MT, Padilla J, Laughlin MH, Thijssen DH. Vascular adaptation to exercise in humans: role of hemodynamic stimuli. Physiol Rev. 2017;97(2):495–528.
9. Tanaka H, Shimizu S, Ohmori F, Muraoka Y, Kumagai M, Yoshizawa M, et al. Increases in blood flow and shear stress to nonworking limbs during incremental exercise. Med Sci Sports Exerc. 2006;38(1):81–5.
10. Simmons GH, Padilla J, Young CN, Wong BJ, Lang JA, Davis MJ, et al. Increased brachial artery retrograde shear rate at exercise onset is abolished during prolonged cycling: role of thermoregulatory vasodilation. J Appl Physiol (1985). 2011;110(2):389–97.
11. Wallace JP. Exercise in hypertension. A clinical review. Sports Med. 2003;33(8):585–98.
12. Durstine JL, Grandjean PW, Davis PG, Ferguson MA, Alderson NL, DuBose KD. Blood lipid and lipoprotein adaptations to exercise: a quantitative analysis. Sports Med. 2001;31(15):1033–62.
13. Birk GK, Dawson EA, Atkinson C, Haynes A, Cable NT, Thijssen DH, et al. Brachial artery adaptation to lower limb exercise training: role of shear stress. J Appl Physiol (1985). 2012;112(10):1653–8.
14. Tinken TM, Thijssen DH, Hopkins N, Dawson EA, Cable NT, Green DJ. Shear stress mediates endothelial adaptations to exercise training in humans. Hypertension. 2010;55(2):312–8.
15. Nigro P, Abe J, Berk BC. Flow shear stress and atherosclerosis: a matter of site specificity. Antioxid Redox Signal. 2011;15(5):1405–14.
16. Libby P, Ridker PM, Maseri A. Inflammation and atherosclerosis. Circulation. 2002;105(9):1135–43.
17. Gimbrone MA Jr, Garcia-Cardena G. Endothelial cell dysfunction and the pathobiology of atherosclerosis. Circ Res. 2016;118(4):620–36.
18. Giroud D, Li JM, Urban P, Meier B, Rutishauer W. Relation of the site of acute myocardial infarction to the most severe coronary arterial stenosis at prior angiography. Am J Cardiol. 1992;69(8):729–32.
19. Libby P. Molecular bases of the acute coronary syndromes. Circulation. 1995;91(11):2844–50.
20. Cheng C, van Haperen R, de Waard M, van Damme LC, Tempel D, Hanemaaijer L, et al. Shear stress affects the intracellular distribution of eNOS: direct demonstration by a novel in vivo technique. Blood. 2005;106(12):3691–8.
21. Cooke JP, Dzau VJ. Nitric oxide synthase: role in the genesis of vascular disease. Annu Rev Med. 1997;48:489–509.
22. Ziegler T, Bouzourene K, Harrison VJ, Brunner HR, Hayoz D. Influence of oscillatory and unidirectional flow environments on the expression of endothelin and nitric oxide synthase in cultured endothelial cells. Arterioscler Thromb Vasc Biol. 1998;18(5):686–92.
23. Lu MH, Chao CF, Tsai SH, Chen JY, Chang LT. Autocrine effects of endothelin on in vitro proliferation of vascular smooth muscle cells from spontaneously hypertensive and normotensive rats. Clin Exp Hypertens. 2006;28(5):463–74.
24. Asakura T, Karino T. Flow patterns and spatial distribution of atherosclerotic lesions in human coronary arteries. Circ Res. 1990;66(4):1045–66.
25. Chatzizisis YS, Coskun AU, Jonas M, Edelman ER, Feldman CL, Stone PH. Role of endothelial shear stress in the natural history of coronary atherosclerosis and vascular remodeling: molecular, cellular, and vascular behavior. J Am Coll Cardiol. 2007;49(25):2379–93.
26. Green DJ, Walsh JH, Maiorana A, Burke V, Taylor RR, O'Driscoll JG. Comparison of resistance and conduit vessel nitric oxide-mediated vascular function in vivo: effects of exercise training. J Appl Physiol. 2004;97(2):749–55.
27. Saternos HC, Almarghalani DA, Gibson HM, Meqdad MA, Antypas RB, Lingireddy A, et al. Distribution and function of the muscarinic receptor subtypes in the cardiovascular system. Physiol Genomics. 2018; https://doi.org/10.1152/physiolgenomics.00062.2017.
28. Ozkor MA, Murrow JR, Rahman AM, Kavtaradze N, Lin J, Manatunga A, et al. Endothelium-derived hyperpolarizing factor determines resting and stimu-

lated forearm vasodilator tone in health and in disease. Circulation. 2011;123(20):2244–53.
29. Newton DJ, Davies J, Belch JJ, Khan F. Role of endothelium-derived hyperpolarising factor in acetylcholine-mediated vasodilatation in skin. Int Angiol. 2013;32(3):312–8.
30. Hambrecht R, Wolf A, Gielen S, Linke A, Hofer J, Erbs S, et al. Effect of exercise on coronary endothelial function in patients with coronary artery disease. N Engl J Med. 2000;342(7):454–60.
31. Zeiher AM, Krause T, Schachinger V, Minners J, Moser E. Impaired endothelium-dependent vasodilation of coronary resistance vessels is associated with exercise-induced myocardial ischemia. Circulation. 1995;91(9):2345–52.
32. Duffy SJ, Castle SF, Harper RW, Meredith IT. Contribution of vasodilator prostanoids and nitric oxide to resting flow, metabolic vasodilation, and flow-mediated dilation in human coronary circulation. Circulation. 1999;100(19):1951–7.
33. Hambrecht R, Hilbrich L, Erbs S, Gielen S, Fiehn E, Schoene N, et al. Correction of endothelial dysfunction in chronic heart failure: additional effects of exercise training and oral L-arginine supplementation. J Am Coll Cardiol. 2000;35(3):706–13.
34. Kubli S, Waeber B, Dalle-Ave A, Feihl F. Reproducibility of laser Doppler imaging of skin blood flow as a tool to assess endothelial function. J Cardiovasc Pharmacol. 2000;36(5):640–8.
35. Bruno RM, Gori T, Ghiadoni L. Endothelial function testing and cardiovascular disease: focus on peripheral arterial tonometry. Vasc Health Risk Manag. 2014;10:577–84.
36. Thijssen DH, Black MA, Pyke KE, Padilla J, Atkinson G, Harris RA, et al. Assessment of flow-mediated dilation in humans: a methodological and physiological guideline. Am J Physiol Heart Circ Physiol. 2011;300(1):H2–12.
37. Green DJ, Dawson EA, Groenewoud HM, Jones H, Thijssen DH. Is flow-mediated dilation nitric oxide mediated?: a meta-analysis. Hypertension. 2014;63(2):376–82.
38. Wray DW, Witman MA, Ives SJ, McDaniel J, Fjeldstad AS, Trinity JD, et al. Progressive handgrip exercise: evidence of nitric oxide-dependent vasodilation and blood flow regulation in humans. Am J Physiol Heart Circ Physiol. 2011;300(3):H1101–H7.
39. Bellien J, Iacob M, Gutierrez L, Isabelle M, Lahary A, Thuillez C, et al. Crucial role of NO and endothelium-derived hyperpolarizing factor in human sustained conduit artery flow-mediated dilatation. Hypertension. 2006;48(6):1088–94.
40. Celermajer DS, Sorensen KE, Gooch VM, Spiegelhalter DJ, Miller OI, Sullivan ID, et al. Non-invasive detection of endothelial dysfunction in children and adults at risk of atherosclerosis. Lancet. 1992;340(8828):1111–5.
41. Tremblay JC, Pyke KE. Flow-mediated dilation stimulated by sustained increases in shear stress: a useful tool for assessing endothelial function in humans? Am J Physiol Heart Circ Physiol. 2018; https://doi.org/10.1152/ajpheart.00534.2017.
42. Vallbracht-Israng KB, Morguet A, Schwimmbeck PL. Correlation of epicardial and systemic flow-mediated vasodilation in patients with atypical angina but no evidence of atherosclerotic disease. Can J Cardiol. 2007;23(13):1054–60.
43. Takase B, Uehata A, Akima T, Nagai T, Nishioka T, Hamabe A, et al. Endothelium-dependent flow-mediated vasodilation in coronary and brachial arteries in suspected coronary artery disease. Am J Cardiol. 1998;82(12):1535–8.
44. Corretti MC, Anderson TJ, Benjamin EJ, Celermajer D, Charbonneau F, Creager MA, et al. Guidelines for the ultrasound assessment of endothelial-dependent flow-mediated vasodilation of the brachial artery: a report of the International Brachial Artery Reactivity Task Force. J Am Coll Cardiol. 2002;39(2):257–65.
45. Halcox JP, Schenke WH, Zalos G, Mincemoyer R, Prasad A, Waclawiw MA, et al. Prognostic value of coronary vascular endothelial dysfunction. Circulation. 2002;106(6):653–8.
46. Fichtlscherer S, Breuer S, Zeiher AM. Prognostic value of systemic endothelial dysfunction in patients with acute coronary syndromes: further evidence for the existence of the "vulnerable" patient. Circulation. 2004;110(14):1926–32.
47. Heitzer T, Schlinzig T, Krohn K, Meinertz T, Munzel T. Endothelial dysfunction, oxidative stress, and risk of cardiovascular events in patients with coronary artery disease. Circulation. 2001;104(22):2673–8.
48. Anderson TJ, Charbonneau F, Title LM, Buithieu J, Rose MS, Conradson H, et al. Microvascular function predicts cardiovascular events in primary prevention: long-term results from the Firefighters and Their Endothelium (FATE) study. Circulation. 2011;123(2):163–9.
49. Matsuzawa Y, Kwon TG, Lennon RJ, Lerman LO, Lerman A. Prognostic value of flow-mediated vasodilation in brachial artery and fingertip artery for cardiovascular events: a systematic review and meta-analysis. J Am Heart Assoc. 2015;4(11):e002270.
50. Neunteufl T, Katzenschlager R, Hassan A, Klaar U, Schwarzacher S, Glogar D, et al. Systemic endothelial dysfunction is related to the extent and severity of coronary artery disease. Atherosclerosis. 1997;129(1):111–8.
51. Poredos P, Orehek M, Tratnik E. Smoking is associated with dose-related increase of intima-media thickness and endothelial dysfunction. Angiology. 1999;50(3):201–8.
52. Meyer AA, Kundt G, Steiner M, Schuff-Werner P, Kienast W. Impaired flow-mediated vasodilation, carotid artery intima-media thickening, and elevated endothelial plasma markers in obese children: the impact of cardiovascular risk factors. Pediatrics. 2006;117(5):1560–7.
53. Imamura M, Biro S, Kihara T, Yoshifuku S, Takasaki K, Otsuji Y, et al. Repeated thermal therapy improves impaired vascular endothelial function in patients

with coronary risk factors. J Am Coll Cardiol. 2001;38(4):1083–8.
54. Ras RT, Streppel MT, Draijer R, Zock PL. Flow-mediated dilation and cardiovascular risk prediction: a systematic review with meta-analysis. Int J Cardiol. 2013;168(1):344–51.
55. Inaba Y, Chen JA, Bergmann SR. Prediction of future cardiovascular outcomes by flow-mediated vasodilatation of brachial artery: a meta-analysis. Int J Cardiovasc Imaging. 2010;26(6):631–40.
56. Pyke KE, Tschakovsky ME. The relationship between shear stress and flow-mediated dilatation: implications for the assessment of endothelial function. J Physiol. 2005;568(Pt 2):357–69.
57. Vlachopoulos C, Xaplanteris P, Aboyans V, Brodmann M, Cifkova R, Cosentino F, et al. The role of vascular biomarkers for primary and secondary prevention. A position paper from the European Society of Cardiology Working Group on peripheral circulation: endorsed by the Association for Research into Arterial Structure and Physiology (ARTERY) Society. Atherosclerosis. 2015;241(2):507–32.
58. Mora S, Cook N, Buring JE, Ridker PM, Lee IM. Physical activity and reduced risk of cardiovascular events: potential mediating mechanisms. Circulation. 2007;116(19):2110–8.
59. Green DJ, O'Driscoll G, Joyner MJ, Cable NT. Exercise and cardiovascular risk reduction: time to update the rationale for exercise? J Appl Physiol (1985). 2008;105(2):766–8.
60. Joyner MJ, Green DJ. Exercise protects the cardiovascular system: effects beyond traditional risk factors. J Physiol. 2009;587(Pt 23):5551–8.
61. Green DJ, Walsh JH, Maiorana A, Best MJ, Taylor RR, O'Driscoll JG. Exercise-induced improvement in endothelial dysfunction is not mediated by changes in CV risk factors: pooled analysis of diverse patient populations. Am J Physiol Heart Circ Physiol. 2003;285(6):H2679–87.
62. Celermajer DS, Sorensen KE, Spiegelhalter DJ, Georgakopoulos D, Robinson J, Deanfield JE. Aging is associated with endothelial dysfunction in healthy men years before the age-related decline in women. J Am Coll Cardiol. 1994;24(2):471–6.
63. Taddei S, Galetta F, Virdis A, Ghiadoni L, Salvetti G, Franzoni F, et al. Physical activity prevents age-related impairment in nitric oxide availability in elderly athletes. Circulation. 2000;101(25):2896–901.
64. DeSouza CA, Shapiro LF, Clevenger CM, Dinenno FA, Monahan KD, Tanaka H, et al. Regular aerobic exercise prevents and restores age-related declines in endothelium-dependent vasodilation in healthy men. Circulation. 2000;102(12):1351–7.
65. Montero D, Walther G, Diaz-Canestro C, Pyke KE, Padilla J. Microvascular dilator function in athletes: a systematic review and meta-analysis. Med Sci Sports Exerc. 2015;47(7):1485–94.
66. Eskurza I, Monahan KD, Robinson JA, Seals DR. Effect of acute and chronic ascorbic acid on flow-mediated dilatation with sedentary and physically active human ageing. J Physiol. 2004;556(Pt 1):315–24.
67. Montero D, Padilla J, Diaz-Canestro C, Muris DM, Pyke KE, Obert P, et al. Flow-mediated dilation in athletes: influence of aging. Med Sci Sports Exerc. 2014;46(11):2148–58.
68. Black MA, Cable NT, Thijssen DH, Green DJ. Impact of age, sex, and exercise on brachial artery flow-mediated dilatation. Am J Physiol Heart Circ Physiol. 2009;297(3):H1109–16.
69. Pierce GL, Eskurza I, Walker AE, Fay TN, Seals DR. Sex-specific effects of habitual aerobic exercise on brachial artery flow-mediated dilation in middle-aged and older adults. Clin Sci (Lond). 2011;120(1):13–23.
70. Hagmar M, Eriksson MJ, Lindholm C, Schenck-Gustafsson K, Hirschberg AL. Endothelial function in post-menopausal former elite athletes. Clin J Sport Med. 2006;16(3):247–52.
71. Kingwell BA, Sherrard B, Jennings GL, Dart AM. Four weeks of cycle training increases basal production of nitric oxide from the forearm. Am J Phys. 1997;272(3 Pt 2):H1070–7.
72. Wang JS. Effects of exercise training and detraining on cutaneous microvascular function in man: the regulatory role of endothelium-dependent dilation in skin vasculature. Eur J Appl Physiol. 2005;93(4):429–34.
73. Shenouda N, Gillen JB, Gibala MJ, MacDonald MJ. Changes in brachial artery endothelial function and resting diameter with moderate-intensity continuous but not sprint interval training in sedentary men. J Appl Physiol (1985). 2017;123(4):773–80.
74. Currie KD, Thomas SG, Goodman JM. Effects of short-term endurance exercise training on vascular function in young males. Eur J Appl Physiol. 2009;107(2):211–8.
75. Tinken TM, Thijssen DH, Black MA, Cable NT, Green DJ. Time course of change in vasodilator function and capacity in response to exercise training in humans. J Physiol. 2008;586(20):5003–12.
76. Green DJ, Smith KJ. Effects of exercise on vascular function, structure, and health in humans. Cold Spring Harb Perspect Med. 2018;8(4):a029819.
77. Laughlin MH. Endothelium-mediated control of coronary vascular tone after chronic exercise training. Med Sci Sports Exerc. 1995;27(8):1135–44.
78. Dinenno FA, Tanaka H, Monahan KD, Clevenger CM, Eskurza I, DeSouza CA, et al. Regular endurance exercise induces expansive arterial remodelling in the trained limbs of healthy men. J Physiol. 2001;534(Pt 1):287–95.
79. Gnasso A, Carallo C, Irace C, De Franceschi MS, Mattioli PL, Motti C, et al. Association between wall shear stress and flow-mediated vasodilation in healthy men. Atherosclerosis. 2001;156(1):171–6.
80. Kamiya A, Togawa T. Adaptive regulation of wall shear stress to flow change in the canine carotid artery. Am J Phys. 1980;239(1):H14–21.

81. Tronc F, Wassef M, Esposito B, Henrion D, Glagov S, Tedgui A. Role of NO in flow-induced remodeling of the rabbit common carotid artery. Arterioscler Thromb Vasc Biol. 1996;16(10):1256–62.
82. Rowley NJ, Dawson EA, Birk GK, Cable NT, George K, Whyte G, et al. Exercise and arterial adaptation in humans: uncoupling localized and systemic effects. J Appl Physiol (1985). 2011;110(5):1190–5.
83. Miyachi M, Tanaka H, Yamamoto K, Yoshioka A, Takahashi K, Onodera S. Effects of one-legged endurance training on femoral arterial and venous size in healthy humans. J Appl Physiol (1985). 2001;90(6):2439–44.
84. Rakobowchuk M, Tanguay S, Burgomaster KA, Howarth KR, Gibala MJ, MacDonald MJ. Sprint interval and traditional endurance training induce similar improvements in peripheral arterial stiffness and flow-mediated dilation in healthy humans. Am J Physiol Regul Integr Comp Physiol. 2008;295(1):R236–42.
85. Clarkson P, Montgomery HE, Mullen MJ, Donald AE, Powe AJ, Bull T, et al. Exercise training enhances endothelial function in young men. J Am Coll Cardiol. 1999;33(5):1379–85.
86. Scholten RR, Spaanderman ME, Green DJ, Hopman MT, Thijssen DH. Retrograde shear rate in formerly preeclamptic and healthy women before and after exercise training: relationship with endothelial function. Am J Physiol Heart Circ Physiol. 2014;307(3):H418–25.
87. Black MA, Green DJ, Cable NT. Exercise prevents age-related decline in nitric-oxide-mediated vasodilator function in cutaneous microvessels. J Physiol. 2008;586(14):3511–24.
88. Higashi Y, Sasaki S, Kurisu S, Yoshimizu A, Sasaki N, Matsuura H, et al. Regular aerobic exercise augments endothelium-dependent vascular relaxation in normotensive as well as hypertensive subjects: role of endothelium-derived nitric oxide. Circulation. 1999;100(11):1194–202.
89. Maiorana A, O'Driscoll G, Cheetham C, Dembo L, Stanton K, Goodman C, et al. The effect of combined aerobic and resistance exercise training on vascular function in type 2 diabetes. J Am Coll Cardiol. 2001;38(3):860–6.
90. Mestek ML, Westby CM, Van Guilder GP, Greiner JJ, Stauffer BL, DeSouza CA. Regular aerobic exercise, without weight loss, improves endothelium-dependent vasodilation in overweight and obese adults. Obesity (Silver Spring). 2010;18(8):1667–9.
91. Walsh JH, Yong G, Cheetham C, Watts GF, O'Driscoll GJ, Taylor RR, et al. Effects of exercise training on conduit and resistance vessel function in treated and untreated hypercholesterolaemic subjects. Eur Heart J. 2003;24(18):1681–9.
92. Hambrecht R, Adams V, Erbs S, Linke A, Krankel N, Shu Y, et al. Regular physical activity improves endothelial function in patients with coronary artery disease by increasing phosphorylation of endothelial nitric oxide synthase. Circulation. 2003;107(25):3152–8.
93. Hambrecht R, Fiehn E, Weigl C, Gielen S, Hamann C, Kaiser R, et al. Regular physical exercise corrects endothelial dysfunction and improves exercise capacity in patients with chronic heart failure. Circulation. 1998;98(24):2709–15.
94. Lewis TV, Dart AM, Chin-Dusting JP, Kingwell BA. Exercise training increases basal nitric oxide production from the forearm in hypercholesterolemic patients. Arterioscler Thromb Vasc Biol. 1999;19(11):2782–7.
95. Allemann Y, Vetter C, Kartal N, Eyer S, Stengel SM, Saner H, et al. Effect of mild endurance exercise training and pravastatin on peripheral vasodilatation of forearm resistance vessels in patients with coronary artery disease. Eur J Cardiovasc Prev Rehabil. 2005;12(4):332–40.
96. Ashor AW, Lara J, Siervo M, Celis-Morales C, Oggioni C, Jakovljevic DG, et al. Exercise modalities and endothelial function: a systematic review and dose-response meta-analysis of randomized controlled trials. Sports Med. 2015;45(2):279–96.
97. Schreuder TH, Green DJ, Nyakayiru J, Hopman MT, Thijssen DH. Time-course of vascular adaptations during 8 weeks of exercise training in subjects with type 2 diabetes and middle-aged controls. Eur J Appl Physiol. 2015;115(1):187–96.
98. Schmidt A, Pleiner J, Bayerle-Eder M, Wiesinger GF, Rodler S, Quittan M, et al. Regular physical exercise improves endothelial function in heart transplant recipients. Clin Transpl. 2002;16(2):137–43.
99. McDermott MM, Ades P, Guralnik JM, Dyer A, Ferrucci L, Liu K, et al. Treadmill exercise and resistance training in patients with peripheral arterial disease with and without intermittent claudication: a randomized controlled trial. JAMA. 2009;301(2):165–74.
100. Desch S, Sonnabend M, Niebauer J, Sixt S, Sareban M, Eitel I, et al. Effects of physical exercise versus rosiglitazone on endothelial function in coronary artery disease patients with prediabetes. Diabetes Obes Metab. 2010;12(9):825–8.
101. Munk PS, Staal EM, Butt N, Isaksen K, Larsen AI. High-intensity interval training may reduce in-stent restenosis following percutaneous coronary intervention with stent implantation: A randomized controlled trial evaluating the relationship to endothelial function and inflammation. Am Heart J. 2009;158(5):734–41.
102. Xing D, Nozell S, Chen YF, Hage F, Oparil S. Estrogen and mechanisms of vascular protection. Arterioscler Thromb Vasc Biol. 2009;29(3):289–95.
103. Green DJ, Hopkins ND, Jones H, Thijssen DH, Eijsvogels TM, Yeap BB. Sex differences in vascular endothelial function and health in humans: impacts of exercise. Exp Physiol. 2016;101(2):230–42.
104. Kannel WB, Hjortland MC, McNamara PM, Gordon T. Menopause and risk of cardiovascular

disease: the Framingham study. Ann Intern Med. 1976;85(4):447–52.
105. Gordon T, Kannel WB, Hjortland MC, McNamara PM. Menopause and coronary heart disease. The Framingham Study. Ann Intern Med. 1978;89(2):157–61.
106. Lerner DJ, Kannel WB. Patterns of coronary heart disease morbidity and mortality in the sexes: a 26-year follow-up of the Framingham population. Am Heart J. 1986;111(2):383–90.
107. Colditz GA, Willett WC, Stampfer MJ, Rosner B, Speizer FE, Hennekens CH. Menopause and the risk of coronary heart disease in women. N Engl J Med. 1987;316(18):1105–10.
108. Taddei S, Virdis A, Ghiadoni L, Mattei P, Sudano I, Bernini G, et al. Menopause is associated with endothelial dysfunction in women. Hypertension. 1996;28(4):576–82.
109. Witteman JC, Grobbee DE, Kok FJ, Hofman A, Valkenburg HA. Increased risk of atherosclerosis in women after the menopause. BMJ. 1989;298(6674):642–4.
110. Moreau KL, Hildreth KL, Meditz AL, Deane KD, Kohrt WM. Endothelial function is impaired across the stages of the menopause transition in healthy women. J Clin Endocrinol Metab. 2012;97(12):4692–700.
111. Virdis A, Ghiadoni L, Pinto S, Lombardo M, Petraglia F, Gennazzani A, et al. Mechanisms responsible for endothelial dysfunction associated with acute estrogen deprivation in normotensive women. Circulation. 2000;101(19):2258–63.
112. Moreau KL, Stauffer BL, Kohrt WM, Seals DR. Essential role of estrogen for improvements in vascular endothelial function with endurance exercise in postmenopausal women. J Clin Endocrinol Metab. 2013;98(11):4507–15.
113. Nyberg M, Egelund J, Mandrup CM, Nielsen MB, Mogensen AS, Stallknecht B, et al. Early postmenopausal phase is associated with reduced prostacyclin-induced vasodilation that is reversed by exercise training: the Copenhagen Women Study. Hypertension. 2016;68(4):1011–20.
114. Nyberg M, Egelund J, Mandrup CM, Andersen CB, Hansen K, Hergel IF, et al. Leg vascular and skeletal muscle mitochondrial adaptations to aerobic high-intensity exercise training are enhanced in the early postmenopausal phase. J Physiol. 2017;595(9):2969–83.
115. Santos-Parker JR, Strahler TR, Vorwald VM, Pierce GL, Seals DR. Habitual aerobic exercise does not protect against micro- or macrovascular endothelial dysfunction in healthy estrogen-deficient postmenopausal women. J Appl Physiol (1985). 2017;122(1):11–9.
116. Bailey TG, Cable NT, Miller GD, Sprung VS, Low DA, Jones H. Repeated warm water immersion induces similar cerebrovascular adaptations to 8 weeks of moderate-intensity exercise training in females. Int J Sports Med. 2016;37(10):757–65.
117. Swift DL, Weltman JY, Patrie JT, Saliba SA, Gaesser GA, Barrett EJ, et al. Predictors of improvement in endothelial function after exercise training in a diverse sample of postmenopausal women. J Womens Health (Larchmt). 2014;23(3):260–6.
118. Casey DP, Pierce GL, Howe KS, Mering MC, Braith RW. Effect of resistance training on arterial wave reflection and brachial artery reactivity in normotensive postmenopausal women. Eur J Appl Physiol. 2007;100(4):403–8.
119. Klonizakis M, Moss J, Gilbert S, Broom D, Foster J, Tew GA. Low-volume high-intensity interval training rapidly improves cardiopulmonary function in postmenopausal women. Menopause. 2014;21(10):1099–105.
120. Moreau KL, Ozemek C. Vascular adaptations to habitual exercise in older adults: time for the sex talk. Exerc Sport Sci Rev. 2017;45(2):116–23.
121. Azadpour N, Tartibian B, Kosar SN. Effects of aerobic exercise training on ACE and ADRB2 gene expression, plasma angiotensin II level, and flow-mediated dilation: a study on obese postmenopausal women with prehypertension. Menopause. 2017;24(3):269–77.
122. Akazawa N, Choi Y, Miyaki A, Tanabe Y, Sugawara J, Ajisaka R, et al. Curcumin ingestion and exercise training improve vascular endothelial function in postmenopausal women. Nutr Res. 2012;32(10):795–9.
123. Bailey TG, Cable NT, Aziz N, Dobson R, Sprung VS, Low DA, et al. Exercise training reduces the frequency of menopausal hot flushes by improving thermoregulatory control. Menopause. 2016;23(7):708–18.
124. Yoshizawa M, Maeda S, Miyaki A, Misono M, Choi Y, Shimojo N, et al. Additive beneficial effects of lactotripeptides intake with regular exercise on endothelium-dependent dilatation in postmenopausal women. Am J Hypertens. 2010;23(4):368–72.
125. Swift DL, Earnest CP, Blair SN, Church TS. The effect of different doses of aerobic exercise training on endothelial function in postmenopausal women with elevated blood pressure: results from the DREW study. Br J Sports Med. 2012;46(10):753–8.
126. Sanders K, Maresh CM, Ballard KD, Creighton BC, Pryor JL, Kraemer WJ, et al. Habitual exercise may maintain endothelium-dependent dilation in overweight postmenopausal women. J Aging Phys Act. 2015;23(1):40–6.
127. Rossow LM, Fahs CA, Thiebaud RS, Loenneke JP, Kim D, Mouser JG, et al. Arterial stiffness and blood flow adaptations following eight weeks of resistance exercise training in young and older women. Exp Gerontol. 2014;53:48–56.
128. Heffernan KS, Fahs CA, Iwamoto GA, Jae SY, Wilund KR, Woods JA, et al. Resistance exercise training reduces central blood pressure and improves microvascular function in African American and white men. Atherosclerosis. 2009;207(1):220–6.

129. Rakobowchuk M, McGowan CL, de Groot PC, Hartman JW, Phillips SM, MacDonald MJ. Endothelial function of young healthy males following whole body resistance training. J Appl Physiol (1985). 2005;98(6):2185–90.
130. Goto C, Higashi Y, Kimura M, Noma K, Hara K, Nakagawa K, et al. Effect of different intensities of exercise on endothelium-dependent vasodilation in humans: role of endothelium-dependent nitric oxide and oxidative stress. Circulation. 2003;108(5):530–5.
131. Spence AL, Carter HH, Naylor LH, Green DJ. A prospective randomized longitudinal study involving 6 months of endurance or resistance exercise. Conduit artery adaptation in humans. J Physiol. 2013;591(5):1265–75.
132. Ramos JS, Dalleck LC, Tjonna AE, Beetham KS, Coombes JS. The impact of high-intensity interval training versus moderate-intensity continuous training on vascular function: a systematic review and meta-analysis. Sports Med. 2015;45(5):679–92.
133. Rakobowchuk M, Harris E, Taylor A, Baliga V, Cubbon RM, Rossiter HB, et al. Heavy and moderate interval exercise training alters low-flow-mediated constriction but does not increase circulating progenitor cells in healthy humans. Exp Physiol. 2012;97(3):375–85.
134. Thijssen DH, Dawson EA, Black MA, Hopman MT, Cable NT, Green DJ. Brachial artery blood flow responses to different modalities of lower limb exercise. Med Sci Sports Exerc. 2009;41(5):1072–9.
135. Pyke KE, Dwyer EM, Tschakovsky ME. Impact of controlling shear rate on flow-mediated dilation responses in the brachial artery of humans. J Appl Physiol (1985). 2004;97(2):499–508.
136. Naylor LH, Carter H, FitzSimons MG, Cable NT, Thijssen DH, Green DJ. Repeated increases in blood flow, independent of exercise, enhance conduit artery vasodilator function in humans. Am J Physiol Heart Circ Physiol. 2011;300(2):H664–9.
137. Carter HH, Spence AL, Atkinson CL, Pugh CJ, Naylor LH, Green DJ. Repeated core temperature elevation induces conduit artery adaptation in humans. Eur J Appl Physiol. 2014;114(4):859–65.
138. Brunt VE, Howard MJ, Francisco MA, Ely BR, Minson CT. Passive heat therapy improves endothelial function, arterial stiffness and blood pressure in sedentary humans. J Physiol. 2016;594(18):5329–42.
139. Ohori T, Nozawa T, Ihori H, Shida T, Sobajima M, Matsuki A, et al. Effect of repeated sauna treatment on exercise tolerance and endothelial function in patients with chronic heart failure. Am J Cardiol. 2012;109(1):100–4.
140. Uematsu M, Ohara Y, Navas JP, Nishida K, Murphy TJ, Alexander RW, et al. Regulation of endothelial cell nitric oxide synthase mRNA expression by shear stress. Am J Phys. 1995;269(6 Pt 1):C1371–8.
141. Woodman CR, Muller JM, Rush JW, Laughlin MH, Price EM. Flow regulation of ecNOS and Cu/Zn SOD mRNA expression in porcine coronary arterioles. Am J Phys. 1999;276(3 Pt 2):H1058–63.
142. Tuttle JL, Nachreiner RD, Bhuller AS, Condict KW, Connors BA, Herring BP, et al. Shear level influences resistance artery remodeling: wall dimensions, cell density, and eNOS expression. Am J Physiol Heart Circ Physiol. 2001;281(3):H1380–9.
143. Wang J, Wolin MS, Hintze TH. Chronic exercise enhances endothelium-mediated dilation of epicardial coronary artery in conscious dogs. Circ Res. 1993;73(5):829–38.
144. Sessa WC, Pritchard K, Seyedi N, Wang J, Hintze TH. Chronic exercise in dogs increases coronary vascular nitric oxide production and endothelial cell nitric oxide synthase gene expression. Circ Res. 1994;74(2):349–53.
145. Dimmeler S, Fleming I, Fisslthaler B, Hermann C, Busse R, Zeiher AM. Activation of nitric oxide synthase in endothelial cells by Akt-dependent phosphorylation. Nature. 1999;399(6736):601–5.
146. Gallis B, Corthals GL, Goodlett DR, Ueba H, Kim F, Presnell SR, et al. Identification of flow-dependent endothelial nitric-oxide synthase phosphorylation sites by mass spectrometry and regulation of phosphorylation and nitric oxide production by the phosphatidylinositol 3-kinase inhibitor LY294002. J Biol Chem. 1999;274(42):30101–8.
147. Hornig B, Maier V, Drexler H. Physical training improves endothelial function in patients with chronic heart failure. Circulation. 1996;93(2):210–4.
148. Trinity JD, Broxterman RM, Richardson RS. Regulation of exercise blood flow: role of free radicals. Free Radic Biol Med. 2016;98:90–102.
149. Cai H. Hydrogen peroxide regulation of endothelial function: origins, mechanisms, and consequences. Cardiovasc Res. 2005;68(1):26–36.
150. Liu Y, Bubolz AH, Mendoza S, Zhang DX, Gutterman DD. H2O2 is the transferrable factor mediating flow-induced dilation in human coronary arterioles. Circ Res. 2011;108(5):566–73.
151. Liu Y, Zhao H, Li H, Kalyanaraman B, Nicolosi AC, Gutterman DD. Mitochondrial sources of H2O2 generation play a key role in flow-mediated dilation in human coronary resistance arteries. Circ Res. 2003;93(6):573–80.
152. Cai H, Harrison DG. Endothelial dysfunction in cardiovascular diseases: the role of oxidant stress. Circ Res. 2000;87(10):840–4.
153. Gryglewski RJ, Palmer RM, Moncada S. Superoxide anion is involved in the breakdown of endothelium-derived vascular relaxing factor. Nature. 1986;320(6061):454–6.
154. Trinity JD, Wray DW, Witman MA, Layec G, Barrett-O'Keefe Z, Ives SJ, et al. Ascorbic acid improves brachial artery vasodilation during progressive handgrip exercise in the elderly through a nitric oxide-mediated mechanism. Am J Physiol Heart Circ Physiol. 2016;310(6):H765–74.
155. Madamanchi NR, Vendrov A, Runge MS. Oxidative stress and vascular disease. Arterioscler Thromb Vasc Biol. 2005;25(1):29–38.

156. Kregel KC, Zhang HJ. An integrated view of oxidative stress in aging: basic mechanisms, functional effects, and pathological considerations. Am J Physiol Regul Integr Comp Physiol. 2007;292(1):R18–36.
157. Kirby BS, Voyles WF, Simpson CB, Carlson RE, Schrage WG, Dinenno FA. Endothelium-dependent vasodilatation and exercise hyperaemia in ageing humans: impact of acute ascorbic acid administration. J Physiol. 2009;587(Pt 9):1989–2003.
158. Wray DW, Nishiyama SK, Harris RA, Zhao J, McDaniel J, Fjeldstad AS, et al. Acute reversal of endothelial dysfunction in the elderly after antioxidant consumption. Hypertension. 2012;59(4):818–24.
159. Taddei S, Virdis A, Ghiadoni L, Salvetti G, Bernini G, Magagna A, et al. Age-related reduction of NO availability and oxidative stress in humans. Hypertension. 2001;38(2):274–9.
160. Ives SJ, Harris RA, Witman MA, Fjeldstad AS, Garten RS, McDaniel J, et al. Vascular dysfunction and chronic obstructive pulmonary disease: the role of redox balance. Hypertension. 2014;63(3):459–67.
161. Levine GN, Frei B, Koulouris SN, Gerhard MD, Keaney JF Jr, Vita JA. Ascorbic acid reverses endothelial vasomotor dysfunction in patients with coronary artery disease. Circulation. 1996;93(6):1107–13.
162. Ting HH, Timimi FK, Boles KS, Creager SJ, Ganz P, Creager MA. Vitamin C improves endothelium-dependent vasodilation in patients with non-insulin-dependent diabetes mellitus. J Clin Invest. 1996;97(1):22–8.
163. Harris RA, Nishiyama SK, Wray DW, Tedjasaputra V, Bailey DM, Richardson RS. The effect of oral antioxidants on brachial artery flow-mediated dilation following 5 and 10 min of ischemia. Eur J Appl Physiol. 2009;107(4):445–53.
164. Dillard CJ, Litov RE, Savin WM, Dumelin EE, Tappel AL. Effects of exercise, vitamin E, and ozone on pulmonary function and lipid peroxidation. J Appl Physiol Respir Environ Exerc Physiol. 1978;45(6):927–32.
165. Hudson MB, Hosick PA, McCaulley GO, Schrieber L, Wrieden J, McAnulty SR, et al. The effect of resistance exercise on humoral markers of oxidative stress. Med Sci Sports Exerc. 2008;40(3):542–8.
166. de Sousa CV, Sales MM, Rosa TS, Lewis JE, de Andrade RV, Simoes HG. The antioxidant effect of exercise: a systematic review and meta-analysis. Sports Med. 2017;47(2):277–93.
167. Donato AJ, Uberoi A, Bailey DM, Wray DW, Richardson RS. Exercise-induced brachial artery vasodilation: effects of antioxidants and exercise training in elderly men. Am J Physiol Heart Circ Physiol. 2010;298(2):H671–8.

7 Exertion-Related Acute Cardiovascular Events: Pathophysiologic Considerations, Risk Modulators, and Prophylactic Interventions

Barry A. Franklin and Peter Kokkinos

Introduction

In 490 BC the Persians were closing in on Athens. The Athenian general Miltiades met the Persian army in a place called Marathon, approximately 26 miles outside Athens. After a fierce battle that led to the defeat of the Persians, a messenger named Pheidippides was summoned to run from the battlefield of Marathon to Athens and deliver the good news to the anxiously waiting Athenians. He reached Athens in ~3 h, delivered his message "Νενικήκαμεν" (we were victorious), and then collapsed and died shortly thereafter. This legendary run gave rise to today's marathon competition.

Although it remains unclear what killed Pheidippides, it is likely that it was an acute cardiac event triggered by extreme exercise in a diseased heart. The modern-day marathon and ultramarathon run by thousands and even millions of runners are proof that we are capable of such physical challenges when trained properly. On the other hand, the occasional exertion-related death of a runner reminds us that vigorous exercise can both protect against and provoke acute cardiovascular events.

Over the years, we have come to the sobering realization that there is an inherent risk of injury when the body is exposed to prolonged and/or high-intensity physical stress, especially when it is unaccustomed. The probability of an exercise-related acute cardiovascular event and its' severity and type are dictated by numerous variables that will be discussed in this chapter.

Cardiovascular Risk of Physical Activity

The increased physiologic and hemodynamic responses that occur during vigorous physical exertion can trigger an acute cardiovascular event in individuals with a diseased or susceptible heart. Numerous studies have documented an increased risk of acute myocardial infarction

B. A. Franklin
Preventive Cardiology and Cardiac Rehabilitation, Department of Cardiovascular Diseases, Beaumont Health and Wellness Center, Royal Oak, MI, USA

Oakland University William Beaumont School of Medicine, Rochester, MI, USA

P. Kokkinos (✉)
Veterans Affairs Medical Center, Department of Cardiology, Washington, DC, USA

Georgetown University School of Medicine, Washington, DC, USA

Department of Kinesiology and Health, Rutgers University, New Brunswick, NJ, USA

George Washington University School of Medicine and Health Sciences, Washington, DC, USA

University of South Carolina, Department of Exercise Science, Arnold School of Public Health, Columbia, SC, USA
e-mail: peter.kokkinos@va.gov

P. Kokkinos, P. Narayan (eds.), *Cardiorespiratory Fitness in Cardiometabolic Diseases*,
https://doi.org/10.1007/978-3-030-04816-7_7

(AMI) and/or sudden cardiac death (SCD) during or shortly after engaging in vigorous physical activity (PA). The etiology of exercise-related cardiovascular events among young and older individuals is generally due to structural cardiovascular abnormalities, most notably hypertrophic cardiomyopathy (HCM), and atherosclerotic cardiovascular disease (CVD), specifically atherosclerotic coronary artery disease (CAD), respectively.

Exercise-Related Cardiovascular Events in Young Individuals

In general, the risk of SCD in young athletes, usually defined as those <40 years of age, is relatively low [1–3]. However, several congenital CVDs have been identified as the cause of exercise-related SCD in young athletes [1–13]. Exercise-related cardiovascular events in young individuals are usually associated with participation in sports. The most frequent pathological findings in this age group are hereditary or congenital cardiovascular anomalies (Table 7.1). Of those, HCM has consistently been reported as the single most common cause of exercise-related SCD, accounting for ~26% to >50% of all events followed by coronary artery anomalies (17%). Atherosclerotic CAD, usually due to genetic abnormalities in low-density lipoprotein (LDL) cholesterol metabolism, accounts for a relatively low percentage of exercise-related cardiovascular events in young athletes [1, 3, 11, 14]. However, differentiating exercise-induced physiological left ventricular hypertrophy (LVH) from HCM may, in some instances, be challenging. A prudent and highly recommended approach is that young athletes with a cardiac wall thickness between 12 and 16 mm should undergo a systematic evaluation by a cardiologist [15].

Table 7.1 Common hereditary or congenital cardiovascular anomalies associated with exertion-related sudden cardiac death in young competitive athletes

Hypertrophic cardiomyopathy (HCM)
Increased cardiac mass (possible HCM)
Aberrant coronary arteries
Other coronary anomalies
Tunneled left anterior descending coronary artery
Idiopathic dilated cardiomyopathy
Ruptured aortic aneurysm
Myocarditis
Aortic valve stenosis
Arrhythmogenic right ventricular dysplasia
Idiopathic myocardial scarring
Mitral valve prolapse
Atrial septal defect
Coarctation of the aorta

In US high school and college athletes (aged, 13–24 years; mean ± SD age 16.9 ± 2.0 for males and 16.2 ± 2.4 for females), the exercise-related death rate was 1 in 133,000 and 1 in 769,000 for males and females, respectively [3]. A relatively higher rate was reported (1 in 33,000) in young but slightly older Italian athletes aged 12–35 (mean ± SD age 23.1 ± 7.0 years) [4]. The higher risk of SCD in young athletes is strongly related to underlying CVDs such as HCM, congenital coronary artery anomalies, arrhythmogenic right ventricular cardiomyopathy, and premature CAD [3, 11, 16].

When comparing competitive athletes to non-athletes, mortality rates were 2.3 versus 0.9 per 100,000 persons per year, respectively, or 2.5-fold higher risk among the athletes. SCD occurred more often in men than in women (2.6 versus 1.1 in 100,000 persons per year, respectively) [4]. Mortality rates in nonathletic men versus nonathletic women were 1.3 versus 0.5 in 100,000 persons per year, respectively. The estimated relative risk among athletes versus nonathletes was 1.95 (CI 1.3 to 2.6; $p < 0.0001$) for males and 2.00 (CI: 0.6–4.9) for females, although statistical significance for females was not attained ($p = 0.15$).

Exercise-Related AMI and SCD in Older Populations

In contrast to younger individuals, the most common cause of exercise-related cardiac arrest or AMI in middle-aged and older individuals is occult or documented atherosclerotic CAD. Several hypotheses have been suggested as triggering mechanisms for plaque rupture, acute coronary thrombosis (Table 7.2), or threatening ventricular arrhythmias (Fig. 7.1). Moreover, it is estimated that ~71% and 85% of individuals in the USA ≥40 and ≥50 years of age, respectively, have subclinical coronary disease [17].

The risk of exercise varies according to the population. In older populations where the prevalence of atherosclerotic CAD is high, the relative risk of SCD during vigorous exercise or physical exertion increases disproportionately [1, 18, 19]. *Nevertheless, the exercise-related absolute risk of a cardiac event remains relatively low, even in older populations.* For example, in the Seattle study, the incidence of cardiac arrest in previously asymptomatic individuals was 25-fold higher than the incidence at rest or during lighter activities. The pattern was similar for exercise-related AMI [18]. In the Rhode Island study, the SCD rate during jogging was 7.6 times higher than during leisure-time or sedentary activities. However, the incidence rate was 1 per year for every 7620 male joggers. This rate was halved (1 per year for every 15,240 joggers), when those with known CAD were excluded [19].

Table 7.2 Potential triggering mechanisms of acute myocardial infarction by strenuous physical exertion

Induces plaque rupture via:
Increased heart rate, blood pressure, and shear forces
Altered coronary artery dimensions
Exercise-induced spasm in diseased artery segments
Renders a fissured plaque more thrombogenic by:
Deepening the fissure
Increasing thrombogenicity
Induces thrombogenesis directly via:
Catecholamine-induced platelet aggregation

A more recent study assessed the incidence and outcomes of cardiac arrest associated with marathon and half-marathon races in the USA from January 1, 2000, to May 31, 2010, in 10.9 million registered runners (mean ± SD age 42 ± 13 years) [20]. Of the 59 cases of cardiac arrest, 42 (71%) were fatal, corresponding to ~4 fatalities per year. The final mile, <5% of the entire marathon distance, accounted for ~50% of the SCDs. The incidence rates of cardiac arrest and SCD during long-distance running races were 1 per 184,000 and 1 per 259,000 participants, respectively. The incidence rate was significantly higher during marathons (1.01 per 100,000 participants) than during half-marathons (0.27 per 100,000 participants) and among men (0.90 per 100,000 participants) than among women (0.16 per 100,000 participants). The investigators concluded that the overall risk of a cardiac event during marathons and half-marathons is relatively low, as compared with other vigorous physical activities. Sufficient postmortem data were available to determine the

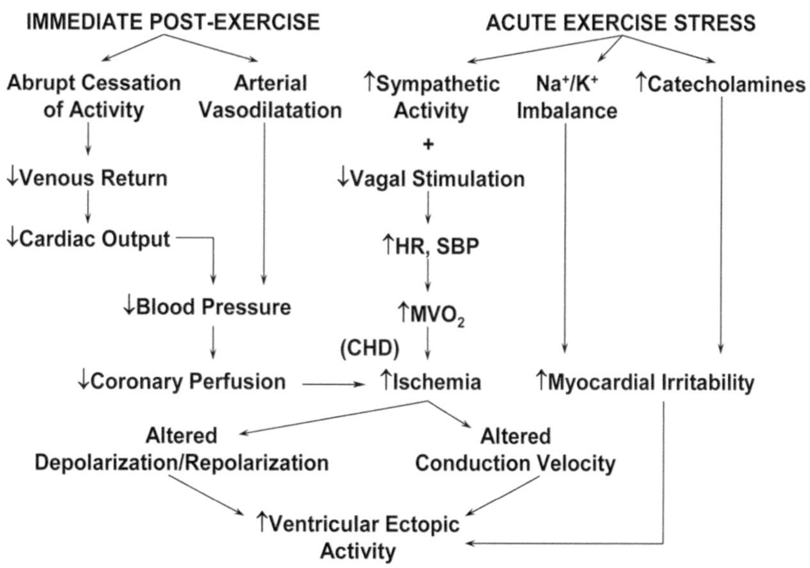

Fig. 7.1 Physiological alterations accompanying acute exercise and recovery and their possible sequelae. HR heart rate, SBP systolic blood pressure, MVO_2, myocardial oxygen consumption, CHD coronary heart disease

likely cause of cardiac arrest in only 31 of the 59 cases (53%). The most frequent clinical and autopsy findings were HCM and atherosclerotic CAD, respectively [20].

In 2017, investigators reported on SCD and cardiac arrest in >9 million triathlon participants over a 30-year period [21]. A total of 135 SCDs occurred, with an incidence of 1.74 per 100,000 participants. This rate was higher than earlier estimates of SCD during the triathlon [22] and exceeded the incidence reported for marathon running [20]. Although women comprised only 15% of the study population, their incidence of cardiovascular events was 3.5-fold less than in men. Most SCDs occurred during the swim segment (67%), whereas the remaining fatalities occurred during bicycling, running, and postrace recovery, 16%, 11%, and 6%, respectively. Of the SCDs whose previous race experience was known (n = 68), 26 (38%) were competing in their first triathlon. Moreover, of the deaths examined at autopsy (n = 61), 27 (44%) had clinically relevant cardiovascular abnormalities, most frequently, atherosclerotic CAD or cardiomyopathy. Overall, men aged ≥40 years were at greatest risk, and on average, the fatalities were ~12 years older than survivors. Collectively, these data suggest that cardiac arrest and SCD during marathon running and triathlon participation occasionally occur and that clinicians evaluating potential race participants should be aware of the heightened risks of HCM and atherosclerotic CAD in this patient population, both of which can often be detected with appropriate medical screening, as well as the increased risk among "first-time" participants. The latter may suggest inadequate preparation or poor training as underlying contributors to some of the exertion-related fatalities [23]. Participants should also be counseled to heed warning signs/symptoms during training and competition [24] and to discontinue exercise and seek medical clearance before resuming PA, since these are often harbingers of exertion-related acute cardiac events. Finally, participants should be advised to avoid sprinting during the final minutes of the race, when complications are most likely to occur [20].

SCD and AMI have also been reported during snow removal and deer hunting [25–27]. In one study, hemodynamic responses and myocardial demands evoked during snow shoveling were similar to those observed in the same subjects during maximal treadmill exercise testing [26]. The highest observed values for heart rate; systolic blood pressure; rate-pressure product; oxygen consumption, expressed as metabolic equivalents (METs; 1 MET = 3.5 mL•kg^{-1}•min^{-1}); and perceived exertion (6–20 scale) during snow shoveling and maximal treadmill testing are shown in Table 7.3. This suggests that the cardiac workload, as signified by the product of heart rate and systolic blood pressure, known as the rate-pressure product [28, 29], of the two activities is similar (322 versus 342 for treadmill testing and snow shoveling, respectively). This transient increase in cardiac demand likely contributes to the disproportionate number of cardiovascular events commonly reported during or soon after snow shoveling [26].

Abrupt, sustained, and marked increases in heart rate, complex arrhythmias, and significant ST-segment depression have also been reported during deer hunting. These findings suggest that the strenuous physical activities associated with deer

Table 7.3 Cardiorespiratory responses during maximal treadmill testing and snow shoveling in sedentary men (n = 10)[a]

Variable	Treadmill testing	Snow shoveling[b]
Heart rate (beats/min)	179 ± 17	175 ± 15
Systolic blood pressure (mm Hg)	181 ± 25	198 ± 17
Rate-pressure product (mm Hg × beats/min × 10^{-2})	322 ± 40	342 ± 34
Oxygen consumption (METs)[c]	9.3 ± 1.8[d]	5.7 ± 0.8
Rating of perceived exertion[e]	17.9 ± 1.5	16.7 ± 1.7

[a]Adapted from Franklin et al. [26]. Results are expressed as mean ± SD
[b]Shoveling rates were self-paced (12 ± 2 loads per minute) during a 10-min bout of work
[c]*METs* metabolic equivalents; 1 MET = 3.5 mL•kg^{-1}•min^{-1}
[d]$p < 0.003$ versus snow shoveling
[e]6–20 scale

hunting, coupled with presumed hyper-adrenergic responses and superimposed environmental stresses (cold air), potentiate the increased risk for cardiovascular events [27].

Although the mechanisms potentially triggering exercise-related acute cardiovascular events are not well-defined, vigorous or high-intensity exercise or physical exertion transiently increases heart rate, systolic blood pressure, and cardiac demands or myocardial oxygen requirements. In the presence of significant CAD that limits coronary blood flow, myocardial ischemia can ensue, triggering malignant ventricular arrhythmias and SCD. Additional causes of exercise-related cardiac events in patients with occult or documented CAD may include coronary plaque rupture, as previously described [30]. These investigators also postulated that the associated myocardial contractions during physical work, along with increased "twisting and bending" of the coronary arteries during each contraction, may contribute to plaque rupture, resulting in AMI and/or SCD.

Most exercise-related deaths in previously asymptomatic adults without a prior history of coronary heart disease are likely due to atherosclerotic plaque rupture in one of the coronary arteries, leading to an acute coronary thrombosis [31]. Exertion-related atherosclerotic plaque rupture has been substantiated by coronary angiography in conditioned and sedentary men with acute coronary syndromes [32], in those shoveling snow [33], and in men with CAD who experienced SCD while engaging in other physically demanding activities [34].

Physical Activity and the Risk of Sudden Cardiac Death

Despite the fact that vigorous PA, particularly when unaccustomed, can trigger acute cardiac events, the evidence overwhelmingly supports that the health benefits of appropriate exercise far outweigh the risks. In addition, the inherent risk of exercise can be further attenuated by maintaining a physically active lifestyle. One widely cited meta-analysis reported a fivefold increased risk of SCD and a 3.5-fold increased risk of AMI during vigorous-intensity PA (≥6 METs). However, these associations were markedly attenuated among persons with high levels of PA [35]. In the Seattle study, the relative risk of cardiac arrest was greatest in the least compared with the most physically active men (56 and 5 times, respectively) [18]. The exercise-related risk of AMI and the modulating role of habitual PA have also been examined in several studies [36–39]. In a US cohort, Mittleman et al. [38] assessed the relative risk of AMI survivors during or within 1 h following exercise. Activities included jogging (30%), yard work such as chopping wood or gardening (52%), and lifting and/or pushing (18%). The relative risk of AMI for the entire cohort was 5.6-fold higher during vigorous exercise compared to less vigorous PA and 18.9 times higher for diabetics. When considering activity status, the risk was 107-fold higher in sedentary individuals (exercising <1 day per week) and declined progressively to 19.4, 8.6, and 2.4 for those exercising 1–2, 3–4, and ≥5 days per week, respectively. This suggests that a sedentary person engaging in unaccustomed, vigorous PA has nearly a 50-fold higher risk of experiencing an exercise-related cardiac event than a person who exercises ~5 times per week. Exercising just one or two times per week cut the risk by >80%.

In a German cohort of 1194 patients (mean age 61 ± 9 years; 74% of whom were men) who survived a MI, the relative risk of MI was 2.1 times higher for those who engaged in vigorous PA defined as ≥6 METs, compared to matched controls. However, the risk was elevated significantly (6.9 times higher) in those engaging in PA <4 times per week, while the risk was only 1.3 times higher in those engaging in PA ≥4 times per week [39]. Similarly, in patients who underwent angioplasty following AMI [37], the overall risk during physical exertion was ten times higher compared to the rest. However, the risk was 30.5 times higher in sedentary individuals, while the risk of those engaging in moderate levels of PA was not raised significantly.

Finally, in the Physicians' Health Study [18, 36], involving a large cohort of male physicians

($n = 21{,}481$), investigators reported a significant transient increase in the relative risk of SCD during and up to 30 min after vigorous exertion. However, the absolute risk of SCD was extremely low during any particular bout of vigorous physical exertion (1 SCD per 1.51 million episodes of exertion). The investigators also concluded that habitual vigorous exercise diminishes the exercise-related risk of SCD.

Collectively, these studies clearly support that vigorous PA is associated with a transient increase in the risk of experiencing an acute cardiac event. The increased risk is further heightened by a sedentary lifestyle and attenuated significantly, but not completely eliminated, by frequently engaging in moderate-to-vigorous PA.

Long-Term Health Benefits and Risks Associated with Exercise

The health benefits of regularly performed structured exercise or leisure-time PA in middle-aged and older individuals, regardless of race, gender, or comorbidities, are well-documented [40–50]. It is also acknowledged that vigorous exercise is associated with a transient increase in the risk of acute cardiac events. However, the risk for those engaging in regular exercises of moderate-to-vigorous intensity and volume is, at the very least, attenuated significantly [16, 19, 20, 36–39]. Therefore, the long-term benefits of exercise outweigh the risk of being sedentary. There is also recognition that health benefits of moderate exercise levels can be eroded and even reversed when high-volume, high-intensity exercise regimens are adopted. Referred to as a U-shaped or reverse J-shaped relationship, this was first hypothesized by Hippocrates who stated that "Exercise in excess is against nature." Accordingly, Paffenbarger et al. [51] noted a progressive decline in death rate when weekly energy expenditure during PA ranged from 500 to 3500 kcal per week. A slight increase in death rates was noted for those exceeding 3500 kcal per week in PA. Recent investigations have also suggested adverse cardiac remodeling and higher cardiovascular mortality with extremely high PA levels [52–55]. Similarly, two recent epidemiologic studies, one in a large cohort ($n = 1119, 239$) of British women [56] and the other in Danish joggers ($n = 1098$) and non-joggers ($n = 3950$) [57], reported a U-shaped relationship between aerobic exercise and cardiovascular morbidity and mortality. However, an important limitation of the former study [56] was the higher smoking prevalence among women participating in daily strenuous exercise (25.6%) as compared with the other exercise groups (13.7% to 15.5%). Moreover, significant methodologic limitations in the Danish study [57] included the low number of subjects in the strenuous jogger group and the fact that inclusion in the non-jogger (control) group allowed participants to walk or bike up to 2 h/week [58]. On the other hand, Arem et al. [59] reported no significant increase in mortality risk with activity levels ≥10 times higher than the minimum guidelines of 75 min of vigorous-intensity or 150 min of moderate-intensity exercise per week, as recommended by The 2008 Physical Activity Guidelines for Americans for "substantial" health benefits. Collectively, given the conflicting data and associated epidemiologic study limitations, it appears premature to conclude that high exercise frequency, intensity, or volumes, as compared with more moderate exercise regimens, may increase cardiovascular risk.

In a cohort of US veterans ($n = 5962$; mean age 56.8 ± 11 years), we found a progressive decline in the incidence of atrial fibrillation with increased levels of cardiorespiratory fitness as determined by age-stratified exercise capacity and no evidence of increase in the group with the highest fitness (9.3 ± 1.2 METs; range, 6.6–14.5). The association trends were similar for those younger than 65 years of age and those 65 years or older [60].

Minimizing the Risk

The risk of exercise-related musculoskeletal injuries and acute cardiovascular events can be minimized, but not eliminated. The goal of any exercise program should be to lower the risk of exercise to an absolute minimum and maximize the benefits. When the exercise-related risk increases, exercise dosage and/or intensity must be re-evaluated and adjusted.

Studies designed to identify and assess the effectiveness of strategies to attenuate the relative and absolute cardiovascular risks of exercise are lacking [16]. Certainly, maintaining adequate fitness appears to be an effective approach in attenuating the risk of exercise-related cardiac events. It is also important that contemporary exercise guidelines are followed. For example, sedentary individuals should not engage in unaccustomed, vigorous high-risk activities and avoid exercising in extreme environmental conditions. Several studies now suggest that snow shoveling and deer hunting are associated with increased cardiovascular events [25–27, 61], probably because these activities are often performed by unfit individuals, in cold temperatures, disproportionately increasing the cardiac demands as substantiated by rate-pressure products that are comparable to or higher than those recorded during peak treadmill exercise while simultaneously lowering the ischemic threshold in some patients [26, 62].

Recommendations to potentially reduce the risk of exercise-related cardiovascular events include: encourage previously sedentary adults to engage in regular, brisk walking programs to move them out of the least fit, least active, "high-risk" cohort; counsel inactive patients/clients to avoid unaccustomed, vigorous-to-near maximal leisure-time, domestic, and recreational physical activity (e.g., racquet sports, water or cross-country skiing, highly competitive sports [basketball], deer hunting, snow shoveling); advocate appropriate warm-up and cool-down procedures; promote education of warning signs/symptoms (e.g., chest pain or pressure, lightheadedness, heart palpitations/arrhythmias, unusual shortness of breath); emphasize strict adherence to prescribed training heart rates and perceived exertion levels (e.g., "fairly light" to "somewhat hard"); and reduce the intensity of exercise under hyperthermic conditions and at altitudes of >1500 m until acclimatized. For example, persons who are not acclimated to heat and who are exposed to temperatures >24 °C experience added heart rate increases of 1 beat per minute

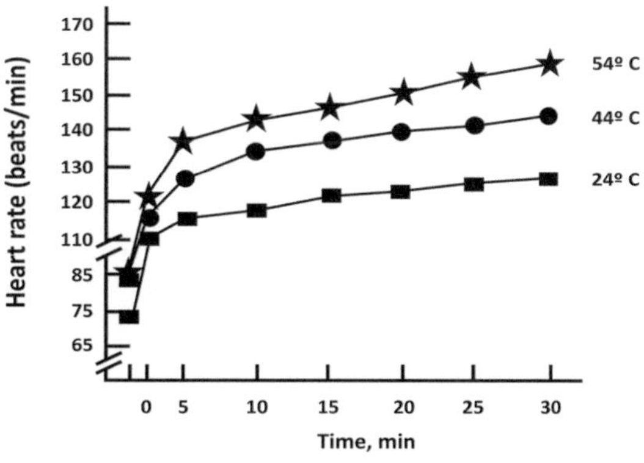

Fig. 7.2 Influence of environmental temperature on heart rate responses at a constant exercise work rate. Heart rate increases approximately 1 beat per minute for each degree Celsius increment in ambient temperature above 24 °C. (Adapted from Pandolf et al. [63])

per °C while exercising and 2–4 beats per minute per °C with concomitant increased humidity (Fig. 7.2) [63].

When previously sedentary individuals initiate an exercise program, it is strongly recommended to begin with a light-to-moderate intensity, specifically 2–3 METs, and gradually increase the intensity of exertion over time (i.e., 2–3 months), to 3–5 METs, provided that they remain asymptomatic. Such recommendations appear prudent since these intensities are below the vigorous PA (≥6 METs) that is commonly associated with the triggering of exercise-related cardiac events [37]. This "progressive transitional phase" should help to reduce the risk of orthopedic/musculoskeletal injury and allow previously sedentary individuals to gradually improve their cardiorespiratory fitness without going through a period during which each bout of vigorous exercise is associated with large spikes in relative cardiovascular risk (Fig. 7.3) [38]. Finally, for individuals with signs/symptoms of myocardial ischemia, which can be highly arrhythmogenic [64], the target heart rate for endurance exercise should be set safely below (≥10 beats per minute) the ischemic electrocardiographic or anginal threshold [65].

Screening selected middle-aged and older individuals before participating in structured exercise and/or PA regimens and younger individuals prior to engaging in sports activities

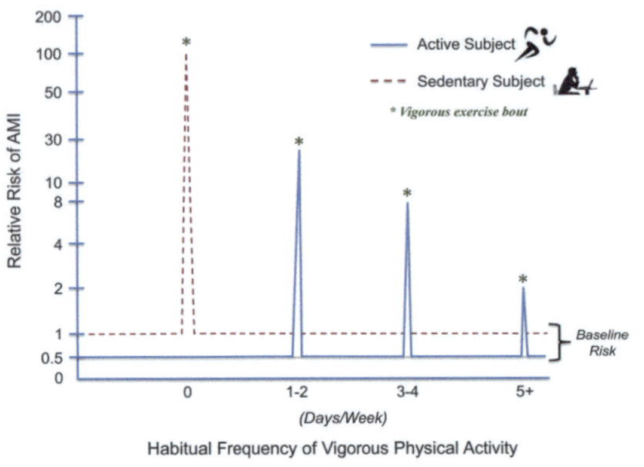

Fig. 7.3 Relative risk of acute myocardial infarction (AMI) at rest and during vigorous physical exertion (≥6 metabolic equivalents) in sedentary and physically active individuals, with specific reference to the habitual frequency of vigorous exertion (days/week). (Adapted from Mittleman et al. [38])

should also be considered [16]. In 2015, the ACSM published revised recommendations for exercise pre-participation screening that eliminated age cutoffs, risk factor profiling, and risk stratification terminology (i.e., low, moderate, high) in their updated screening algorithm [66]. The new algorithm focused on four major variables: (1) the individual's current level of PA; (2) known cardiovascular, metabolic, or renal disease (CMRD) or signs/symptoms suggestive of disease; (3) the desired or anticipated exercise intensity; and (4) the potential hazards of unaccustomed, high-intensity PA. These characteristics have been identified as important modulators of exercise-related acute cardiovascular events. The term "medical clearance" replaced specific recommendations for a medical/physical examination with or without exercise testing, as it was felt these evaluations should be at the clinician's discretion. Moreover, patients with pulmonary disease, per se, are no longer automatically referred for medical clearance to exercise, perhaps with the exception of chronic obstructive pulmonary disease which, in current or former smokers, often serves as an independent predictor of cardiovascular risk [67]. The new recommendations can be succinctly summarized by four points:

- Physically active asymptomatic individuals without known CMRD may continue their usual moderate- or vigorous-intensity exercise and progress gradually as tolerated according to contemporary ACSM guidelines. Those who develop signs or symptoms of CMRD should immediately discontinue exercise and seek medical clearance before resuming exercise of any intensity.
- Physically active asymptomatic individuals with known CMRD who have been recently (previous 12 months) medically cleared may continue a moderate-intensity exercise program, unless they develop signs or symptoms, which require immediate cessation of exercise and medical reassessment.
- Physically inactive individuals without known CMRD may begin light-to-moderate-intensity exercise without medical clearance and, provided they remain asymptomatic, progress gradually in intensity as recommended by current ACSM guidelines.
- Physically inactive individuals with known CMRD or signs/symptoms that are suggestive of these diseases should seek medical clearance before starting an exercise program, regardless of the intensity.

Finally, an important distinction regarding the exercise-related health benefits and risks in young versus older individuals should be emphasized. Engaging in regular exercise of moderate-to-vigorous intensity improves cardiorespiratory fitness and confers health benefits for older, healthy individuals and those with occult or documented CAD. Ultimately, the exercise-related health benefits invariably outweigh the associated cardiovascular risks. In contrast, vigorous-to-high-intensity exercise in younger individuals with hereditary or congenital structured cardiovascular abnormalities does not improve the condition and may trigger threatening and sometimes fatal arrhythmias in a diseased or susceptible heart. Accordingly, these individuals should only engage in low-to-moderate-intensity exercise, since higher-intensity exercise may be proscribed [16].

Exercise Intensity and Duration

Few specific data are available regarding the intensity of exercise and the associated risks. High-volume, high-intensity exercise training regimens and competition are generally associated with a higher risk for cardiovascular complications and musculoskeletal injury. There is also little information on exercise duration and the incidence of injury. In one study, the rate of cardiac arrest was higher during marathons (1.01 per 100,000; 95% CI, 0.72–1.38) than during half-marathons (0.27; 95% CI, 0.17–0.43) [20]. Cardiac arrests appear to cluster in the latter stages of a marathon (around the 20-mile mark), with ~50% of the SCDs occurring during the final mile or at the finish line [68].

Use of Cardioprotective Medications Prior to Exercise

Although there are no definitive data indicating that cardioprotective medications prevent exercise-related acute cardiovascular events, it has been suggested that distance runners at risk, that is, those with evidence of subclinical coronary disease (e.g., elevated coronary artery calcium) [69–72], may benefit from taking targeted medications, specifically low-dose, uncoated pre-race aspirin [73, 74], to reduce the elevated, transient risk for atherothrombosis, causing vulnerable plaques to morph into culprit lesions of acute coronary thrombosis [75, 76]. The rationale for this recommendation stems from the fact that there has been more than a twofold increase in race-related cardiac arrests since 2005 [20], that most middle-aged and older individuals have subclinical CAD [17], that asymptomatic distance runners commonly show elevated inflammatory and hemostatic markers during races [77, 78], and that aspirin, which also likely inhibits epinephrine-induced platelet aggregation, has been conclusively shown to prevent first myocardial infarctions in healthy men [79]. Nevertheless, in the Myocardial Infarction Onset Study [38], the relative risk of triggering AMI by heavy physical exertion was not significantly different between aspirin users and nonusers. Similarly, Kim et al. [20] concluded that taking aspirin before participating in marathons or half-marathons has limited efficacy, since acute plaque rupture and thrombosis did not appear to be an important cause of race-related cardiac arrest. Although Albano et al. [80] reported acute coronary thrombosis in three male athletes in good physical condition without known atherosclerotic CVD after completing the 2011 Boston Marathon, it was unclear whether any of these runners used prophylactic pre-race aspirin administration.

Based on these data and other recent reports [81–85], the International Marathon Medical Directors Association has suggested that the lifetime benefit of reducing cardiac events and improving survival through distance running [86–88] can be enhanced by attenuating the transient heightened risk of SCD during distance races and competition [38, 89] via pre-race aspirin administration for men >40 years with approval by their physician, after considering the associated risks for gastrointestinal bleeding or allergy [90].

In addition, taking short-acting beta-blockers before strenuous exercise has been suggested as a complementary cardioprotective intervention [91], by reducing the rate-pressure product [28, 29], shear forces, and associated cardiac demands during distance training and competition (Fig. 7.4). Tofler et al. [92] reported that peak and average heart rates during standardized bouts of physical exertion were significantly lower 30 min after ingestion of a beta-blocker (propranolol, 10 mg) and aspirin (100 mg) than during a control period (118 ± 21 versus 132 ± 16 bpm, $p = 0.016$; and 86 ± 12 versus 96 ± 12 bpm, $p = 0.007$). Using the Thrombolysis in Myocardial Infarction Phase II (TIMI II) database, researchers concluded that beta-blockers appear to provide the most compelling evidence for protection against physical stress [93]. With pending results of a prospective

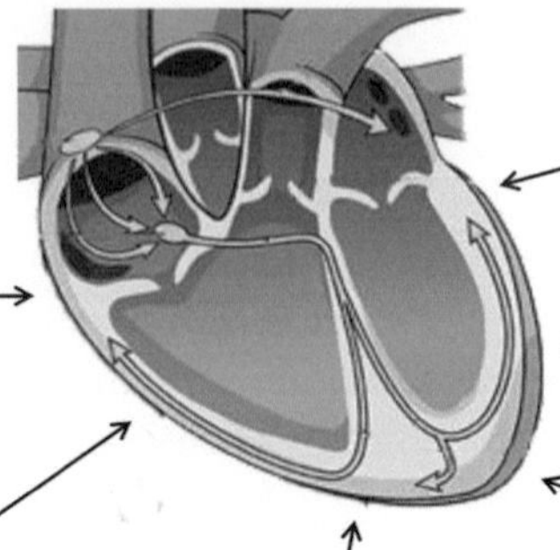

Fig. 7.4 Mechanisms by which taking short-acting beta-blockers prior to vigorous physical activity may decrease the risk of exercise-related acute cardiovascular events

Table 7.4 Potential cardioprotective effects of regular physical activity

Anti-atherosclerotic	Psychological	Anti-thrombotic	Anti-ischemic	Antiarrhythmic
Increase HDL-cholesterol Insulin sensitivity	Social support	Fibrinolysis	Coronary flow EPCs and CACs Nitric oxide	Vagal tone HR variability
Decrease Total cholesterol LDL-cholesterol Blood pressure Inflammation Adiposity	Depression Stress	Platelet adhesiveness Fibrinogen Blood viscosity	Myocardial O_2 demand Endothelial dysfunction	Adrenergic activity

HDL high-density lipoprotein, *EPCs* endothelial progenitor cells, *CACs* cultured/circulating angiogenic cells, O_2 oxygen, *LDL* low-density lipoprotein, *HR* heart rate

randomized trial specifically in distance runners, in aggregate, these data suggest that pre-race ingestion of aspirin, the only pharmacologic agent with a class 1A recommendation for prehospital administration in the event of an acute coronary syndrome, and prophylactic beta-blockade may be helpful in preventing the triggering of exercise-related acute cardiovascular events.

Conclusions

Although regular moderate-to-vigorous exercise or habitual PA reduces the likelihood of exertion-related acute cardiac events, vigorous activity can also acutely increase the risk of SCD and AMI in susceptible persons. Exercise-associated acute cardiac events generally occur in individuals with known or occult CVD. Hereditary or congenital cardiovascular abnormalities are predominantly responsible for cardiac events in young individuals, whereas atherosclerotic CAD is primarily responsible for these events in middle-aged and older adults. The absolute rate of exercise-related SCD is extremely low and varies with the prevalence of disease in the study population. The incidence of both AMI and SCD is greatest in habitually sedentary individuals who perform unaccustomed, vigorous-to-high-intensity exercise. Prodromal symptoms during training and/or competition are often harbingers of exertion-related nonfatal and fatal acute cardiovascular events. Maintaining cardiorespiratory fitness through regular PA may help to reduce the likelihood of exercise-related cardiovascular complications in persons with known or occult atherosclerotic CAD, likely due to antiatherosclerotic, antithrombotic, anti-ischemic, and antiarrhythmic mechanisms (Table 7.4). Intriguing data also suggest pre-race ingestion of aspirin, short-acting beta-blockers, or both, may be helpful in reducing the number of acute cardiovascular events reported each year during or immediately after high-volume, high-intensity endurance training or competition. The essential feature of a safe and effective exercise regimen is a gradual progression during which an individual remains below an intensity that evokes abnormal signs or symptoms. These considerations should help physicians and allied health professionals to put the "risk of exercise" in proper perspective.

Acknowledgment The authors thank Brenda White for her assistance with the preparation of this manuscript.

References

1. Maron BJ. Sudden death in young athletes. N Engl J Med. 2003;349(11):1064–75.
2. Maron BJ, Roberts WC, McAllister HA, Rosing DR, Epstein SE. Sudden death in young athletes. Circulation. 1980;62(2):218–29.
3. Van Camp SP, Peterson RA. Cardiovascular complications of outpatient cardiac rehabilitation programs. JAMA. 1986;256(9):1160–3.
4. Corrado D, Thiene G, Nava A, Rossi L, Pennelli N. Sudden death in young competitive athletes: clinicopathologic correlations in 22 cases. Am J Med. 1990;89(5):588–96.
5. Davis JA, Cecchin F, Jones TK, Portman MA. Major coronary artery anomalies in a pediatric population: incidence and clinical importance. J Am Coll Cardiol. 2001;37(2):593–7.
6. Drory Y, Turetz Y, Hiss Y, Lev B, Fisman EZ, Pines A, et al. Sudden unexpected death in persons less than 40 years of age. Am J Cardiol. 1991;68(13):1388–92.
7. Furlanello F, Bettini R, Cozzi F, Del Favero A, Disertori M, Vergara G, et al. Ventricular arrhythmias and sudden death in athletes. Ann N Y Acad Sci. 1984;427:253–79.
8. Liberthson RR. Sudden death from cardiac causes in children and young adults. N Engl J Med. 1996;334(16):1039–44.
9. Maron BJ. Cardiovascular risks to young persons on the athletic field. Ann Intern Med. 1998;129(5):379–86.
10. Maron BJ, Gohman TE, Aeppli D. Prevalence of sudden cardiac death during competitive sports activities in Minnesota high school athletes. J Am Coll Cardiol. 1998;32(7):1881–4.
11. Maron BJ, Shirani J, Poliac LC, Mathenge R, Roberts WC, Mueller FO. Sudden death in young competitive athletes. Clinical, demographic, and pathological profiles. JAMA. 1996;276(3):199–204.
12. Thiene G, Nava A, Corrado D, Rossi L, Pennelli N. Right ventricular cardiomyopathy and sudden death in young people. N Engl J Med. 1988;318(3):129–33.
13. Thiene G, Pennelli N, Rossi L. Cardiac conduction system abnormalities as a possible cause of sudden death in young athletes. Hum Pathol. 1983;14(8):704–9.
14. Maron BJ, Doerer JJ, Haas TS, Tierney DM, Mueller FO. Sudden deaths in young competitive athletes: analysis of 1866 deaths in the United States, 1980–2006. Circulation. 2009;119(8):1085–92.
15. Rawlins J, Bhan A, Sharma S. Left ventricular hypertrophy in athletes. Eur J Echocardiogr. 2009;10(3):350–6.
16. Thompson PD, Franklin BA, Balady GJ, Blair SN, Corrado D, Estes NA 3rd, et al. Exercise and acute cardiovascular events placing the risks into perspective: a scientific statement from the American Heart Association Council on Nutrition, Physical Activity, and Metabolism and the Council on Clinical Cardiology. Circulation. 2007;115(17):2358–68.
17. Tuzcu EM, Kapadia SR, Tutar E, Ziada KM, Hobbs RE, McCarthy PM, et al. High prevalence of coronary atherosclerosis in asymptomatic teenagers and young adults: evidence from intravascular ultrasound. Circulation. 2001;103(22):2705–10.
18. Siscovick DS, Weiss NS, Fletcher RH, Lasky T. The incidence of primary cardiac arrest during vigorous exercise. N Engl J Med. 1984;311(14):874–7.
19. Thompson PD, Funk EJ, Carleton RA, Sturner WQ. Incidence of death during jogging in Rhode Island from 1975 through 1980. JAMA. 1982;247(18):2535–8.
20. Kim JH, Malhotra R, Chiampas G, d'Hemecourt P, Troyanos C, Cianca J, et al. Cardiac arrest during long-distance running races. N Engl J Med. 2012;366(2):130–40.
21. Harris KM, Creswell LL, Haas TS, Thomas T, Tung M, Isaacson E, et al. Death and cardiac arrest in the U.S. triathlon participants, 1985 to 2016: a case series. Ann Intern Med. 2017;167(8):529–35.
22. Harris KM, Henry JT, Rohman E, Haas TS, Maron BJ. Sudden death during the triathlon. JAMA. 2010;303(13):1255–7.
23. Sanchis-Gomar F, Santos-Lozano A, Garatachea N, Pareja-Galeano H, Fiuza-Luces C, Joyner MJ, Lucia A. My patient wants to perform strenuous endurance exercise. What's the right advice? Int J Cardiol. 2015;197:248–53.
24. Thompson PD, Stern MP, Williams P, Duncan K, Haskell WL, Wood PD. Death during jogging or running. A study of 18 cases. JAMA. 1979;242(12):1265–7.
25. Franklin BA, George P, Henry R, Gordon S, Timmis GC, O'Neill WW. Acute myocardial infarction after manual or automated snow removal. Am J Cardiol. 2001;87(11):1282–3.
26. Franklin BA, Hogan P, Bonzheim K, Bakalyar D, Terrien E, Gordon S, et al. Cardiac demands of heavy snow shoveling. JAMA. 1995;273(11):880–2.
27. Haapaniemi S, Franklin BA, Wegner JH, Hamar S, Gordon S, Timmis GC, et al. Electrocardiographic responses to deer hunting activities in men with and without coronary artery disease. Am J Cardiol. 2007;100(2):175–9.
28. Jorgensen CR, Wang K, Wang Y, Gobel FL, Nelson RR, Taylor H. Effect of propranolol on myocardial oxygen

consumption and its hemodynamic correlates during upright exercise. Circulation. 1973;48(6):1173–82.
29. Kitamura K, Jorgensen CR, Gobel FL, Taylor HL, Wang Y. Hemodynamic correlates of myocardial oxygen consumption during upright exercise. J Appl Physiol. 1972;32(4):516–22.
30. Black A, Black MM, Gensini G. Exertion and acute coronary artery injury. Angiology. 1975;26(11):759–83.
31. Davies MJ, Thomas AC. Plaque fissuring--the cause of acute myocardial infarction, sudden ischaemic death, and crescendo angina. Br Heart J. 1985;53(4):363–73.
32. Ciampricotti R, Deckers JW, Taverne R, el Gamal M, Relik-van Wely L, Pool J. Characteristics of conditioned and sedentary men with acute coronary syndromes. Am J Cardiol. 1994;73(4):219–22.
33. Hammoudeh AJ, Haft JI. Coronary-plaque rupture in acute coronary syndromes triggered by snow shoveling. N Engl J Med. 1996;335(26):2001.
34. Burke AP, Farb A, Malcom GT, Liang Y, Smialek JE, Virmani R. Plaque rupture and sudden death related to exertion in men with coronary artery disease. JAMA. 1999;281(10):921–6.
35. Dahabreh IJ, Paulus JK. Association of episodic physical and sexual activity with triggering of acute cardiac events: systemic review and meta-analysis. JAMA. 2011;305(12):1225–33.
36. Albert CM, Mittleman MA, Chae CU, Lee IM, Hennekens CH, Manson JE. Triggering of sudden death from cardiac causes by vigorous exertion. N Engl J Med. 2000;343(19):1355–61.
37. Giri S, Thompson PD, Kiernan FJ, Clive J, Fram DB, Mitchel JF, et al. Clinical and angiographic characteristics of exertion-related acute myocardial infarction. JAMA. 1999;282(18):1731–6.
38. Mittleman MA, Maclure M, Tofler GH, Sherwood JB, Goldberg RJ, Muller JE. Triggering of acute myocardial infarction by heavy physical exertion. Protection against triggering by regular exertion. Determinants of Myocardial Infarction Onset Study Investigators. N Engl J Med. 1993;329(23):1677–83.
39. Willich SN, Lewis M, Löwel H, Arntz HR, Schubert F, Schröder R. Physical exertion as a trigger of acute myocardial infarction. Triggers and mechanisms of Myocardial Infarction Study Group. N Engl J Med. 1993;329(23):1684–90.
40. Kokkinos P. Physical activity and cardiovascular disease prevention: current recommendations. Angiology. 2008;59(2 Suppl):26S–9S.
41. Kokkinos P, Faselis C, Myers J, Sui X, Zhang J, Tsimploulis A, et al. Exercise capacity and risk of chronic kidney disease in US veterans: a cohort study. Mayo Clin Proc. 2015;90(4):461–8.
42. Kokkinos P, Manolis A, Pittaras A, Doumas M, Giannelou A, Panagiotakos DB, et al. Exercise capacity and mortality in hypertensive men with and without additional risk factors. Hypertension. 2009;53(3):494–9.
43. Kokkinos P, Myers J. Exercise and physical activity: clinical outcomes and applications. Circulation. 2010;122(16):1637–48.
44. Kokkinos P, Myers J, Faselis C, Panagiotakos DB, Doumas M, Pittaras A, et al. Exercise capacity and mortality in older men: a 20-year follow-up study. Circulation. 2010;122(8):790–7.
45. Kokkinos P, Myers J, Kokkinos JP, Pittaras A, Narayan P, Manolis A, et al. Exercise capacity and mortality in black and white men. Circulation. 2008;117(5):614–22.
46. Kokkinos P, Myers J, Nylen E, Panagiotakos DB, Manolis A, Pittaras A, et al. Exercise capacity and all-cause mortality in African American and Caucasian men with type 2 diabetes. Diabetes Care. 2009;32(4):623–8.
47. Kokkinos PF, Faselis C, Myers J, Narayan P, Sui X, Zhang J, et al. Cardiorespiratory fitness and incidence of major adverse cardiovascular events in US veterans: a cohort study. Mayo Clin Proc. 2017;92(1):39–48.
48. Kokkinos PF, Faselis C, Myers J, Panagiotakos D, Doumas M. Interactive effects of fitness and statin treatment on mortality risk in veterans with dyslipidaemia: a cohort study. Lancet. 2013;381(9864):394–9.
49. Myers J, Prakash M, Froelicher V, Do D, Partington S, Atwood JE. Exercise capacity and mortality among men referred for exercise testing. N Engl J Med. 2002;346(11):793–801.
50. Mora S, Redberg RF, Cui Y, Whiteman MK, Flaws JA, Sharrett AR, et al. Ability of exercise testing to predict cardiovascular and all-cause death in asymptomatic women: a 20-year follow-up of the lipid research clinics prevalence study. JAMA. 2003;290(12):1600–7.
51. Paffenbarger RS Jr, Hyde RT, Wing AL, Hsieh CC. Physical activity, all-cause mortality, and longevity of college alumni. N Engl J Med. 1986;314(10):605–13.
52. Drca N, Wolk A, Jensen-Urstad M, Larsson SC. Atrial fibrillation is associated with different levels of physical activity levels at different ages in men. Heart. 2014;100(13):1037–42.
53. Mons U, Hahmann H, Brenner H. A reverse J-shaped association of leisure time physical activity with prognosis in patients with stable coronary heart disease: evidence from a large cohort with repeated measurements. Heart. 2014;100(13):1043–9.
54. O'Keefe JH, Patil HR, Lavie CJ, Magalski A, Vogel RA, McCullough PA. Potential adverse cardiovascular effects from excessive endurance exercise. Mayo Clin Proc. 2012;87(6):587–95.
55. Oxborough D, Birch K, Shave R, George K. "Exercise-induced cardiac fatigue"--a review of the echocardiographic literature. Echocardiography. 2010;27(9):1130–40.
56. Armstrong ME, Green J, Reeves GK, Beral V, Cairns BJ, Millon Women Study Collaborators. Frequent physical activity may not reduce vascular disease risk as much as moderate activity: large prospective study of women in the United Kingdom. Circulation. 2015;131(8):721–9.
57. Schnohr P, O'Keefe JH, Marott JL, Lange P, Jensen GB. Dose of jogging and long-term mortality: the Copenhagen City Heart Study. J Am Coll Cardiol. 2015;65(5):411–9.

58. Maessen MFH, Hopman MTE, Verbeek ALM, Eijsvogels TMH. Dose of jogging: mortality versus longevity. J Am Coll Cardiol. 2015;65(24):2672–3.
59. Arem H, Moore SC, Patel A, Hartge P, Berrington de Gonzalez A, Visvanathan K, et al. Leisure time physical activity and mortality: a detailed pooled analysis of the dose-response relationship. JAMA Intern Med. 2015;175(6):959–67.
60. Faselis C, Kokkinos P, Tsimploulis A, Pittaras A, Myers J, Lavie CJ, et al. Exercise capacity and atrial fibrillation risk in veterans: a cohort study. Mayo Clin Proc. 2016;91(5):558–66.
61. Franklin BA, Bonzheim K, Gordon S, Timmis GC. Snow shoveling: a trigger for acute myocardial infarction and sudden coronary death. Am J Cardiol. 1996;77(10):855–8.
62. Juneau M, Johnstone M, Dempsey E, Waters DD. Exercise-induced myocardial ischemia in a cold environment. Effect of antianginal medications. Circulation. 1989;79(5):1015–20.
63. Pandolf KB, Cafarelli E, Noble BJ, Metz KF. Hyperthermia: effect on exercise prescription. Arch Phys Med Rehabil. 1975;56(12):524–6.
64. Hoberg E, Schuler G, Kunze B, Obermoser AL, Hauer K, Mautner HP, et al. Silent myocardial ischemia as a potential link between lack of premonitoring symptoms and increased risk of cardiac arrest during physical stress. Am J Cardiol. 1990;65(9):583–9.
65. American College of Sports Medicine. Guidelines for exercise testing and prescription. 7th ed. Baltimore: Lippincott Williams & Wilkins; 2005.
66. Riebe D, Franklin BA, Thompson PD, Garber CE, Whitfield GP, Magal M, et al. Updating ACSM's recommendations for exercise preparticipation health screening. Med Sci Sports Exerc. 2015;47(11):2473–9.
67. de Barros e Silva PG, Califf RM, Sun JL, McMurray JJ, Holman R, Haffner S, et al. Chronic obstructive pulmonary disease and cardiovascular risk: insights from the NAVIGATOR trial. Int J Cardiol 2014;176(3):1126–8.
68. Redelmeier DA, Greenwald JA. Competing risks of mortality with marathons: retrospective analysis. BMJ. 2007;335(7633):1275–7.
69. Carr JJ, Jacobs DR Jr, Terry JG, Shay CM, Sidney S, Liu K, et al. Association of coronary artery calcium in adults aged 32 to 46 years with incident coronary heart disease and death. JAMA Cardiol. 2017;2(4):391–9.
70. Möhlenkamp S, Leineweber K, Lehmann N, Braun S, Roggenbuck U, Perrey M, et al. Coronary atherosclerosis burden, but not transient troponin elevation, predicts long-term outcome in recreational marathon runners. Basic Res Cardiol. 2014;109(1):391. https://doi.org/10.1007/s00395-013-0391-8.
71. Tsiflikas I, Thomas C, Fallmann C, Schabel C, Mangold S, Ketelsen D, et al. Prevalence of subclinical coronary artery disease in middle-aged, male marathon runners detected by cardiac CT. Rofo. 2015;187(7):561–8.
72. Merghani A, Maestrini V, Rosmini S, Cox AT, Dhutia H, Bastiaenan R, et al. Prevalence of subclinical coronary artery disease in masters endurance athletes with a low atherosclerotic risk profile. Circulation. 2017;136(2):126–37.
73. Siegel AJ. Prerace aspirin to protect susceptible runners from cardiac arrest during marathons: is opportunity knocking? Open Heart. 2015;2(1):e000102. https://doi.org/10.1136/openhrt-2014-000102.
74. Siegel AJ, Noakes TD. Can pre-race aspirin prevent sudden cardiac death during marathons? Br J Sports Med. 2017;51(22):1579–81.
75. Libby P, Crea F. Clinical implications of inflammation for cardiovascular primary prevention. Eur Heart J. 2010;31(7):777–83.
76. Maddox TM, Stanislawski MA, Grunwald GK, Bradley SM, Ho PM, Tsai TT, et al. Nonobstructive coronary artery disease and risk of myocardial infarction. JAMA. 2014;312(17):1754–63.
77. Siegel AJ, Stec JJ, Lipinska I, Van Cott EM, Lewandrowski KB, Ridker PM, et al. Effect of marathon running on inflammatory and hemostatic markers. Am J Cardiol. 2001;88(8):918–20.
78. Huskens D, Roest M, Remijn JA, Konings J, Kremers RM, Bloemen S, et al. Strenuous exercise induces a hyperreactive rebalanced hemostatic state that is more pronounced in men. Thromb Haemost. 2016;115(6):1109–19.
79. Steering Committee of the Physicians' Health Study Research Group. Final report on the aspirin component of the ongoing Physicians' Health Study. N Engl J Med. 1989;321(3):129–35.
80. Albano AJ, Thompson PD, Kapur NK. Acute coronary thrombosis in Boston marathon runners. N Engl J Med. 2012;366(2):184–5.
81. Pignone M, Alberts MJ, Colwell JA, Cushman M, Inzucchi SE, Mukherjee D, et al. Aspirin for primary prevention of cardiovascular events in people with diabetes. J Am Coll Cardiol. 2010;55(25):2878–86.
82. Siegel AJ. Pheidippides redux: reducing risk for acute cardiac events during marathon running. Am J Med. 2012;125(7):630–5.
83. Walkey AJ. Preventing cardiovascular complications of acute infection: a missed opportunity? Circulation. 2014;129(13):1375–7.
84. Halvorsen S, Andreotti F, ten Berg JM, Cattaneo M, Coccheri S, Marchioli R, et al. Aspirin therapy in primary cardiovascular disease prevention: a position paper of the European Society of Cardiology Working Group on Thrombosis. J Am Coll Cardiol. 2014;64(3):319–27.
85. Smith DL, Horn GP, Woods J, Ploutz-Snyder R, Fernhall B. Effect of aspirin supplementation on hemostatic responses in firefighters aged 40 to 60 years. Am J Cardiol. 2016;118(2):275–80.
86. Lee DC, Pate RR, Lavie CJ, Sui X, Church TS, Blair SN. Leisure-time running reduces all-cause and cardiovascular mortality risk. J Am Coll Cardiol. 2014;64(5):472–81.
87. Aengevaeren VL, Mosterd A, Braber TL, Prakken NHJ, Doevendans PA, Grobbee DE, et al. Relationship between lifelong exercise volume and

coronary atherosclerosis in athletes. Circulation. 2017;136(2):138–48.
88. Lee DC, Brellenthin AG, Thompson PD, Sui X, Lee IM, Lavie CJ. Running as a key lifestyle medicine for longevity. Prog Cardiovasc Dis. 2017;60(1):45–55.
89. Smyth A. O'Donnell M, Lamelas P, Teo K, Rangarajan S, Yusuf S. Physical activity and anger or emotional upset as triggers of acute myocardial infarction: the INTERHEART Study. Circulation 2016;134(1):1059–1067.
90. Siegel AJ. IMMDA Advisory, 2015: pre-race aspirin to prevent heart attack and/or cardiac arrest during long distance running. Available at: immda.org/wp-content/uploads/2015/08/Spring-2015-Pre-race-ASA.pdf. Accessed 19 June 2018.
91. Shaw E, Tofler GH, Buckley T, Bajorek B, Ward M. Therapy for triggered acute risk prevention: a study of feasibility. Heart Lung Circ. 2009;18(5):347–52.
92. Tofler GH, Spinaze M, Shaw E, Buckley T. Therapy for triggered acute risk prevention in subjects at increased cardiovascular risk. Am J Cardiol. 2013;111(12):1755–8.
93. Tofler GH, Muller JE, Stone PH, Forman S, Solomon RE, Knatterud GL, et al. Modifiers of timing and possible triggers of acute myocardial infarction in the thrombolysis in myocardial infarction phase II (TIMI II) study group. J Am Coll Cardiol. 1992;20(5):1049–55.

8 Exercise and Blood Pressure Control in Hypertension

Hayley V. MacDonald and Linda S. Pescatello

Abbreviations

1RM	One-repetition maximum
ACC	American College of Cardiology
ACSM	American College of Sports Medicine
AHA	American Heart Association
BP	Blood pressure
CO	Cardiac output
CVD	Cardiovascular disease
DBP	Diastolic blood pressure
Ex R_x	Exercise prescription
FIT	Frequency, intensity, and time
FITT-VP	Frequency, intensity, time, type, volume, and progression
HIIT	High-intensity interval training
HR	Heart rate
IHG	Isometric handgrip
JNC 7	The Seventh Report of the Joint National Committee on Prevention, Detection, Evaluation, and Treatment of High Blood Pressure
JNC 8	The Eighth Report of the Joint National Committee on Prevention, Detection, Evaluation, and Treatment of High Blood Pressure
MAP	Mean arterial pressure
PEH	Postexercise hypotension
RPE	Rating of perceived exertion
RT	Resistance training
SBP	Systolic blood pressure
TPR	Total peripheral resistance
USA	United States
$\dot{V}O_2$ max	Maximal oxygen consumption
$\dot{V}O_2$ peak	Peak oxygen consumption
$\dot{V}O_2R$	Oxygen consumption reserve

H. V. MacDonald (✉)
Department of Kinesiology, The University of Alabama, Tuscaloosa, AL, USA
e-mail: hvmacdonald@ua.edu

L. S. Pescatello
Department of Kinesiology, University of Connecticut, Storrs, CT, USA

Introduction

Hypertension Is a Major Public Health Problem

Hypertension is the most common, costly, and modifiable cardiovascular disease (CVD) risk factor in the United States (USA) and world [1–3]. Among 195 countries and territories, high systolic blood pressure (SBP) is the *leading* global risk factor and has accounted for 10.5 million deaths and 212.1 million years of life lost over the past two decades [3]. In the United States, the number of hypertension-related deaths increased 62% from the year 2000 to 2013 (i.e., from 245,220 to 396,675 deaths) [4]. The estimated direct and indirect cost of hypertension is

P. Kokkinos, P. Narayan (eds.), *Cardiorespiratory Fitness in Cardiometabolic Diseases*,
https://doi.org/10.1007/978-3-030-04816-7_8

$51.2 billion, and this figure is projected to increase to $274 billion by the year 2030 [1]. For these reasons, the Department of Health and Human Services established hypertension as a high-priority, leading health indicator within the Healthy People 2020 national objectives by aiming to (a) increase the proportion of adults with hypertension whose blood pressure (BP) is under control by 18% and (b) reduce the proportion of adults diagnosed with hypertension by 10% by the year 2020 [5]. Similarly, the World Health Organization has established a series of key targets to reduce the risk of premature death from CVD and stroke by 25% by the year 2025 ("25 by 25") [6]. One of the key targets, and arguably the most impactful, is reducing the global prevalence of SBP >140 mmHg by 25%.

Early diagnosis, including accurate and repetitive BP measurements using standard professional methodology and procedures, and effective antihypertensive therapeutic interventions are essential for meeting the Healthy People 2020 national objectives. Untreated and poorly controlled hypertension contributes to and accelerates pathological processes that lead to increased risk of CVD, shorter life expectancy free of CVD, more years lived with CVD, and increased of risk of mortality [2, 7–9]. Adoption of a healthy lifestyle is fundamental for the primary prevention, treatment, and control of hypertension. Given that the relationship between BP and CVD risk is linear, continuous, and consistent, early and aggressive lifestyle intervention is critical in order to prevent or delay the rapid, progressive rise in BP [2, 10, 11].

Definition and Key Concepts

Hypertension is a health condition defined by a transitory or sustained elevation of systemic arterial BP to a level likely to induce cardiovascular damage or result in other adverse health consequences [12]. Since the 2003 publication of the Seventh Report of the Joint National Committee on Prevention, Detection, Evaluation, and Treatment of High BP (JNC 7) [13], several large-scale epidemiological studies and meta-analyses [9, 11, 14–18] have clearly and consistently shown increased cardiovascular risk at BP levels far below those used to define hypertension traditionally (i.e., resting SBP ≥140 mmHg or diastolic BP [DBP] ≥90 mmHg [13]). Starting at 115/75 mmHg, cardiovascular risk doubles for every 20 mmHg increase in SBP or 10 mmHg in DBP [9, 11]. Therefore, the American College of Cardiology (ACC) and the American Heart Association (AHA), with support from other professional societies, published the 2017 Guideline for the Prevention, Detection, Evaluation, and Management of High BP in Adults [10], a long-awaited update to the JNC 7 [13].

The most noteworthy change in the 2017 ACC/AHA guideline is the recommendation to use *lower* SBP and DBP thresholds to define hypertension among the general population (Table 8.1). These guidelines also recommend

Table 8.1 Blood pressure thresholds and classification scheme according to the 2017 American College of Cardiology/American Heart Association Guideline [10]

BP threshold (mmHg)			2017 ACC/AHA
Systolic BP		Diastolic BP	Classification scheme[a, b]
<120	and	<80	Normal BP (*normal BP*)
120–129	and	<80	Elevated BP (*prehypertension*)
130–139	or	80–89	Stage 1 hypertension (*prehypertension*)
140–159	or	90–99	Stage 2 hypertension (*stage 1 hypertension*)
≥160	or	≥ 100	Stage 2 hypertension (*stage 2 hypertension*)

BP blood pressure, *ACC/AHA* American College of Cardiology/American Heart Association
[a]Individuals with differing systolic BP and diastolic BP classifications should be designated to the higher BP category
[b]The BP classification scheme corresponding to the Seventh Report of the Joint National Committee (JNC 7) on Prevention, Detection, Evaluation, and Treatment of High BP [13] is provided in parentheses

incorporating the estimated 10-year risk of atherosclerotic CVD (determined by the ACC/AHA Pooled Cohort Equations [19]) *in addition* to resting BP to guide antihypertensive medication treatment decisions. Accordingly, hypertension is now defined as a resting SBP of 130 mmHg or greater, a resting DBP of 80 mmHg or greater, taking antihypertensive medication, being told by a physician or health professional on at least two occasions that one has high BP, or any combination of these criteria [10]. Using this definition, ≈103 million Americans (46%) [10, 20] and approximately 1.4 billion adults (31%) worldwide [21] have hypertension. Of note, this global estimate is based on the previous definition of hypertension (i.e., SBP or DBP of ≥140 mmHg or ≥90 mmHg, respectively [13]) and, thus, underestimates the global burden of hypertension as defined in the 2017 ACC/AHA guideline.

In addition to redefining hypertension, the 2017 ACC/AHA guideline eliminated the term "prehypertension" (SBP ranging from 120 to 139 mmHg and/or DBP ranging from 80 to 89 mmHg) introduced in the JNC 7 [13]. Instead, they include a BP category termed "elevated BP," defined as resting SBP ranging from 120 to 129 mmHg *and* DBP <80 mmHg [10]. There is substantial evidence from individual epidemiological studies and meta-analyses of these data that show a graded and progressive rise in cardiovascular risk as BP levels increase from normal BP, to elevated BP, to stage 1 hypertension [10]. Hence, elevated BP, like prehypertension, represents an opportunity for increased awareness and intervention so that individuals with this condition can delay or prevent incident hypertension through the adoption of healthy lifestyle interventions, such as participation in regular exercise [10, 11, 22–25].

In approximately 90% of cases, the etiology of hypertension is unknown, and it is called essential, idiopathic, or primary hypertension. Systemic hypertension with a known cause is referred to as secondary or inessential hypertension. Systemic hypertension primarily involves disorders and diseases of the renal, endocrine, or nervous systems, such as kidney disease, Cushing's syndrome, and Guillain-Barre Syndrome, respectively. Other causes of secondary hypertension are obstructive sleep apnea, tumors, or drug-induced.

Although essential hypertension and secondary hypertension are the major classifications of hypertension, several other descriptive terms are used to define various types of hypertension [10]:

- Isolated systolic hypertension is defined as SBP of 130 mmHg or greater and DBP of less than 90 mmHg.
- White coat hypertension is characterized by elevated BP readings when measured in the physician's office (or other clinical setting) but normal BP when measured outside of the physician's office using ambulatory or home BP monitoring.
- Masked hypertension is characterized by normal BP readings when measured in the physician's office (or other clinical setting) but elevated BP when measured outside of the physician's office using ambulatory or home BP monitoring. There are three subtypes of masked hypertension: morning, daytime (stress-induced), and nocturnal hypertension [26].
- Pulmonary hypertension is characterized by elevated pulmonary arterial pressure accompanied by dyspnea, fatigue, syncope, and/or substernal chest pain.
- Resistant hypertension is defined as the failure to achieve goal BP in patients who are adhering to maximum doses of an appropriate three-drug regimen that includes a diuretic. Resistant hypertension may be caused by improper BP assessments, volume overload (i.e., fluid retention, excess sodium intake), drug-induced (i.e., side effect of a prescription medication), lifestyle habits (e.g., diet, excessive alcohol intake), or other identifiable causes of hypertension (i.e., secondary hypertension) (for an expanded discussion on resistant hypertension and cardiorespiratory fitness, see Chap. 7).

- Malignant hypertension is defined by markedly elevated BP levels (i.e., SBP >200 mmHg and/or DBP >140 mmHg) due to papilledema, a condition of optic nerve swelling that is secondary to elevated intracranial pressure [27].

Pathophysiology

BP is a highly heterogeneous, quantitative trait that serves as a biomarker of hypertension. Many physiologic factors have been implicated in the pathogenesis and maintenance of elevated BP that include (but are not limited to) activation of the sympathetic nervous and renin-angiotensin-aldosterone systems, endothelial dysfunction, and vascular structural changes [28–31]. The regulation of BP is a sophisticated and multifaceted process as it is modulated by intermediary phenotypes associated with renal, hormonal, vascular, peripheral, and central adrenergic pathways. BP regulation is further complicated by the fact that these intermediary phenotypes are controlled by complex, sometimes redundant, interwoven mechanisms, including BP itself [32, 33]. According to Ohm's law, mean arterial pressure (MAP) is the product of cardiac output (CO) and total peripheral resistance (TPR): MAP = CO × TPR. Therefore, the pathogenic mechanisms leading to hypertension must increase TPR, CO, or both [34]. Once hypertension has been established, it is commonly characterized by elevated TPR and a lower or normal CO [34].

Essential hypertension, as detected by resting (brachial) BP levels, tends to develop gradually, emphasizing the importance of prevention and early diagnosis. Essential hypertension tends to cluster in families and represents a collection of genetically based diseases and syndromes with several underlying inherited biochemical abnormalities. Factors considered important in the genesis of essential hypertension include family history, genetic predispositions, salt sensitivity, imbalances in the major BP regulatory systems that favor vasoconstriction over vasodilation, and their interaction with environmental factors. Several lifestyle-related factors have been commonly implicated in the development of hypertension and include obesity, physical inactivity, and excessive salt intake. The relationship among these modifiable factors is complex, with several overlapping mechanisms of action. Indeed, even modest alterations in these lifestyle-related factors can elicit reductions in SBP ranging from 2 to 20 mmHg [10].

Early manifestations of essential hypertension such as autonomic dysfunction (diminished parasympathetic and increased sympathetic tone) are present far before noticeable elevations in BP occur [31] (see Davis et al. [35] and Grassi et al. [36] for detailed reviews on autonomic and hemodynamic disturbances that occur with hypertension). In the presence of other CVD risk factors (e.g., obesity and dyslipidemia), early markers of dysfunction are often exacerbated, and the pathophysiologic progression toward fully developed hypertension is accelerated [28, 37]. Thus, elevations in CO, normal TPR, and enhanced endothelium-dependent dilation characterize the early (developmental) stages of essential hypertension. As elevations in BP progress toward essential hypertension, it becomes better characterized by normal CO, elevated TPR, endothelial dysfunction, and left ventricular hypertrophy – alterations that reflect the adverse hemodynamic and vascular changes that arise from chronically elevated peripheral resistance [34].

Chronic elevations in peripheral resistance may be related to neurohumoral mechanisms (e.g., increases in circulating levels of epinephrine), myogenic autoregulation, structural changes in small arteries, or a combination of these factors [31]. Poiseuille's law states that resistance is *inversely* related to the vessel radius of the fourth power [34]; thus, functional or structural changes in arterial lumen size or radius are major determinants of TPR. Decreases in lumen size or radius will increase TPR, which in turn aids in the maintenance of persistent elevations in BP and, subsequently, hypertension (for detailed reviews see Safar et al. [38] and Laurent et al. [39]). Sustained elevations in pressure exert greater vessel wall stress that, overtime, induce alterations in the vessel properties and wall composition that favor mechanobiological responses that attempt to reduce wall stress (i.e., vascular thickening and structural stiffening). However, these compensatory mechanisms eventually fail, and endothelial dysfunction ensues. Of note, changes in vascular structure and function have traditionally been viewed as either the *cause* or the *consequence* of elevated BP. More recent perspectives suggest that, based on the totality of available evidence, vascular stiffness is *both* a cause and a consequence of hypertension [40].

Hypertension, if untreated, contributes to and accelerates the pathological processes that lead to premature death from heart disease, stroke, and renal failure [41]. Hypertension damages the endothelium, which predisposes the individual to atherosclerosis and other vascular pathologies. Hypertension-induced vascular damage can lead to stroke and transient ischemic attacks as well as end-stage renal disease. Chronic elevations in BP increase afterload on the heart and thus the mechanical stress or workload of the heart. In response to these stressors (and other neurohormonal factors), the left ventricle may undergo distinct structural changes or *maladaptation* that include increased left ventricular wall thickness and wall mass and decreased chamber size. Collectively, these alterations characterize a condition known as concentric left ventricular hypertrophy [42–45]. Concentric left ventricular hypertrophy is an antecedent to chronic heart failure and is an independent risk factor for other types of CVD, such as coronary heart disease and stroke [42, 46, 47].

Epidemiological Evidence of the Scope of the Hypertension (Prevalence and Incidence)

Several definitions of hypertension exist in the literature, resulting in slight variations in hypertension prevalence and control rates [48, 49]. The importance of utilizing a clear and consistent definition of hypertension is essential to guiding diagnosis, treatment, control, and surveillance of hypertension. As such, the definition of hypertension and adult BP categories published in the 2017 ACC/AHA guideline will be the BP classification scheme incorporated in this chapter (Table 8.1) [10].

Hypertension affects ≈103 million (45.6%) adults living in the United States [10, 20], an additional 31 million newly diagnosed Americans when compared to prior estimates using the JNC 7 definition of hypertension (i.e., ≈72 million or 31.9% of US adults) [13, 20]. Despite a higher prevalence of hypertension in the United States under the new guideline, the majority of newly diagnosed adults can be treated with lifestyle modifications (e.g., diet and exercise) without concomitant pharmacological intervention. Like JNC 7 [13], the 2017 ACC/AHA guideline [10] recommends that pharmacological treatment be initiated among the general population when resting SBP or DBP levels exceed 140 mmHg or 90 mmHg, respectively, or among those with stage 1 hypertension (Table 8.1) with high CVD risk (i.e., patients with known CVD, diabetes mellitus, or chronic kidney disease, or estimated CVD risk >10%). Accordingly, there is a small increase (1.9%) in the proportion of US adults who are recommended pharmacological therapy under the 2017 ACC/AHA guideline compared to the JNC 7 (36.2% vs. 34.3%) [20].

Another ≈27 million US adults (≈12%) have elevated BP [20]. This means more than half (≈60%) of the adult population in the United States – approximately ≈130 million Americans – have high BP (i.e., elevated BP to established stage 1 or 2 hypertension). Individuals with elevated BP are at increased risk for developing hypertension, additional CVD risk factors, heart disease, and stroke [10, 37, 50]. The rate of progression from elevated BP to hypertension can occur rapidly (within a 5-year period) [1, 9, 51, 52] and is positively and strongly associated with age, baseline BP, and comorbidities [53, 54].

The prevalence of hypertension increases substantially with age, with 77% and 82% of US adults ≥65 and ≥75 yr of age, respectively, having hypertension compared to ≈36% of adults <55 yr of age [10, 55]. Among adults ≥50 yr of age, the lifetime risk of developing hypertension approaches 90% [1, 10, 53]. The prevalence of hypertension also varies by racial/ethnic populations and sexes living in the United States [1, 10]:

- Non-Hispanic whites 20 yr or older, 47% of men and 41% of women
- Non-Hispanic Asians 20 yr or older, 45% of men and 36% of women
- Non-Hispanic blacks 20 yr or older, 59% of men and 56% of women
- Hispanic Americans 20 yr or older, 44% of men and 42% of women

On average, blacks have the highest prevalence of hypertension of all other races [1, 10]. For adults 45 years of age without hypertension, the 40-year risk of developing hypertension was 93% for blacks, 92% for Hispanic, 86% for white, and 84% for Chinese adults [10]. Compared to whites, blacks develop hypertension earlier in life, their BP is higher over their lifetime, and among those with hypertension, blacks are more likely to have resistant hypertension than whites and Hispanics (19.0% vs. 13.5% and 11.2%, respectively) [1, 56]. Despite similar awareness and treatment rates as whites, blacks experience more severe hypertension and greater difficulty in achieving BP control due to reduced effectiveness of some antihypertensive medications, resulting in 1.5 times greater risk of heart failure, 1.8 times greater risk of fatal strokes, and 4.2 times greater risk of end-stage renal disease [1].

Hypertension is one of the most common primary diagnoses in the United States (≈34% of all office-based physician visits by adults in 2013 were related to hypertension care [57, 58]) and is the leading cause for medication prescriptions among adults >50 yr [59, 60]. Overall, population estimates of awareness, treatment, and control of hypertension in the United States have increased overtime, but the rate of improvement has plateaued in recent years [55, 61]. In contrast, the prevalence of hypertension has remained unchanged for more than a decade [61]. The most recent estimates show that among adults ≥20 yr of age with hypertension, 84.1% were aware of their condition, 76.0% were receiving treatment for their high BP, and 52% were properly controlled (BP control was higher, 69%, among those currently being treated) [1], which falls short of the Healthy People 2020 target of controlling 61.2% of all adults with hypertension [61]. A recent paper by Quindry and Franklin [62] nicely summarizes the independent and interrelated cardioprotective effects of exercise and pharmacotherapies prescribed to treat CVDs and related risk factors. The authors put forth the notion that in order to effectively reduce the prevalence and burden of CVD, contemporary therapies must include *both* adjunctive exercise and lifestyle interventions in addition to pharmacological agents. Indeed, if the prevalence and control of hypertension were improved by increasing the use of lifestyle-based antihypertensive therapies, such as exercise, as a primary or complementary treatment strategy, our society would experience substantial health and economic benefits.

Epidemiologic Association Between Cardiorespiratory Fitness and Hypertension

The preventive benefits of physical activity on all-cause mortality and the onset of CVD risk factors have been documented in many large-scale prospective studies and are summarized in several recent reviews [63–72]. These data clearly and consistently demonstrate that physical activity and cardiorespiratory fitness are inversely and independently associated with cardiovascular morbidity and mortality among both healthy and clinical populations (e.g., adults with CVD), independent of sex/gender and race/ethnicity. Accumulating evidence from prospective cohort studies show that, on average, every one metabolic equivalent increase in cardiorespiratory fitness is associated with a 10–25% reduction in mortality risk [66, 71–73], with the least fit individuals (i.e., <5 metabolic equivalents) experiencing the greatest reduction in risk.

The cardioprotective benefits of physical activity are expansive, but for the purposes of this chapter, we will focus our discussion on the relation between cardiorespiratory fitness and hypertension. Several recent studies have added to a growing body of evidence that shows baseline cardiorespiratory fitness is an important predictor of incident hypertension, such that higher levels of baseline physical activity and cardiorespiratory fitness are associated with a lower risk of incident hypertension among men and women [63, 72, 74–77]. More recent investigations have added to our understanding of this relationship by examining longitudinal patterns in cardiorespiratory fitness and incident hypertension [78–80]. Collectively, these studies support that improvements in cardiorespiratory fitness throughout one's lifetime are associated with the lowest risk of incident hypertension. Similarly, longitudinal patterns that result in higher levels of cardiorespiratory fitness being maintained later in life are also associated with lower risk of incident hypertension [79].

In addition to the cardioprotective effects of physical fitness, several studies also support that higher levels of muscular fitness (i.e., muscular strength and endurance) confer similar protective effects both *independently* and *jointly* with high levels of cardiorespiratory fitness. Moreover, higher levels of muscular fitness are associated with lower risk of developing CVD risk factors, including hypertension [81–83], CVDs, and all-cause mortality [84–89]. Among those with hypertension, higher levels of muscle strength were inversely associated with mortality, independent of cardiorespiratory fitness [85, 90]. Reductions in mortality risk were even greater among individuals with high levels of muscular strength *and* cardiorespiratory fitness. These findings underscore the importance of including both aerobic and resistance exercises in the Ex R_x for individual adults with hypertension [23, 24, 91].

To summarize, there is overwhelming evidence to support that cardiorespiratory fitness may be the single best predictor of cardiovascular morbidity and mortality among the general population and those with established hypertension. In fact, a recent Scientific Statement published by the AHA advocated that cardiorespiratory fitness be considered a clinical vital sign and that it be assessed as part of routine practice among healthy and clinical populations [72]. Increases in cardiorespiratory fitness and the maintenance of such improvements favorably modulate the age-related progressive increase in arterial stiffness [92], BP, and, ultimately, the development of hypertension [63, 66, 78, 79]. Among those with hypertension, higher levels of cardiorespiratory fitness are associated with reduced BP and left ventricular hypertrophy regression, which in turn may slow the progression of hypertension to more severe forms [63, 64]. In addition, when the types and quantity of physical activities and/or structured exercises required to improve cardiorespiratory and muscular fitness levels are executed appropriately, additional coexisting CVD risk factors (e.g., obesity, dyslipidemia) may experience favorable effects, resulting in even greater health benefits [63–65, 67, 68, 70, 72, 81, 83, 90, 93, 94].

The Antihypertensive Effects of Exercise

Participation in regular exercise is a key modifiable determinant of hypertension and is recognized as a cornerstone therapy for the primary prevention, treatment, and control of high BP [10, 11, 22–25]. Meta-analyses of randomized controlled, intervention trials have concluded that regular, aerobic exercise lowers resting BP 5–7 mmHg, while dynamic resistance exercise lowers resting BP 2–3 mmHg among individuals with hypertension [91, 95]. The magnitude of these BP reductions following aerobic and resistance exercise can lower CVD risk by 20–30% and 6–14%, respectively [9, 10, 13, 96]. Furthermore, aerobic exercise can lower BP by a magnitude that rivals those obtained with first-line antihypertensive medications [13, 96–98]. Exercising as little as 1 day per week is as effective (or even more so) than pharmacotherapy for reducing all-cause mortality among those with hypertension [99]. In addition, when lifestyle modifications are executed appropriately, coexisting CVD risk factors may also experience benefits, translating to an even greater reduction in overall cardiovascular risk. Indeed, a recent meta-analysis of major exercise and drug trials showed no statistically detectable difference between exercise and drug interventions for the secondary prevention of coronary heart disease and prediabetes, and physical activity interventions were more effective than drug interventions for the secondary prevention of stroke mortality [100].

For these reasons the 2017 ACC/AHA guideline [10], JNC 7 [13], 2014 Evidence-Based Guidelines for the Management of High Blood Pressure in Adults (JNC 8) [101], AHA/ACC 2013 Lifestyle Work Group [25], European Society of Hypertension and European Society of Cardiology [102], Canadian Hypertension Education Program [103], and the ACSM [23] universally endorse aerobic exercise for the primary prevention and treatment of hypertension. Although the recommended exercise prescription (Ex R_x) for individuals with hypertension in terms of the *f*requency (how often?), *i*ntensity (how hard?), *t*ime (how long?), *t*ype (what kind?), *v*olume (how much?), and *p*rogression (or FITT-VP) principle varies slightly across the various aforementioned organizational guidelines (Table 8.2), the general consensus is that adults with elevated BP to established hypertension should participate in 30–60 min/d of moderate-intensity aerobic exercise on most, if not all, days of the week to total 150 min/wk of exercise (or more) supplemented by moderate-intensity dynamic resistance training (RT) on 2–3 d/wk [91].

It should be noted that these recommendations are limited by methodological quality of the studies upon which the evidence is based [91, 104]. Major limitations in the current state of the literature include small sample sizes, assessing study populations with normal and elevated BP rather than hypertension, not accounting for major confounders to the BP response to exercise that include timing of the last bout of exercise and detraining effects, and lack of standard protocols for the assessment of BP and the exercise intervention. As a result of these limitations, the effectiveness of exercise as antihypertensive lifestyle therapy among individuals with hypertension has been underestimated [91, 95, 105]. Furthermore, large randomized clinical trials that examine both the acute and chronic BP lowering effects of exercise among diverse populations are needed before professional organizations can definitively determine the optimal Ex R_x for individuals with hypertension. New and emerging research are highlighted later in this chapter, as such studies may serve to fine-tune exercise prescription among individuals with hypertension.

Presently, the ACSM recommends the following *FITT-VP* Ex R_x for individuals with hypertension (Table 8.3) [24]:

- *F*requency: For aerobic exercise, on most, preferably all days of the week supplemented by resistance exercise 2–3 d/wk and flexibility exercise 2–3 d/wk.
- *I*ntensity: Moderate (i.e., 40–<60% oxygen consumption reserve [$\dot{V}O_2R$] or 11–14 on a scale of 6 [no exertion] to 20 [maximal exertion] level of physical exertion [106] or an intensity that causes noticeable increases in heart rate [HR] and breathing) for aerobic exercise, moderate-to-vigorous (60–80% of one-repetition maximum [1RM]) for resistance, and stretch to the point of feeling tightness or slight discomfort for flexibility.
- *T*ime: For aerobic exercise, a minimum of 30 min or up to 60 min/d for continuous or accumulated aerobic exercise. If intermittent, begin with a minimum of 10 min bouts.
- *T*ype: For aerobic exercise, emphasis should be placed on prolonged, rhythmic activities using large muscle groups such as walking, cycling, or swimming. Dynamic resistance exercise may supplement aerobic exercise and should consist of at least one set of 8–12 repetitions of 8–10 different exercises targeting the major muscle groups. For flexibility, hold each muscle 10–30 s for 2–4 repetitions per muscle group. Balance (neuromotor) exercise training 2–3 d/wk is also recommended as adjuvant exercise in individuals at high risk for fall (i.e., older adults) and is likely to benefit younger adults as well.
- *V*olume: To total at least 150 min/wk or 700–2000 kcal/wk of moderate-intensity aerobic exercise.
- *P*rogression: Progress gradually, avoiding large increases in any of the components of the FITT. Increase exercise duration over the first 4–6 wk and then increase frequency, intensity, and time (or some combination of these) to achieve the recommended volume of 700–2000 kcal/wk over the next 4–8 months. Progression may be individualized based on tolerance and preference in a conservative manner.

Table 8.2 The existing professional exercise recommendations among adults with hypertension

FITT of the Ex R_x	Professional committee/organization JNC 8 [101] and AHA/ACC Lifestyle Work Group [25]	JNC 7 [13]	AHA Scientific Statement [161]	ACSM Position Stand [23]	ESH/ESC [102]	2016 CHEP [103]	2017 ACC/AHA Guideline [10]
*F*requency (how often?)	3–4 d/wk ≥12 wk	5–7 d/wk (most days)	5–7 d/wk (most days)	5–7 d/wk	5–7 d/wk	4–7 d/wk and habitual activity	5–7 d/wk (most days)
*I*ntensity (how hard?)	Moderate to vigorous[a]		Moderate to vigorous[a]	Moderate[a]	Moderate[a]	Moderate[a]	Moderate to vigorous[a]
*T*ime (how long?)	40 min/d	≥30 min/d	150 min/wk	30–60 min/d (single or multiple ≥ 10 min bouts)	≥30 min/d	30–60 min/d (accumulation)	90–150 min/wk
*T*ype (what kind?) *Primary*	Aerobic exercise	Aerobic exercise	Aerobic exercise	Aerobic exercise	Aerobic exercise	Aerobic exercise	Aerobic exercise
Evidence rating	High[b]/Grade B[b], COR IIa, LOE A[c]		COR I, LOE A[c]	LOE A[d] LOE B[d]	COR I, LOE A–B	LOE Grade D[e]	COR I, LOE A[c]
Adjuvant			RT	RT[a] 2–3 d•wk^{-1}	RT[a] 2–3 d/wk	RT, Isometric (Handgrip) RT	RT, Isometric RT 3 d/wk
Evidence rating			COR IIa, LOE B[c]	LOE B[f, d]		LOE Grade D[e]	COR I, LOE A[c]

Reprinted from Pescatello LS et al. [104], with permission from Elsevier

Shaded boxes indicate information was missing or not reported in original report. *ACC* American College of Cardiology, *ACSM* American College of Sports Medicine, *AE* aerobic exercise, *AHA* American Heart Association, *CHEP* Canadian Hypertension Education Program, *COR* class of recommendation, indicates the *strength* of the recommendation, *ESH* European Society of Hypertension, *ESC* European Society of Cardiology, *Ex* R_x exercise prescription, *FITT* *f*requency, *i*ntensity, *t*ime, and *t*ype, *LOE* level of evidence, rates the *quality* of scientific evidence, *JNC* 7 Seventh Report of the Joint National Committee, *JNC* 8 Eighth Report of the Joint National Committee, *RT* dynamic resistance training (unless specified otherwise), $\dot{V}O_2R$ oxygen consumption reserve

[a]Moderate intensity, 40–59% $\dot{V}O_2R$ or an intensity that causes noticeable increases in heart rate and breathing; 60–80% of 1RM for RT; vigorous (or high) intensity, ≥60% $\dot{V}O_2R$ or an intensity that causes substantial increases in heart rate and breathing

[b]Evidence statement (LOE), *AE lowers blood pressure (BP)*, high; evidence recommendation (COR), *FIT* (*f*requency, *i*ntensity, *t*ime) *of the Ex* R_x *to lower BP*, Grade B or moderate (COR IIa, LOE A)[c]

[c]AHA criteria to evaluate the COR and LOE [10, 161]

[d]Strength of evidence (COR): *immediate effects of AE* (i.e., *postexercise hypotension*), Category B; *long-term effects of AE* (i.e., *chronic effects*), Category A; *FIT of the Ex* R_x *to lower BP*, Category B

[e]Strength of evidence (LOE) ranges from Grade A to D *(strongest to weakest evidence)* [103]; *AE recommendations for individuals with normal BP to prevent hypertension or for individuals with hypertension to reduce BP*, Grade D; *for individuals with normal BP or stage 1 hypertension, resistance exercise* (i.e., *RT, isometric handgrip RT*) *does not adversely influence BP*, Grade D; *higher intensities of exercise are not more effective*, Grade D

[f]*Immediate effects of RT*, COR C[c]

Table 8.3 The current exercise prescription for adults with hypertension [23, 24]

FITT-VP principle of the Ex R_x	ACSM recommendations
*F*requency (how often?)	5–7 d/wk
*I*ntensity (how hard?)[a]	Moderate (40–<60% $\dot{V}O_2R$ or 12–13 on a scale of 6 [no exertion] to 20 [maximal exertion] level of physical exertion or an intensity that causes noticeable increases in heart rate and breathing)
*T*ime (how long?)	≥30–60 min/d; one continuous bout or multiple bouts of at least 10 min each
*T*ype (what kind?) *Primary*	Aerobic exercise; prolonged, rhythmic activities using large muscle groups (e.g., walking, cycling, swimming)
Adjuvant 1	Muscle strengthening *F:* 2–3 d/wk (non-consecutive) *I:* Moderate-to-vigorous-intensity (60–80% of 1RM); major muscle groups *T:* 8–10 exercises; 2–4 set of 8–12 repetitions
Adjuvant 2	Flexibility *F:* ≥2–3 d/wk *I:* Stretch to the point of feeling tightness or slight discomfort *T:* ≥10 min/d; ≥4 repetitions per muscle group; hold each static stretch for 10–30 s
Adjuvant 3[b]	Neuromotor *F:* ≥2–3 d/wk *I:* undetermined *T:* ≥20–30 min/d
*V*olume (how much?)[c]	≥150 min/wk or 700–2000 kcal/wk
*P*rogression	Progress gradually, avoiding large increases in any of the components of the Ex R_x; increase exercise duration over first 4–6 wk and then increase frequency, intensity, and time (or some combination of these) to achieve recommended quantity and quality of exercise over next 4–8 months

Note. ACSM American College of Sports Medicine, *FITT f*requency, *i*ntensity, *t*ime, *t*ype, *v*olume, and *p*rogression of exercise, *Ex R_x* exercise prescription; 1*RM* one-repetition maximum, $\dot{V}O_2R$ oxygen consumption reserve

[a]Vigorous-intensity aerobic exercise (i.e., ≥60% $\dot{V}O_2R$ or ≥14 on a scale of 6–20 [106]) may elicit greater and more extensive benefits and may be introduced after exercise preparticipation health screening and gradual progression

[b]Balance (neuromotor) training is recommended for older adults, individuals who are at substantial risk of falling, and is likely to benefit younger adults as well

[c]For greater and more extensive benefits, progress exercise volume to total 60 min/d and 300 min/wk of moderate intensity

The Relationship Between the Blood Pressure Effects of Acute (i.e., Postexercise Hypotension) and Chronic Exercise (i.e., Exercise Training)

Physiological responses to acute or short-term exercise translate into functional adaptations that occur during and persist for some time after an isolated exercise session, a phenomenon termed the last bout effect. It has been previously hypothesized that frequent repetition of these acute exercise sessions produces more permanent structural adaptations, forming the exercise training response. These persistent alterations in structure and function remain for as long as the training regimen is continued and then dissipate quickly, returning to pretraining values [107]. Several recently published studies support the notion that the reductions in BP experienced immediately following a single bout of exercise are similar in magnitude to those experienced after exercise training, an observation that suggests the BP benefits attributed to chronic exercise are largely the result of *postexercise hypotension* or PEH [22, 108–110]. PEH describes the immediate, short-term reductions in BP following acute exercise and persists for up to 24 h after the exercise bout [24].

The relationship between the BP response to acute and chronic exercise has yet to be fully elucidated; however, they appear to be related [22, 108–115]. Initial studies examining whether PEH could be used to predict the BP response to aerobic exercise training reported moderate to large correlations between the acute and chronic SBP (r = 0.66–0.89) and DBP (r = 0.66–0.75) responses [110–112]. Since then, researchers have published similar observations for dynamic resistance (r = 0.47–0.74 for SBP, r = 0.45–0.80 for DBP) [110, 114, 115] and isometric resistance (SBP only: r = 0.0.58 for handgrip, r = ≈0.77 for leg) [109, 113] exercise ($P < 0.05$ for all). Collectively, these studies support the notion that the BP response to exercise training is largely a function of PEH.

However, it should be noted that 20–25% of individuals with hypertension do not experience reductions in BP to acute or chronic exercise [23]. Some individuals may even experience *increases* in BP as a result of exercise training [116], albeit this is far less common and not consistently reported [117]. Therefore, PEH has great potential to be used as a health screening tool to identify individuals with hypertension that will (likely) respond favorably to exercise as a nonpharmacologic, lifestyle-based therapy to control their high BP. Further research in a larger, more diverse sample of adults with hypertension is needed to substantiate this premise.

The next section will overview the effects of *acute* (i.e., immediate, short-term, or PEH) and *chronic* (i.e., long-term or training) aerobic, resistance (dynamic and isometric), and concurrent exercise on BP among individuals with hypertension. When appropriate, new and emerging research will be presented that has the potential to alter the way in which exercise may be prescribed to prevent, treat, and control hypertension.

Interventional Evidence of Aerobic (Endurance) Exercise and Blood Pressure Effects

Acute, Immediate, or Short-Term Effects, or Postexercise Hypotension

The BP reductions following acute exercise are immediate but short-term, persisting for up to 24 h after the exercise bout [24]. This response is termed postexercise hypotension or PEH and is an *expected* physiological response to exercise [22, 23, 91, 108, 118–120]. For this reason, individuals with hypertension are encouraged to exercise on most days of the week in order to benefit from the acute effects of aerobic exercise on BP [23, 24]. The BP response to acute aerobic exercise has been summarized in several reviews [108, 121–125], concluding that a single bout of aerobic exercise lowers resting SBP 6–11 mmHg and DBP 4–5 mmHg among adults with high BP and that the magnitude of PEH depends on several factors, including the characteristics of the sample and the intensity and duration of the aerobic exercise performed.

Despite the considerable range in the magnitude of PEH reported in these reviews, the general overall consensus supports that the magnitude of BP reductions resulting from acute aerobic exercise is most pronounced in individuals who stand to benefit the most (i.e., individuals with higher BP compared to normal BP) [23, 24, 124–127]. Short (10–15 min) and long (30–40 min) bouts of aerobic exercise performed continuously at a constant intensity (i.e., workload) or in intervals elicit PEH, independent of exercise intensity [91, 108]. However, there is accumulating evidence to suggest that BP benefits may be maximized when acute aerobic exercise is performed at more vigorous levels of physical exertion (i.e., the magnitude of the BP reductions is intensity-dependent) [91, 108]. New and emerging evidence regarding the relationship between aerobic exercise intensity and PEH will be discussed in the sections that follow.

A limited number of studies have directly compared aspects of the FIT of an acute aerobic exercise intervention on PEH among adults with hypertension [91, 104]. As a result, it remains unclear which factors, that is, aerobic exercise intensity, duration, the total work performed [128], or how the exercise is conducted (i.e., continuous, interval, intermittent or fractionized), are more influential in determining magnitude and duration of PEH. New and emerging evidence regarding the acute effects of aerobic exercise, and its application to the current Ex R_x for hypertension, will be discussed next.

Eicher and colleagues [129] published one of the first studies showing that the illustrated magnitude of the BP reductions resulting from acute aerobic exercise occurs as a direct function of intensity such that the greater the intensity, the greater the BP reduction [91]. Briefly, Eicher et al. [129] examined the antihypertensive effects of three bouts of acute aerobic exercise performed at light (40% of VO_{2max}), moderate (60% of VO_{2max}), and vigorous (100% of VO_{2max}) intensity in men with elevated BP to stage 1 hypertension ($n = 45$). The authors found that BP decreased by 1.5/0.6 mmHg for every 10% increase in relative VO_{2max}, suggesting that more vigorous levels of physical exertion lowered BP to a greater extent than lower levels of physical exertion for individuals willing and able to tolerate more intense levels of exercise [129].

More recent investigations have focused on whether PEH is modulated by *how* the aerobic exercise is performed (i.e., single bout of continuous exercise vs. multiple bouts spread intermittently throughout the day). Bhammar et al. [130] compared the effects of fractionized aerobic exercise (3 × 10 min bouts) spread throughout the day (morning, midday, and afternoon) and a single bout of continuous exercise (1 × 30 min bout) performed at 60–65% of VO_{2peak} on ambulatory BP among 11 individuals with elevated BP. Bhammar et al. concluded that fractionized exercise was as effective as continuous exercise in eliciting PEH, reducing SBP 3–4 mmHg compared to control throughout the day until the following morning. Less is known about the antihypertensive effects of very short (<10 min) bouts of aerobic exercise. Miyashita et al. [131] compared the BP response to 30 min of running at 70% of VO_2max performed in either a single continuous bout (1 × 30 min) or multiple, very short bouts (10 × 3 min) among seven young men with elevated BP. Miyashita et al. reported reductions in SBP of 6 and 8 mmHg, respectively, that persisted for 24 h after the bout ($Ps < 0.01$). Taken together, these studies suggest that short (10 min) and very short (3 min) bouts of intermittent aerobic exercise interspersed throughout the day elicit PEH and that the antihypertensive effects of short and very short bouts of moderate-to-vigorous-intensity aerobic exercise are similar in magnitude and duration to those observed following a single bout of continuous aerobic exercise of the same intensity [130, 131].

In summary, a single, isolated session of aerobic exercise results in an immediate reduction in BP on the order of 5–7 mmHg among individuals with hypertension (i.e., PEH), with the greatest reductions occurring among those with the highest BP (i.e., upwards of 8–11 mmHg) [23, 91, 124–127]. PEH is a low-threshold phenomenon in terms of exercise duration as short (≈10 min) and now very short (<10 min) durations of exercise produce PEH [130, 132–134]. However, the minimum duration needed to produce the effect is dependent on the intensity of the exercise [131] and, at this time, remains to be determined. New and emerging research indicates that exercise intensity is an important determinant of PEH such that increasing levels of exertion lower BP in a dose-response pattern [91, 125, 129, 135] and that short bouts of exercise accumulated across a day can have the same beneficial impact on BP as one continuous bout of exercise [125, 130, 131].

Chronic, Training, or Long-Term Effects

Meta-analyses of studies investigating the antihypertensive effect of chronic aerobic exercise training among individuals with hypertension have concluded that dynamic aerobic or endurance exercise training reduces resting office and 24-h ambulatory BP 5–7 mmHg [136–139] and 3–4 mmHg [140, 141], respectively, among individuals with high BP. Of note, the participants in these meta-analyses were generally white and/or middle-aged, limiting the generalizability of the results to more diverse populations [95]. Nonetheless, one clear pattern that has emerged from these meta-analyses is that resting BP is lower due to aerobic exercise training and that the magnitude of the reduction is greatest for those with the highest BP.

Of the meta-analyses conducted to date, most have failed to provide insight into how population characteristics and/or the FIT of the exercise intervention moderate the BP effects of aerobic (endurance) exercise training [95, 104, 108, 141], with the exception of two [98, 142]. Briefly, Whelton et al. [98] examined a large group ($n = 2419$) of racially/ethnically diverse patients ($n = 1935$ whites; $n = 391$ Asians; and $n = 93$ blacks) and reported BP reductions of 3/3 mmHg for whites, 6/7 mmHg for Asians, and 11/3 mmHg for blacks [98]. More recently, Cornelissen and Smart [142] examined the effect of aerobic exercise training lasting at least 4 wk in duration on resting BP and identified several moderators related to characteristics of the sample and the aerobic exercise intervention. Briefly, the authors found that samples consisting of all men experienced BP reductions that were greater in magnitude than those of all women (3–5 mmHg vs. 1 mmHg), concluding that sex may influence the BP response to exercise training. They also found that the magnitude of training-induced BP reductions was greater among studies that implemented exercise training programs lasting <24 wk than ≥24 wk (3–6 mmHg vs. 1–2 mmHg), involved aerobic exercise sessions lasting 30–45 min/session, and accumulated a weekly exercise volume of <210 min compared to a weekly volume ≥210 min. Last, aerobic exercise intensity appeared to alter the BP response to training such that BP reductions were greatest with moderate-to-vigorous-intensity aerobic exercise training compared to lower intensity aerobic exercise (4–5/2–3 mmHg vs. ≈1 mmHg) [142].

A growing body of new and emerging evidence suggests that high-intensity interval training (HIIT), characterized by brief periods of very high-intensity aerobic exercise (>90% of VO_2max) separated by recovery periods of lower-intensity exercise or rest [143], may be superior to continuous, moderate-intensity aerobic exercise in lowering BP. Indeed, a recent review found that HIIT resulted in greater BP benefit for individuals with hypertension than normal BP (8 mmHg vs. 3 mmHg, respectively) [91]. HIIT holds promise for some people with hypertension because it allows individuals to perform brief periods of vigorous-intensity exercise that would not be tolerable for longer periods of time. In addition, HIIT can also yield an equal amount of work (i.e., energy expenditure) compared to continuous, moderate-intensity exercise in a shorter amount of time [91, 143–145]. Additional investigations involving more diverse samples with hypertension are warranted.

In summary, the BP reductions experienced after aerobic exercise training appear to be equivalent in magnitude to those observed with PEH (i.e., 5–7 mmHg) [136, 137, 139], supporting the notion that BP reductions following chronic exercise or exercise training are largely a function of PEH. Furthermore, as with PEH, the magnitude of the BP reductions with exercise training appears to be greatest in those with the highest BP [136–139, 141], and exercise intensity appears to be an important moderator of the BP response to aerobic exercise training, with BP reductions occurring in a dose-response fashion [142]. HIIT shows promise as a viable alternative to the current ACSM Ex R_x recommendations for hypertension; however, further investigation is warranted among individuals with hypertension to more definitively determine the benefit-to-risk ratio of exercising at vigorous intensity among a population that is predisposed to heightened CVD risk [91, 143] (for an expanded discussion on the risks associated with exercise, see Chap. 25). Last, the FITT components of the aerobic exercise training intervention (i.e., the duration, intensity, and weekly volume of exercise) and population characteristics (i.e., sex, race/ethnicity) appear to moderate the BP response to aerobic exercise training and warrant confirmation in future randomized controlled trials [98, 142].

Interventional Evidence of Dynamic Resistance Exercise and Blood Pressure Effects

Dynamic resistance exercise involves both a lifting and lowering phase that occurs during each repetition against an external resistance, or load does not change. These phases of muscular activity correspond to the shortening and lengthening of the involved muscle group. It was previously thought that individuals with hypertension should avoid resistance exercise due to reports of marked elevations in BP while exercising [146] and following the Valsalva maneuver [147]. Indeed, increases in BP as high as 480/350 mmHg have been recorded among bodybuilders during a single bout of heavy resistance exercise performed at or above 80% of 1RM until concentric failure [146]. However, such BP surges are known to return to initial values within 10 s of the last repetition of each set [146], and to the best of our knowledge, it remains to be answered whether brief elevations in BP of this magnitude are harmful. In fact, there is an established, but growing, body of literature that shows muscular strength is inversely associated with CVD and all-cause mortality [85, 90, 148, 149], incident hypertension, and prevalence of other adverse cardiometabolic health outcomes [81–83, 90].

Acute, Immediate, or Short-Term Effects, or Postexercise Hypotension

An increasing number of studies [150–155] as well as reviews and meta-analyses [122, 123, 125, 156] are reporting immediate reductions in BP following acute dynamic resistance exercise that persist for several hours after the bout or PEH. Furthermore, the magnitude of these reductions appears to be the greatest among those with the highest BP. Indeed, a recent meta-analysis [156] of 30 acute dynamic resistance exercise studies (81 interventions) involving 646 adults with normal BP to established hypertension concluded that dynamic resistance exercise elicited PEH to a greater extent among samples with hypertension ($n = 141$) compared to samples with normal BP ($n = 505$) (9/5–6 mmHg vs. 3/3 mmHg, respectively) ($P < 0.01$). This same meta-analysis also identified several moderator patterns related to the FIT of the dynamic resistance exercise intervention that will be discussed as new and emerging research below.

A limited number of studies have examined aspects of the FIT of an acute resistance exercise intervention on PEH, and when they have, the results have been mixed. For example, some studies have shown that high-intensity (80% of 1RM) acute resistance exercise results in greater BP reductions than light-moderate-intensity (50% of 1RM) resistance exercise (≈34/16 mmHg vs. ≈24/7 mmHg) [150, 151], while other studies have reported reductions of similar magnitude following light- (40% of 1RM) and high (80% of 1RM)-intensity acute resistance exercise (14/1–2 mmHg) [152].

More consistent evidence seems to support that the volume of resistance exercise (i.e., the number of exercises, repetitions, and sets of a given exercise) more so than the intensity moderates the magnitude of PEH. For example, Scher et al. [155] examined the effect of low versus high volume on PEH among 16 older adults with treated hypertension (130/76 mmHg). All subjects performed 1 set of 20 repetitions at light intensity (40% of 1RM) at each station in the 10-exercise circuit; however, the number of total circuits (laps) differed such that subjects completed two sessions that consisted of low (1 lap; 20 min) and high (2 laps; 40 min) volume. The authors reported that both low and high volumes of resistance exercise elicited PEH for 60 min in the laboratory compared to control (Ps < 0.05), but the magnitude of these reductions was greater after high- rather than low-volume resistance exercise (10/7 mmHg vs. 8/6 mmHg, respectively) ($P < 0.05$). Interestingly, only high-volume resistance exercise reduced awake and 24-h ambulatory SBP compared to control, and again, these reductions were greater than those observed after lower volumes of resistance exercise (Ps < 0.05).

Two recent meta-analyses seem to confirm these observations. Cassonatto et al. [156] reported that the magnitude of PEH was greater following a bout of resistance exercise that involved larger muscle groups (targeted with either single- or multi-joint movements) than smaller muscle groups (SBP only: 3–5 mmHg vs. 1–2 mmHg) ($P < 0.05$), and in a separate meta-analysis, Carpio-Rivera et al. [125] found that PEH magnitude was associated with the number of exercises performed in a given session ($r = -0.20$) and the number of sets performed per exercise ($r = -0.47$) (Ps ≤ 0.01) such that a greater number of resistance exercises and sets per exercise elicited greater reductions in BP.

To summarize, acute resistance exercise can lead to remarkable surges in BP while exercising;

however, whether this phenomenon is harmful to overall cardiovascular health is unknown [146]. In fact, most of the studies involving individuals with hypertension have reported immediate reductions in BP following a single bout of dynamic resistance exercise that appear to be clinically meaningful and comparable to the magnitude of PEH resulting from acute aerobic exercise among individuals with hypertension (i.e., ≈5–10 mmHg vs. 5–7 mmHg, upwards of 8–11 mmHg based on new and emerging research presented in this chapter) [150–155]. Similar to the BP benefits resulting from acute and chronic aerobic exercise, BP reductions following acute dynamic resistance exercise appear to be more pronounced in individuals who stand to benefit the most (i.e., those with higher BP compared to normal BP) [125, 156, 157]. At this time, it is unclear whether other patient characteristics or aspects of the FIT of the acute resistance exercise intervention influence PEH.

Chronic, Training, or Long-Term Effects

Until recently, the general consensus from randomized controlled trials and meta-analyses [95, 158] has been that dynamic RT lowers resting BP, but to a lesser degree than aerobic exercise training (i.e., 2–3 mmHg vs. 5–7 mmHg). A major limitation of earlier meta-analyses resided in the fact that the majority of included studies involved white and/or middle-aged adults with normal BP and elevated BP, limiting the generalizability of the results to more ethnically diverse populations and, importantly, to those with hypertension [95].

Recent investigations, and meta-analyses of these newly published studies, have shown that BP reductions following dynamic RT are similar to those resulting from aerobic exercise training. For example, Mota et al. [154] found that 16 wk of moderate-intensity (i.e., 70% of 1RM) dynamic RT reduced resting BP 14/4 mmHg among women with treated hypertension. Likewise, Moraes et al. [159] reported that 12 wk of moderate-intensity (60% of 1RM) dynamic RT reduced resting BP 16/12 mmHg among men with hypertension. Most recently, we meta-analyzed 64 controlled studies (71 interventions) involving middle-aged adults (n = 2344), the majority of who were white (57%) with elevated BP (126/76 mmHg) [158]. On average, we found that dynamic RT interventions of moderate intensity, performed 2–3 d/wk for 14 wk, elicited BP reductions of ≈3/2 mmHg. However, subsequent moderator analyses revealed dynamic RT elicited greater BP reductions among individuals with hypertension (6/5 mmHg) and elevated BP (3/3 mmHg) compared to normal BP (0/1 mmHg).

Of note, we found that the antihypertensive effects of dynamic RT were moderated by race/ethnicity, such that among nonwhite samples with hypertension, BP was reduced 14/10 mmHg, a magnitude that is approximately twice that reported following aerobic exercise training (i.e., 5–7 mmHg) [158]. These promising findings suggest that, for some populations, dynamic RT elicits BP reductions comparable to or greater than those achieved with aerobic exercise training, and for those patients (i.e., nonwhite samples with hypertension), dynamic resistance exercise may serve as a viable stand-alone antihypertensive lifestyle therapeutic option [158].

Presently, professional committees/organizations recommend that individuals with hypertension engage in moderate-intensity, *dynamic* resistance exercise 2–3 d/wk as a supplement to aerobic exercise training. Upon more careful scrutiny of the literature [91] and the new findings by MacDonald et al. [158], there is suggestive evidence that dynamic resistance exercise can be an alternative stand-alone exercise modality option for patients with hypertension. These findings are consistent with the new and emerging evidence regarding the acute effects of dynamic resistance exercise presented in the previous section. Additional randomized controlled, intervention trials are needed to determine if these novel findings prove to be true and to better understand what FIT features of the dynamic RT program would yield the greatest BP benefit.

In summary, it has long been thought that dynamic RT reduces BP ≈ 2–3 mmHg. However, new and emerging research has demonstrated that dynamic resistance exercise has an even more beneficial influence on BP among those diagnosed with hypertension (i.e., ≈5–6 mmHg, upwards of ≈10–14 mmHg) [158–160]. Additionally, of the few meta-analyses that have explored the influence of population characteristics, they have shown that initial BP levels and race/ethnicity can influence the magnitude of reductions experienced after dynamic RT and warrant additional investigation [158]. Based on the available evidence, it is unclear whether other aspects of the FIT of the Ex R_x influence the magnitude of BP reductions following dynamic RT.

Interventional Evidence of Isometric Resistance Exercise and Blood Pressure Effects

Isometric resistance exercise involves sustained contraction against an immovable load or resistance with no (or minimal) change in length of the involved muscle group. To date, two different forms of isometric resistance exercise have been evaluated in terms of their effectiveness to lower BP: isometric handgrip (IHG) and isometric leg exercise. Currently, the ACSM and other professional committees/organizations (Table 8.2) do not provide guidelines on isometric resistance exercise for adults with hypertension due to the limited evidence supporting its effectiveness to lower high BP [23, 24]. In 2013, a Scientific Statement from the AHA featured IHG as a potentially effective adjunctive alternative therapy for lowering BP but stated there were inconsistent or inclusive data regarding its efficacy as antihypertensive therapy at the time [161]. Additional studies have been published since then, and two professional committees/organizations [10, 103] included IHG exercise as another potentially viable exercise-based therapeutic option for adults with hypertension in their most recent treatment guidelines (Table 8.2). Despite these recent endorsements, significant gaps in the current state of knowledge regarding the effects of isometric exercise on resting BP remain. Furthermore, there are fewer well-controlled isometric exercise interventions compared to aerobic and dynamic resistance exercise, especially among those involving adults with hypertension [142, 162, 163].

Acute, Immediate, or Short-Term Effects, or Postexercise Hypotension

The antihypertensive effects of isometric exercise among adults with hypertension have primarily been evaluated in terms of their long-term or chronic BP benefit [162, 164, 165]. A limited number of studies have evaluated PEH following a single bout of isometric exercise among adults with hypertension [166–170] and with mixed results.

Two studies [169, 170] observed PEH following a single bout of IHG exercise, reporting reductions in ambulatory SBP of 5.4 mmHg over 7 hours under conditions of daily living [169] and office SBP reductions ranging from 14.4 to 18.7 mmHg during 60 min of recovery in the laboratory [170]. In contrast, three studies did not observe PEH following a single bout of IHG exercise [166–168]. Reasons for the discrepancies observed among these studies are not completely clear but appear to be the result of differences in study design (e.g., ambulatory vs. laboratory assessment of PEH) and patient clinical characteristics (e.g., age, baseline BP, race/ethnicity, physical activity level, among others). Of note, the study of Ash et al. [166] is the only study to date to directly compare the magnitude and duration of PEH (laboratory/office BP and ambulatory BP over 19 h) after acute IHG exercise with acute aerobic exercise in the same group of adults with elevated BP to stage 1 hypertension (n = 27). Using a randomized controlled crossover design, Ash et al. [166] reported that aerobic exercise induced a clinically meaningful reduction in ambulatory BP compared to non-exercise control (4–6 mmHg) over awake hours, while IHG failed to elicit PEH. In addition to differences in experimental study design, Ash et al.'s [166] participants were sedentary, with low cardiorespiratory fitness, elevated to stage 1 hypertension, not receiving antihypertensive medication, and obese, and the majority (56%) were African-Americans – a major contrast to the study participants reporting favorable BP effects following IHG exercise (i.e., participants were physically active, with average cardiorespiratory fitness, normal BP, or normal BP levels controlled with antihypertensive medication, of normal weight, and mostly Caucasian) [162, 164, 169, 170].

In summary, there is a lack of compelling evidence at this time to support that acute isometric resistance exercise, particularly IHG exercise, elicits PEH among adults with elevated to established hypertension.

Chronic, Training, or Long-Term Effects

As previously stated, the majority of isometric resistance exercise studies including adults with hypertension have examined the long-term or chronic BP effects [162, 164, 165, 171, 172]. Based on the findings from two recent meta-analyses [162, 164], IHG training consisting of four sets × 2 min unilateral IHG contractions at 30% MVC performed 3 d/wk for 8 wk or longer reduced resting BP 4–5/5–6 mmHg among adults with hypertension ($n = 61$), all of whom were on medication. Carlson et al. [164] and Inder et al. [162] also found that IHG training significantly reduced resting BP among adults with normal BP ($n = 162$ and $n = 217$). Interestingly, both meta-analyses reported that SBP was reduced to a greater extent among adults with normal BP compared to those with hypertension, while the opposite was true for DBP: 7.8/3.1 mmHg versus 4.3/5.5 mmHg [164] and 5.4/2.9 mmHg versus 4.5/5.5 mmHg [162], respectively. Both meta-analyses were unable to explain the larger reductions in SBP among the adults with normal BP compared to adults with hypertension, and the reverse pattern observed for DBP. Furthermore, the small sample of participants with hypertension were derived from the same three studies [173–175] in both meta-analyses. Their sample of adults with hypertension ($n = 61$) is much smaller in size than the samples of adults with hypertension in meta-analyses investigating aerobic [142], dynamic resistance [158] and combined aerobic and dynamic resistance [176] exercise training. For these reasons, any conclusions made about the antihypertensive benefits of isometric RT should be made with caution.

Despite earlier claims of superior BP-lowering effects resulting from isometric resistance exercise, not all investigations have come to a similar conclusion. Moreover, few studies have directly compared the BP response to isometric RT with aerobic or dynamic resistance exercise, modalities that are currently recognized as primary or adjuvant lifestyle therapy for adults with hypertension. Of interest are three recently published studies [166, 172, 177] that evaluated the long-term or chronic changes in resting and ambulatory BP induced by isometric RT compared to aerobic exercise training, which is universally endorsed for the primary prevention and treatment of hypertension. Collectively, these studies [166, 172, 177] reported that aerobic exercise training significantly reduced office (≈4–10/3–4 mmHg) [172, 177] and ambulatory BP over waking hours (≈5.5–8/4.4–5 mmHg) [166, 172] post- compared to pre-intervention, while IHG training did not.

To summarize, earlier studies and meta-analyses of these studies suggest that isometric resistance exercise may reduce resting BP on average 4–5/5–6 mmHg among adults with hypertension. However, the majority of isometric resistance exercise studies have included either young, healthy white men with normal BP or older, white men with well-controlled hypertension through pharmacological agents [163, 178]; women and racial/ethnic minorities have been consistently underrepresented in this literature. Although once promising, more recent research questions the effectiveness of isometric RT as antihypertensive therapy.

Interventional Evidence of Concurrent Exercise and Blood Pressure Effects

Concurrent exercise is defined as aerobic and resistance exercise being performed in close proximity to each other (i.e., in a single exercise session or within a couple hours of one another) [104, 179]. The ACSM does not currently provide any guidelines on concurrent exercise for adults with hypertension due to the limited number of studies that have investigated the acute and chronic effects of concurrent exercise on BP among adults with hypertension. However, based on the new and emerging evidence that will be discussed in the sections that follow, it appears that concurrent exercise may be as effective as aerobic exercise as antihypertensive therapy among individuals with hypertension [91].

Acute, Immediate, or Short-Term Effects, or Postexercise Hypotension

In comparison to the aerobic and dynamic resistance exercise literature, fewer studies have investigated the acute effects of concurrent (*combined* aerobic and resistance) exercise among adults with high BP [104, 108, 179]. Collectively, these studies reported BP reductions ranging from 6 to 12 mmHg for SBP and 3 to 17 mmHg for DBP, respectively [179–184]. Based on the limited number of small studies conducted to date, it is likely premature to comment on the population or FIT characteristics that may modulate the duration and magnitude of PEH following acute concurrent exercise. At this time, however, no clear moderator patterns have emerged in relation to the intervention characteristics such as the concurrent exercise intensity, volume, or the order of the aerobic and resistance exercise components and the magnitude and duration of PEH.

For example, a single bout of concurrent exercise consisting of moderate-to-vigorous-intensity aerobic exercise and moderate-intensity resistance exercise (70–75% of 1RM) lowered BP 6–11/3–5 mmHg and remained lowered for 60–90 min following the bout [180, 182, 183]. Similarly, acute concurrent exercise consisting of moderate-to-vigorous-intensity aerobic exercise and low-intensity resistance exercise (40–50% of 1RM) lowered BP by 7–12/3–17 mmHg for 30–180 min following the bout [181, 184]. Tibana et al. [180] observed a similar effect when investigating the influence of moderate-intensity aerobic exercise (30 min at 70% of HR reserve) followed by either low- (1 set) or high (3 sets)-volume resistance exercise (8–12 repetitions for 6 exercises at 80% of 10RM workload) among 16 women with normal to high BP. They reported that SBP was reduced 7–9 mmHg compared to control for 90 min following both concurrent exercise sessions. Lastly, the order of the aerobic and resistance exercise components within the concurrent exercise session does not appear to influence PEH among adults with hypertension. Menêses et al. [184] found that aerobic exercise (30 min at 50–60% of HR reserve) performed before or after dynamic resistance exercise (3 sets of 10 repetitions for 7 exercises at 50% of 1RM) elicited PEH among 19 middle-aged women with controlled hypertension (130/68 mmHg), and the magnitude of these reductions was not different between conditions (7–8/3 mmHg).

In contrast to the concurrent exercise variables discussed thus far, *how* the concurrent exercise session is performed (i.e., single bout vs. multiple bouts interspersed throughout the day) does appear to modulate PEH. In a recent study, Azevêdo et al. [182] investigated the effects of concurrent exercise (3 sets of 10 repetitions for 4 exercises at 75% of 8RM workload followed by 20 min of moderate-to-vigorous-intensity aerobic exercise) performed in a single bout (in the morning *or* evening) compared to fractionized (spread throughout the day, in the morning, *and* in the evening) on PEH among 11 middle-aged women with hypertension. The authors found that a single session of concurrent exercise performed in the morning *or* evening, but not fractionized throughout the day, reduced SBP 10.7 mmHg and 6.3 mmHg compared to control. Furthermore, reductions in SBP were greater following a single bout of concurrent exercise performed in the morning compared to fractionized concurrent exercise (−10.7 mmHg vs. +3.3 mmHg, respectively).

To summarize, a single bout of concurrent exercise elicits PEH among middle-aged to older adults with high BP, and the magnitude of these reductions appears to be similar to those observed after aerobic exercise. Moreover, based on the limited number of small studies conducted to date, the currently available data does not suggest that PEH is modulated by aspects of the acute concurrent exercise intervention (i.e., exercise intensity, volume, or the order of the aerobic and resistance exercise components). However, further investigation is warranted among larger samples of adults with hypertension to determine whether aspects of the FIT of the acute concurrent exercise intervention influence PEH. At this time, it is unclear whether patient characteristics influence PEH.

Chronic, Training, or Long-Term Effects

The results of several recent meta-analyses and concurrent exercise training studies suggest that concurrent exercise may be as effective as aerobic exercise as antihypertensive therapy among individuals with hypertension [91, 176]. Briefly, Hayashino et al. [185] performed a meta-analysis of 42 trials, 14 of which were concurrent exercise training trials involving middle-aged adults with type 2 diabetes mellitus and hypertension (36%). The authors reported BP reductions of 1.7/2.3 mmHg following aerobic training, 2.8/2.3 mmHg following dynamic RT, and 3.2/1.9 mmHg following concurrent exercise training, with no statistically significant differences among the three modalities [185]. Cornelissen and Smart [142] reported similar findings in their meta-analysis of 93 trials, such that BP was reduced 3.5/2.5 mmHg following aerobic exercise training (105 interventions), 1.8/3.2 mmHg following dynamic resistance exercise training (29 interventions), and 2.2 mmHg (SBP only) following concurrent exercise training (14 interventions). Once again, no differences were noted among the three modality groups.

Most recently, Corso et al. [176] pooled 68 trials (76 interventions) and examined the influence of concurrent exercise training on BP. The authors found, on average, concurrent exercise training performed 3 d/wk at moderate intensity (aerobic, 55% of VO_2max; resistance, 60% of 1RM), ≈60 min/d for 20 wk, significantly reduced BP by 3.2/2.5 mmHg. However, among trials of higher study quality that examined BP as the primary outcome, individuals with hypertension experienced BP reductions as great as 9.2/7.7 mmHg [176]. BP reductions of this magnitude are clinically meaningful and, if confirmed, could result in an expansion of the existing professional exercise recommendations for hypertension to include concurrent exercise training. Interestingly, as stated within the ACSM's current exercise recommendations [23], individuals with hypertension would almost *always* be engaging in concurrent exercise training (i.e., aerobic exercise supplemented by dynamic RT). Therefore, it is imperative that future trials better explore the combined influence of aerobic and dynamic resistance exercise as antihypertensive lifestyle therapy among individuals with hypertension to determine whether patient characteristics or aspects of the FIT of the Ex R_x influence the BP response to chronic concurrent exercise.

In summary, new and emerging research examining the influence of aerobic exercise training in combination with dynamic RT (i.e., concurrent exercise training) is promising as it appears that concurrent exercise may elicit chronic BP reductions similar in magnitude to those seen after aerobic exercise training [91, 176, 179]. However, future randomized controlled trials are needed before concurrent exercise training can be integrated in the Ex R_x for individuals with hypertension.

Mechanisms of Exercise-Induced Blood Pressure Changes

An isolated bout of aerobic, and now, based on new and emerging evidence, dynamic resistance and concurrent exercise, elicits immediate reductions in BP of 5–7 mmHg among individuals with hypertension that persist for up to 24 h or PEH [10, 24]. The precise mechanisms responsible for PEH are not clear. However, it is unlikely that PEH is the result of a single underlying mechanism given the complexity of BP regulation and the multifactorial pathogenesis of hypertension. Rather, PEH represents a collection of complex hemodynamic adjustments that occur in response to and in recovery from exercise, and these adjustments are driven by several highly coordinated and controlled mechanisms [29,

186]. Arterial pressure is determined by CO and TPR; thus, the mechanisms that mediate acute and chronic exercise-induced BP reductions can be further discussed in terms of their individual determinants: HR and stroke volume (CO) and the degree of vasoconstriction or vasodilation of individual vascular beds (TPR).

PEH following acute aerobic exercise is characterized by a reduction in vascular resistance resulting from peripheral vasodilation. This sustained postexercise vasodilation is mediated by combined central neural mechanisms (arterial baroreflex resetting) and local vasodilatory mechanisms [186]. PEH following acute dynamic resistance exercise, in contrast, is characterized by an attenuation in CO resulting from reduced stroke volume and increase in vascular resistance [186]. The underlying mechanisms of PEH, hemodynamic adjustments (e.g., regional vascular changes), and autonomic contributions (e.g., baroreflex resetting) are better documented following aerobic than resistance exercise. However, differences in the mechanisms that underlie PEH may be related to changes in cardiac sympathetic activation and/or arterial baroreflex sensitivity, as well as local vasodilatory controls.

BP reductions observed with exercise training are primarily the result of reductions in TPR. Although exercise training can alter HR and stroke volume, the net effect on resting CO is minimal among healthy populations. Peripheral resistance is mediated by neurohumoral and structural adaptations such as increased vasodilatory factors (e.g., nitric oxide), decreased vasoconstrictor factors (e.g., norepinephrine), increased vessel diameter, and/or increased vessel distensibility [29, 34] (for an expanded discussion on exercise and the endothelium, see Chap. 3). Therefore, reductions in TPR after acute exercise appear to be predominately the result of exercise-induced alterations involving the sympathetic nervous and renin-angiotensin systems and their influence on vascular, renal, and baroreceptor function [29, 118–120]. Frequent repetition of acute exercise bouts produces more permanent structural adaptations and persistent alterations in function, leading to long-term reductions in BP (i.e., the exercise training response).

Clinical Implications and New Advances in Exercise Prescription for Optimizing Blood Pressure Benefits

The FITT Ex R_x recommendations that follow are based upon the new and emerging findings discussed in this chapter as they related to the current consensus of knowledge regarding the effects of acute and chronic aerobic, dynamic resistance, and concurrent exercise on hypertension as presented in this chapter. The modified Ex R_x we propose below is summarized in Table 8.4:

*F*requency:

- Aerobic exercise should be performed on most, preferably all, days of the week (i.e., 5–7 d/wk) in combination with dynamic resistance exercise 2–3 d/wk on non-consecutive days.
- A combination of aerobic and dynamic resistance exercise can be performed on separate days (i.e., *combined* aerobic and resistance exercise) or during the same exercise session (i.e., *concurrent* exercise).
- Aerobic and resistance exercise should be supplemented by flexibility exercise 2–3 d/wk.

This recommendation is made due to the well-established immediate and sustained BP lowering effects of acute aerobic exercise or PEH [22, 23, 91, 108, 118–120, 124–126, 129, 130], and the new and emerging evidence that supports acute dynamic resistance [150–153, 155–157] and concurrent [179–184] exercise can elicit PEH to a similar magnitude as aerobic exercise among adults with hypertension. Put simply, BP is lower on days when individuals with hypertension exercise than the days they do not exercise.

Table 8.4 The modified exercise prescription for adults with hypertension based on new and emerging evidence [91, 104]

FITT-VP principle of the Ex R_x	Modified ACSM recommendations
*F*requency (how often?)	Aerobic exercise: 5–7 d/wk Dynamic resistance exercise: ≥2–3 d/wk (non-consecutive) A combination of aerobic and dynamic resistance exercise can be performed on separate days (i.e., *combined* aerobic and resistance exercise) or during the same exercise session (i.e., *concurrent* exercise) *What's new*: The addition of dynamic resistance as another viable stand-alone antihypertensive therapeutic option
*I*ntensity (How hard?)[a]	Aerobic exercise: moderate-to-vigorous (40–≥60% of $\dot{V}O_2R$ or 12–≥14 on a scale of 6 [no exertion] to 20 [maximal exertion] level of physical exertion or an intensity that causes noticeable increases in heart rate and breathing) Dynamic resistance exercise: moderate (60–80% of 1RM or 12–14 on a scale of 6 [no exertion] to 20 [maximal exertion] level of physical exertion) Concurrent exercise: a combination of moderate-to-vigorous-intensity aerobic exercise and moderate-intensity resistance exercise as described above *What's new*: The expansion of the recommendation for aerobic exercise intensity to include higher levels of physical exertion (i.e., vigorous-intensity aerobic exercise)
*T*ime (how long?)	Aerobic exercise: ≥30–60 min/d; one continuous bout or multiple bouts of ≥10 min (moderate intensity) or ≥ 3–10 min (vigorous intensity, i.e., ≥60% of $\dot{V}O_2R$) each Dynamic resistance exercise: 8–10 exercises; 1–4 sets of 8–12 repetitions Concurrent exercise: ≥20–30 min/d of aerobic exercise and dynamic resistance exercise consisting of 4–8 exercises; 1–3 sets of 8–12 repetitions *What's new*: The inclusion of multiple "very short bouts" (i.e., 3–10 min), performed at vigorous intensity, that can be interspersed throughout the day Specific recommendations regarding the aerobic and resistance exercises when performed concurrently in a single exercise session
*T*ype (what kind?) *Primary*	Aerobic exercise: prolonged, rhythmic activities using large muscle groups (e.g., walking, cycling, swimming) performed continuously at a constant intensity or with repeated bouts alternating between high and low (≥70% vs. <40% of $\dot{V}O_2R$) intensity (i.e., *interval exercise*) Dynamic resistance exercise: a combination of multi- and single-joint exercises targeting the major muscle groups of the upper and lower body using traditional or circuit resistance training Concurrent exercise: a combination of the aerobic and resistance exercises described above performed in any order (i.e., aerobic exercise can be performed before *or* after resistance exercise) *What's new*: The recommendation for the type of aerobic exercise has been expanded to include interval exercise Specific recommendations regarding the order of aerobic and resistance exercises when performed concurrently in a single exercise session
Adjuvant 1	Flexibility *F:* ≥2–3 d/wk *I:* Stretch to the point of feeling tightness or slight discomfort *T:* ≥10 min/d; ≥4 repetitions per muscle group; hold each static stretch for 10–30 s

(continued)

Table 8.4 (continued)

FITT-VP principle of the Ex R_x	Modified ACSM recommendations
Adjuvant 2[b]	Neuromotor *F:* ≥2–3 d/wk *I:* undetermined *T:* ≥20–30 min/d
*V*olume (how much?)[c]	≥150 min/wk or 700–2000 kcal/wk of *total* aerobic and resistance exercise
*P*rogression	Progress gradually, avoiding large increases in any of the components of the Ex R_x; increase exercise duration over first 4–6 wk and then increase frequency, intensity, and time (or some combination of these) to achieve recommended quantity and quality of exercise over next 4–8 months

ACSM American College of Sports Medicine, *FITT* *f*requency, *i*ntensity, *t*ime, *t*ype, *v*olume, and *p*rogression of exercise; *Ex R_x* exercise prescription, 1*RM* one-repetition maximum, $\dot{V}O_2R$ oxygen consumption reserve

[a]Vigorous-intensity aerobic exercise (i.e., ≥60% of $\dot{V}O_2R$ or ≥ 14 on a scale of 6–20 [106]) appears to elicit greater and more extensive benefits than lower levels of physical exertion for individuals who are willing and able to tolerate more intense levels of exercise and may be introduced after exercise preparticipation health screening and gradual progression

[b]Balance (neuromotor) training is recommended for older adults, individuals who are at substantial risk of falling, and is likely to benefit younger adults as well

[c]For greater and more extensive benefits, progress exercise volume to total 60 min/d and 300 min/wk of moderate-to-vigorous intensity

Also, individuals with hypertension are often overweight to obese and have additional CVD risk factors (i.e., insulin resistance, dyslipidemia, the metabolic syndrome) [28, 37, 50]. Therefore, large amounts of caloric expenditure should be emphasized [24] while maintaining lean mass, muscular strength, and function [108].

*I*ntensity:

- Aerobic exercise: Moderate-to-vigorous intensity (i.e., 40–≥60% $\dot{V}O_2R$; 12–≥14 rating of perceived physical exertion on the Borg 6–20 scale [106]) or an intensity that causes noticeable increases in HR and breathing
- Dynamic resistance exercise: moderate-intensity (60–80% of 1RM; 12–14 rating of perceived physical exertion on the Borg 6–20 scale [106])

Due to the growing evidence that greater BP reductions can be achieved with greater levels of physical exertion [22, 91, 125, 129, 135], the aerobic exercise intensity recommendation has been expanded to include vigorous intensity if the patient or client is willing and able to tolerate higher levels of physical exertion. For dynamic resistance and concurrent exercise, it appears that moderate-intensity resistance exercise is efficacious for reducing BP among adults with hypertension [150–152, 155, 157, 159].

*T*ime:

- Aerobic exercise: 30–60 min/d of continuous or intermittent (i.e., fractionized) exercise. If intermittent, bouts should be ≥10 min (moderate-intensity exercise) or ≥3–10 min (vigorous-intensity exercise, i.e., >60–80% $\dot{V}O_2R$) in duration depending on the level of physical exertion and accumulate to total 30–60 min/d.
- Dynamic resistance exercise: should consist of at least 1 set of 8–12 repetitions for 8–10 exercises targeting the major muscle groups.
- Concurrent exercise: ≥20–30 min/d of continuous aerobic exercise and dynamic resistance exercise consisting of at least 1 set of 8–12 repetitions for 4–8 exercises targeting the major muscle groups.

This recommendation is consistent with existing evidence that PEH is a low-threshold phenomenon regarding the time (duration) of the acute aerobic exercise bout but has been expanded to consider the interaction between time and intensity. When several short bouts of aerobic exercise are interspersed throughout the day,

PEH offers a viable therapeutic lifestyle option for BP control among individuals with high BP [125, 130, 131]. Bouts of at least 10 min are recommended for moderate-intensity aerobic exercise, while bouts of <10 min (i.e., ≥3–10 min) may be recommended for more vigorous-intensity aerobic exercise. At this time, there is no compelling evidence to support that intermittent or fractionized resistance or concurrent exercise [182] can offer the same PEH benefit reported with a single, continuous bout of resistance or concurrent exercise, respectively.

*T*ype:

- For aerobic exercise, emphasis should be placed on prolonged, rhythmic activities using large muscle groups such as walking, cycling, or swimming. Aerobic activities can be performed continuously at a constant intensity or in repeated bouts alternating between high and low (≥70% vs. <40% $\dot{V}O_2R$) intensity (i.e., *interval exercise*).
- For dynamic resistance exercise, emphasis should be placed on multi- and single-joint exercises that target the major muscle groups of the upper and lower body. Resistance exercises can be performed using a conventional or circuit (i.e., lighter weights, higher repetitions, with minimal rest between exercises) RT protocol.
- For concurrent exercise, a combination of the aerobic and resistance exercises described above can be performed in the same exercise session, in any order (i.e., aerobic exercise can be performed before *or* after resistance exercise).
- For older adults or individuals who are at substantial risk of falling, neuromotor (balance) training 2–3 d/wk is also recommended as adjuvant exercise.

Aerobic exercise training has consistently been shown to lower BP among adults with hypertension, and now, new and emerging research supports that dynamic resistance and concurrent exercise training can elicit comparable BP reductions. Therefore, we have expanded this recommendation to include dynamic resistance exercise and concurrent exercise as viable stand-alone antihypertensive therapy that should be performed in addition to aerobic exercise. Consistent with our expanded recommendation for aerobic exercise intensity, we have also modified this recommendation to include interval aerobic exercise. BP reductions following aerobic interval training (e.g., HIIT) are similar to or exceed those observed with continuous, constant-intensity aerobic exercise [91, 132, 135, 143]. Furthermore, interval exercise allows adults with hypertension to experience the health and BP benefits associated with higher levels of physical exertion that would not be tolerable with longer duration exercise [91, 143–145]. The recommendation for dynamic resistance exercise has been expanded with specific information regarding the RT protocol. Existing as well as new and emerging evidence has shown that adults with hypertension experience similar BP benefit with conventional and circuit resistance exercise [108, 158]. Finally, there is no strong evidence to support that the order of the aerobic and resistance exercise performed in a single concurrent exercise session influences PEH or the BP reductions that occur with training.

Special Considerations

- Consideration should be given to the level of BP control, recent changes in antihypertensive drug therapy, medication-related adverse effects, the presence of target organ disease and other comorbidities, and age. Adjustments to the Ex R_x should be made accordingly. In general, progression should be gradual, avoiding large increases in any of the FITT components of the exercise prescription, especially intensity.
- An exaggerated BP response to relatively low exercise intensities and at HR levels <85% of the age-predicted maximum HR is likely to occur in some individuals, even after resting BP is controlled with antihypertensive medication (<130 and <80 mmHg). In some cases, an exercise test may be beneficial to establish the exercise HR corresponding to the exaggerated BP in these individuals.

- Exercise is contraindicated if resting SBP exceeds 200 mmHg or DBP exceeds 110 mmHg.
- When exercising, it is prudent to maintain a SBP less than 220 mmHg and/or DBP less than 105 mmHg.
- Although vigorous-intensity aerobic exercise is not necessarily contraindicated in patients with hypertension, moderate-intensity aerobic exercise is generally recommended to optimize the benefit-to-risk ratio.
- Individuals with hypertension are often overweight or obese. The Ex R_x should focus on increasing caloric expenditure coupled with reducing caloric intake to facilitate weight reduction and minimize weight gain (see Chap. 11).
- Inhaling and breath holding while engaging in the actual lifting of a weight (i.e., Valsalva maneuver) can result in extremely high BP responses, dizziness, and even fainting. Thus, such practice should be avoided during resistance exercise.
- Individuals taking antihypertensive medications should be monitored during and after exercise for potential adverse interactions with exercise (see Table A.1 in the ACSM's Guidelines for Exercise Testing and Prescription [24] for a comprehensive summary of the effect of antihypertensive medications at rest and in response to exercise).
- β-Blockers and diuretics may adversely affect thermoregulatory function or increase the predisposition to hypoglycemia in certain individuals. Individuals taking β-blockers and diuretics should be well informed about signs and symptoms of heat intolerance and/or hypoglycemia and should be educated on how to make prudent modifications in their exercise routine to prevent adverse events.
- β-Blockers may also attenuate the HR response to exercise, while α-blockers, calcium channel blockers, and vasodilators may lead to sudden excessive reductions in postexercise BP. Therefore, an adequate cooldown may be especially important for patients taking these medications.
- Given that the BP lowering effects of exercise are immediate (i.e., a physiological response termed PEH), individuals should be educated about these immediate BP benefits to possibly enhance adherence.

Gaps in the Literature and Future Research Needs in the Exercise Prescription for Hypertension

It should be noted that these recommendations are limited by methodological quality of the studies upon which the evidence is based [91, 95]. Major limitations in the current state of the literature include small sample sizes, assessing study populations with normal BP rather than hypertension, not accounting for major confounders to the BP response to exercise that include timing of the last bout of exercise and detraining effects, and lack of standard protocols for the assessment of BP and the exercise intervention. As a result of these limitations, the effectiveness of exercise as antihypertensive lifestyle therapy among individuals with hypertension has been underestimated [91, 95, 105]. Furthermore, large randomized clinical trials that examine both the acute and chronic BP lowering effects of exercise among diverse populations are needed before professional organizations can definitively determine the optimal Ex R_x for individuals with hypertension.

Key Points

- Hypertension is the most common, modifiable, and costly CVD risk factor.
- Adults with hypertension are encouraged to engage in 30 min/d (or more) of moderate-intensity aerobic exercise on most, if not all, days of the week in addition to moderate-intensity dynamic resistance exercise 2–3 d/wk to total 150 min/wk of total exercise (or more) to prevent and control high BP (Table 8.4).
- The antihypertensive effects of acute and chronic aerobic exercise are a low-duration

phenomenon with intermittent durations appearing as effective as continuous durations in lowering BP.

- Exercise intensity is an important moderator of the antihypertensive effects of acute and chronic aerobic exercise with individuals with the highest BP experiencing the greatest BP benefit. Furthermore, vigorous-intensity exercise appears to elicit greater and more extensive benefits than lower levels of physical exertion for individuals who are willing and able to tolerate more intense levels of exercise and may be introduced after exercise preparticipation health screening and gradual progression (Table 8.4).
- Acute resistance exercise may result in marked elevations in BP while exercising; however, these BP surges appear to immediately decrease back to levels below that of baseline; the magnitude of the BP reductions is clinically meaningful and is most pronounced in individuals who stand to benefit the most (i.e., those with higher BP compared to normal BP).
- It has long been thought that dynamic RT reduces BP ≈ 2–3 mmHg. However, new and emerging research has demonstrated that dynamic RT has an even more beneficial influence on BP among those diagnosed with hypertension, reductions that are comparable to or greater than those achieved with aerobic exercise training. Based on this new and emerging research, we recommend that adults with hypertension perform dynamic RT *in addition to* aerobic exercise as stand-alone antihypertensive lifestyle therapy (Table 8.4).
- New and emerging research also indicates that aerobic and resistance exercise performed *concurrently* reduces BP to levels similar to that of aerobic exercise training. Future research is needed to confirm these findings.
- Despite the volume of literature on exercise and hypertension, there remains a critical need to identify patient and FITT exercise interventions' characteristics that influence the BP response to acute and chronic exercise so that exercise can be more precisely prescribed as antihypertensive therapy.

Conclusions

Hypertension is one of the most important CVD risk factors due to its high prevalence and significant medical costs [1, 2]. Indeed, hypertension affects approximately 46% of adults in the United States (≈103 million) [10, 20] and more than 31% of adults worldwide (>1.4 billion) [21]. Both the 2017 ACC/AHA guideline [10] and the ACSM [23] recommend aerobic exercise supplemented by dynamic resistance exercise as initial lifestyle therapy for individuals with hypertension because it lowers BP 5–7 mmHg and 2–3 mmHg, respectively, among those with hypertension. BP reductions of this magnitude can decrease the risk of developing CVD by 20–30% and rival those obtained with first-line antihypertensive medications [9, 10, 13, 96] as well as with other types of lifestyle therapy. New and emerging research has shown dynamic resistance and concurrent exercise to elicit BP reductions comparable to or greater than those achieved with aerobic exercise training and may serve as viable stand-alone antihypertensive therapeutic options for some patients. We have expanded the current exercise recommendations for hypertension in Table 8.4 to include this, as well as the other new and emerging research discussed in this chapter. Future research that addresses the existing research gaps is needed to confirm these findings.

References

1. Benjamin EJ, Blaha MJ, Chiuve SE, Cushman M, Das SR, Deo R, et al. Heart disease and stroke statistics-2017 update: a report from the American Heart Association. Circulation. 2017;135(10):e146–603. https://doi.org/10.1161/CIR.0000000000000485.
2. Olsen MH, Angell SY, Asma S, Boutouyrie P, Burger D, Chirinos JA, et al. A call to action and a lifecourse strategy to address the global burden of raised blood pressure on current and future generations: the lancet commission on hypertension. Lancet. 2016;388(10060):2665–712.
3. GBD 2016 Risk Factors Collaborators. Global, regional, and national comparative risk assessment of 84 behavioural, environmental and occupational, and metabolic risks or clusters of risks, 1990-2016: a

systematic analysis for the global burden of disease study 2016. Lancet. 2017;390(10100):1345–422.
4. Kung HC, Xu J. Hypertension-related mortality in the United States, 2000–2013. NCHS Data Brief. Hyattsville: National Center for Health Statistics; 2015. No.: 193.
5. Office of Disease Prevention and Health Promotion. Heart disease and stroke. Healthy people 2020 [Internet]. 2016. Available from https://www.healthypeople.gov/2020/topics-objectives/topic/heart-disease-and-stroke
6. Sacco RL, Roth GA, Reddy KS, Arnett DK, Bonita R, Gaziano TA, et al. The heart of 25 by 25: achieving the goal of reducing global and regional premature deaths from cardiovascular diseases and stroke: a modeling study from the American Heart Association and world heart federation. Circulation. 2016;133(23):e674–90.
7. WHO. A global brief on hypertension: silent killer, global public health crisis. Geneva: WHO Press, World Health Organization; 2013. No.: WHO/DCO/WHD/2013.2.
8. Franco OH, Peeters A, Bonneux L, de Laet C. Blood pressure in adulthood and life expectancy with cardiovascular disease in men and women: life course analysis. Hypertension. 2005;46(2):280–6.
9. Lewington S, Clarke R, Qizilbash N, Peto R, Collins R. Prospective Studies Collaboration. Age-specific relevance of usual blood pressure to vascular mortality: a meta-analysis of individual data for one million adults in 61 prospective studies. Lancet. 2002;360(9349):1903–13.
10. Whelton P, Carey R, Aronow W, Casey D, Collins K, Himmelfarb CD, et al. 2017 ACC/AHA/AAPA/ABC/ACPM/AGS/APhA/ASH/ASPC/NMA/PCNA guideline for the prevention, detection, evaluation, and management of high blood pressure in adults: a report of the American College of Cardiology/American Heart Association task force on clinical practice guidelines [published online November 13, 2017]. Hypertension.
11. Forouzanfar MH, Liu P, Roth GA, Ng M, Biryukov S, Marczak L, et al. Global burden of hypertension and systolic blood pressure of at least 110 to 115 mmHg, 1990-2015. JAMA. 2017;317(2):165–82.
12. Stedman TL. Stedman's medical dictionary. 28th ed. Philadelphia: Lippincott Williams & Wilkins; 2006.
13. Chobanian AV, Bakris GL, Black HR, Cushman WC, Green LA, Izzo JL Jr, et al. Seventh report of the joint national committee on prevention, detection, evaluation, and treatment of high blood pressure. Hypertension. 2003;42(6):1206–52.
14. Huang Y, Su L, Cai X, Mai W, Wang S, Hu Y, et al. Association of all-cause and cardiovascular mortality with prehypertension: a meta-analysis. Am Heart J. 2014;167(2):160–168.e1.
15. Rapsomaniki E, Timmis A, George J, Pujades-Rodriguez M, Shah AD, Denaxas S, et al. Blood pressure and incidence of twelve cardiovascular diseases: lifetime risks, healthy life-years lost, and age-specific associations in 1.25 million people. Lancet. 2014;383(9932):1899–911.
16. Guo X, Zhang X, Guo L, Li Z, Zheng L, Yu S, et al. Association between pre-hypertension and cardiovascular outcomes: a systematic review and meta-analysis of prospective studies. Curr Hypertens Rep. 2013;15(6):703–16.
17. Huang Y, Wang S, Cai X, Mai W, Hu Y, Tang H, et al. Prehypertension and incidence of cardiovascular disease: a meta-analysis. BMC Med. 2013;11:177. https://doi.org/10.1186/1741-7015-11-177.
18. Wang S, Wu H, Zhang Q, Xu J, Fan Y. Impact of baseline prehypertension on cardiovascular events and all-cause mortality in the general population: a meta-analysis of prospective cohort studies. Int J Cardiol. 2013;168(5):4857–60.
19. Goff DC Jr, Lloyd-Jones DM, Bennett G, Coady S, D'Agostino RB, Gibbons R, et al. 2013 ACC/AHA guideline on the assessment of cardiovascular risk: a report of the American College of Cardiology/American Heart Association task force on practice guidelines. Circulation. 2014;129(25 Suppl 2):S49–73.
20. Muntner P, Carey RM, Gidding S, Jones DW, Taler SJ, Wright JT Jr, et al. Potential US population impact of the 2017 ACC/AHA high blood pressure guideline. Circulation. 2018;137(2):109–18. https://doi.org/10.1161/CIRCULATIONAHA.117.032582.
21. Mills KT, Bundy JD, Kelly TN, Reed JE, Kearney PM, Reynolds K, et al. Global disparities of hypertension prevalence and control: a systematic analysis of population-based studies from 90 countries. Circulation. 2016;134(6):441–50.
22. Pescatello LS, MacDonald HV, Johnson BT. Chapter 1. the effects of aerobic exercise on hypertension: current consensus and emerging research. In: Pescatello LS, editor. Effects of exercise on hypertension: from cells to physiological systems. Cham: Springer International Publishing; 2015. p. 3–24.
23. Pescatello LS, Franklin BA, Fagard R, Farquhar WB, Kelley GA, Ray CA, et al. American College of Sports Medicine position stand: exercise and hypertension. Med Sci Sports Exerc. 2004;36(3):533–53.
24. Riebe D, American College of Sports Medicine. ACSM's guidelines for exercise testing and prescription. 10th ed. Philadelphia: Wolters Kluwer/Lippincott Williams & Wilkins Health; 2017. p. 480.
25. Eckel RH, Jakicic JM, Ard JD, de Jesus JM, Houston Miller N, Hubbard VS, et al. 2013 AHA/ACC guideline on lifestyle management to reduce cardiovascular risk: a report of the American College of Cardiology/American Heart Association task force on practice guidelines. J Am Coll Cardiol. 2014;63(25 Pt B):2960–84.
26. Kario K. Essential manual of 24 hour blood pressure management from morning to nocturnal hypertension. Oxford: John Wiley & Sons; 2015. p. 150.
27. Cremer A, Amraoui F, Lip G, Morales E, Rubin S, Segura J, et al. From malignant hypertension to hypertension-MOD: a modern definition for an old

but still dangerous emergency. J Hum Hypertens. 2016;30(8):463–6.
28. Oparil S, Zaman MA, Calhoun DA. Pathogenesis of hypertension. Ann Intern Med. 2003;139(9):761–76.
29. Sabbahi A, Arena R, Elokda A, Phillips SA. Exercise and hypertension: uncovering the mechanisms of vascular control. Prog Cardiovasc Dis. 2016;59(3):226–34.
30. Mitchell GF. Arterial stiffness and hypertension. Hypertension. 2014;64(1):13–8.
31. Fernandez C, Sander GE, Giles TD. Prehypertension: defining the transitional phenotype. Curr Hypertens Rep. 2016;18(1):2. https://doi.org/10.1007/s11906-015-0611-8.
32. Carretero OA, Oparil S. Essential hypertension. Part I: Definition and etiology. Circulation. 2000;101(3):329–35.
33. Joyner MJ, Limberg JK. Blood pressure regulation: every adaptation is an integration? Eur J Appl Physiol. 2014;114(3):445–50.
34. Kaplan N. Primary hypertension: pathogenesis. In: Kaplan N, Flynn J, editors. Kaplan's clinical hypertension. 9th ed. Philadelphia: Lippincott Williams & Wilkins; 2006. p. 50–121.
35. Davis JT, Rao F, Naqshbandi D, Fung MM, Zhang K, Schork AJ, et al. Autonomic and hemodynamic origins of prehypertension: central role of heredity. J Am Coll Cardiol. 2012;59(24):2206–16.
36. Grassi G, Mark A, Esler M. The sympathetic nervous system alterations in human hypertension. Circ Res. 2015;116(6):976–90.
37. Safar ME, Balkau B, Lange C, Protogerou AD, Czernichow S, Blacher J, et al. Hypertension and vascular dynamics in men and women with metabolic syndrome. J Am Coll Cardiol. 2013;61(1):12–9.
38. Safar ME, Blacher J, Jankowski P. Arterial stiffness, pulse pressure, and cardiovascular disease-is it possible to break the vicious circle? Atherosclerosis. 2011;218(2):263–71.
39. Laurent S, Boutouyrie P. The structural factor of hypertension: large and small artery alterations. Circ Res. 2015;116(6):1007–21.
40. Humphrey JD, Harrison DG, Figueroa CA, Lacolley P, Laurent S. Central artery stiffness in hypertension and aging: a problem with cause and consequence. Circ Res. 2016;118(3):379–81.
41. Lackland DT. Controlling hypertension to prevent target organ damage: perspectives from the world hypertension league president. Ethn Dis. 2016;26(3):267–70.
42. Oktay AA, Lavie CJ, Milani RV, Ventura HO, Gilliland YE, Shah S, et al. Current perspectives on left ventricular geometry in systemic hypertension. Prog Cardiovasc Dis. 2016;59(3):235–46.
43. Drazner MH. The progression of hypertensive heart disease. Circulation. 2011;123(3):327–34.
44. MacMahon S, Peto R, Collins R, Godwin J, Cutler J, Sorlie P, et al. Blood pressure, stroke, and coronary heart disease: part 1, prolonged differences in blood pressure: prospective observational studies corrected for the regression dilution bias. Lancet. 1990;335(8692):765–74.
45. Santos M, Shah AM. Alterations in cardiac structure and function in hypertension. Curr Hypertens Rep. 2014;16(5):428. https://doi.org/10.1007/s11906-014-0428-x.
46. Katholi RE, Couri DM. Left ventricular hypertrophy: major risk factor in patients with hypertension: Update and practical clinical applications. Int J Hypertens. 2011;2011:495349.
47. Bombelli M, Facchetti R, Carugo S, Madotto F, Arenare F, Quarti-Trevano F, et al. Left ventricular hypertrophy increases cardiovascular risk independently of in-office and out-of-office blood pressure values. J Hypertens. 2009;27(12):2458–64.
48. Crim MT, Yoon SS, Ortiz E, Wall HK, Schober S, Gillespie C, et al. National surveillance definitions for hypertension prevalence and control among adults. Circ Cardiovasc Qual Outcomes. 2012;5(3):343–51.
49. Whelton PK. The elusiveness of population-wide high blood pressure control. Annu Rev Public Health. 2015;36(1):109–30.
50. Chapman MJ, Sposito AC. Hypertension and dyslipidaemia in obesity and insulin resistance: Pathophysiology, impact on atherosclerotic disease and pharmacotherapy. Pharmacol Ther. 2008;117(3):354–73.
51. Fields LE, Burt VL, Cutler JA, Hughes J, Roccella EJ, Sorlie P. The burden of adult hypertension in the United States 1999 to 2000: a rising tide. Hypertension. 2004;44(4):398–404.
52. Muntner P, Woodward M, Mann DM, Shimbo D, Michos ED, Blumenthal RS, et al. Comparison of the framingham heart study hypertension model with blood pressure alone in the prediction of risk of hypertension: the multi-ethnic study of atherosclerosis. Hypertension. 2010;55(6):1339–45.
53. Vasan RS, Larson MG, Leip EP, Kannel WB, Levy D. Assessment of frequency of progression to hypertension in non-hypertensive participants in the Framingham heart study: a cohort study. Lancet. 2001;358(9294):1682–6.
54. De Marco M, de Simone G, Roman MJ, Chinali M, Lee ET, Russell M, et al. Cardiovascular and metabolic predictors of progression of prehypertension into hypertension: the strong heart study. Hypertension. 2009;54(5):974–80.
55. Nwankwo T, Yoon SS, Burt V, Gu Q. Hypertension among adults in the United States: National health and nutrition examination survey, 2011-2012. NCHS Data Brief. 2013;133:1–8.
56. Sim JJ, Bhandari SK, Shi J, Liu IL, Calhoun DA, McGlynn EA, et al. Characteristics of resistant hypertension in a large, ethnically diverse hypertension population of an integrated health system. Mayo Clin Proc. 2013;88(10):1099–107.
57. Ashman JJ, Rui P, Schappert SM. Age differences in visits to office-based physicians by adults with hypertension: United states, 2013. NCHS Data

Brief. Hyattsville, MD: National Center for Health Statistics; 2016. No.: 263.
58. Hing E, Rui P, Palso K. National ambulatory medical care survey: 2013 state and national summary tables [Internet]. 2017; Available at: http://www.cdc.gov/nchs/ahcd/ahcd_products.htm.
59. Staessen JA, Wang JG, Birkenhager WH. Outcome beyond blood pressure control? Eur Heart J. 2003;24(6):504–14.
60. Kantor ED, Rehm CD, Haas JS, Chan AT, Giovannucci EL. Trends in prescription drug use among adults in the United States from 1999–2012. JAMA. 2015;314(17):1818–31. https://doi.org/10.1001/jama.2015.13766.
61. Egan BM, Li J, Hutchison FN, Ferdinand KC. Hypertension in the united states, 1999 to 2012: progress toward healthy people 2020 goals. Circulation. 2014;130(19):1692–9.
62. Quindry JC, Franklin BA. Cardioprotective exercise and pharmacologic interventions as complementary antidotes to cardiovascular disease. Exerc Sport Sci Rev. 2018;46(1):5–17.
63. Kokkinos P. Cardiorespiratory fitness, exercise, and blood pressure. Hypertension. 2014;64(6):1160–4.
64. Lavie CJ, Arena R, Swift DL, Johannsen NM, Sui X, Lee DC, et al. Exercise and the cardiovascular system: clinical science and cardiovascular outcomes. Circ Res. 2015;117(2):207–19.
65. Lee DC, Brellenthin AG, Thompson PD, Sui X, Lee IM, Lavie CJ. Running as a key lifestyle medicine for longevity. Prog Cardiovasc Dis. 2017;60(1):45–55.
66. Sui X, Sarzynski MA, Lee DC, Kokkinos PF. Impact of changes in cardiorespiratory fitness on hypertension, dyslipidemia and survival: an overview of the epidemiological evidence. Prog Cardiovasc Dis. 2017;60(1):56–66.
67. Kokkinos P. The impact of exercise and physical fitness on blood pressure, left ventricular hypertrophy, and mortality among individuals with prehypertension and hypertension. In: Pescatello LS, editor. Effects of exercise on hypertension. Cham: Springer International Publishing; 2015. p. 87–102.
68. Harber MP, Kaminsky LA, Arena R, Blair SN, Franklin BA, Myers J, et al. Impact of cardiorespiratory fitness on all-cause and disease-specific mortality: Advances since 2009. Prog Cardiovasc Dis. 2017;60(1):11–20.
69. Swift DL, Johannsen NM, Earnest CP, Newton RL Jr, McGee JE, Church TS. Cardiorespiratory fitness and exercise training in African Americans. Prog Cardiovasc Dis. 2017;60(1):96–102.
70. Myers J, McAuley P, Lavie CJ, Despres JP, Arena R, Kokkinos P. Physical activity and cardiorespiratory fitness as major markers of cardiovascular risk: their independent and interwoven importance to health status. Prog Cardiovasc Dis. 2015;57(4):306–14.
71. Shiroma EJ, Lee IM. Physical activity and cardiovascular health: lessons learned from epidemiological studies across age, gender, and race/ethnicity. Circulation. 2010;122(7):743–52.
72. Ross R, Blair SN, Arena R, Church TS, Despres JP, Franklin BA, et al. Importance of assessing cardiorespiratory fitness in clinical practice: a case for fitness as a clinical vital sign: a scientific statement from the American Heart Association. Circulation. 2016;134(24):e653–99.
73. Kokkinos P, Myers J. Exercise and physical activity: clinical outcomes and applications. Circulation. 2010;122(16):1637–48.
74. Carnethon MR, Evans NS, Church TS, Lewis CE, Schreiner PJ, Jacobs DR Jr, et al. Joint associations of physical activity and aerobic fitness on the development of incident hypertension: coronary artery risk development in young adults. Hypertension. 2010;56(1):49–55.
75. Chase NL, Sui X, Lee DC, Blair SN. The association of cardiorespiratory fitness and physical activity with incidence of hypertension in men. Am J Hypertens. 2009;22(4):417–24.
76. Jae SY, Babu AS, Yoon ES, Kurl S, Laukkanen JA, Choi YH, et al. Impact of cardiorespiratory fitness and risk of systemic hypertension in nonobese versus obese men who are metabolically healthy or unhealthy. Am J Cardiol. 2017;120(5):765–8.
77. Juraschek SP, Blaha MJ, Whelton SP, Blumenthal R, Jones SR, Keteyian SJ, et al. Physical fitness and hypertension in a population at risk for cardiovascular disease: the henry ford ExercIse testing (FIT) project. J Am Heart Assoc. 2014;3(6):e001268. https://doi.org/10.1161/JAHA.114.001268.
78. Liu J, Sui X, Lavie CJ, Zhou H, Park YM, Cai B, et al. Effects of cardiorespiratory fitness on blood pressure trajectory with aging in a cohort of healthy men. J Am Coll Cardiol. 2014;64(12):1245–53.
79. Sui X, Sarzynski MA, Lee D, Lavie CJ, Zhang J, Kokkinos PF, et al. Longitudinal patterns of cardiorespiratory fitness predict the development of hypertension among men and women. Am J Med. 2017;130(4):469.e2–76.e2.
80. Chow L, Eberly LE, Austin E, Carnethon M, Bouchard C, Sternfeld B, et al. Fitness change effects on midlife metabolic outcomes. Med Sci Sports Exerc. 2015;47(5):967–73.
81. Crump C, Sundquist J, Winkleby MA, Sundquist K. Interactive effects of physical fitness and body mass index on the risk of hypertension. JAMA Intern Med. 2016;176(2):210–6.
82. Maslow AL, Sui X, Colabianchi N, Hussey J, Blair SN. Muscular strength and incident hypertension in normotensive and prehypertensive men. Med Sci Sports Exerc. 2010;42(2):288–95.
83. Vaara JP, Fogelholm M, Vasankari T, Santtila M, Hakkinen K, Kyrolainen H. Associations of maximal strength and muscular endurance with cardiovascular risk factors. Int J Sports Med. 2014;35(4):356–60.
84. Andersen K, Rasmussen F, Held C, Neovius M, Tynelius P, Sundstrom J. Exercise capacity and muscle strength and risk of vascular disease and arrhythmia in 1.1 million young swedish men: cohort study. BMJ. 2015;351:h4543.

85. Artero EG, Lee DC, Ruiz JR, Sui X, Ortega FB, Church TS, et al. A prospective study of muscular strength and all-cause mortality in men with hypertension. J Am Coll Cardiol. 2011;57(18):1831–7.
86. Crump C, Sundquist J, Winkleby MA, Sundquist K. Aerobic fitness, muscular strength and obesity in relation to risk of heart failure. Heart. 2017;103(22):1780–7.
87. Karlsen T, Nauman J, Dalen H, Langhammer A, Wisloff U. The combined association of skeletal muscle strength and physical activity on mortality in older women: the HUNT2 study. Mayo Clin Proc. 2017;92(5):710–8.
88. Ruiz JR, Sui X, Lobelo F, Morrow JR Jr, Jackson AW, Sjostrom M, et al. Association between muscular strength and mortality in men: prospective cohort study. BMJ. 2008;337:a439.
89. Stamatakis E, Lee IM, Bennie J, Freeston J, Hamer M, O'Donovan G, et al. Does strength promoting exercise confer unique health benefits? a pooled analysis of eleven population cohorts with all-cause, cancer, and cardiovascular mortality endpoints. Am J Epidemiol. 2018;187:1102–12.
90. Artero EG, Lee DC, Lavie CJ, Espana-Romero V, Sui X, Church TS, et al. Effects of muscular strength on cardiovascular risk factors and prognosis. J Cardiopulm Rehabil Prev. 2012;32(6):351–8.
91. Pescatello LS, MacDonald HV, Lamberti L, Johnson BT. Exercise for hypertension: a prescription update integrating existing recommendations with emerging research. Curr Hypertens Rep. 2015;17(11):87. https://doi.org/10.1007/s11906-015-0600-y.
92. Gando Y, Murakami H, Kawakami R, Yamamoto K, Kawano H, Tanaka N, et al. Cardiorespiratory fitness suppresses age-related arterial stiffening in healthy adults: a 2-year longitudinal observational study. J Clin Hypertens (Greenwich). 2016;18(4):292–8.
93. Lavie CJ, De Schutter A, Parto P, Jahangir E, Kokkinos P, Ortega FB, et al. Obesity and prevalence of cardiovascular diseases and prognosis-the obesity paradox updated. Prog Cardiovasc Dis. 2016;58(5):537–47.
94. Nauman J, Stensvold D, Coombes JS, Wisløff U. Cardiorespiratory fitness, sedentary time, and cardiovascular risk factor clustering. Med Sci Sports Exerc. 2016;48(4):625–32.
95. Johnson BT, MacDonald HV, Bruneau ML Jr, Goldsby TU, Brown JC, Huedo-Medina TB, et al. Methodological quality of meta-analyses on the blood pressure response to exercise: a review. J Hypertens. 2014;32(4):706–23.
96. ALLHAT Officers and Coordinators for the ALLHAT Collaborative Research Group. Major outcomes in high-risk hypertensive patients randomized to angiotensin-converting enzyme inhibitor or calcium channel blocker vs diuretic: the antihypertensive and lipid-lowering treatment to prevent heart attack trial (ALLHAT). JAMA. 2002;288(23):2981–97.
97. Whelton PK, He J, Appel LJ, Cutler JA, Havas S, Kotchen TA, et al. Primary prevention of hypertension: clinical and public health advisory from the national high blood pressure education program. JAMA. 2002;288(15):1882–8.
98. Whelton SP, Chin A, Xin X, He J. Effect of aerobic exercise on blood pressure: a meta-analysis of randomized, controlled trials. Ann Intern Med. 2002;136(7):493–503.
99. Brown RE, Riddell MC, Macpherson AK, Canning KL, Kuk JL. The joint association of physical activity, blood-pressure control, and pharmacologic treatment of hypertension for all-cause mortality risk. Am J Hypertens. 2013;26(8):1005–10.
100. Naci H, Ioannidis JP. Comparative effectiveness of exercise and drug interventions on mortality outcomes: metaepidemiological study. BMJ. 2013;347:f5577.
101. James PA, Oparil S, Carter BL, Cushman WC, Dennison-Himmelfarb C, Handler J, et al. 2014 evidence-based guideline for the management of high blood pressure in adults: report from the panel members appointed to the eighth joint national committee (JNC 8). JAMA. 2013;311(5):507–20.
102. Mancia G, Fagard R, Narkiewicz K, Redon J, Zanchetti A, Bohm M, et al. 2013 ESH/ESC practice guidelines for the management of arterial hypertension. Blood Press. 2014;23(1):3–16.
103. Leung AA, Nerenberg K, Daskalopoulou SS, McBrien K, Zarnke KB, Dasgupta K, et al. Hypertension Canada's 2016 Canadian hypertension education program guidelines for blood pressure measurement, diagnosis, assessment of risk, prevention, and treatment of hypertension. Can J Cardiol. 2016;32(5):569–88.
104. Pescatello LS, MacDonald HV, Ash GI, Lambert LM, Farquhar WB, Arena R, et al. Assessing the existing professional exercise recommendations for hypertension: a review and recommendations for future research priorities. Mayo Clin Proc. 2015;90(6):801–12.
105. Pescatello LS, Corso LML, MacDonald HV, Thompson PDT, Taylor BA, Panza GA, et al. Small sample sizes confound understanding of cardiometabolic responses to exercise. Exerc Sport Sci Rev. 2017;45(3):173–80. https://doi.org/10.1249/JES.0000000000000115.
106. Borg G. Perceived exertion as an indicator of somatic stress. Scand J Rehabil Med. 1970;2(2):92–8.
107. Moker EA, Bateman LA, Kraus WE, Pescatello LS. The relationship between the blood pressure responses to exercise following training and detraining periods. PLoS One. 2014;9(9):e105755.
108. MacDonald HV, Pescatello LS. Exercise prescription for hypertension: new advances for optimizing blood pressure benefits. In: Watson RR, Zibadi S, editors. Lifestyle in heart health and disease. 1st ed. London: Academic Press; 2018. p. 115–36.
109. Somani YB, Baross AW, Brook RD, Milne KJ, McGowan CL, Swaine IL. Acute response to a 2-minute isometric exercise test predicts the blood pressure-lowering efficacy of isometric

resistance training in young adults. Am J Hypertens. 2018;31(3):362–8.
110. Wegmann M, Hecksteden A, Poppendieck W, Steffen A, Kraushaar J, Morsch A, et al. Postexercise hypotension as a predictor for long-term training-induced blood pressure reduction: a large-scale randomized controlled trial. Clin J Sport Med. 2017; https://doi.org/10.1097/JSM.0000000000000475.
111. Hecksteden A, Grutters T, Meyer T. Association between postexercise hypotension and long-term training-induced blood pressure reduction: a pilot study. Clin J Sport Med. 2013;23(1):58–63.
112. Liu S, Goodman J, Nolan R, Lacombe S, Thomas SG. Blood pressure responses to acute and chronic exercise are related in prehypertension. Med Sci Sports Exerc. 2012;44(9):1644–52.
113. Devereux GR, Wiles JD, Howden R. Immediate post-isometric exercise cardiovascular responses are associated with training-induced resting systolic blood pressure reductions. Eur J Appl Physiol. 2015;115(2):327–33.
114. Tibana RA, de Sousa NM, da Cunha ND, Pereira GB, Thomas SG, Balsamo S, et al. Correlation between acute and chronic 24-hour blood pressure response to resistance training in adult women. Int J Sports Med. 2015;36(1):82–9.
115. Moreira SR, Cucato GG, Terra DF, Ritti-Dias RM. Acute blood pressure changes are related to chronic effects of resistance exercise in medicated hypertensives elderly women. Clin Physiol Funct Imaging. 2016;36(3):242–8.
116. Bouchard C, Blair SN, Church TS, Earnest CP, Hagberg JM, Hakkinen K, et al. Adverse metabolic response to regular exercise: is it a rare or common occurrence? PLoS One. 2012;7(5):e37887.
117. Leifer ES, Mikus CR, Karavirta L, Resnick BD, Kraus WE, Hakkinen K, et al. Adverse cardiovascular response to aerobic exercise training: is this a concern? Med Sci Sports Exerc. 2016;48(1):20–5.
118. Luttrell MJ, Halliwill JR. Recovery from exercise: vulnerable state, window of opportunity, or crystal ball? Front Physiol. 2015;6:204.
119. Kenney MJ, Seals DR. Postexercise hypotension. key features, mechanisms, and clinical significance. Hypertension. 1993;22(5):653–64.
120. Halliwill JR, Buck TM, Lacewell AN, Romero SA. Postexercise hypotension and sustained postexercise vasodilatation: what happens after we exercise? Exp Physiol. 2013;98(1):7–18.
121. MacDonald JR. Potential causes, mechanisms, and implications of post exercise hypotension. J Hum Hypertens. 2002;16(4):225–36.
122. Cardoso CG Jr, Gomides RS, Queiroz AC, Pinto LG, da Silveira LF, Tinucci T, et al. Acute and chronic effects of aerobic and resistance exercise on ambulatory blood pressure. Clinics (Sao Paulo). 2010;65(3):317–25.
123. Gomes Anunciacao P, Doederlein PM. A review on post-exercise hypotension in hypertensive individuals. Arq Bras Cardiol. 2011;96(5):e100–9.
124. Oliveira Marques-Silvestre AC, do Socorro Brasileiro-Santos M, Sarmento de Oliveira A, Thiago Maciel da Silva F, da Cruz Santos A, da Cruz Santos A. Magnitude of acute aerobic post-exercise hypotension: a systematic review of randomized trials. Motricidade. 2014;10(3):99–111.
125. Carpio-Rivera E, Moncada-Jimenez J, Salazar-Rojas W, Solera-Herrera A. Acute effects of exercise on blood pressure: a meta-analytic investigation. Arq Bras Cardiol. 2016;106(5):422–33.
126. Ciolac EG, Guimaraes GV, D'Avila VM, Bortolotto LA, Doria EL, Bocchi EA. Acute aerobic exercise reduces 24-h ambulatory blood pressure levels in long-term-treated hypertensive patients. Clinics (Sao Paulo). 2008;63(6):753–8.
127. Pescatello LS, Kulikowich JM. The aftereffects of dynamic exercise on ambulatory blood pressure. Med Sci Sports Exerc. 2001;33(11):1855–61.
128. Jones H, George K, Edwards B, Atkinson G. Is the magnitude of acute post-exercise hypotension mediated by exercise intensity or total work done? Eur J Appl Physiol. 2007;102(1):33–40.
129. Eicher JD, Maresh CM, Tsongalis GJ, Thompson PD, Pescatello LS. The additive blood pressure lowering effects of exercise intensity on post-exercise hypotension. Am Heart J. 2010;160(3):513–20.
130. Bhammar DM, Angadi SS, Gaesser GA. Effects of fractionized and continuous exercise on 24-h ambulatory blood pressure. Med Sci Sports Exerc. 2012;44(12):2270–6.
131. Miyashita M, Burns SF, Stensel DJ. Accumulating short bouts of running reduces resting blood pressure in young normotensive/pre-hypertensive men. J Sports Sci. 2011;29(14):1473–82.
132. Ciolac EG, Guimaraes GV, Avila VM D, Bortolotto LA, Doria EL, Bocchi EA. Acute effects of continuous and interval aerobic exercise on 24-h ambulatory blood pressure in long-term treated hypertensive patients. Int J Cardiol. 2009;133(3):381–7.
133. Guidry MA, Blanchard BE, Thompson PD, Maresh CM, Seip RL, Taylor AL, et al. The influence of short and long duration on the blood pressure response to an acute bout of dynamic exercise. Am Heart J. 2006;151(6):1322.e5–12.
134. MacDonald JR, MacDougall JD, Hogben CD. The effects of exercise duration on post-exercise hypotension. J Hum Hypertens. 2000;14(2):125–9.
135. Santana HA, Moreira SR, Asano RY, Sales MM, Cordova C, Campbell CS, et al. Exercise intensity modulates nitric oxide and blood pressure responses in hypertensive older women. Aging Clin Exp Res. 2013;25(1):43–8.
136. Cornelissen VA, Fagard RH. Effects of endurance training on blood pressure, blood pressure-regulating mechanisms, and cardiovascular risk factors. Hypertension. 2005;46(4):667–75.
137. Kelley GA, Kelley KA, Tran ZV. Aerobic exercise and resting blood pressure: a meta-analytic review of randomized, controlled trials. Prev Cardiol. 2001;4(2):73–80.

138. Kelley GA, Kelley KS, Tran ZV. Walking and resting blood pressure in adults: a meta-analysis. Prev Med. 2001;33(2 Pt 1):120–7.
139. Fagard RH. Physical fitness and blood pressure. J Hypertens Suppl. 1993;11(5):S47–52.
140. Cornelissen VA, Buys R, Smart NA. Endurance exercise beneficially affects ambulatory blood pressure: a systematic review and meta-analysis. J Hypertens. 2013;31(4):639–48.
141. Sosner P, Guiraud T, Gremeaux V, Arvisais D, Herpin D, Bosquet L. The ambulatory hypotensive effect of aerobic training: a reappraisal through a meta-analysis of selected moderators. Scand J Med Sci Sports. 2017;27(3):327–41.
142. Cornelissen VA, Smart NA. Exercise training for blood pressure: a systematic review and meta-analysis. J Am Heart Assoc. 2013;2(1):e004473.
143. Kessler HS, Sisson SB, Short KR. The potential for high-intensity interval training to reduce cardiometabolic disease risk. Sports Med. 2012;42(6):489–509.
144. Gibala MJ, Little JP, Macdonald MJ, Hawley JA. Physiological adaptations to low-volume, high-intensity interval training in health and disease. J Physiol. 2012;590(5):1077–84.
145. Batacan RB Jr, Duncan MJ, Dalbo VJ, Tucker PS, Fenning AS. Effects of high-intensity interval training on cardiometabolic health: a systematic review and meta-analysis of intervention studies. Br J Sports Med. 2017;51(6):494–503.
146. MacDougall JD, Tuxen D, Sale DG, Moroz JR, Sutton JR. Arterial blood pressure response to heavy resistance exercise. J Appl Physiol (1985). 1985;58(3):785–90.
147. Porth CJ, Bamrah VS, Tristani FE, Smith JJ. The valsalva maneuver: mechanisms and clinical implications. Heart Lung. 1984;13(5):507–18.
148. Crump C, Sundquist J, Winkleby MA, Sundquist K. Interactive effects of aerobic fitness, strength, and obesity on mortality in men. Am J Prev Med. 2017;52(3):353–61.
149. Volaklis KA, Halle M, Meisinger C. Muscular strength as a strong predictor of mortality: a narrative review. Eur J Intern Med. 2015;26(5):303–10.
150. Brito Ade F, de Oliveira CV, Santos Mdo S, Santos AC. High-intensity exercise promotes postexercise hypotension greater than moderate intensity in elderly hypertensive individuals. Clin Physiol Funct Imaging. 2014;34(2):126–32.
151. de Freitas BA, Brasileiro-Santos Mdo S, Coutinho de Oliveira CV, Sarmento da Nobrega TK, Lucia de Moraes Forjaz C, da Cruz Santos A. High-intensity resistance exercise promotes postexercise hypotension greater than moderate intensity and affects cardiac autonomic responses in women who are hypertensive. J Strength Cond Res. 2015;29(12):3486–93.
152. Cavalcante PA, Rica RL, Evangelista AL, Serra AJ, Figueira A Jr, Pontes FL Jr, et al. Effects of exercise intensity on postexercise hypotension after resistance training session in overweight hypertensive patients. Clin Interv Aging. 2015;10:1487–95.
153. Moraes MR, Bacurau RF, Casarini DE, Jara ZP, Ronchi FA, Almeida SS, et al. Chronic conventional resistance exercise reduces blood pressure in stage 1 hypertensive men. J Strength Cond Res. 2012;26(4):1122–9.
154. Mota MR, Oliveira RJ, Terra DF, Pardono E, Dutra MT, de Almeida JA, et al. Acute and chronic effects of resistance exercise on blood pressure in elderly women and the possible influence of ACE I/D polymorphism. Int J Gen Med. 2013;6:581–7.
155. Scher LM, Ferriolli E, Moriguti JC, Scher R, Lima NK. The effect of different volumes of acute resistance exercise on elderly individuals with treated hypertension. J Strength Cond Res. 2011;25(4):1016–23.
156. Casonatto J, Goessler KF, Cornelissen VA, Cardoso JR, Polito MD. The blood pressure-lowering effect of a single bout of resistance exercise: a systematic review and meta-analysis of randomised controlled trials. Eur J Prev Cardiol. 2016;23(16):1700–14.
157. Melo CM, Alencar Filho AC, Tinucci T, Mion D Jr, Forjaz CL. Postexercise hypotension induced by low-intensity resistance exercise in hypertensive women receiving captopril. Blood Press Monit. 2006;11(4):183–9.
158. MacDonald HV, Johnson BT, Huedo-Medina TB, Livingston J, Forsyth KC, Kraemer WJ, et al. Dynamic resistance training as stand-alone antihypertensive lifestyle therapy: a meta-analysis. J Am Heart Assoc. 2016;5(10) https://doi.org/10.1161/JAHA.116.003231.
159. Moraes MR, Bacurau RF, Simoes HG, Campbell CS, Pudo MA, Wasinski F, et al. Effect of 12 weeks of resistance exercise on post-exercise hypotension in stage 1 hypertensive individuals. J Hum Hypertens. 2012;26(9):533–9.
160. Mota MR, de Oliveira RJ, Dutra MT, Pardono E, Terra DF, Lima RM, et al. Acute and chronic effects of resistive exercise on blood pressure in hypertensive elderly women. J Strength Cond Res. 2013;27(12):3475–80.
161. Brook RD, Appel LJ, Rubenfire M, Ogedegbe G, Bisognano JD, Elliott WJ, et al. Beyond medications and diet: alternative approaches to lowering blood pressure: a scientific statement from the American Heart Association. Hypertension. 2013;61(6):1360–83.
162. Inder JD, Carlson DJ, Dieberg G, McFarlane JR, Hess NC, Smart NA. Isometric exercise training for blood pressure management: a systematic review and meta-analysis to optimize benefit. Hypertens Res. 2016;39(2):88–94.
163. Millar PJ, McGowan CL, Cornelissen VA, Araujo CG, Swaine IL. Evidence for the role of isometric exercise training in reducing blood pressure: potential mechanisms and future directions. Sports Med. 2014;44(3):345–56.

164. Carlson DJ, Dieberg G, Hess NC, Millar PJ, Smart NA. Isometric exercise training for blood pressure management: a systematic review and meta-analysis. Mayo Clin Proc. 2014;89(3):327–34.
165. Hurley BF, Hanson ED, Sheaff AK. Strength training as a countermeasure to aging muscle and chronic disease. Sports Med. 2011;41(4):289–306.
166. Ash GI, Taylor BA, Thompson PD, MacDonald HV, Lamberti L, Chen MH, et al. The antihypertensive effects of aerobic versus isometric handgrip resistance exercise. J Hypertens. 2017;35(2):291–9.
167. Goessler K, Buys R, Cornelissen VA. Low-intensity isometric handgrip exercise has no transient effect on blood pressure in patients with coronary artery disease. J Am Soc Hypertens. 2016;10(8):633–9.
168. Olher Rdos R, Bocalini DS, Bacurau RF, Rodriguez D, Figueira A Jr, Pontes FL Jr, et al. Isometric handgrip does not elicit cardiovascular overload or post-exercise hypotension in hypertensive older women. Clin Interv Aging. 2013;8:649–55.
169. van Assche T, Buys R, de Jaeger M, Coeckelberghs E, Cornelissen VA. One single bout of low-intensity isometric handgrip exercise reduces blood pressure in healthy pre- and hypertensive individuals. J Sports Med Phys Fitness. 2017;57(4):469–75.
170. Souza LR, Vicente JB, Melo GR, Moraes VC, Olher RR, Sousa IC, et al. Acute hypotension after moderate-intensity handgrip exercise in hypertensive elderly people. J Strength Cond Res. 2018;32(10):2971–7.
171. Carlson DJ, Inder J, Palanisamy SK, McFarlane JR, Dieberg G, Smart NA. The efficacy of isometric resistance training utilizing handgrip exercise for blood pressure management: a randomized trial. Medicine (Baltimore). 2016;95(52):e5791.
172. Goessler KF, Buys R, VanderTrappen D, Vanhumbeeck L, Cornelissen VA. A randomized controlled trial comparing home-based isometric handgrip exercise versus endurance training for blood pressure management. J Am Soc Hypertens. 2018;12:285–93.
173. Badrov MB, Horton S, Millar PJ, McGowan CL. Cardiovascular stress reactivity tasks successfully predict the hypotensive response of isometric handgrip training in hypertensives. Psychophysiology. 2013;50(4):407–14.
174. Stiller-Moldovan C, Kenno K, McGowan CL. Effects of isometric handgrip training on blood pressure (resting and 24 h ambulatory) and heart rate variability in medicated hypertensive patients. Blood Press Monit. 2012;17(2):55–61.
175. Taylor AC, McCartney N, Kamath MV, Wiley RL. Isometric training lowers resting blood pressure and modulates autonomic control. Med Sci Sports Exerc. 2003;35(2):251–6.
176. Corso LM, MacDonald HV, Johnson BT, Farinatti P, Livingston J, Zaleski AL, et al. Is concurrent training efficacious antihypertensive therapy? A meta-analysis. Med Sci Sports Exerc. 2016;48(12):2398–406.
177. Pagonas N, Vlatsas S, Bauer F, Seibert FS, Zidek W, Babel N, et al. Aerobic versus isometric handgrip exercise in hypertension: a randomized controlled trial. J Hypertens. 2017;35(11):2199–206.
178. McGowan CL, Proctor DN, Swaine I, Brook RD, Jackson EA, Levy PD. Isometric handgrip as an adjunct for blood pressure control: a primer for clinicians. Curr Hypertens Rep. 2017;19(6):51. 017-0748-8.
179. MacDonald HV, Farinatti PV, Lamberti LM, Pescatello LS. Chapter 3. the effects of concurrent exercise on hypertension: current consensus and emerging research. In: Pescatello LS, editor. Effects of exercise on hypertension: from cells to physiological systems. Cham: Springer International Publishing; 2015. p. 47–86.
180. Tibana RA, Nascimento Dda C, de Sousa NM, de Almeida JA, Moraes MR, Durigan JL, et al. Similar hypotensive effects of combined aerobic and resistance exercise with 1 set versus 3 sets in women with metabolic syndrome. Clin Physiol Funct Imaging. 2015;35(6):443–50.
181. Anunciacao PG, Farinatti PT, Goessler KF, Casonatto J, Polito MD. Blood pressure and autonomic responses following isolated and combined aerobic and resistance exercise in hypertensive older women. Clin Exp Hypertens. 2016;38(8):710–4.
182. Azevedo LM, de Souza AC, Santos LE, Miguel Dos Santos R, de Fernandes MO, Almeida JA, et al. Fractionated concurrent exercise throughout the day does not promote acute blood pressure benefits in hypertensive middle-aged women. Front Cardiovasc Med. 2017;4:6.
183. Dos Santos ES, Asano RY, Gomes Filho I, Nilson Lima L, Panelli P, Nascimento DD, et al. Acute and chronic cardiovascular response to 16 weeks of combined eccentric or traditional resistance and aerobic training in elderly hypertensive women: a randomized controlled trial. J Strength Cond Res. 2014;28(11):3073–84.
184. Meneses AL, Forjaz CL, de Lima PF, Batista RM, Monteiro MD, Ritti-Dias RM. Influence of endurance and resistance exercise order on the post-exercise hemodynamic responses in hypertensive women. J Strength Cond Res. 2015;29(3):612–8.
185. Hayashino Y, Jackson JL, Fukumori N, Nakamura F, Fukuhara S. Effects of supervised exercise on lipid profiles and blood pressure control in people with type 2 diabetes mellitus: a meta-analysis of randomized controlled trials. Diabetes Res Clin Pract. 2012;98(3):349–60.
186. Romero SA, Minson CT, Halliwill JR. The cardiovascular system after exercise. J Appl Physiol. 2017;122(4):925–32.

Role of Physical Activity, Exercise, and Cardiorespiratory Fitness in the Management of Resistant Hypertension

9

Puneet Narayan and Anubhav Kumar

Abbreviations

ABPM	Ambulatory blood pressure monitor
BP	Blood pressure
CKD	Chronic kidney disease
CRF	Cardiorespiratory fitness
CVD	Cardiovascular disease
DM2	Type 2 diabetes mellitus
ETT	Exercise tolerance test
HIIT	High-intensity interval training
hs-CRP	High-sensitivity C-reactive protein
HTN	Hypertension
LVH	Left ventricular hypertrophy
METs	Metabolic equivalents
OSA	Obstructive sleep apnea
PA	Physical activity
PWV	Pulse wave velocity

Introduction

Hypertension (HTN) is the most common treatable risk factor for cardiovascular (CV) disease. Lowering blood pressure (BP) has been the most pivotal intervention in decreasing CV morbidity and mortality not just in patients with isolated HTN but also in hypertensives with comorbidities like type 2 diabetes mellitus (DM2), dyslipidemia, chronic kidney disease (CKD), and other established CV diseases like coronary artery disease and cerebrovascular disease.

The direct association between BP levels and CV events has been known since the initial Framingham Heart Study reports in the 1950s showing a strong association between HTN and outcomes including myocardial infarction, congestive heart failure, strokes, and kidney disease [1]. The benefit of lowering BP with medications to improve CV outcomes and mortality has been recognized since Dr. Edward Freis' landmark Department of Veterans Affairs Cooperative Study [2]. Great advances have been made since then in managing HTN with resulting improved outcomes. However, there remains a group of treated hypertensives that continues to be at high risk in spite of these advances. These are patients with resistant HTN in whom either BP remains uncontrolled ≥130/80 mm of Hg despite being treated simultaneously with optimal dosages of ≥3 antihypertensive medications, one of which is a diuretic, or in whom BP may be controlled but who require ≥4 or more antihypertensive agents. It should be noted that this is the new definition of resistant HTN per the latest guidelines formulated in 2017, prior to which resistant HTN was said to be present when BP was ≥140/90 using the above parameters [3]. Whether this lack of control is a result of poor drug combinations or non-compliance, the fact remains that

P. Narayan (✉) · A. Kumar
Clinical Research Institute of Northern Virginia, Burke, VA, USA

P. Kokkinos, P. Narayan (eds.), *Cardiorespiratory Fitness in Cardiometabolic Diseases*,
https://doi.org/10.1007/978-3-030-04816-7_9

approximately 15–30% of the treated HTN population can be classified as having resistant HTN [4]. Patients with resistant HTN remain at an even higher risk for CV outcomes, renal outcomes, and all-cause mortality compared to patients who do not have resistant HTN [5] and have been a focus of the HTN community for the past several years. This increased CV risk due to resistant HTN has been shown in many studies. Daugherty et al., for example, reported that adverse CV outcomes were 50% higher in the resistant HTN group, driven mostly by chronic kidney disease [5]. In general, however, it is estimated that there is an over twofold higher risk of CV events in patients with resistant HTN compared to all patients being newly treated for HTN [3]. In one study the all-cause mortality was 40% higher in women with apparent resistant HTN compared to the nonresistant cohort [6]. Additionally, getting BP under control with polypharmacy does not necessarily afford the expected protection against CV outcomes in resistant hypertensive patients. This was evident in a large Kaiser Permanente study which showed that the highest number of events occurred in the group of patients in whom BP was controlled but with four or more antihypertensive medications. This group of patients indeed had an even worse outcome than the group of patients who had uncontrolled BP with three antihypertensive medications [7].

Thus it is imperative to investigate interventions other than drug therapy to determine if additional methods can be identified which could help improve prognosis of patients with resistant HTN. Modalities other than medications have been studied in RH with mixed results. Some of these have been invasive procedures aiming to modify neurogenic or hormonal factors known to adversely impact BP. However, two such interventions, carotid baroreceptor stimulation and renal nerve denervation, were found to be either not widely applicable [8] or ineffective in controlled double blind randomized trials [9].

The impact of cardiorespiratory fitness (CRF) on BP has been studied in varied populations including normotensives, prehypertensives, and hypertensives [10]. Regularly performed exercise leading to improvements in CRF has been shown to lower blood pressure in patients with prehypertension, HTN, and even resistant HTN [10]. Large and well-conducted epidemiologic studies have also shown an inverse and graded association between CRF and mortality in the general hypertensive population [11]. However, it is not known if increased CRF can attenuate mortality risk in patients with resistant HTN. This chapter will discuss the factors associated with and those that predispose to the development of RH and factors that make BP more resistant to treatment, together with the impact of physical activity (PA), exercise, and CRF on lowering BP, morbidity, and mortality in patients with resistant HTN.

Factors Associated with Resistant Hypertension

Resistant HTN can be present in patients without any additional factors; however, certain conditions are likely to be associated with it [12]. Conditions commonly associated with a higher prevalence of resistant HTN are older age, obesity, smoking, obstructive sleep apnea (OSA), DM2, left ventricular hypertrophy (LVH), and CKD. However, there are several other factors and conditions that can render HTN difficult to control including use of excessive sodium, alcohol, certain medications, and secondary forms of HTN associated with endocrine disorders, central nervous system tumors, and coarctation of aorta [13]. An effort should always be made to identify the treatable forms of HTN during initial evaluation of all hypertensive patients based on history, physical examination, and focused laboratory testing and imaging. It has been shown that addressing these risk factors for resistant HTN helps in lowering BP and the benefits of exercise in these populations have been substantiated by several studies, albeit not all in patients with resistant HTN. The next section focuses on the effect of physical activity (PA), exercise training, and/or CRF on certain risk factors of resistant HTN.

Effect of PA and CRF on Risk Factors for Resistant Hypertension

Age

RH is most common in older hypertensives [12]. In this group uncontrolled systolic BP is the main problem. Additionally, older hypertensives generally have other risk factors which increase the susceptibility to develop RH. Even in the absence of additional risk factors, aging contributes to arterial stiffness and decreased aortic compliance [12, 14], which predispose to additional cardiovascular risks. Studies of effect of exercise on central hemodynamics in elderly patients with RH are not available; however, McDonnell et al. [15] have demonstrated that regular exercise is associated with lower systolic BP, diastolic BP, and large artery stiffness in older individuals. A limitation in treating elderly patients with HTN, especially in situations requiring polypharmacy for several concomitant illnesses, is the risk of orthostatic hypotension, which predisposes to syncope, falls, and injuries. Taking this into consideration, the role of moderate- to high-intensity exercise to facilitate control of BP and thereby decrease the requirement for pharmacological therapy is critical in elderly hypertensives. Beneficial effects of exercise in elderly have been validated by many studies, and it is recommended that exercise be implemented in elderly to manage HTN [16–23].

Obstructive Sleep Apnea

It has been long known that OSA increases the risk of CV events. Association of OSA with HTN is also well established, and it is recommended that patients with treatment-resistant HTN be screened for OSA [24]. Increased arterial stiffness has been shown to be present in patients with OSA even in the absence of HTN. In a study of 1921 subjects, patients with moderate to severe OSA had higher brachial-ankle pulse wave velocity at baseline, and severity of OSA predicted future severity of arterial stiffness [25]. There are several other pathological changes precipitated by OSA which can facilitate the development of RH. Some of these changes are secondary to periods of hypoxia caused by OSA leading to activation of endothelin and sympathetic nervous systems [26, 27], which can lead to the development of RH. Exercise intervention studies in OSA patients with RH are lacking; however, regularly performed aerobic exercises have been shown to decrease BP in hypertensive patients with OSA [24].

Diabetes Mellitus

Diabetic patients have a higher risk of having RH. A number of pathophysiologic processes could be contributing to it. Elia et al. [28] in a prospective study reported that DM2 patients had significantly higher pulse wave velocity (PWV) compared to nondiabetics. This risk was nine times higher in uncontrolled diabetics than in nondiabetics. As stated above hypertensive LVH is a risk factor for RH. Coexistence of DM2 with HTN further increases the risk for increase in LV mass, LV dysfunction, and arterial stiffness [29]. While exercise intervention studies focusing only on diabetic patients with RH are not available, exercise training in diabetic hypertensives has been reported to improve not just BP and diabetic control but also endothelial function and left ventricular diastolic function [30]. In a meta-analysis reviewing the effects of supervised exercise on BP and lipid levels in high-risk diabetic patients with HTN and dyslipidemia, 42 trials with 2808 patients were included. Results showed that structured exercise was associated with lowering of systolic BP, diastolic BP, and low-density lipoprotein cholesterol and an increase in high-density lipoprotein cholesterol [31]. Exercise intervention studies in diabetics with RH should be a field for future research.

Left Ventricular Hypertrophy

LVH is a known risk factor of poorer cardiovascular outcomes and mortality in hypertensives. Risk of having resistant HTN is higher in hypertensives who have LVH [12]. Fernando et al. reported that regression of electrocardiographic LVH in patients with RH is protective against a composite endpoint of cardiovascular events, CV mortality, and all-cause mortality [32]. Studies in RH with LVH have shown that exercise training can help lower BP, decrease medication requirement, and even lead to regression of LVH in some cases. In a study of 46 African-American patients with severe HTN and LVH, patients were assigned to a 16-week exercise training or a control group. Exercise training was effective in lowering BP, decreasing antihypertensive medications, and decreasing LVH [33]. No exercise related or other adverse events were noted in the study. These patients were on multiple antihypertensive medications, and several met the criteria for RH. Based on these studies, it is evident that exercise has a role in managing patients with RH and regression of LVH in these patients results in improved CV and mortality outcomes.

Chronic Kidney Disease

RH is commonly seen in patients with CKD. There are several factors in CKD patients with RH that can make BP difficult to control including sodium and water retention. Arterial stiffness is also enhanced in patients with CKD; hence the increase in volume from sodium and water retention is not able to be accommodated adequately. This effect is further exacerbated in CKD patients since eGFR is decreased and the increased volume cannot be handled appropriately. Aortic stiffness, which is seen with aging in hypertensives, is further enhanced by the presence of CKD, together with aortic calcification. These changes result in an increase in pulse pressure, PWV, central aortic pressures, and risk of developing LVH. These are known features of patients with RH which are further exacerbated by the presence of CKD. Arterial stiffness and calcification have additional adverse CV effects. Baroreceptor compensatory reflexes may be blunted in patients with decreased carotid compliance secondary to local structural changes, leading to rise in BP and limiting efforts to control it [12]. It is known that it is difficult to control blood pressure in the presence of CKD with most patients requiring three or more antihypertensive medications for control [34]. While exercise has been shown to benefit several conditions that are associated with and/or predispose to the risk of developing CKD as discussed above, not all studies have shown a favorable effect of exercise training in lowering BP in CKD hypertensives. In a group of 150 patients with stage 2–4 CKD and HTN without DM2, Barcellos et al. randomized 76 patients to exercise and 74 to a control group, with a primary aim of assessing change in eGFR and secondary aims of studying effects on weight, systolic BP, diastolic BP, functional capacity, and metabolic parameters [35]. Following 16 weeks of aerobic and resistance training, no between-group differences were noted in BP, eGFR, body weight, or lipid profile. Significant improvements were, however, noted in hs-CRP, fasting glucose, and functional capacity in the exercise group. In another small study of 11 diabetic, obese patients with stage 2–4 CKD on medical management, 7 patients were randomized to aerobic exercise [36]. The exercise consisted of 6 weeks of exercise training preceding 18 weeks of supervised home exercise. At the end of this 24-week study, only a nonsignificant decrease in systolic BP was noted. While in these studies the effect on BP was disappointing, it should not discourage future research to study the role of PA, exercise, and CRF in the management of these patients. This is especially important since no specific, large-scale studies have been done to prospectively assess the role of exercise training or CRF in managing RH in CKD patients and this field remains open for future research in these high-risk patients.

Central Aortic Pressures in Resistant Hypertension

Several risk factors associated with a higher prevalence of resistant HTN are also associated with structural changes in the aorta which lead to increase in central aortic blood pressures [12]. Increasing age leads to stiffening of the aorta [14] which is associated with decreased compliance and distensibility. Changes in distensibility of the aorta with age are likely secondary to decreases in elastic fibers and increase in collagen [37] and vascular smooth muscle cells [38].

It has been long known that in patients on antihypertensive therapy, cardiovascular risk remains elevated if central blood pressures are not controlled even if brachial pressures are within normal limits. In the Conduit Artery Function Evaluation (CAFE) study, the effects of two different combinations of antihypertensive therapies on changes in central aortic pulse pressures and hemodynamics were compared in 2199 patients to assess the impact on outcomes. At the end of follow-up, control of brachial systolic BP was similar in both groups, but central aortic pressure was lower in the group treated with amlodipine with possible addition of perindopril versus those treated with atenolol with possible addition of bendroflumethiazide. Lower central aortic pulse pressure was found to be significantly and directly associated with cardiovascular outcomes and renal events [39]. In a meta-analysis of 17 studies with a total of 15,877 patients who had a mean follow-up 7.7 years, predictive value of aortic PWV for CV events and all-cause mortality was assessed [40]. Authors reported that in patients with high PWV, the relative risk of total CV events was 2.26 (95% confidence interval: 1.89–2.70, 14 studies). Cardiovascular mortality was 2.02 (95% confidence interval: 1.68 to 2.42, 10 studies) and all-cause mortality 1.90 (95% confidence interval: 1.61 to 2.24, 11 studies). Patients with HTN and other established cardiovascular diseases had an even higher relative risk of cardiovascular event rate and mortality with increased aortic PWV. An increase of 1 m/s in aortic PWV increased the risks for all endpoints by 14–15%, and with a 1 standard deviation increase in aortic PWV, the risk for all endpoints rose by 42–42%. There are no long-term, prospective, randomized studies in this population to assess the long-term effect of exercise on abnormal aortic pressure indices in patients with RH. However, a study utilizing high-intensity interval training (HIIT) in high-risk hypertensive patients has shown some benefit as described in the next section.

High-Intensity Interval Training in Resistant Hypertension

The recommendations for PA and exercise to improve the risk factors of CV disease are PA spread over a several days per week to equal about 200 min per week. These recommendations are based on the beneficial effects of exercise on outcomes as assessed by PA questionnaires and/or objectively measured CRF. However, some studies have shown that shorter durations of higher-intensity exercise may help high-risk patients by having a favorable effect on central aortic pressures. Elevated central aortic pressure is an independent predictor of poorer outcomes in hypertensive patients, and it is known to be elevated in patients with resistant HTN [41]. In 50 high-risk patients with metabolic syndrome, effects of durations and frequencies of high-intensity interval training (HIIT) on aortic pressure were assessed. It was reported that only 4 min of HIIT, performed thrice a week, with a weekly volume of 12 min, performed for 16 weeks, was able to decrease aortic reservoir pressure [42]. Effects of HIIT in RH have not been explored and remain an open factor to investigate in future research.

Effect of Exercise and CRF on Resistant Hypertension

Effect of exercise in lowering BP has been evaluated by some investigators. In these studies, the prior definition to define RH was used which was BP of ≥140/90 mm Hg despite treatment with adequate dosages of three or more antihypertensive medications, one of which is a diuretic or requiring a regimen of four or more medications for control and not the new cutoff of ≥130/80 mm Hg. Dimeo et al. evaluated ambulatory BP and pulse wave analysis to assess arterial compliance and cardiac index in 50 patients with RH. Patients were randomized to exercise for 8–12 weeks on a treadmill or to a control group. Exercise intensity was monitored by serum lactate levels with a target of 2.0 ± 0.5 mmol/L. Exercise was effective in significantly lowering ambulatory daytime systolic and diastolic BP, and this reduction was seen during exertion as well. Exercise training also resulted in increased exercise capacity based on changes in maximal oxygen uptake and lactate curves. This study, however, did not show any change in arterial compliance and cardiac index [43].

In an interesting trial, Guimaraes et al. studied the effect of exercising in heated water on 24-h ambulatory BP parameters in patients with RH [44]. A total of 32 patients met the protocol enrollment criteria, of whom 16 were randomized to heated water exercise and 16 to a control group. Patients randomized to the active arm exercised for 60 min, thrice a week for 12 weeks in a pool heated to 32 °C, by walking and performing calisthenic exercises. No change in activity was recommended for the control group. In the control group, there was a significant increase noted in 24-h systolic and diastolic BP and daytime and nighttime diastolic BP. In contrast, in the active group, heated pool exercises significantly decreased office BP by 36/12 mm Hg together with a significant decrease in 24-h daytime and nighttime systolic BP and diastolic BP parameters.

Effect of CRF on Mortality in Patients with Resistant Hypertension

The protective effect of exercise against mortality in the general hypertensive patients has been shown in many studies. A review of literature which included 48,625 men and 47,625 women, with a minimum 1 year of follow-up, showed that both cardiovascular and all-cause mortality were inversely related to PA in all the studies. The authors reported that hypertensives who participated in any level of PA had a 16–67% reduced risk of CV mortality, whereas the inactive group had an over twofold increase risk of mortality [45].

The effect of PA, exercise, and CRF on mortality in patients with RH has not been evaluated in prospective, randomized, controlled studies. However, the association of CRF with all-cause mortality in patients with RH was studied by our group in African-American patients with RH [46]. From a group of 9968 patients, 1276 men were identified as having RH based on the prior definition of BP ≥140/90 mm Hg on three antihypertensive medications, one of which was a diuretic or use of >4 antihypertensive medications. All these patients had undergone an exercise tolerance test (ETT) at the Department of Veterans Affairs Medical Center in Washington, DC. To eliminate the confounding effect of age on exercise capacity, patients were categorized in four age-specific CRF groups according to the peak metabolic equivalents (METs) reached on a standard Bruce protocol. The mean follow-up was 9.5 ± 4.2 years during which an inverse relationship was noted between all-cause mortality and CRF, with mortality being the highest in the least-fit group and slowest in the high-fit group. In comparison to the least-fit group, mortality was 21% lower in the low-fit group, 36% lower in the moderate-fit group, and 62% lowest in the high-fit group (Fig. 9.1). This reduction was statistically significant in the moderate- and high-fit groups. With an increase in each MET in exercise capacity, the mortality rate decreased by 18%. This study did have limitations in that it included only African-Americans, male patients who had access to full, unrestricted medical management under the Veterans Affairs Medical Center umbrella. Thus, the results may not be generalizable to females, non-veterans, and patients of other racial backgrounds. Another limitation was that the analysis was based on data collected at baseline, and any changes in medications, level of CRF, and other lifestyle factors could not be taken into consideration. Nonetheless, these findings are gratifying considering the difficulty in altering the risk of CV events and all-cause mortality in RH patients, despite medical therapy as discussed earlier in this chapter. The study population had multiple CV risk factors

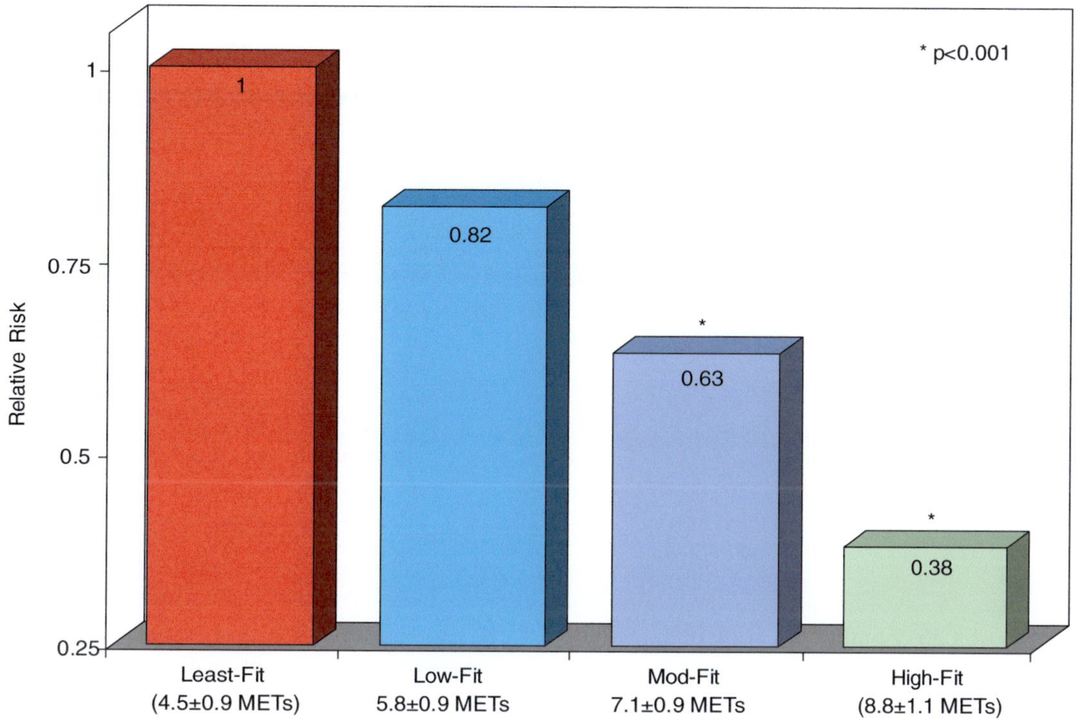

Fig. 9.1 Mortality risk according to fitness categories in patients with resistant hypertension

Table 9.1 Clinical characteristics of survivors deceased during follow-up

	Alive	Dead	*p*-value
n	1274	412	
Age in years	59.6 ± 9.7	61.0 ± 10.2	<0.001
Males, %	94.9	97.0	0.023
BMI in kg/m²	30.9 ± 5.4	29.4 ± 5.6	0.001
Heart rate (beats/min)	71.0 ± 13.5	72.4 ± 14.3	0.07
Systolic BP (mm Hg)	134.2 ± 18.4	140.7 ± 22.7	<0.001
Diastolic BP (mm Hg)	80.5 ± 11.4	79.9 ± 12.1	0.35
Peak METs	6.8 ± 1.8	5.8 ± 1.6	<0.001
Duration of hypertension (years)	4.5 ± 4.4	2.6 ± 2.9	<0.001
Alcohol/substance abuse, *n* (%)	373(23.3)	19 (22.6)	0.50
Smokers, *n* (%)	258 (21.4)	134 (27.7	0.004
Diabetics, *n* (%)	198 (20.5)	194 (27.0)	0.001
CKD/HIV, *n* (%)	344 (22.8)	48 (27.4)	0.42
MACE, *n* (%)	314 (20.6)	78 (48.8)	<0.001

(Table 9.1) and still benefited from having improved CRF.

The study also revealed a statistically lower systolic BP in the high-fit group (Table 9.2) which is an important finding, considering the difficulty in controlling BP in this group of patients.

It is also noteworthy that the METs achieved by the moderate-fit and high-fit groups were only 7.1 + 0.9 METs and 8.8 + 1.1 METs, respectively (Fig. 9.1).

This is a level that is likely to be easily achieved by most patients with RH as it is equiva-

Table 9.2 Clinical characteristics of participants according to fitness categories

	Least-fit	Low-fit	Moderate-fit	High-fit	*p*-value
n	396	439	492	359	
Age in years	60.9 ± 10.6	61.0 ± 10.2	60.3 ± 9.6	60.2 ± 10.2	0.55
Males, %	94.9	97.0	97.6	98.6	
Race					0.88
African-Americans, n (%)	310 (78.3)	344 (78.4)	391 (79.5)	277 (77.2)	
White/other n (%)	86 (21.7	95 (21.6)	101 (20.5)	82 (22.8)	
BMI in kg/m^2	31.9 ± 6.7	30.9 ± 5.2	30.1 ± 4.8	28.9 ± 4.7	<0.001
Heart rate per minute	75.0 ± 14.7	72.6 ± 13.7	69.8 ± 12.8	67 ± 712.5	0.001
Systolic BP (mmHg)	138.5 ± 21.1	138.3 ± 20.6	134.2 ± 18.5	131.8 ± 17.8	<0.001
Diastolic BP (mmHg)	80.9 ± 12.7	80.4 ± 11.7	80.2 ± 11.1	79.9 ± 10.9	0.63
Peak METs	4.5 ± 0.9	5.8 + 0.9	7.1 ± 0.9	8.8 ± 1.1	<0.001
Duration of HTN (years)	4.1 ± 3.8	3.7 ± 3.8	4.6 ± 4.5	4.1 ± 4.2	0.004
Alcohol/substance abuse, *n* (%)	15 (3.8)	23 (5.2)	28 (5.7)	18 (5.0)	0.62
Smokers, *n* (%)	142 (35.9)	117 (26.7)	139 (28.3)	85 (23.7)	0.002
Diabetics, *n* (%)	202 (51.0)	194 (44.2)	199 (40.4)	123 (34.3)	<0.001
CKD/HIV, *n* (%)	38 (9.6)	54 (12.3)	51 (10.4)	32 (8.9)	0.42
MACE, *n* (%)	55 (13.9)	52 (11.8)	35 (7.5)	16 (4.5)	<0.001

lent to just a 30–40-min brisk walk on most days of the week. To date no pharmacological study has shown an impact on mortality in RH population. Hence, it is gratifying to have a study supporting the inverse association of improved CRF with all-cause mortality in a subset of patients with RH. Future studies will likely validate the findings of this study and make the results generalizable to the general resistant hypertensive population.

Summary and Conclusions

RH is a disease that often defies control even with polypharmacy. This lack of BP control, at times, may be a pseudo-resistance to treatment, since it could be because of inadequate dosages or poor combinations of antihypertensive medications, non-compliance with therapy, or unhealthy lifestyles that interfere with BP control. Nevertheless, the result is that resistant hypertensives remain a high-risk population. They disproportionately utilize healthcare funds due to cost of medications, need for more frequent medical evaluations, and management of sequelae of RH. As discussed above it is not uncommon for these patients to have additional CV risk factors and comorbidities, like DM2, dyslipidemia, CKD, LVH, and obesity, which further increase the risk of future CV events. Increasing CRF has been shown to improve many of these coexisting cardiovascular indices and their related outcomes, in several studies [46, 47].

The role of improving CRF in complicated hypertensive patients is pivotal in managing not only HTN but also coexisting risk factors and conditions. As discussed above the degree of fitness, as measured by CRF, to realize CV and mortality, benefits are achievable for most patients, being equivalent to a 30–40-min brisk walk on most days of the week. This simple habit will have a beneficial effect not just on BP but also on other coexisting cardiovascular risk factors and decrease the global burden of CV outcomes including all-cause mortality. To date several studies have endorsed the role of PA, exercise, and CRF in decreasing morbidity and mortality in hypertensives with and without coexisting conditions. Such large, prospective, randomized, long-term studies are lacking in RH. Available studies, however, have verified the role of PA and exercise training in positively modifying the pathological vascular changes that are seen in RH including increased PWV and high central aortic pressure. Exercise training has been shown to regress LVH in patients with resistant HTN. Lastly, there is a strong inverse relationship between CRF and all-cause mortality in patients with RH.

Collectively data presented in this chapter establish the significant role of improving physical fitness in decreasing morbidity and all-cause mortality in patients with RH. It is thus imperative that efforts should be made by healthcare professionals to consider providing physical activity and exercise guidance as critical as prescribing medications. They should inform their patients that the best probability of controlling their BP and, perhaps, decreasing their dependence on medications is by adopting a healthy lifestyle. This is an important factor to be considered since RH patients not only require polypharmacy for HTN but also for concomitant medical conditions, like DM2, CKD, CV diseases, and dyslipidemia. Physicians should, however, emphasize to patients adopting positive changes in levels of PA and/or exercise that these changes have to be sustained long term, essentially life long, because benefits of exercise, just like of medications, are only realized with regular use.

References

1. Kagan A, Gordon T, Kannel WB, Dawber TR. Blood pressure and its relation to coronary heart disease in the Framingham study; hypertension volume VII. Drug action, epidemiology and hemodynamics. In: Proceedings of the Council for High Blood Pressure Research, American Heart Association. New York: American Heart Association; 1959. p. 53–81.
2. Principal Investigator, Freis E. Effects of treatment on morbidity and mortality in hypertension: II. Results in patients with diastolic blood pressure averaging 90 through 114 mmHg. JAMA. 1970;213:1143–51.
3. Whelton PK, Carey RM, Aronow WS, Casey DE Jr, Collins KJ, Dennison Himmelfarb C, DePalma SM, Gidding S, Jamerson KA, Jones DW, MacLaughlin EJ, Muntner P, Ovbiagele B, Smith SC Jr, Spencer CC, Stafford RS, Taler SJ, Thomas RJ, Williams KA Sr, Williamson JD, Wright JT Jr. 2017 ACC/AHA/AAPA/ABC/ACPM/AGS/APhA/ASH/ASPC/NMA/PCNA guideline for the prevention, detection, evaluation, and management of high blood pressure in adults: executive summary. J Am Coll Cardiol. 2017;71:2199. https://doi.org/10.1016/j.jacc.2017.11.005.
4. Pimenta E, Calhoun DA. Resistant hypertension: incidence, prevalence and prognosis. Circulation. 2012;125(13):1594–6.
5. Daugherty SL, Powers JD, Magid DJ, Tavel HM, Masoudi FA, Margolis KL, O'Connor PJ, Selby JV, Ho PM. Incidence and prognosis of resistant hypertension in hypertensive patients. Circulation. 2012;125(13):1635–42. https://doi.org/10.1161/CIRCULATIONAHA.111.068064. Epub 2012 Feb 29.
6. Smith SM, Huo T, Gong Y, Handberg E, Gulati M, Merz CN, Pepine CJ, Cooper-DeHoff RM. Mortality risk associated with resistant hypertension among women: analysis from three prospective cohorts encompassing the Spectrum of Women's heart disease. J Womens Health (Larchmt). 2016;25(10):996–1003.
7. Sim JJ, Bhandari SK, Shi J, Reynolds K, Calhoun DA, Kalantar-Zadeh K, Jacobsen SJ. Comparative risk of renal, cardiovascular, and mortality outcomes in controlled, uncontrolled resistant, and non-resistant hypertension. Kidney Int. 2015;88(3):622–32.
8. Zhang J, Zhou S, Xua G. Carotid baroreceptor stimulation: a potential solution for resistant hypertension. Interv Neurol. 2014;2(3):118–22.
9. Bhatt DL, Kandzari DE, O'Neill WW, D'Agostino R, Flack JM, Katzen BT, Leon MB, Liu M, Mauri L, Negoita M, Sidney A, Cohen SA, Oparil S, Rocha-Singh K, Townsend RR, Bakris GL, for the SYMPLICITY HTN-3 investigators. A controlled trial of renal denervation for resistant hypertension. N Engl J Med. 2014;370:1393–401.
10. Ben-Sira D, Oliveira JMF. Hypertension in aging: physical activity as primary prevention. Eur Rev Aging Phys Act. 2007;4:85–9.
11. Faselis C, Doumas M, Pittaras A, Narayan P, Myers J, Tsimploulis A, Kokkinos P. Exercise capacity and all-cause mortality in male veterans with hypertension aged ≥70 years. Hypertension. 2014;64:30–5.
12. Williams B. The aorta and resistant hypertension. JACC. 2009;53(5):452–4. https://doi.org/10.1016/j.jacc.2008.10.027.
13. Pimenta E, Gaddam KK, Oparil S. Mechanisms and treatment of resistant hypertension. J Clin Hypertens. 2008;10(3):239–44.
14. Meyer ML, Tanaka H, Palta P, et al. Correlates of segmental pulse wave velocity in older adults: the atherosclerosis risk in communities (ARIC) study. Am J Hypertens. 2016;29:114–22.
15. McDonnell BJ, Maki-Petaja KM, Munnery M, Yasmin Wilkinson IB, Cockcroft JR, McEniery CM. Habitual exercise and blood pressure: age dependency and underlying mechanisms. Am J Hypertens. 2013;26(3):334–41.
16. Kelley GA, Kelley KS. Progressive resistance exercise and resting blood pressure: a meta-analysis of randomized controlled trials. Hypertension. 2000;35:838–43.
17. Xin X, He J, Frontini MG, et al. Effects of alcohol reduction on blood pressure: a meta-analysis of randomized control trials. Hypertension. 2001;38:1112–7.

18. Hagberg JM, Park JJ, Brown MD. The role of exercise training in the treatment of hypertension: an update. Sports Med. 2000;30:193–206.
19. Hamdorf PA, Penhall RK. Walking with its training effects on the fitness and activity patterns of 79-91 year old females. Aust NZ J Med. 1999;29:22–8.
20. Brandão Rondon MU, Alves MJ, Braga AM, et al. Postexercise blood pressure reduction in elderly hypertensive patients. J Am Coll Cardiol. 2002;39:676–82.
21. Kelley GA, Kelley KS. Aerobic exercise and resting blood pressure in older adults: a meta-analysis review of randomized controlled trials. J Gerontol Ser A Biol Med Sci. 2001;56:M298–303.
22. Huang G, Thompson CJ, Osness WH. Influence of a 10-week controlled exercise program on resting blood pressure in sedentary older adults. J Appl Res. 2006;6:188–95.
23. Toth PP. Short-term aerobic exercise in the elderly promotes blood pressure reduction. J Appl Res. 2006;6:186–7.
24. Mancia G, Laurent S, Gabiti-Rosei E, et al. Reappraisal of European guidelines on hypertension management: a European society of hypertension task force document. J Hypertens. 2009;27:2121–58.
25. Kim J, Lee SK, Yoon DW, Shin C. Obstructive sleep apnoea is associated with progression of arterial stiffness independent of obesity in participants without hypertension: a KoGES prospective cohort study. Sci Rep. 2018;8(1):8152. https://doi.org/10.1038/s41598-018-26587-y.
26. Phillips BG, Narkiewicz K, Pesek CA, et al. Effects of obstructive sleep apnea on endothelin-1 and blood pressure. J Hypertens. 1999;17(1):61–6.
27. Khan A, Patel NK, O'Hearn DJ, Khan S. Resistant hypertension and obstructive sleep apnea. Int J Hypertens. 2013;2013:193010.
28. Elias MF, Crichton GE, Dearborn PJ, Robbins MA, Abhayaratna WP. Associations between type 2 diabetes mellitus and arterial stiffness: a prospective analysis based on the maine-syracuse study. Pulse (Basel). 2018;5(1–4):88–98. https://doi.org/10.1159/000479560.
29. Devereux RB, Roamn MJ, Paraniacas M, et al. Impact of diabetes on cardiac structure and function: the strong heart study. Circulation. 2000;101:2271–6.
30. Stewart KJ. Exercise training and the cardiovascular consequences of type 2 diabetes and hypertension: plausible mechanisms for improving cardiovascular health. JAMA. 2002;288(13):1622–31.
31. Hayashino Y, Jackson JL, Fukumori N, Nakamura F, Fukuhara S. Effects of supervised exercise on lipid profiles and blood pressure control in people with type 2 diabetes mellitus: a meta-analysis of randomized controlled trials. Diabetes Res Clin Pract. 2012;98(3):349–60. https://doi.org/10.1016/j.diabres.2012.10.004. Epub 2012 Oct 29.
32. Fernando GF, Cardosa CRL, Fiszman R, Muxfeldt S. Prognostic impact of baseline and serial changes in electrocardiographic left ventricular hypertrophy in resistant hypertension. Am Heart J. 2010;159(5):833–40.
33. Kokkinos PF, Narayan P, Colleran JA, Pittaras A, Notargiacomo A, Reda D, Papademetrious V. Effects of regular exercise on blood pressure and left ventricular hypertrophy in African American men with severe hypertension. N Engl J Med. 1995;333:1462–7.
34. Keane WF, Eknoyan G. Proteinuria, albuminuria, risk, assessment, detection, elimination (PARADE): a position paper of the National Kidney Foundation. Am J Kidney Dis. 1999;33:1004–10.
35. Barcellos FC, Del Vecchio FB, Reges A, Mielke G, Santos IS, Umpierre D, Bohlke M, Hallal PC. Exercise in patients with hypertension and chronic kidney disease: a randomized controlled trial. J Hum Hypertens. 2018;32:397. https://doi.org/10.1038/s41371-018-0055-0.
36. Leehey DJ, Moinuddin I, Bast JP, Qureshi S, Jelinek CS, Cooper C, Edwards LC, Smith BM, Collins EG. Aerobic exercise in obese diabetic patients with chronic kidney disease: a randomized and controlled pilot study. Cardiovasc Diabetol. 2009;8:62. https://doi.org/10.1186/1475-2840-8-62.
37. Fritze O, Romero B, Schleicher M, et al. Age-related changes in the elastic tissue of the human aorta. J Vasc Res. 2012;49:77–86.
38. Amento EP, Ehsani N, Palmer H, et al. Cytokines and growth factors positively and negatively regulate interstitial collagen gene expression in human vascular smooth muscle cells. Arterioscler Thromb. 1991;11:1223–30.
39. The CAFE Investigators, CAFE Steering Committee and Writing Committee, Williams B, Lacy PS, Thom SM, Cruickshank K, Stanton A, Collier D, Hughes AD, Thurston H, O'Rourke M, for the Anglo-Scandinavian Cardiac Outcomes Trial (ASCOT) Investigators. Differential impact of blood pressure–lowering drugs on central aortic pressure and clinical outcomes. Principal results of the conduit artery function evaluation (CAFE) study. Circulation. 2006;113:1213–25.
40. lachopoulos C, Aznaouridis K, Stefanadis C. Prediction of cardiovascular events and all-cause mortality with arterial stiffness: a systematic review and meta-analysis. J Am Coll Cardiol. 2010;55(13):1318–27.
41. O'Rourke MF, Safar ME, Adji A. Resistant hypertension and central aortic pressure. J Hypertens. 2014;32(3):699–701.
42. Ramosa JS, Dalleckb LC, Ramosc MV, Fabio Borranid F, Robertsa L, Gomersalla S, Beethama KS, Diasa KA, Keatinga SE, Fassetta RG, Sharmanf JF, Coombes JS. 12 min/week of high-intensity interval training reduces aortic reservoir pressure in individuals with metabolic syndrome: a randomized trial. J Hypertens. 2016;34:1977–87.
43. Dimeo F, Pagonas N, Seibert F, Arndt R, Zidek W, Westhoff TH. Aerobic exercise reduces blood pressure in resistant hypertension. Hypertension. 2012;60:653–8.

44. Guimaraes GV, de Barros Cruz LG, Fernandes-Silva MM, Dorea EL, Bocchi EA. Heated water-based exercise training reduces 24-hour ambulatory blood pressure levels in resistant hypertensive patients: a randomized controlled trial (HEx trial). Int J Cardiol. 2014;172(2):434–41. https://doi.org/10.1016/j.ijcard.2014.01.100. Epub 2014 Jan 24.
45. Rossi A, Dikareva A, Bacon SL, Daskalopoulou SS. The impact of physical activity on mortality in patients with high blood pressure: a systematic review. J Hypertens. 2012;30(7):1277–88.
46. Narayan P, Doumas M, Kumar A, Faselis CJ, Myers JN, Pittaras A, Kokkinos PF. Impact of cardiorespiratory fitness on mortality in black male veterans with resistant systemic hypertension. Am J Cardiol. 2017;120(9):1568–71. https://doi.org/10.1016/j.amjcard.2017.07.055. Epub 2017 Jul 31.
47. Myers J, Prakash M, Froelicher V, et al. Exercise capacity and mortality among men referred for exercise testing. N Engl J Med. 2002;346:793–801.

Physical Activity, Blood Pressure, and Cardiac Structure and Function

10

Peter Kokkinos, Puneet Narayan, and Andreas Pittaras

Introduction

Chronic increases in the hemodynamic burden lead to compensatory responses and cardiac adaptations specific to the demands imposed upon the myocytes, ultimately leading to an increase in left ventricular mass (LVM) and left ventricular hypertrophy (LVH) [1]. Specifically, pressure overload imposed by a chronically or intermittently elevated blood pressure (BP) more commonly leads to increased cardiac wall thickness and LVM and reduced left ventricular (LV) chamber size, a condition known as concentric LVH [2–5]. Further characterization of concentric LVH is a ratio of LV wall thickness to diastolic diameter > 0.42, referred to as "relative wall thickness" [6]. Conversely, volume overload is consistent with eccentric LVH characterized by relatively large LV chamber size and relative wall thickness within normal limits (≤0.42) [7, 8]. A third pattern has also been identified, characterized by an increase in relative wall thickness, but not LVM. This pattern is known as concentric remodeling [8–10]. Cardiac parameters and classification of cardiac hypertrophy are presented in Table 10.1.

Table 10.1 Classification of left ventricular hypertrophy

LV mass index (gm/m^2)	Males, ≤115 Females, ≤95	Males, >115 Females, >95
Relative wall thickness		
≤0.42	Normal geometry	Eccentric hypertrophy
>0.42	Concentric remodeling	Concentric hypertrophy

Adapted from Lang et al. [6]

The presence of LVH caused by hypertension-induced increase in afterload, especially when characterized by concentric geometry is a strong and independent risk factor of future cardiac events and all-cause mortality. The risk of cardiovascular morbid events, including sudden cardiac

P. Kokkinos (✉)
Veterans Affairs Medical Center, Department of Cardiology, Washington, DC, USA

Georgetown University School of Medicine, Washington, DC, USA

Department of Kinesiology and Health, Rutgers University, New Brunswick, NJ, USA

George Washington University School of Medicine and Health Sciences, Washington, DC, USA

University of South Carolina, Department of Exercise Science, Arnold School of Public Health, Columbia, SC, USA
e-mail: peter.kokkinos@va.gov

P. Narayan
Clinical Research Institute of Northern Virginia, Burke, VA, USA

A. Pittaras
Department of Cardiology, GW University, Veteran Affairs Medical Center, Washington, DC, USA

P. Kokkinos, P. Narayan (eds.), *Cardiorespiratory Fitness in Cardiometabolic Diseases*,
https://doi.org/10.1007/978-3-030-04816-7_10

death, increases threefold in these patients [4, 11, 12]. Conversely, LVH regression is associated with a significant reduction in cardiovascular events and death [13–16]. Concentric LVH regression occurs with reductions in resting BP achieved by most antihypertensive agents. The degree of regression is directly related to the degree of BP reduction, further supporting, at least in part, that the stimulus for concentric LVH is pressure overload [17–20].

The Athlete's Heart: A Historical Perspective

Acute and chronic increases in physical work or exercise also impose an increased demand on the cardiovascular system. Accordingly, acute and chronic cardiac adaptations occur to compensate for the increased workload. This chapter focuses on the chronic cardiac adaptations resulting from chronic exposure to vigorous aerobic and resistanceexercises.

Exercise-related cardiac adaptations, including chamber enlargement, bradycardia, and arrhythmias resulting from chronic and vigorous exercise or physical activity in general endured by athletes have been described since the late 1800s and continue to intrigue clinicians and scientists. Early reports of an enlarged heart were noted in Harvard University rowers [21], elite Nordic skiers [22], and Boston Marathon runners [23, 24]. These findings were largely viewed as beneficial cardiac adaptations in response to exercise-indused icreased hemodynamic demand [23, 24].

The development of the electrocardiogram (ECG) made it possible to also reveal abnormalities in the electrical activity of the heart [25–30]. More recently, advances in echocardiography and magnetic resonance imaging have led to a more comprehensive understanding of the athlete's heart. In a landmark study of Olympic-caliber athletes, no adverse cardiac events of cardiac function during 8.6 ± 3 years of intense training were observed [31]. In general, the prevailing concept is still that the cardiac structural and functional adaptations resulting from chronic, rigorous, but not unwarranted exercises are physiological and do not lead to adverse cardiac events or compromised cardiac function [31].

Exercise-related structural and functional cardiac adaptations are specific to the mode and intensity of the activity. Aerobic or endurance exercises are characterized by low-to-moderate intensity and long-duration activities (i.e., long-distance running or swimming). Most of the energy demands of such activities are provided by the aerobic energy-generating processes. Conversely, high-intensity, short-duration activities (i.e., 100-yard dash, resistance or strength training) derive most of the energy demands via the anaerobic pathways (glycolysis) and are known as anaerobic [23]. The acute cardiovascular responses to these two types of activities differ considerably. Consequently, prolonged exposure to either of these also results in considerably different chronic adaptations.

Aerobic Activities and LVH

Aerobic exercises of adequate duration and intensity lead to cardiac remodeling that includes increases in left and right ventricular chamber dimensions; left atrial cavity size, with normal systolic and diastolic function. In 947 Italian Olympic athletesengaging in a very rigorous training involving both aerobic/resistance exercises, LV wall thickness was ≤13 mm, and only 15 rowers and 1 cyclist (1.7%) exceeded 13 mm [32]. Similarly, in 3000 highly trained British athletes, only 1.5% exhibited cardiac wall thickness >12 mm for males and >11 mm for females and in all cases with chamber enlargement [33]. Others have reported LV wall thickness beyond 13 mm in some individuals engaging in extreme exercises such as ultramarathon running and highly trained cyclists [34–36]. Collectively, it appears that the physiological limit of exercise-induced LV wall thickness even with extreme exercise is 16 mm [37–39], and LV wall thickness exceeding 16 mm is likely pathological [39–42].

As stated, these chronic cardiac adaptations are considered normal physiologic responses to the increased hemodynamic demand of the particular sport, exercise, or physical activity. They are not associated with diastolic dysfunction, arrhythmias, or adverse prognosis, manifestation observed in hypertension-induced LVH [7, 8, 31]. There is also evidence that the aforementioned cardiac adaptations regress quickly when training is discontinued for 3 or more months [41, 43–45].

Resistance Exercises and LVH

Resistance exercises typically represented by weight training are predominantly anaerobic in nature. Some misunderstanding persists as to whether strength or resistance training alone results in concentric LVH [32]. Resistance exercises are associated with increased LV wall thicknesses, often disproportionate relative to cavity size. However, absolute values uncorrected for body surface area usually remain within the accepted normal range of ≤12 mm. It is important to mention that most sports or daily activities are comprised of both aerobic and anaerobic types of activities. Consequently, structural and functional cardiac adaptations reflect the combined demands of the particular sport or activity. This is most evident in elite athletes participating in sports such as cycling, rowing, and swimming that incorporate both aerobic and resistance components. These athletes have the most extreme increase in both LV wall thickness and cavity size [32]. It is also important to emphasize that an increase in either alone (wall thickness or LV diastolic dimension) will not be physiologically desirable. LV chamber dilatation without comparable increase in wall thickness will lead to an inappropriate increase in wall tension that is detrimental to the heart [45].

Pathological LVH in Athletes

LV wall thickness between 13 and 16 mm observed in some highly trained athletes, especially those engaging in sports requiring a combination of aerobic and isometric/resistance activities, may be within the physiological limits of exercise-induced LV wall thickness and present no health risks. However, a differentiation between exercise-induced physiological LVH and hypertrophic cardiomyopathy (HCM), the most leading cause of exercise-related sudden cardiac death in young athletes [42], can be challenging. A prudent approach and highly recommended is that an athlete with wall thickness between 12 and 16 mm should have a systematic evaluation by a cardiologist [41]. Clinical characteristics indicating a pathological LVH in athletes are presented in Table 10.2.

Table 10.2 Clinical characteristics indicative of pathological LVH in athletes with left ventricular wall thickness between 13 and 16 mm

Symptoms	Unexplained syncope, particularly during exercise Palpitations Shortness of breath disproportionate to the exercise performed Dizziness Chest pain
Family history	HCM in a first-degree relative
Demographics	Age, 16 years old Female sex Participation in purely isometric sport Small body surface area
Echocardiography	Left ventricular wall thickness > 16 mm Asymmetrical septal hypertrophy Small left ventricular cavity diameter in end-diastole Presence of systolic anterior motion of the mitral valve leaflet and associated left ventricular outflow obstruction Abnormal indices of diastolic function
12-lead ECG	Pathological Q-waves ST segment depression Left bundle branch block T-wave inversions in the lateral/inferior leads
Cardiopulmonary exercise testing	Peak VO_2 max, 50 mL/kg/min or <120% of age-predicted maximum
Cardiac MRI	Demonstration of apical hypertrophy Demonstration of significant myocardial fibrosis with gadolinium enhancement
Detraining	Failure of regression of left ventricular hypertrophy

Adapted from Rawlins et al. [41]

Exercise-Induced LVH and Arrhythmogenicity

Exercise-induced arrhythmogenicity in certain conditions [46] and higher prevalence of atrial fibrillation (AF) in middle-aged and older elite athletes participating in long-term high-intensity physical activity (PA), as compared with the general population, have been reported [47–53]. This association does not appear to be directly related to the magnitude of exercise-induced physiologic LVH [45, 54]. It is more directly related to intensity as well as number of hours or days spent per week engaged in vigorous PA [47, 48, 51, 53]. However, these arrhythmias are usually abolished or substantially reduced after relatively brief periods of deconditioning [45].

Conversely, when we examined the role of moderate exercise intensities on AF in 5962 middle-aged and older veterans, we noted that increased cardiorespiratory fitness (CRF) had a protective effect. Specifically, we noted an inverse and graded association between AF incidence and CRF. The AF risk was 21% lower for each 1-MET increase in exercise capacity. Compared with the least fit individuals, the risk was 20% lower for moderately fit, 45% for fit, and 63% for highly fit individuals [55]. Similar trends were observed for those younger than 65 years and those 65 years or older. These findings suggest that CRF achieved by moderate-intensity exercise prevents the incidence of AF regardless of age.

Exercise Training, BP, and LVH regression

Relatively small reductions in BP achieved by antihypertensive therapy lead to substantial health benefits and mortality risk reduction [56–59]. LVH regression proportional to the degree of BP reduction [17–20] contributes in part to the these health benefits [13–16]. Exercise-related BP reduction of approximately 4–10 mmHg in systolic BP and 3–8 mmHg in diastolic BP for individuals with stage 1 hypertension regardless of age or gender has been documented by well-controlled studies [60–64]. It is reasonable to assume that similar exercise-induced reductions in BP should lead to similar health benefits, including LVH regression. Large and well-conducted epidemiologic studies have reported a significant, inverse, and graded association between CRF as indicated by exercise capacity and mortality risk in hypertensive individuals and those with high normal resting BP [65–70].

The effects of exercise-related BP reduction on LVH regression have not been studied extensively. However, most interventional studies support that the exercise-induced BP results in LVH regression in patients with LVH [71–76].

We randomly assigned 46 African-American men with resistant hypertension (35–76 years of age) to 16 weeks of supervised aerobic exercise training exercise plus antihypertensive medication (23 men) or antihypertensive medication alone (23 men). After 16 weeks the exercise group exhibited 7/5 mm Hg reduction in systolic and diastolic BP, respectively, while diastolic BP in the control group increased by 2 mmHg. In addition, LV wall thickness, LVM, and the LVM index decreased significantly after 16 weeks in patients who exercised, whereas there was no significant change in the non-exercisers [73]. In another randomized, controlled trial, 82 overweight participants (45 women and 37 men) were assigned to supervised aerobic exercise only, a behavioral weight management program that included exercise or a waiting-list control group for 6 months. BP fell by 7/6 mmHg for systolic and diastolic BP, respectively, in the weight management group and by 3/4 mmHg in the aerobic exercise group. In addition, participants in the intervention groups exhibited significant decreases in LV wall thickness and a trend toward a decrease in LVM index, relative to the control group [72]. Significant reductions in cardiac wall thickness and LVM index were also reported in 16 hypertensive patients after 24 weeks of aerobic exercise [76] and a trend toward lower LVM in middle-aged hypertensive males and females with aerobic exercise training [71]. Similarly, significant BP and LV wall thickness and LVM index reductions were noted in 11 middle-aged hypertensives engaging in approximately 6 months of aerobic exercise. The reduction in resting systolic BP correlated significantly with a regression of concentric remodeling. There were no BP or cardiac changes in the controls [75]. Finally, in the HARVEST study [74], BP declined during a median follow-up of 8.3 years in physically active individuals (n = 173) and increased slightly in the sedentary group (n = 281). Physically active individuals were less likely to develop LVH than their sedentary counterparts.

In contrast, no changes in LV were observed in 23 obese individuals with a mean baseline BP 131/84 mmHg, despite significant reductions in BP [77]. Similarly, no structural or functional cardiac changes were noted after 24 weeks of aerobic exercise and resistance training in 51 overweight and obese individuals with untreated baseline systolic BP of 130–150 mmHg or diastolic BP 85–99 mmHg [78].

However, there are several deficiencies in the two studies that make their conclusions questionable. First, in the study by Reid et al. [77], a closer scrutiny of the findings reveal that LVM index in the exercise group decreased by approximately 8% (153 g/m^2 to 141 g/m^2 for baseline and post exercise, respectively) and increased by approximately 10% (141 g/m^2 to 155 g/m^2 for baseline and post exercise, respectively) in the control group. Moreover, cardiac wall thickness decreased after exercise, although statistical significance was not achieved, perhaps due to relatively small number of patients studied (n = 7). The investigators also reported the exercise group had significantly greater wall thickness at baseline, and this was the only group to show a reduction in wall thickness after 12 weeks of exercise. Collectively, these findings support a trend toward exercise-induced cardiac remodeling occurred, but statistical significance was not achieved, perhaps due to a small number of study participants.

In the other study [78], it is clear as to how many of the participants were truly hypertensive, since the baseline BP range was 130–150 mmHg systolic or diastolic BP 85–99 mmHg. Moreover, based on baseline LVM index normal values (63.6 g/m^2), LVH was absent. Thus, it is reasonable to assume that exercise or any other intervention cannot "fix" what is not broken. The exercise intervention was also a mixture of both strength and aerobic training. The cardiovascular responses and chronic adaptations to these two types of activities differ considerably, and strength training is likely to result LV wall thickness rather than LVH regression [32]. Collectively, the limited evidence regarding the effects of exercise on cardiac remodeling supports that LVH regression is likely to occur, if proper exercise is implemented in populations with LVH. However, more studies are needed to confirm these findings.

Exercise Blood Pressure and LVH

As noted, the degree of LVH regression is proportional to the degree of BP reduction with pharmacologic therapies [17–20]. A meta-analysis of four clinical trials assessing echocardiographic regression of LVH reported only 8% LVH regression [19]. Others reported different effects among antihypertensive medication classes on LVM reduction. Specifically, LVM index reduction was 13% with angiotensin II receptor antagonists; 11% with calcium antagonists; 10% with ACE inhibitors; 8% with diuretics; and 6% with beta-blockers [79]. The degree of exercise-induced LVH regression is comparable to what has been reported by most pharmacotherapies [80]. However, the exercise-related reduction in BP was substantially lower than the reported 26.6/16.6 mmHg with pharmacotherapies [81]. For example, in our study, resting blood pressure was lowered by 7/5 mmHg, an average reduction in BP observed with exercise [60–64], reflecting a 12.3% reduction in LVM index. This LVH reduction is similar to the 13% reduction achieved by angiotensin II receptor antagonists and over two times higher to that achieved by beta-blockers, resulting from a reduction in BP of approximately 13% for all antihypertensive medication [79]. Based on these data is 1% LVM index regression for every 1% reduction in BP. In our study, systolic BP was lowered by approximately 5% (138/88 ± 10/7 mmHg at baseline to

131/83 ± 15/8 mmHg post exercise), yet LVH regression was 12.3%, approximately 2.5% regression per 1% reduction in BP. This suggests that exercise-induced LVH regression may be modulated not only by a lower resting BP but other factors. A closer look at our data revealed that 16 weeks of exercise training resulted in a significantly lower exercise BP at the submaximal and peak exercise workloads, compared to baseline BP at the same submaximal and peak workloads. Specifically, exercise systolic BP was 27 mmHg lower (14%) at three METs, 32 mmHg lower (15%) at five METs, and 20 mmHg (9%) lower at peak exercise [73, 82, 83]. Since the metabolic demand of most daily activities falls within 3–5 METs [23, 24], these findings support that the systolic BP during most daily activities will be substantially lower following aerobic exercise training. Consequently, the daily hemodynamic load and metabolic demands of the myocardium in these individuals would also be substantially lower. Furthermore, we can assume that the reduced hemodynamic load may have played a far greater role in the regression of LVH than the resting BP. This assumption is further supported by the strong association noted between the BP responses at the submaximal workload of approximately 4–5 METs and LVH in 790 middle-aged individuals with BP < 140/90 mmHg [69, 84] who underwent echocardiographic studies, 24 h ambulatory BP monitoring, and a standard exercise treadmill test (Bruce protocol). LVM index, daytime BP, and exercise systolic BP at the workload of approximately 4–5 METs were significantly lower in moderate- and high-fit individuals compared to the low-fit. A systolic BP threshold of ≥150 mmHg at the exercise intensity of 4–5 METs was identified as the exercise systolic BP threshold, beyond which the risk for LVH increased fourfold for every 10 mmHg rise in systolic BP. When the cohort was stratified based on the exercise systolic BP <150 mmHg and ≥150 mmHg, comparisons between the two groups showed all cardiac parameters are more favorable in the group with systolic BP < 150 mmHg. It is also important to emphasize that the resting BP between the two groups was similar, suggesting that the impetus for LVH was systolic BP during physical work, such as daily activities. This is further supported by the similarity between systolic BP of 148 ± 12 mmHg at the workload of 4–5 METs and daytime ambulatory systolic BP 144 ± 11 mmHg for individuals in the same cohort [84]. Thus, the association between systolic BP during physical exertion and LVM [69, 84] suggests that the daily exposure to relatively high systolic BP (≥150 mmHg) provides the impetus for an increase in LVM even among normotensive individuals. Similar findings have been reported in a relatively smaller cohort (n = 49) individuals with hypertension at the exercise workload of approximately seven METs. Systolic BP at this workload was directly and independently associated with cardiac wall thickness and LVM index. This association was stronger than the association noted with office BP and 24 h ambulatory systolic BP [85].

Collectively these findings support that aerobic exercise training lowers the systolic BP response during absolute and maximal workloads. Consequently, systolic BP response during daily activities is less likely to exceed the threshold of 15 mmHg, suggested as the stimulus that will elicit LV mass increase.

Vigorous Exercise in Patients with Hypertension-Induced LVH

The long-term effects of rigorous exercise such as that demanded by competitive sports (basketball, soccer, etc.) and even noncompetitive activities (long-distance running, cycling, weight training, etc.) on cardiac structure and function in individuals with hypertension-induced LVH have not been studied. It is likely that high-intensity activities impose an excessive demand on the cardiovascular system and perpetuate further maladaptations. Therefore, such activities should be avoided. Instead, the recommendations of the American College of Sports Medicine and the American Heart Association of low-to-moderate intensity aerobic exercise (brisk walk) of approximately 30 min per day, most if not all days of the week, should be encouraged by healthcare providers [86–88]. Such exercise is safe for almost all ages and populations with comorbidities [73] and has been shown to have a favorable effect on the traditional and novel cardiovascular risk factors [61], including LVH regression [73].

Conclusions

Chronic exercises of adequate intensity, duration, and volume impose an increase in the hemodynamic load. As a result, cardiac adaptations ensue specific to the type of exercise and demand imposed to accommodate the increased hemodynamic load. The exercise-related cardiac adaptations are not associated with diastolic dysfunction, arrhythmias, or adverse prognosis, manifestations observed in hypertension-induced LVH.

Emerging evidence supports that the strongest impetus for cardiac adaptations is the systolic BP during daily activities. This hemodynamic load threshold for cardiac adaptations is reflected by an exercise systolic BP of approximately ≥150 mmHg at the workload of approximately 4–5 METs (first stage of the Bruce protocol). Moderate-intensity aerobic training lowers exercise systolic BP at absolute and maximal workloads. The lower systolic BP leads to a relatively lower hemodynamic load during daily activities, ultimately lowering the stimulus for LV mass increase.

Vigorous training usually endured by athletes leads to increased LV wall thickness that usually does not exceed 13 mm. However, in some athletes engaging high levels of vigorous training that involves both isotonic and isometric/resistance exercises, LV wall thickness may exceed 13 mm and be as high as 16 mm. In these cases, a differentiation between exercise-induced physiological LVH and the existence of HCM, the most leading cause of exercise-related sudden cardiac death in young athletes, should be made by a trained cardiologist.

Perhaps the time has come to refer to exercise-induced cardiac structural adaptations that lead to improved cardiac efficiency and ultimately accommodate the imposed physiologic demand as *eutrophic*. Conversely, *hypertrophic* cardiac adaptations should be considered exclusively those imposed by pathophysiologic conditions (hypertension, cardiac injury, HCM) and encroach upon cardiac efficiency, ultimately leading to compromised cardiac dysfunction and even death.

Considering that most exercise-related health outcomes occur with moderate-intensity exercises, it is recommended that prolonged, high-intensity, and high-volume exercises with inadequate rest periods between exercising days should be avoided, especially by older populations. Although specific guidelines are hard to implement, a brisk walk to a slow jog at the exercise intensity of 12–16 min per mile, 4–6 days weekly for 150–200 min per week is adequate for optimal health benefits.

References

1. Lorell BH, Carabello BA. Left ventricular hypertrophy: pathogenesis, detection, and prognosis. Circulation. 2000;102(4):470–9.
2. Cohn JN, Ferrari R, Sharpe N. Cardiac remodeling–concepts and clinical implications: a consensus paper from an international forum on cardiac remodeling. Behalf of an International Forum on Cardiac Remodeling. J Am Coll Cardiol. 2000;35(3):569–82.
3. Ganau A, Devereux RB, Roman MJ, de Simone G, Pickering TG, Saba PS, et al. Patterns of left ventricular hypertrophy and geometric remodeling in essential hypertension. J Am Coll Cardiol. 1992;19(7):1550–8.
4. Levy D, Salomon M, D'Agostino RB, Belanger AJ, Kannel WB. Prognostic implications of baseline electrocardiographic features and their serial changes in subjects with left ventricular hypertrophy. Circulation. 1994;90(4):1786–93.
5. Levy D, Garrison RJ, Savage DD, Kannel WB, Castelli WP. Prognostic implications of echocardiographically determined left ventricular mass in the Framingham Heart Study. N Engl J Med. 1990;322(22):1561–6.
6. Lang RM, Bierig M, Devereux RB, Flachskampf FA, Foster E, Pellikka PA, et al. Recommendations for chamber quantification: a report from the American Society of Echocardiography's Guidelines and Standards Committee and the Chamber Quantification Writing Group, developed in conjunction with the European Association of Echocardiography, a branch of the European Society of Cardiology. J Am Soc Echocardiogr. 2005;18(12):1440–63.
7. Frohlich ED, Apstein C, Chobanian AV, Devereux RB, Dustan HP, Dzau V, et al. The heart in hypertension. N Engl J Med. 1992;327(14):998–1008.

8. Drazner MH. The progression of hypertensive heart disease. Circulation. 2011;123(3):327–34.
9. Khouri MG, Peshock RM, Ayers CR, de Lemos JA, Drazner MH. A 4-tiered classification of left ventricular hypertrophy based on left ventricular geometry: the Dallas heart study. Circ Cardiovasc Imaging. 2010;3(2):164–71.
10. Sehgal S, Drazner MH. Left ventricular geometry: does shape matter? Am Heart J. 2007;153(2):153–5.
11. Verdecchia P, Schillaci G, Borgioni C, Ciucci A, Gattobigio R, Zampi I, et al. Prognostic value of a new electrocardiographic method for diagnosis of left ventricular hypertrophy in essential hypertension. J Am Coll Cardiol. 1998;31(2):383–90.
12. Verdecchia P, Schillaci G, Borgioni C, Ciucci A, Gattobigio R, Zampi I, et al. Prognostic value of left ventricular mass and geometry in systemic hypertension with left ventricular hypertrophy. Am J Cardiol. 1996;78(2):197–202.
13. Devereux RB, Wachtell K, Gerdts E, Boman K, Nieminen MS, Papademetriou V, et al. Prognostic significance of left ventricular mass change during treatment of hypertension. JAMA. 2004;292(19):2350–6.
14. Pierdomenico SD, Cuccurullo F. Risk reduction after regression of echocardiographic left ventricular hypertrophy in hypertension: a meta-analysis. Am J Hypertens. 2010;23(8):876–81.
15. Larstorp AC, Okin PM, Devereux RB, Olsen MH, Ibsen H, Dahlof B, et al. Regression of ECG-LVH is associated with lower risk of new-onset heart failure and mortality in patients with isolated systolic hypertension; the LIFE study. Am J Hypertens. 2012;25(10):1101–9.
16. Okin PM, Devereux RB, Jern S, Kjeldsen SE, Julius S, Nieminen MS, et al. Regression of electrocardiographic left ventricular hypertrophy during antihypertensive treatment and the prediction of major cardiovascular events. JAMA. 2004;292(19):2343–9.
17. Mathew J, Sleight P, Lonn E, Johnstone D, Pogue J, Yi Q, et al. Reduction of cardiovascular risk by regression of electrocardiographic markers of left ventricular hypertrophy by the angiotensin-converting enzyme inhibitor ramipril. Circulation. 2001;104(14):1615–21.
18. Muiesan ML, Salvetti M, Monteduro C, Bonzi B, Paini A, Viola S, et al. Left ventricular concentric geometry during treatment adversely affects cardiovascular prognosis in hypertensive patients. Hypertension. 2004;43(4):731–8.
19. Verdecchia P, Angeli F, Borgioni C, Gattobigio R, de Simone G, Devereux RB, et al. Changes in cardiovascular risk by reduction of left ventricular mass in hypertension: a meta-analysis. Am J Hypertens. 2003;16(11 Pt 1):895–9.
20. Muiesan ML, Salvetti M, Rizzoni D, Castellano M, Donato F, Agabiti-Rosei E. Association of change in left ventricular mass with prognosis during long-term antihypertensive treatment. J Hypertens. 1995;13(10):1091–5.
21. Darling EA. Observations on the sterilization of catgut. J Boston Soc Med Sci. 1899;3(10):269–73.
22. Henschen S. Skidlauf und skidwettlauf: eine medizinische sportstudie. Mitt Med Klin Upsala. 1899;2:15.
23. White PD. The pulse after a marathon race. JAMA. 1918;71:1047–8.
24. White PD. Bradycardia in athletes, especially long distance runners. JAMA. 1942;120:642.
25. Arstila M, Koivikko A. Electrocardiographic and vectorcardiographic signs of left and right ventricular hypertrophy in endurance athletes. J Sports Med Phys Fitness. 1966;6(3):166–75.
26. Chignon JC, Distel R, Courtois B, Leclerq J, Andrivet R. Orientation of the analysis of electrical tracings regarding athletes. J Sports Med Phys Fitness. 1969;9(4):241–4.
27. Gott PH, Roselle HA, Crampton RS. The athletic heart syndrome. Five-year cardiac evaluation of a champion athlete. Arch Intern Med. 1968;122(4):340–4.
28. Hanne-Paparo N, Wendkos MH, Brunner D. T wave abnormalities in the electrocardiograms of top-ranking athletes without demonstrable organic heart disease. Am Heart J. 1971;81(6):743–7.
29. Hunt EA. Electrocardiographic study of 20 champion swimmers before and after 110-yard sprint swimming competition. Can Med Assoc J. 1963;88:1251–3.
30. Van Ganse W, Versee L, Eylenbosch W, Vuylsteek K. The electrocardiogram of athletes. Comparison with untrained subjects. Br Heart J. 1970;32(2):160–4.
31. Pelliccia A, Kinoshita N, Pisicchio C, Quattrini F, Dipaolo FM, Ciardo R, et al. Long-term clinical consequences of intense, uninterrupted endurance training in olympic athletes. J Am Coll Cardiol. 2010;55(15):1619–25.
32. Pelliccia A, Maron BJ, Spataro A, Proschan MA, Spirito P. The upper limit of physiologic cardiac hypertrophy in highly trained elite athletes. N Engl J Med. 1991;324(5):295–301.
33. Sharma S, Maron BJ, Whyte G, Firoozi S, Elliott PM, McKenna WJ. Physiologic limits of left ventricular hypertrophy in elite junior athletes: relevance to differential diagnosis of athlete's heart and hypertrophic cardiomyopathy. J Am Coll Cardiol. 2002;40(8):1431–6.
34. Fagard RH. Impact of different sports and training on cardiac structure and function. Cardiol Clin. 1997;15(3):397–412.
35. Nagashima J, Musha H, Takada H, Murayama M. New upper limit of physiologic cardiac hypertrophy in Japanese participants in the 100-km ultramarathon. J Am Coll Cardiol. 2003;42(9):1617–23.
36. Rodriguez Reguero JJ, Iglesias Cubero G, de la Iglesia Lopez J, Terrados N, Gonzalez V, Cortina R, et al. Prevalence and upper limit of cardiac hypertrophy in professional cyclists. Eur J Appl Physiol Occup Physiol. 1995;70(5):375–8.
37. Basavarajaiah S, Wilson M, Whyte G, Shah A, McKenna W, Sharma S. Prevalence of hypertrophic

cardiomyopathy in highly trained athletes: relevance to pre-participation screening. J Am Coll Cardiol. 2008;51(10):1033–9.
38. Pluim BM, Zwinderman AH, van der Laarse A, van der Wall EE. The athlete's heart. A meta-analysis of cardiac structure and function. Circulation. 2000;101(3):336–44.
39. Spirito P, Pelliccia A, Proschan MA, Granata M, Spataro A, Bellone P, et al. Morphology of the "athlete's heart" assessed by echocardiography in 947 elite athletes representing 27 sports. Am J Cardiol. 1994;74(8):802–6.
40. Basavarajaiah S, Boraita A, Whyte G, Wilson M, Carby L, Shah A, et al. Ethnic differences in left ventricular remodeling in highly-trained athletes relevance to differentiating physiologic left ventricular hypertrophy from hypertrophic cardiomyopathy. J Am Coll Cardiol. 2008;51(23):2256–62.
41. Rawlins J, Bhan A, Sharma S. Left ventricular hypertrophy in athletes. Eur J Echocardiogr. 2009;10(3):350–6.
42. Maron BJ. Sudden death in young athletes. N Engl J Med. 2003;349(11):1064–75.
43. Basavarajaiah S, Wilson M, Junagde S, Jackson G, Whyte G, Sharma S, et al. Physiological left ventricular hypertrophy or hypertrophic cardiomyopathy in an elite adolescent athlete: role of detraining in resolving the clinical dilemma. Br J Sports Med. 2006;40(8):727–9; discussion 9.
44. Pelliccia A, Maron BJ, De Luca R, Di Paolo FM, Spataro A, Culasso F. Remodeling of left ventricular hypertrophy in elite athletes after long-term deconditioning. Circulation. 2002;105(8):944–9.
45. Maron BJ, Pelliccia A. The heart of trained athletes: cardiac remodeling and the risks of sports, including sudden death. Circulation. 2006;114(15):1633–44.
46. Harper RW, Mottram PM. Exercise-induced right ventricular dysplasia/cardiomyopathy–an emerging condition distinct from arrhythmogenic right ventricular dysplasia/cardiomyopathy. Heart Lung Circ. 2009;18(3):233–5.
47. Abdulla J, Nielsen JR. Is the risk of atrial fibrillation higher in athletes than in the general population? A systematic review and meta-analysis. Europace. 2009;11(9):1156–9.
48. Aizer A, Gaziano JM, Cook NR, Manson JE, Buring JE, Albert CM. Relation of vigorous exercise to risk of atrial fibrillation. Am J Cardiol. 2009;103(11):1572–7.
49. Baldesberger S, Bauersfeld U, Candinas R, Seifert B, Zuber M, Ritter M, et al. Sinus node disease and arrhythmias in the long-term follow-up of former professional cyclists. Eur Heart J. 2008;29(1):71–8.
50. Karjalainen J, Kujala UM, Kaprio J, Sarna S, Viitasalo M. Lone atrial fibrillation in vigorously exercising middle aged men: case-control study. BMJ. 1998;316(7147):1784–5.
51. Molina L, Mont L, Marrugat J, Berruezo A, Brugada J, Bruguera J, et al. Long-term endurance sport practice increases the incidence of lone atrial fibrillation in men: a follow-up study. Europace. 2008;10(5):618–23.
52. Mont L, Ruiz-Granell R, Martinez JG, Carmona JR, Fidalgo M, Cobo E, et al. Impact of anti-tachycardia pacing on atrial fibrillation burden when added on top of preventive pacing algorithms: results of the prevention or termination (POT) trial. Europace. 2008;10(1):28–34.
53. Heidbuchel H, Anne W, Willems R, Adriaenssens B, Van de Werf F, Ector H. Endurance sports is a risk factor for atrial fibrillation after ablation for atrial flutter. Int J Cardiol. 2006;107(1):67–72.
54. Biffi A, Maron BJ, Di Giacinto B, Porcacchia P, Verdile L, Fernando F, et al. Relation between training-induced left ventricular hypertrophy and risk for ventricular tachyarrhythmias in elite athletes. Am J Cardiol. 2008;101(12):1792–5.
55. Faselis C, Kokkinos P, Tsimploulis A, Pittaras A, Myers J, Lavie CJ, et al. Exercise capacity and atrial fibrillation risk in veterans: a cohort study. Mayo Clin Proc. 2016;91(5):558–66.
56. Chobanian AV, Bakris GL, Black HR, Cushman WC, Green LA, Izzo JL Jr, et al. The seventh report of the joint national committee on prevention, detection, evaluation, and treatment of high blood pressure: the JNC 7 report. JAMA. 2003;289(19):2560–72.
57. Collins R, Peto R, Godwin J, MacMahon S. Blood pressure and coronary heart disease. Lancet. 1990;336(8711):370–1.
58. Collins R, Peto R, MacMahon S, Hebert P, Fiebach NH, Eberlein KA, et al. Blood pressure, stroke, and coronary heart disease. Part 2, Short-term reductions in blood pressure: overview of randomised drug trials in their epidemiological context. Lancet. 1990;335(8693):827–38.
59. MacMahon S, Peto R, Cutler J, Collins R, Sorlie P, Neaton J, et al. Blood pressure, stroke, and coronary heart disease. Part 1, Prolonged differences in blood pressure: prospective observational studies corrected for the regression dilution bias. Lancet. 1990;335(8692):765–74.
60. Cornelissen VA, Fagard RH. Effects of endurance training on blood pressure, blood pressure-regulating mechanisms, and cardiovascular risk factors. Hypertension. 2005;46(4):667–75.
61. Kokkinos P, Myers J. Exercise and physical activity: clinical outcomes and applications. Circulation. 2010;122(16):1637–48.
62. Pescatello LS, Franklin BA, Fagard R, Farquhar WB, Kelley GA, Ray CA, et al. American College of Sports Medicine position stand. Exercise and hypertension. Med Sci Sports Exerc. 2004;36(3):533–53.
63. Huai P, Xun H, Reilly KH, Wang Y, Ma W, Xi B. Physical activity and risk of hypertension: a meta-analysis of prospective cohort studies. Hypertension. 2013;62(6):1021–6.
64. Whelton SP, Chin A, Xin X, He J. Effect of aerobic exercise on blood pressure: a meta-analysis of randomized, controlled trials. Ann Intern Med. 2002;136(7):493–503.

65. Blair SN, Kohl HW 3rd, Barlow CE, Gibbons LW. Physical fitness and all-cause mortality in hypertensive men. Ann Med. 1991;23(3):307–12.
66. Faselis C, Doumas M, Panagiotakos D, Kheirbek R, Korshak L, Manolis A, et al. Body mass index, exercise capacity, and mortality risk in male veterans with hypertension. Am J Hypertens. 2012;25(4):444–50.
67. Kokkinos P, Manolis A, Pittaras A, Doumas M, Giannelou A, Panagiotakos DB, et al. Exercise capacity and mortality in hypertensive men with and without additional risk factors. Hypertension. 2009;53(3):494–9.
68. Kokkinos P, Myers J, Doumas M, Faselis C, Manolis A, Pittaras A, et al. Exercise capacity and all-cause mortality in prehypertensive men. Am J Hypertens. 2009;22(7):735–41.
69. Kokkinos P, Pittaras A, Narayan P, Faselis C, Singh S, Manolis A. Exercise capacity and blood pressure associations with left ventricular mass in prehypertensive individuals. Hypertension. 2007;49(1):55–61.
70. Myers J, Prakash M, Froelicher V, Do D, Partington S, Atwood JE. Exercise capacity and mortality among men referred for exercise testing. N Engl J Med. 2002;346(11):793–801.
71. Baglivo HP, Fabregues G, Burrieza H, Esper RC, Talarico M, Esper RJ. Effect of moderate physical training on left ventricular mass in mild hypertensive persons. Hypertension. 1990;15(2 Suppl):I153–6.
72. Hinderliter A, Sherwood A, Gullette EC, Babyak M, Waugh R, Georgiades A, et al. Reduction of left ventricular hypertrophy after exercise and weight loss in overweight patients with mild hypertension. Arch Intern Med. 2002;162(12):1333–9.
73. Kokkinos PF, Narayan P, Colleran JA, Pittaras A, Notargiacomo A, Reda D, et al. Effects of regular exercise on blood pressure and left ventricular hypertrophy in African-American men with severe hypertension. N Engl J Med. 1995;333(22):1462–7.
74. Palatini P, Visentin P, Dorigatti F, Guarnieri C, Santonastaso M, Cozzio S, et al. Regular physical activity prevents development of left ventricular hypertrophy in hypertension. Eur Heart J. 2009;30(2):225–32.
75. Turner MJ, Spina RJ, Kohrt WM, Ehsani AA. Effect of endurance exercise training on left ventricular size and remodeling in older adults with hypertension. J Gerontol A Biol Sci Med Sci. 2000;55(4):M245–51.
76. Rinder MR, Spina RJ, Peterson LR, Koenig CJ, Florence CR, Ehsani AA. Comparison of effects of exercise and diuretic on left ventricular geometry, mass, and insulin resistance in older hypertensive adults. Am J Physiol Regul Integr Comp Physiol. 2004;287(2):R360–8.
77. Reid CM, Dart AM, Dewar EM, Jennings GL. Interactions between the effects of exercise and weight loss on risk factors, cardiovascular haemodynamics and left ventricular structure in overweight subjects. J Hypertens. 1994;12(3):291–301.
78. Stewart KJ, Ouyang P, Bacher AC, Lima S, Shapiro EP. Exercise effects on cardiac size and left ventricular diastolic function: relationships to changes in fitness, fatness, blood pressure and insulin resistance. Heart. 2006;92(7):893–8.
79. Klingbeil AU, Schneider M, Martus P, Messerli FH, Schmieder RE. A meta-analysis of the effects of treatment on left ventricular mass in essential hypertension. Am J Med. 2003;115(1):41–6.
80. Dahlof B, Devereux RB, Kjeldsen SE, Julius S, Beevers G, de Faire U, et al. Cardiovascular morbidity and mortality in the Losartan Intervention For Endpoint reduction in hypertension study (LIFE): a randomised trial against atenolol. Lancet. 2002;359(9311):995–1003.
81. Dahlof B, Sever PS, Poulter NR, Wedel H, Beevers DG, Caulfield M, et al. Prevention of cardiovascular events with an antihypertensive regimen of amlodipine adding perindopril as required versus atenolol adding bendroflumethiazide as required, in the Anglo-Scandinavian Cardiac Outcomes Trial-Blood Pressure Lowering Arm (ASCOT-BPLA): a multicentre randomised controlled trial. Lancet. 2005;366(9489):895–906.
82. Kokkinos P, Chrysohoou C, Panagiotakos D, Narayan P, Greenberg M, Singh S. Beta-blockade mitigates exercise blood pressure in hypertensive male patients. J Am Coll Cardiol. 2006;47(4):794–8.
83. Kokkinos PF, Narayan P, Fletcher RD, Tsagadopoulos D, Papademetriou V. Effects of aerobic training on exaggerated blood pressure response to exercise in African-Americans with severe systemic hypertension treated with indapamide +/− verapamil +/− enalapril. Am J Cardiol. 1997;79(10):1424–6.
84. Kokkinos P, Pittaras A, Manolis A, Panagiotakos D, Narayan P, Manjoros D, et al. Exercise capacity and 24-h blood pressure in prehypertensive men and women. Am J Hypertens. 2006;19(3):251–8.
85. Lim PO, Donnan PT, MacDonald TM. Blood pressure determinants of left ventricular wall thickness and mass index in hypertension: comparing office, ambulatory and exercise blood pressures. J Hum Hypertens. 2001;15(9):627–33.
86. Nelson ME, Rejeski WJ, Blair SN, Duncan PW, Judge JO, King AC, et al. Physical activity and public health in older adults: recommendation from the American College of Sports Medicine and the American Heart Association. Med Sci Sports Exerc. 2007;39(8):1435–45.
87. Nelson ME, Rejeski WJ, Blair SN, Duncan PW, Judge JO, King AC, et al. Physical activity and public health in older adults: recommendation from the American College of Sports Medicine and the American Heart Association. Circulation. 2007;116(9):1094–105.
88. American College of Sports M, Chodzko-Zajko WJ, Proctor DN, Fiatarone Singh MA, Minson CT, Nigg CR, et al. American College of Sports Medicine position stand. Exercise and physical activity for older adults. Med Sci Sports Exerc. 2009;41(7):1510–30.

Physical Activity, Cardiorespiratory Fitness, and the Diabetes Spectrum

11

Eric S. Nylén and Peter Kokkinos

Abbreviations

ADA	American Diabetes Association
CRF	Cardiorespiratory fitness
CVD	Cardiovascular disease
DM1	Type 1 diabetes mellitus
DM2	Type 2 diabetes mellitus
GDM	Gestational diabetes mellitus
GLUT4	Glucose transporter 4
HgbA1c	Glycosylated hemoglobin A1c
HIIT	High-intensity interval training
IGT	Impaired glucose tolerance
IR	Insulin resistance
VO_2max	Maximal oxygen uptake
MVPA	Moderate-vigorous physical activity
NNT	Numbers needed to treat
RT	Resistance training

E. S. Nylén
Department of Endocrinology, VAMC and George Washington University School of Medicine, Washington, DC, USA

P. Kokkinos (✉)
Veterans Affairs Medical Center, Department of Cardiology, Washington, DC, USA

Georgetown University School of Medicine, Washington, DC, USA

Department of Kinesiology and Health, Rutgers University, New Brunswick, NJ, USA

George Washington University School of Medicine and Health Sciences, Washington, DC, USA

University of South Carolina, Department of Exercise Science, Arnold School of Public Health, Columbia, SC, USA
e-mail: peter.kokkinos@va.gov

Introduction

Approaching the centennial of the discovery of insulin that launched a paradigm shift in the medical management of diabetes [1], the disease has subsequently burgeoned into one of the dominant epidemics worldwide along with the global increase in obesity [2]. The long-term complications of this noncommunicable chronic illness include being the leading cause of end-stage renal failure, adult-onset blindness, and non-traumatic amputations. Atherosclerotic CVD is the leading cause of morbidity and mortality among individuals with diabetes and is the major cause of disability, reduced quality of life, and premature death [3, 4]. Despite the revolutionary impact of insulin, the critical and complementary role of physical activity was recognized just a few years later by van Noorden and Isaak in 1927 [5] which in turn was preceded by the concept of maximal oxygen consumption during peak exercise [6]. Currently, there exists a widely appreciated clinical conundrum; i.e., although exercise and improved fitness significantly ameliorate many of the complex pathophysiology pathways of dysglycemia, achieving enhanced fitness is a challenge to the dominant societal sedentary trends such that its therapeutic utilization is poorly executed and/or adhered to. Indeed, subjects with diabetes appear to be particularly sedentary [7] and exhibit reduced measured cardiorespiratory fitness (CRF), irrespective of duration or lack of complications [8–10]. Since

P. Kokkinos, P. Narayan (eds.), *Cardiorespiratory Fitness in Cardiometabolic Diseases*,
https://doi.org/10.1007/978-3-030-04816-7_11

CRF and/or PA status is a stronger predictor of mortality than any other risk factors [11, 12], the current chapter explores the role of exercise, exercise intolerance, and fitness in the prevention and management of diabetes.

Pathophysiology

Diabetes is broadly classified into type 1 diabetes (DM1) and type 2 diabetes (DM2). In the case of DM2, it is preceded by a prediabetic state which is defined as impaired glucose tolerance, impaired fasting glucose, and/or an intermediate HgbA1c concentration (5.7–6.4%). The prediabetic state progresses to overt diabetes in about 11% annually, and the lifetime risk approximates 70%. DM2, which constitutes the majority of subjects with diabetes, is characterized by combined IR and the development of hyperglycemia when insulin secretion becomes abnormal as the pancreatic β-cells are unable to counter decreased insulin action, a secretory β-cell defect characterized by an initial first-phase decline followed by progressive decline due to reduction in β-cell mass [13].

In contrast, the pathophysiology of DM1 involves pancreatic islet-cell autoimmunity with T-cell-mediated destruction of β-cells wherein autoantibodies target the 65 kDa glutamic acid decarboxylase, insulinoma-associated protein 2, zinc transporter 8, and/or insulin itself. These are DM1 biomarkers and are present months to years before the onset of symptoms and can therefore be used to identify and study individuals who are at risk of developing DM1. Despite the different pathophysiologic backgrounds, a minority of DM1 patients has some remaining β-cell function and can exhibit IR [14].

The hallmark pathology in both DM1 and DM2 is the development of microvascular disease leading to retinopathy, nephropathy, and neuropathy, pathologies that are amenable to improvement with glycemic control [15]. Diabetes also increases the risk for macrovascular CVD which is the leading cause of mortality, albeit much less responsive to optimized glycemic management [4, 16]. Moreover, although the overall prevalence of CVD has decreased in the last 10 years, there still persists an excess of mortality from diabetes-related CVD emphasizing the role for additional risk factor reduction.

Metabolic glucose homeostasis at rest involves glucose uptake by muscle that is insulin-sensitive furnishing muscle glycogen. During exercise, however, muscle contractions increase glucose uptake from the circulation that is not reliant on insulin and which supplements ongoing intramuscular glycogenolysis [17]. In muscle there exist several glucose transporters, the dominant being glucose transporter 4 (GLUT4) whose translocation is responsive to both insulin and muscle contractions [18]. In DM2 the insulin-responsive GLUT4 is impaired [19]; however, exercise augmentation of GLUT4 abundance is still intact along with glucose uptake from the circulation [18]. Accordingly, studies clearly show that exercise improves insulin sensitivity and improves IR in diabetes most likely via changes in GLUT4 and vascular reactivity [20–22].

On a cellular level and highlighted in Dr. Gidlund's chapter, mitochondrial dysfunction, whether due to decreased activity, abnormal size, or decreased biogenesis, has been implicated in the pathophysiology of DM2, and these organelles are highly responsive to the stimulus created by muscle contraction and exercise and have a direct link to insulin action/inaction. For example, in vivo mitochondrial function, content, and glucose disposal were restored following 12 weeks of exercise training (with 13% increased VO_2max) [23].

The Physical Activity Spectrum and Exercise Intolerance

Physical activity typically refers to "the expenditure of energy above that of the resting state by contraction of skeletal muscle to produce bodily movement," while exercise is "a type of physical activity that involves planned, structured and repetitive bodily movement performed for the purpose of improving physical fitness" [24].

Physical activity or exercise can be classified broadly as aerobic or anaerobic. Aerobic activities or exercises consist of repetitive, relatively low-intensity, and long-duration movements that utilize large muscle groups and derive most of the energy requirements via the aerobic pathways with the main substrate being fatty acids. Anaerobic activities or exercises are those defined by relatively high intensities and short duration that derive most of the energy requirements for such activities via the anaerobic pathways where the substrate is glucose. Chronic exposure to either aerobic or anaerobic activities leads to significant increases in the capacity of respective system (aerobic or anaerobic) to meet the energy demands of the working muscles. Specifically, chronic exposure to aerobic exercises of adequate intensity and duration leads to increased aerobic capacity or cardiorespiratory fitness (CRF). The maximal capacity of the cardiorespiratory system to deliver oxygen to the working muscles and the capacity of these muscles to utilize it is referred to as maximal oxygen consumption (VO_2max). Direct assessment of VO_2 max is the most accurate and reproducible method. However, this direct assessment is labor-intensive and cost prohibitive. Thus, indirect assessments of CRF, although not as accurate, have been established and used extensively, especially for large cohorts and diseased populations [6, 25]. CRF is typically reported as metabolic equivalents (METs), with one MET defined as the amount of oxygen consumption at rest (3.5 ml O_2/kg/min).

In parallel with the emergence of affluent type of socioeconomic development, physical inactivity and obesity have dramatically increased in the latter half of the twentieth century, both of which have been shown to be strong and independent risk factors for associations to diabetes (mostly DM2) and its related comorbidities [26]. The *International Diabetes Federation Diabetes Atlas* estimates that in 2017, there were 425 million patients with diabetes worldwide which is expected to rise to 629 million people by 2045 [27]. In the USA, approximately 33.5 million people had diabetes in 2017 with a prevalence of 13.3%, with about 11% of them undiagnosed [28], and approximately 5% of people with diabetes have DM1 [29].

The association between PA and health has been firmly established in multiple studies including those with diabetes which has generated several volume-focused guidelines [30, 31], promoting moderate vigorous physical activity (MVPA) for 150 min/week, typically performed at greater than ~45% of VO_2 max. The amount of MVPA approximating ≥3 METs has been shown to reduce the health risks associated with numerous chronic illnesses and their prevention. Thus, the relationship between measured CRF and all-cause mortality is inverse and dose-dependent [32]. However, it is well established that the majority of current human activity occurs in a spectrum of activities not aimed for fitness. For example, there is a host of non-exercise PA such as walking, etc. that nevertheless impact favorably on the incidence of DM2 [33]. However, measuring CRF is still a stronger predictor of outcome than self-reported PA [34].

Most humans spend the majority of time being sedentary, i.e., "physical activity levels less than those required for optimal health and prevention of premature death" contributing to the rise in chronic illnesses [35], i.e., energy expenditure in the range of 1–1.5 METs [36]. It has, furthermore, been pointed out that the underlying pathophysiological pathways of sedentary inactivity are not necessarily the opposite of those involved with PA and fitness. A dose-response phenomenon can be achieved by capturing the degree of sedentary behavior using television viewing as a proxy of noncontractile activity with all-cause and CVD mortality [37, 38]. Importantly, the amount of sedentary sitting time is independent of the time spent performing exercise [39], and it is proposed that the physiological mechanisms leading to adverse outcomes being sedentary are independent from MVPA [40]. Being sedentary (measured as additional 2 h per day watching TV) also increased relative risk of developing DM2 using a meta-analysis approach [41].

Subjects with DM2 appear to be particularly prone to sedentary behavior as reported in the Medical Expenditure Panel Survey, where the majority of subjects with diabetes were given instructions about exercise by health professionals but only 31% of those with no diabetes received similar information [42]. However, only a minority of those with diabetes reported being physically active, while a majority of those without diabetes were physically active [43]. Indeed, subjects with diabetes in addition to being sedentary have reduced CRF, not related to the duration of the disease or subsequent complications [44]. As a consequence of certain vascular abnormalities (i.e., decreased VO_2 peak and slowed kinetics for oxygen uptake), subjects with diabetes exhibit exercise intolerance with subnormal CRF (Table 11.1, Fig. 11.1) [8, 44]. The 2016 American Diabetes Association's position statement on physical activity/exercise and diabetes encompasses not only exercise promotion but also includes specific recommendations to reduce and interrupt prolonged sitting [31].

Cardiorespiratory Fitness and Risk of Developing Diabetes

Several epidemiological studies report an inverse association between PA and the incidence of DM2 and support the protective role of MVPA against the development of DM2 [45]. A similar relationship of an inverse association between measured CRF and the incidence of DM2 has also been reported [46–49], supported by meta-analysis

Table 11.1 Examples of possible causes of exercise intolerance in subjects with diabetes

Abnormality	Reference #
Abnormal oxygen uptake	[8, 44]
Lower VO_2max at baseline	[44]
Abnormal/low numbers of mitochondria	[129]
Autonomic neuropathy/abnormal heart rate recovery	[130]
Decreased cardiac perfusion	[131]
Dehydration	[132]
Degenerative joint disease/poor mobility	[133]
Endothelial dysfunction	[44]
Hyperglycemia	[134]
Insulin resistance	[135]
Obesity	[44]
Left ventricular dysfunction (overt and/or subclinical)	[136]
Metformin	[67]
Muscle weakness	[111]
Sarcopenia	[106]
Statin therapy	[82, 84]

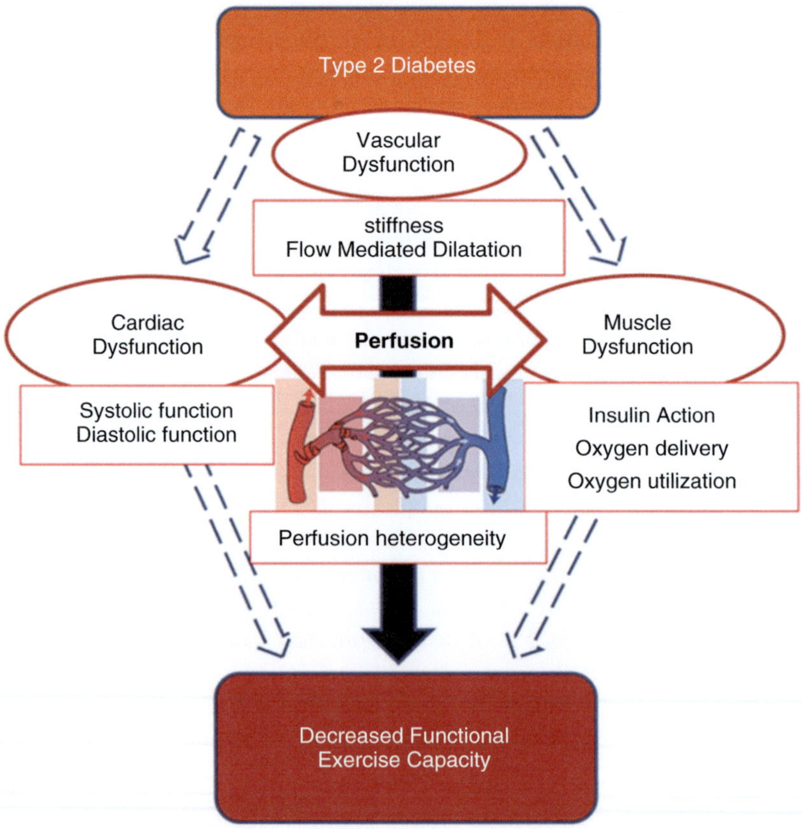

Fig. 11.1 Schematic representation of some of the cardiovascular abnormalities associated with exercise intolerance in subjects with type 2 diabetes. (Figure as originally published in Wahl et al. [146])

where the incidence was independent of several common risk factors of DM2 and where 1-MET higher CRF level decreased DM2 incidence by 5% [50]. Cardiorespiratory fitness is generally known to decrease with age, and when CRF was measured on several occasions over a 20-year period, there was a significantly higher incidence of DM2 in those with the most substantial decline in CRF [51]. In another study where CRF was measured on several occasions, those with consistently elevated CRF had a decreased risk of developing DM2 by 28%, whereas there was no protective effect from a transiently elevated CRF [52].

Obesity is also a very strong risk factor for diabetes. Although the relative role of fitness across the spectrum of obesity and diabetes risk is not fully resolved, promoting increased fitness may be more effective than weight control in the obese compared to overweight persons to decrease the risk of obesity [53]. Although both a reduced CRF and a higher BMI are independently associated with DM2 incident, when considered simultaneously, CRF attenuated but did not eliminate the increased risks of DM2 associated with overweight and obesity in both men and women [54, 55].

Cardiorespiratory Fitness Intervention and Diabetes Prevention

There are now multiple prospective randomized studies using lifestyle programs with MVPA that convincingly show the importance of enhanced fitness in preventing DM2 and mortality. Those with IGT and early DM2 in the Malmö feasibility study underwent a 1-year intervention including supervised exercise and nutritional advice followed by analysis after an additional 5 years. The results showed that those with IGT and early DM2 had normalized their glucose tolerance by 52% and 23%, respectively [56]. In the Da Qing study, following randomization of the IGT subjects, those receiving (minor) exercise promotion had the most significant reduction in the development of DM2 by 42–46% over 6 years [57]. In the 20-year follow-up of this study, the effect persisted despite the intervention having been discontinued [58]. In the Finnish Diabetes Prevention Study (DPS), with combined intense lifestyle program (diet and exercise), the mean follow-up was 3.2 years, and the relative risk reduction to DM2 was 58% [59]. The follow-up of DPS was performed 13 years later showing a persistent reduction in DM2 incidence [60]. The Diabetes and Prevention Program (DPP) was similar in design to DPS but recruited more subjects over a shorter time of observation (2.8 years) [61]. The results were similar to DPS as well, with a 58% relative risk reduction after 4 years and continuation of an active lifestyle significantly reduced the incidence of DM2 over 10 years where the diabetes risk was reduced by 34% in the original intensive lifestyle intervention group [62]. During a mean follow-up of 15 years, diabetes incidence was reduced by 27% in the lifestyle intervention group and 18% in those treated with metformin [63]. Interestingly, at 15 years, men had a substantially higher prevalence of microvascular complications than women, and there was no improvement in microvascular outcomes in men. However, in women the lifestyle intervention was associated with a 21% reduction in aggregate microvascular outcomes compared with placebo [63]. A significant reduction in severe diabetic retinopathy was observed in the long-term follow-up of the Da Qing trial [58]. The DPP also established that the prediabetes state, if persistent, increases the risk of CVD, whereas resolution of prediabetes reduced the risk of both DM2 and CVD [64].

In terms of preventing DM2, the NNT in both the lifestyle arms of DPS and the DPP was about 5–7 [61, 65]. The DPP also included a randomized arm wherein subjects used metformin. Although there was a risk reduction of new-onset DM2 with metformin, it was intermediary between lifestyle and control, and, furthermore, similar use of metformin in the Indian Diabetes Prevention Study revealed no additional benefit by adding metformin to the lifestyle arm [66]. Another finding in the metformin arm of DPP was that remission to normoglycemia was less likely when subjects were exposed to metformin compared to the active lifestyle intervention arm, and combining metformin to exercise may impede benefits [64, 67].

Though lifestyle intervention has become a routine recommendation for patients with prediabetes, there is a paucity of data regarding mortality outcomes. The Da Qing follow-up study, however, showed a significant decrease in cardiovascular and all-cause mortality [68]. Cardiorespiratory fitness was a strong modulator of survival in another large relatively healthy prediabetic cohort [69]. We have also reported a strong inverse and graded association between CRF and mortality risk with a 13% decrease for every 1-MET increase in fitness in an elderly and more comorbid and sedentary population [70].

Women with gestational diabetes mellitus (GDM), defined as any degree of hyperglycemia recognized for the first time during pregnancy, are also at higher risk of developing DM2. The presence of GDM predicts a lower CRF in the offspring 16 years later [71]. Using a combined lifestyle approach appears to reduce the risk of developing GDM based on data from 23 randomized control trials [72]. A more dedicated exercise approach in early pregnancy has also been shown to be effective in significantly preventing GDM along with reduced gestational weight gain in obese subjects, and the ADA currently recommends moderate PA as part of any management plan, provided clearance from medical or obstetrical problem [31, 73, 74].

In general, systematic reviews and meta-analysis support that comprehensive lifestyle interventions are effective in lowering the incidence of DM2 in high-risk patients [75]. In addition, the efficacy of lifestyle interventions to reduced diabetes incidence was sustained for several years successfully, while the success of glucose-lowering medications was short-lived [76]. Finally, observational studies and several meta-analyses of randomized controlled trials of statins have reported unfavorable glycemic homeostasis [77] and higher dose-related risk for developing DM2 in those treated with statins compared to placebo or standard care [78, 79]. Evidence from large epidemiologic studies strongly support an inverse, independent, and graded association between CRF and risk for developing certain chronic illnesses including DM2 [54, 55, 61]. We have also shown that both statin therapy and increased CRF were independently associated with lower mortality risk in those treated and not treated with statins [80]. Additionally, the combination of statin therapy and increased CRF was more effective in lowering mortality risk than either alone [80, 81]. However, the impact of increased CRF on the development of DM2 in statin-treated patients has not been examined. Furthermore, some [82, 83] but not all studies [84–86] suggest that improvements in CRF in response to exercise training may be blunted by statin therapy.

In one study, the interaction between CRF and DM2 incidence was assessed in 4092 dyslipidemic patients (age = 58.8 ± 10.9 years) treated with statins and 3001 patients (age = 57.2 ± 11.2 years) not treated with statins [87]. The DM2 incidence was 24% higher in statin-treated compared to non-statin-treated patients. CRF was inversely related to DM2 incidence. For every 1-MET increase in exercise capacity, the adjusted risk for developing DM2 declined by 6% ($p < 0.001$). Comparisons across quartiles of fitness categories (least-fit to high-fit) revealed that the adjusted risk for developing DM2 declined progressively with increasing fitness and was 34% lower for high-fit individuals when compared to those in the least-fit category.

Furthermore, to assess the impact of CRF on the risk for developing DM2, we used the non-statin-treated cohort as the reference group and compared it with the aforementioned fitness categories of the statin-treated cohort. We found that DM2 incidence was significantly elevated (50% higher) for individuals in the least-fit and low-fit (22% higher) categories. For the moderate and high-fit individuals, the risk was similar to those not treated with statins (Fig. 11.2). These findings suggest that the risk of DM2 incidence in dyslipidemic patients treated with statins may be significantly attenuated by moderate increases in CRF.

Cardiorespiratory Fitness and Diabetes Management

As presciently noted by Isaak and van Noorden, enhanced PA was and continues to be a cornerstone of diabetes prevention and management [5], albeit it presents a significant challenge to efficiently implement [88]. Subjects with diabetes

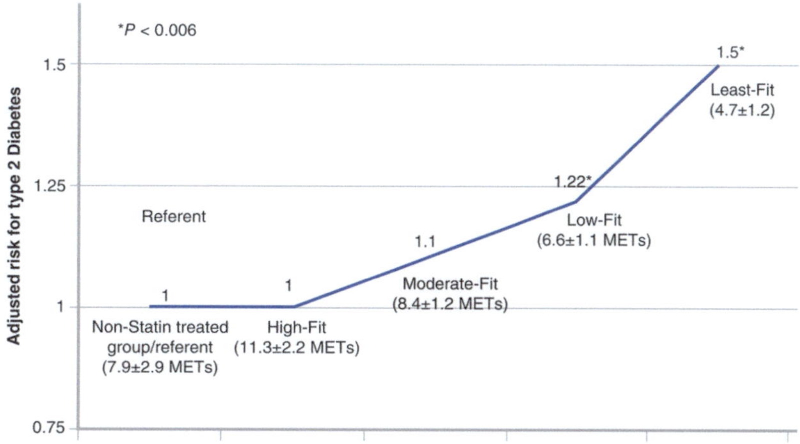

Fig. 11.2 Incidence of DM2 according to cardiorespiratory fitness status in dyslipidemic patients treated with statins as compared to those not treated with statins. (Modified from Kokkinos et al. [87])

have an approximately two- to fourfold increased likelihood of experiencing CVD, and peak exercise METs is the strongest predictor of death in healthy and those with various CVD risks including diabetes [11, 12, 89]. Importantly, higher fitness levels reduce mortality independent of BMI and age [90–93]. In general, habitual aerobic exercise, even at modest levels (<6 METs), improves insulin sensitivity and reduces HgbA1c by approximately 0.7% without change in weight [94–97]. For example, a week of aerobic exercise results in improved whole-body insulin sensitivity primarily as a result of enhanced insulin sensitivity in peripheral tissues via a non-insulin-dependent response. Focusing on measured CRF, a detailed review of 9 randomized trials revealed an improvement in VO_2max by ~12% over 20 weeks when 132 DM2 subjects with early diabetes (4.1 years) exercised at 50–75% of VO_2max [98]. Moreover, higher exercise intensity produced an augmented response in VO_2max also seen when tracking improvements in HbgA1c. These impressive effects are, however, short with the acute effect lasting about 24 h. Optimally, subjects with diabetes should engage in regular PA on a daily basis, and the shorter the exposure to PA, the higher the effort is needed to get the same effect on insulin sensitivity. Similar glycemic results from our own experience in sedentary elderly DM2 veterans with high degree of comorbidity using multiple medications are shown in Figs. 11.3, 11.4, 11.5, and 11.6.

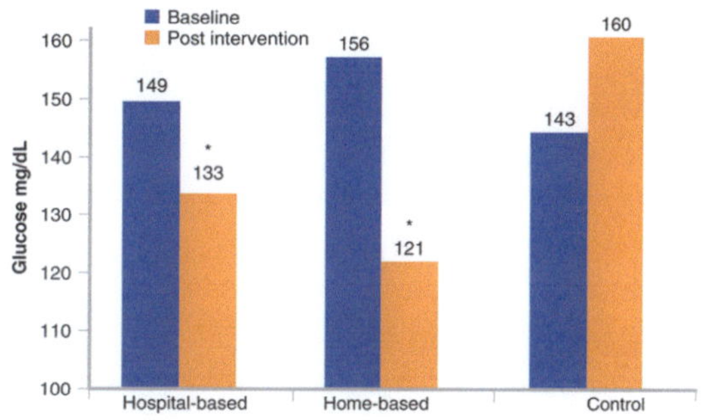

Fig. 11.3 Changes in glucose levels after 12 weeks of supervised (hospital-based; $n = 454$) exercise or non-supervised (home-based; $n = 86$) exercise and controls ($n = 192$) ($^*p < 0.05$)

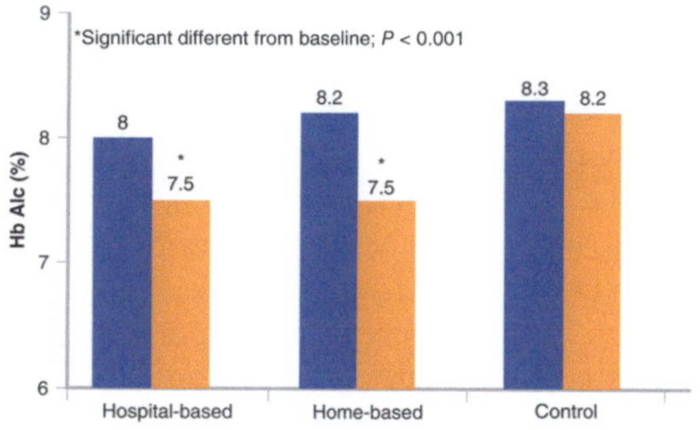

Fig. 11.4 Changes in HbA1c levels after 12 weeks of supervised (hospital-based; $n = 349$) exercise or non-supervised (home-based; $n = 58$) exercise and controls ($n = 81$)

Nevertheless, a recent large prospective lifestyle study sponsored by the National Institutes of Health was prematurely stopped after failing

Figs. 11.5 and 11.6 Changes in fasting blood glucose (Fig. 11.5) and HgbA1c (Fig. 11.6) following 12 weeks participation in a lifestyle program consisting of nutritional advice and combined aerobic and resistance training in 488 sedentary veterans with DM2. The mean change in cardiorespiratory fitness (METs) was 20%; and weight decreased by 2%. Red graph = baseline; green graph = after 12 weeks

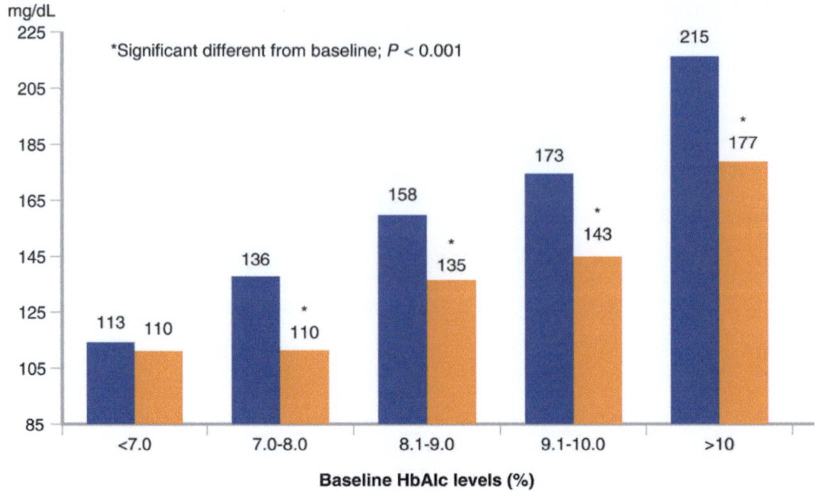

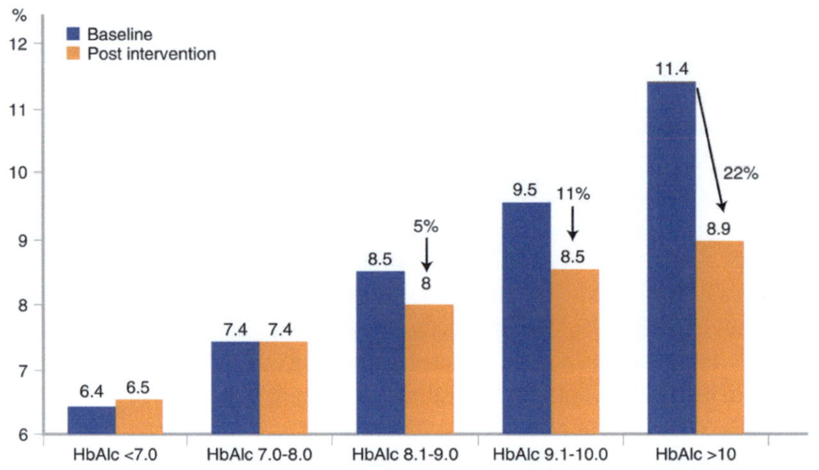

to show CVD benefits of an intensive lifestyle program [99, 100]. The Look AHEAD study tested the hypothesis that an intensive multi-component lifestyle program would reduce the incidence of CVD outcomes and improve other health parameters, including CVD risk and metabolic aspects, in overweight and/or obese DM2 subjects. The goals were to maintain at least a 7% weight loss and gradually get at least 175 minutes per week of moderate-intensity PA being active at least 5 times per week. In this study, CRF improved significantly in the first year [101]. Although there was no reduction in CVD risk, those who lost at least 10% of their body-weight had a 20% lower risk of the primary outcome (adjusted HR 0.80) and a 21% lower risk of secondary outcome (adjusted HR 0.79); however, change in fitness was not significantly associated with a change in the primary outcome. There were several problems with this study. First, the CVD event rate was very low (0.07% per year). Thus, there was a very low overall rate in both the intervention and control groups. Second, the improvements of ~1 METs achieved in the first year of the trial was probably too low considering the low fitness baseline which is below the METs threshold for age [102]. Moreover, there was a rapid decline in METs in the second year such that these subjects tracked from rapidly going from unfit to slightly more fit back to unfit in 2 years which has previously shown not to be of benefit [52]. Post hoc analysis revealed that those that actually achieved at least two METs above baseline showed an improvement in secondary outcomes [103]. Another benefit shown by this study was that higher weekly MVPA was associated with greater long-term weight loss and weight maintenance [99], a phenomenon supported in a different study using more mechanistic methodology [104].

There was also an interesting equivalency intervention study designed to test whether a lifestyle intervention (aerobic and resistance exercise training) results in equivalent glycemic control compared with standard care among adults with DM2 diagnosed for about 5–6 years. A secondary aim was to assess if lifestyle intervention ultimately leads to a reduction in glucose-lowering medication [105]. The study was designed so that the treatment target for glycemic control was 6.5% HbA1c level. If this target was reached, the glucose-lowering medication dose was halved. If the HbA1c level was unchanged or lower at the following medical consultation, the glucose-lowering medication was discontinued. If HbA1c level exceeded 7.5%, the glucose-lowering medication was increased according to the pre-specified algorithm.

The investigators reported that the lifestyle intervention compared with standard care resulted in a change in glycemic control that did not meet the criterion for equivalence but was in a direction consistent with benefit.

Although this conclusion may be viewed as disappointing, a closer look at the study reveals several noteworthy findings. First, HbA1c in the standard care group increased substantially above baseline values at 3 and 6 months of follow-up and was back to baseline (6.74% vs 6.66%) at the end of study (12 months). Glycemic control was undoubtedly achieved by increases in glucose-lowering medication in approximately 44% of the participants.

Conversely, in the lifestyle group, HA1c was substantially lower from baseline at 3 and 6 months, began an upward trend at 9 months, but was still lower than baseline levels and 12 months (6.65% vs 6.34%). Glucose-lowering medication was reduced in 73% of participants and eliminated in over 56%.

Given the aforementioned findings, the reported failure of the lifestyle intervention group to achieve statistical equivalence should not overshadow the fact that exercise intervention reduced glucose-lowering medication in 73% of the participants, eliminated medication in 56% of them, and achieved a substantially more favorable glycemic control. Thus, one can argue that the more salient finding of this study was that lifestyle intervention (i.e., exercise) achieved a favorable glucose control even when medication was withdrawn or reduced in a large number of the participants. This level of glucose control was matched only by using substantially more glucose-lowering medication in the standard care group.

In addition to aerobic approaches to fitness in DM2, the role of resistance training (RT) has regained acceptance with the recognition that these subjects are becoming older, are often obese, have high degree of sedentarism, and are frequently sarcopenic [106]. Indeed, older adults with DM2 have greater muscle mass loss, reduced upper and lower body strength, increased visceral adiposity, and increased disability [107–109]. Poorly controlled DM2 patients have, in addition, poor capillary recruitment during skeletal contraction [110]. Not surprisingly, the largest effect of RT is on the musculoskeletal measurements such as muscle strength [111], but RT can also significantly improve insulin sensitivity, glycemic control including HbA1c, increase fat-free mass, reduce the requirement for diabetes medications, reduce abdominal adiposity, and improve cardiovascular risk markers [112–114]. Overall resistance exercise training is a promising strategy to promote overall metabolic health in individuals with T2D via improvements in muscle mitochondrial performance and increases in muscle mass that may positively impact insulin responsiveness and glucose control [115].

A strategy of combining aerobic and RT appears to enhance metabolic control in DM2 compared to either activity alone [116, 117]. Studies have reported that the combination of aerobic plus RT has additive benefits on glucose control and can achieve greater reductions in DM2 incidence than the use of a single exercise modality. Thus, current guidelines for DM2 prevention and management recommend at least 150 min per week of MVPA and an additional two (ideally three) resistance sessions per week (at least 60 min) [118]. A systematic meta-analysis of the combination approach (diet + aerobic exercise + RT) to prevent diabetes concluded that there was a modest weight loss and small improvements in glycemic control, fitness, and dietary intake [119]. It should be noted that there is also evidence for the positive effect of breaking up of prolonged sedentary time with light walking with improved glycemic parameters [120]. In addition, the response to exercise is different depending on the duration of DM2; those with long-standing DM2 have more extreme exercise intolerance, muscle weakness, and sarcopenia and may benefit more from RT.

Newer exercise approaches beyond MVPA and sedentary breaks such as HIIT may improve adherence by reducing the amount of time dedicated to fitness and may also enhance glycemia and CRF [121]. For those medically cleared for more exhaustive exercise, subjects perform repeated short bursts of maximal activity near 90% of VO_2max which is interspersed with recovery periods, but the total time is considerably shortened and saving time. A meta-analysis shows improved glycemic response to HIIT compared to MVP [122].

Despite the impressive health impact of enhanced CRF, it is widely recognized that there is heterogeneity in exercise response in subjects with diabetes both metabolically as well as changes in CRF. Moreover, perhaps as many as 15–20% of subjects undergoing exercise training do not respond metabolically as would be expected [123]. There may also be genetic variants that could be important in predicting CRF responsiveness [124]. Another concern regards the aforementioned exercise intolerance and the negative interaction between the ubiquitous use of statins and PA and the diabetogenic risk of statins [125, 126]. Although some studies show a reduced VO_2 max with the use of statins [127], the combination of fitness and statin enhances survival [128], and the risk of developing diabetes from statins is potently modulated by improved CRF [87]. In addition, several other factors including cardiometabolic, neuromuscular, and joint factors alone or in combination may contribute to exercise intolerance [129–136]. A complete list of factors that may contribute to exercise intolerance is presented in Table 11.1.

Conclusion

Poor CRF is a well-established independent predictor of CVD and overall mortality among subjects with prediabetes, DM1, and DM2. Increased PA and higher CRF confer metabolic health benefits for DM2 patients in proportion to the level of fitness independent of BMI. Although the role and metabolic impact of exercise in subjects with DM1 is dynamic and complex, a recent systematic review and meta-analysis of subjects enrolled in exercise training revealed improvements in insulin requirement, waist circumference, BMI, VO_2 max, and LDL cholesterol in DM1 patients [137]. Increases in PA patterns have thus emerged as an integral part of the prevention and management supported by a multitude of reproducible randomized studies confirming the strong link to enhanced CRF.

From the pioneering studies of transportation workers by Morris [138] to state-of-the-art discovery of novel exercise-related phosphoproteome signaling pathways [139] and the genetics predicting CRF [140], exercise science has made impressive advances with recent involvement by National Institutes of Health into uncovering molecular transducers of exercise [141]. Stemming the epidemics of chronic illnesses such as diabetes spectrum disorders present significant implementation challenges; however, the crux being adherence, therapeutic regimens should be designed to improve CRF in a society where a profound lifestyle shift has taken place dominated by non-exercise PA and sedentary behaviors. Being a modifiable risk factor, there is no doubt that a healthcare provider prescription for enhanced fitness is an essential start perhaps aided by using CRF as a vital sign [142]. Promoting a lifestyle of PA must also involve progressive societal and political engagement via education and support for alternatives to transportation, creating more appropriate indoor and outdoor architecture while also being mindful of harm from emerging exposure risks from pollution [143].

Finally, the excessive economic burden of diabetes must be considered. In the latest 2017 assessment of the healthcare costs of DM performed by the American Diabetes Association, the incurred medical expenditure is approximately 2.3 times higher than those without diabetes, an increase by 26% since 2012 [144]. According to a recently published economic analysis of the Veterans Exercise Testing Study [145], the care cost was inversely associated with CRF. Specifically, the healthcare cost for subjects in the least-fit quartile was approximately \$14,662 ($p < 0.001$) higher per patient per year compared with those in the fittest quartile, after controlling for potential confounding variables. Each 1-MET higher increment in fitness was associated with a \$1592 annual reduction in healthcare costs (5.6% lower cost per MET), and each higher quartile of fitness was associated with a \$4163 annual cost reduction per patient. Although this study did not directly assess the healthcare cost of diabetic patients, considering the relatively low CRF characteristic of DM2 patients, improving CRF is likely to lower the healthcare cost in this populations.

References

1. Banting FG, Best CH, Collip JB, Campbell WR, Fletcher AA. Pancreatic extracts in the treatment of diabetes mellitus. Can Med Assoc J. 1922;12:141–6.
2. World Health Organization. Global status report on noncommunicable diseases 2010. Geneva: World Health Organization; 2011.
3. American Diabetes Association. Cardiovascular disease and risk management. Diabetes Care. 2017;40:S75–87.
4. Morrish NJ, Wang SL, Stevens LK, Fuller JH, Keen H. Mortality and causes of death in the WHO multinational study of vascular disease in diabetes. Diabetologia. 2001;44(Suppl 2):S14–21.
5. Katsch D. Work therapy for diabetes patients. Die Arbeitstherapie der Zuckerkranken. Erg Physikal Diat Ther. 1939;1:1–36.
6. Hill AV, Long CNH, Lupton H. Muscular exercise, lactic acid and the supply and utilization of oxygen. Pt. 1-III. Proc R Soc. 1924;96:438.
7. Henson J, Dunstan DW, Davies MJ, Yates T. Sedentary behaviour as a new behavioural target in the prevention and treatment of type 2 diabetes. Diabetes Metab Res Rev. 2016;32(Suppl 1):213–20.
8. Green S, Egana M, Baldi JC, Lamberts R, Regensteiner JG. Cardiovascular control during exercise in type 2 diabetes mellitus. J Diabetes Res. 2015;2015:654204.
9. Leite SA, Monk AM, Upham PA, Bergenstal RM. Low cardiorespiratory fitness in people at risk for type 2 diabetes: early marker for insulin resistance. Diabetol Metab Syndr. 2009;1:1–6.
10. Fang ZY, Sharman J, Prins JB, Marwick TH. Determinants of exercise capacity in patients with type 2 diabetes. Diabetes Care. 2005;28:1643–8.
11. Wei M, Gibbons LW, Kampert JB, Nichaman MZ, Blair SN. Low cardiorespiratory fitness and physical inactivity as predictors of mortality in men with type 2 diabetes. Diabetes Care. 2000;132:605–11.
12. Myers J, Prakash M, Froelicher V, Do D, Partington S, Atwood JE. Exercise capacity and mortality among men referred for exercise testing. N Engl J Med. 2002;346:793–801.
13. Butler AE, Janson J, Bonner-Weir S, Ritzel R, Rizza RA, Butler PC. β-Cell deficit and increased beta-cell apoptosis in humans with type 2 diabetes. Diabetes. 2003;52:102–10.
14. Priya G, Kalra S. A review of insulin resistance in type 1 diabetes: is there a place for adjunctive metformin? Diabetes Ther. 2017;9:349. https://doi.org/10.1007/s13300-017-0333-9.
15. Barrett EJ, Liu Z, Khamaisi M, King GL, Klein R, Klein BEK, et al. Diabetic microvascular disease: an endocrine society scientific statement. J Clin Endocrinol Metab. 2017;102(12):4343–410.
16. Skyler JS, Bergenstal R, Bonow RO, et al. Intensive glycemic control and the prevention of cardiovascular events: implications of the ACCORD, ADVANCE, and VA diabetes trials: a position statement of the American Diabetes Association and a scientific statement of the American College of Cardiology Foundation and the American Heart Association. Diabetes Care. 2009;32:187–92.
17. Jensen TE, Richter EA. Regulation of glucose and glycogen metabolism during and after exercise. J Physiol. 2012;590(Pt 5):1069–76.
18. Coderre L, Kandror KV, Vallega G, Pilch PF. Identification and characterization of an exercise-sensitive pool of glucose transporters in skeletal muscle. J Biol Chem. 1995;270:27584–8.
19. Cline GW, Petersen KF, Krssak M, Shen J, Hundal RS, Trajanoski Z, et al. Impaired glucose transport as a cause of decreased insulin-stimulated muscle glycogen synthesis in type 2 diabetes. N Engl J Med. 1999;341:240–6.
20. Goodyear LJ, Kahn BB. Exercise, glucose transport, and insulin sensitivity. Annu Rev Med. 1998;49:235–61.
21. Richter EA, Hargreaves M. Exercise, GLUT4, and skeletal muscle glucose uptake. Physiol Rev. 2013;93:993–1017.

22. Prior SJ, Goldberg AP, Ortmyer HK, Chin ER, Chen D, Blumenthal JD, Ryan AS. Increased skeletal muscle capillarization independently enhances insulin sensitivity in older adults after exercise training and detraining. Diabetes. 2015;64:3386–95.
23. Meex RCR, Schrauwen-Hinderling VB, Moonen-Kornips E, Schaart G, Mensink M, Phielix E, et al. Restoration of muscle mitochondrial function and metabolic flexibility in type 2 diabetes by exercise training is paralleled by increased myocellular fat storage and improved insulin sensitivity. Diabetes. 2010;59:572–9.
24. Yardley JE, Alberga A, Kenny GP, Sigal RJ. Lifestyle issues: exercise. In: Holt RIG, Cockram CS, Flyvbjerg A, Goldstein BJ, editors. Textbook of diabetes. 4th ed. London: Wiley-Blackwell; 2010. p. 358–79.
25. Laukkanen JA, Kurl S, Salonen JT. Cardiorespiratory fitness and physical activity as risk predictors of future atherosclerotic cardiovascular diseases. Curr Atheroscler Rep. 2002;4:468–76.
26. Sullivan PW, Morrato EH, Ghushchyan V, Wyatt HR, Hill JO. Obesity, inactivity, and the prevalence of diabetes and diabetes-related cardiovascular comorbidities in the U.S., 2000–2002. Diabetes Care. 2005;28:1599–603.
27. IDF Atlas 2017 – 8th ed. http://www.diabetesatlas.org/resources/2017-atlas.html.
28. Selvin E, Wang D, Lee A, Bergenstal RM, Coresh J. Identifying trends in undiagnosed diabetes in U.S. adults by using confirmatory definition. Ann Int Med. 2017;167:769–76.
29. CDC. www.cdc.gov/diabetes/basics/type1.html.
30. U.S. Department of Health and Human Services. 2008 Physical activity guidelines for Americans. Washington, DC: U.S. Government Printing Office; 2008.
31. Colberg SR, Sigal RJ, Yardley JE, Riddell MC, Dunstan DW, Dempsey PC, et al. Physical activity/exercise and diabetes: a position statement of the American Diabetes Association. Diabetes Care. 2016;39:2065–79.
32. Blair SN, Kohl HW 3rd, Paffenbarger RS Jr, Clark DG, Cooper KH, Gibbons LW. Physical fitness and all-cause mortality: a prospective study of healthy men and women. JAMA. 1989;262:2395–401.
33. Weinstein AR, Sesso HD, Lee IM, Cook NR, Manson JE, Buring JE, Gaziano JM. Relationship of physical activity vs body mass index with type 2 diabetes in women. JAMA. 2004;292:1188–94.
34. Swift DL, Lavie CJ, Johannsen NM, Arena R, Earnest CP, O'Keefe JH, et al. Physical activity, cardiorespiratory fitness, and exercise training in primary and secondary coronary prevention. Circ J. 2013;77:281–92.
35. Booth FW, Roberts CK, Thyfault JP, Ruegsegger GN, Toedebusch RG. Role of inactivity in chronic diseases. Physiol Rev. 2017;97:1351–402.
36. Owen N, Leslie E, Salmon J, Fotheringham MJ. Environmental determinants of physical activity and sedentary behavior. Exerc Sport Sci Rev. 2000;28:153–8.
37. Dunstan DW, Barr EL, Healy GN, Salmon J, Shaw JE, Balkau B, et al. Television viewing time and mortality: the Australian Diabetes, Obesity and Lifesyle Study (AusDiab). Circulation. 2010;121:384–91.
38. Hu FB, Li TY, Colditz GA, Willett WC, Manson JE. Television watching and other sedentary behaviors in relation to risk of obesity and type 2 diabetes mellitus in women. JAMA. 2003;289:1785–91.
39. Thyfault JP, Du M, Kraus WE, Levine JA, Booth FW. Physiology of sedentary behavior and its relationship to health outcomes. Med Sci Sports Exerc. 2015;47:1301–5.
40. Craft LL, Zderic TW, Gapstur SM, Vaniterson EH, Thomas DM, Siddique J, Hamilton MT. Evidence that women meeting physical activity guidelines do not sit less: an observational inclinometry study. Int J Behav Nutr Phys Act. 2012 Oct 4;9:122. https://doi.org/10.1186/1479-5868-9-122.
41. Hamilton MT, Hamilton DG, Zderic TW. Sedentary behavior as a mediator of type 2 diabetes. Med Sport Sci. 2014;60:11–26.
42. Morrato EH, Hill JO, Wyatt HR, Ghushchyan V, Sullivan PW. Are health care professionals advising patients with diabetes or at risk for developing diabetes to exercise more? Diabetes Care. 2006;29:543–8.
43. Morrato EH, Hill JO, Wyatt HR, Ghushchyan V, Sullivan PW. Physical activity in US adults with diabetes and at risk of diabetes. Diabetes Care. 2003;30:203–9.
44. Reusch JE, Bridenstine M, Regensteiner JG. Type 2 diabetes mellitus and exercise impairment. Rev Endocr Metab Disord. 2013;14:77–86.
45. Helmrich SP, Ragland DR, Leung RW, Paffenbarger RS. Physical activity and reduced occurrence of non insulin dependent diabetes mellitus. New Engl J Med. 1991;325:147–52.
46. Wei M, Gibbons LW, Mitchell TL, Kampert JB, Lee CD, Blair SN. The association between cardiorespiratory fitness and impaired fasting glucose and type 2 diabetes mellitus in men. Ann Intern Med. 1999;130:89–96.
47. Sawada SS, Lee IM, Muto T, Matuszaki K, Blair SN. Cardiorespiratory fitness and the incidence of type 2 diabetes: prospective study of Japanese men. Diabetes Care. 2003;26:2918–22.
48. Sui X, Hooker SP, Lee IM, et al. A prospective study of cardiorespiratory fitness and risk of type 2 diabetes in women. Diabetes Care. 2008;31:550–5.
49. Crump C, Sundquist J, Winkleby MA, Sieh W, Sundquist K. Physical fitness among Swedish military conscripts and long-term risk for type 2 diabetes mellitus: a cohort study. Ann Intern Med. 2016;164:577–82.
50. Zaccardi F, O'Donovan G, Webb DR, Yates T, Kurl S, Khunti K, et al. Cardiorespiratory fitness and risk of type 2 diabetes mellitus: a 23-year cohort study and a meta-analysis of prospective studies. Atherosclerosis. 2015;243:131–7.

51. Carnethon MR, Sternfeld B, Schreiner PJ, Jacobs DR Jr, Lewis CE, Liu K, Sidney S. Association of 20-year changes in cardiorespiratory fitness with incident type 2 diabetes: the coronary artery risk development in young adults (CARDIA) fitness study. Diabetes Care. 2009;32:1284–8.
52. Momma H, Sawada SS, Lee IM, Gando Y, Kawakami R, Terada S, et al. Consistently high level of cardiorespiratory fitness and incidence of type 2 diabetes. Med Sci Sports Exerc. 2017;49:2048–55.
53. Holtermann A, Gyntelberg F, Bauman A, Thorsten Jensen M. Cardiorespiratory fitness, fatness and incident diabetes. Diabetes Res Clin Pract. 2017;134:113–20.
54. Sui X, Hooker SP, Lee IM, Church TS, Colabianchi N, Lee CD, et al. A prospective study of cardiorespiratory fitness and risk of type 2 diabetes in women. Diabetes Care. 2008;31:550–5.
55. Lee DC, Sui X, Lee IM, Church TS, Blair SN. Associations of cardiorespiratory fitness and obesity with risks of impaired fasting glucose and type 2 diabetes in men. Diabetes Care. 2009;32:257–62.
56. Eriksson KF, Lindgarde F. Prevention of type 2 (non-insulin-dependent) diabetes mellitus by diet and physical exercise. The 6-year Malmo feasibility study. Diabetologia. 1991;34:891–8.
57. Pan XR, Li GW, Hu YH, Wang JX, Yang WY, An ZX, et al. Effects of diet and exercise in preventing NIDDM in people with impaired glucose tolerance. The Da Qing IGT and Diabetes Study. Diabetes Care. 1997;20:537–44.
58. Gong Q, Gregg EW, Wang J, An Y, Zhang P, Yang W, Li H, et al. Long-term effects of a randomised trial of a 6-year lifestyle intervention in impaired glucose tolerance on diabetes-related microvascular complications: the China Da Qing Diabetes Prevention Outcome Study. Diabetologia. 2011;54:300–7.
59. Lindström J, Louheranta A, Mannelin M, Rastas M, Salminen V, Eriksson J, et al. The Finnish Diabetes Prevention Study (DPS): lifestyle intervention and 3-year results on diet and physical activity. Diabetes Care. 2003;26:3230–6.
60. Lindström J, Peltonen M, Eriksson JG, Ilanne-Parikka P, Aunola S, Keinänen-Kiukaanniemi S, et al., Finnish Diabetes Prevention Study (DPS). Improved lifestyle and decreased diabetes risk over 13 years: long-term follow-up of the randomised Finnish Diabetes Prevention Study (DPS). Diabetologia. 2013;56:284–93.
61. Knowler WC, Barrett-Connor E, Fowler SE, Hamman RF, Lachin JM, Walker EA, Nathan DM. Reduction in the incidence of type 2 diabetes with lifestyle intervention or metformin. N Engl J Med. 2002;346:393–403.
62. Knowler WC, Fowler SE, Hamman RF, et al. Diabetes Prevention Program Research Group. 10-year follow-up of diabetes incidence and weight loss in the Diabetes Prevention Program Outcomes Study. Lancet. 2009;374:1677–86.
63. Diabetes Prevention Program Research Group. Long-term effects of lifestyle intervention or metformin on diabetes development and microvascular complications over 15-year follow-up: the Diabetes Prevention Program Outcomes Study. Lancet Diabetes Endocrinol. 2015;3:866–75.
64. Perreault L, Pan Q, Mather KJ, Watson KE, Hamman RF, Kahn SE. Effect of regression from prediabetes to normal glucose regulation on long-term reduction in diabetes risk: results from the Diabetes Prevention Program Outcomes Study. Lancet. 2012;379:2243–51.
65. Tuomilehto J, Lindstrom J, Eriksson JG, Valle TT, Hamalainen H, Ilanne-Parikka P, et al. Prevention of type 2 diabetes mellitus by changes in lifestyle among subjects with impaired glucose tolerance. N Engl J Med. 2001;344:1343–50.
66. Ramachandran A, Snehalatha C, Mary S, Mukesh B, Bhaskar AD, Vijay V, Indian Diabetes Prevention Programme (IDPP). The Indian Diabetes Prevention Programme shows that lifestyle modification and metformin prevent type 2 diabetes in Asian Indian subjects with impaired glucose tolerance (IDPP-1). Diabetologia. 2006;49:289–97.
67. Malin SK, Braun B. Impact of metformin on exercise-induced metabolic adaptations to lower type 2 diabetes risk. Exerc Sport Sci Rev. 2016;44:4–11.
68. Li G, Zhang P, Wang J, An Y, Gong Q, Gregg EW, et al. Cardiovascular mortality, all-cause mortality, and diabetes incidence after lifestyle intervention for people with impaired glucose tolerance in the Da Qing Diabetes Prevention Study: a 23-year follow-up study. Lancet Diabetes Endocrinol. 2014;2:474–80.
69. McAuley PA, Artero EG, Sui X, Lavie CJ, Almeida MJ, Blair SN. Fitness, fatness, and survival in adults with prediabetes. Diabetes Care. 2014;37:529–36.
70. Nylen ES, Ni D, Myers J, Chang M, Plunkett MT, Kokkinos P. Cardiorespiratory fitness impact on all-cause mortality in prediabetic veterans. J Endocrinol Metab. 2015;5:215–9.
71. Tikanmäki M, Tammelin T, Vääräsmäki M, Sipola-Leppänen M, Miettola S, Pouta A, et al. Prenatal determinants of physical activity and cardiorespiratory fitness in adolescence – Northern Finland Birth Cohort 1986 study. BMC Public Health. 2017;17:346.
72. Shepherd E, Gomersall JC, Tieu J, Han S, Crowther CA, Middleton P. Combined diet and exercise interventions for preventing gestational diabetes mellitus. Cochrane Database Syst Rev. 2017;11:CD010443.
73. Wang C, Wei Y, Zhang X, Zhang Y, Xu Q, Sun Y, et al. A randomized clinical trial of exercise during pregnancy to prevent gestational diabetes mellitus and improve pregnancy outcome in overweight and obese pregnant women. Am J Obstet Gynecol. 2017;216:340–51.
74. Koivusalo SB, Rönö K, Klemetti MM, Roine RP, Lindström J, Erkkola M, et al. Gestational diabetes mellitus can be prevented by lifestyle intervention: the Finnish gestational diabetes prevention study

(RADIEL): a randomized controlled trial. Diabetes Care. 2016;39:24–30.
75. Schellenberg ES, Dryden DM, Vandermeer B, Ha C, Korownyk C. Lifestyle interventions for patients with and at risk for type 2 diabetes. Ann Intern Med. 2013;159:543–51.
76. Haw JS, Galaviz KI, Straus AN, Kowalski AJ, Magee MJ, Weber MB, et al. Long-term sustainability of diabetes prevention approaches: a systematic review and meta-analysis of randomized clinical trials. JAMA Intern Med. 2017;177:1808. https://doi.org/10.1001/jamainternmed.2017.6040.
77. Bellia A, Rizza S, Lombardo MF, et al. Deterioration of glucose homeostasis in type 2 diabetic patients one year after beginning of statins therapy. Atherosclerosis. 2012;223:197–203.
78. Carter AA, Gomes T, Camacho X, Juurlink DN, Shah BR, Mamdani MM. Risk of incident diabetes among patients treated with statins: population based study. BMJ. 2013;346:f2610.
79. Preiss D, Seshasai SR, Welsh P, et al. Risk of incident diabetes with intensive-dose compared with moderate-dose statin therapy: a meta-analysis. JAMA. 2011;305:2556–64.
80. Kokkinos PF, Faselis C, Myers J, Panagiotakos D, Doumas M. Interactive effects of fitness and statin treatment on mortality risk in veterans with dyslipidaemia: a cohort study. Lancet. 2013;381:394–9.
81. Nylen ES, Faselis C, Kheirbek R, Myers J, Panagiotakos D, Kokkinos P. Statins modulate the mortality risk associated with obesity and cardiorespiratory fitness in diabetics. J Clin Endocrinol Metab. 2013;98:3394–401.
82. Mikus CR, Boyle LJ, Borengasser SJ, et al. Simvastatin impairs exercise training adaptations. J Am Coll Cardiol. 2013;62:709–14.
83. Muraki A, Miyashita K, Mitsuishi M, Tamaki M, Tanaka K, Itoh H. Coenzyme Q10 reverses mitochondrial dysfunction in atorvastatin-treated mice and increases exercise endurance. J Appl Physiol. 2012;113:479–86.
84. Thompson PD, Panza G, Zaleski A, Taylor B. Statin-associated side effects. J Am Coll Cardiol. 2016;67:2395–410.
85. Franklin BA, Lavie CJ. Impact of statins on physical activity and fitness: ally or adversary? Mayo Clin Proc. 2015;90:1314–9.
86. Williams PT, Thompson PD. Effects of statin therapy on exercise levels in participants in the National Runners' and Walkers' health study. Mayo Clin Proc. 2015;90:1338–47.
87. Kokkinos P, Faselis C, Narayan P, Myers J, Nylen E, Sui X, et al. Cardiorespiratory fitness and incidence of type 2 diabetes in United States veterans on statin therapy. Am J Med. 2017;130:1192–8.
88. Praet SF, van Loon LJ. Exercise therapy in type 2 diabetes. Acta Diabetol. 2009;46:263–78.
89. Haffner SM, Lehto S, Ronnemaa T, Pyoala K, Laakso M. Mortality from coronary heart disease in subjects with type 2 diabetes and in non-diabetic subjects with and without prior myocardial infarction. N Engl J Med. 1998;339:229–34.
90. Church TS, Cheng YJ, Earnest CP, Barlow CE, Gibbons LW, et al. Exercise capacity and body composition as predictors of mortality among men with diabetes. Diabetes Care. 2004;27:83–8.
91. McAuley PA, Myers JN, Abella JP, Tan SY, Froelicher VF. Exercise capacity and body mass as predictors of mortality among male veterans with type 2 diabetes. Diabetes Care. 2007;30:1539–43.
92. Kokkinos P, Myers J, Nylen E, Panagiotakos DB, Manolis A, Pittaras A, et al. Exercise capacity and all-cause mortality in African American and Caucasian men with type 2 diabetes. Diabetes Care. 2009;32:623–8.
93. Nylen ES, Kokkinos P, Myers J, Faselis C. Prognostic effect of exercise capacity on mortality in older adults with diabetes mellitus. J Am Geriatr Soc. 2010;58:1850–4.
94. Schneider SH, Amorosa LF, Khachadurian AK, Ruderman NB. Studies on the mechanism of improved glucose control during regular exercise in type 2 (non-insulin-dependent) diabetes. Diabetologia. 1984;26:355.
95. Mayer-Davis EJ, D'Agostino R Jr, Karter AJ, Haffner SM, Rewers MJ, Saad M, Bergman RN. Intensity and amount of physical activity in relation to insulin sensitivity: the Insulin Resistance Atherosclerosis Study. JAMA. 1998;279:669–74.
96. Boule NG, Haddad E, Kenny GP, Wells GA, Sigal RJ. Effects of exercise on glycemic control and body mass in type 2 diabetes mellitus; a meta-analysis of controlled clinical trials. JAMA. 2001;286:1218–27.
97. Winnick JJ. Short-term aerobic exercise training in obese humans with type 2 diabetes mellitus improves whole-body insulin sensitivity through gains in peripheral, not hepatic insulin sensitivity. J Clin Endocrinol Metab. 2008;93:771–8.
98. Boule NG, Kenny GP, Haddad E, Wells GA, Sigal RJ. Meta-analysis of the effects of structured exercise training on cardiorespiratory fitness in type 2 diabetes mellitus. Diabetologia. 2003;46:1071–81.
99. The Look AHEAD Research Group. Cardiovascular effects of intensive lifestyle intervention in type 2 diabetes. New Engl J Med. 2013;369:145–54.
100. Look AHEAD Research Group, Gregg EW, Jakicic JM, Blackburn G, Bloomquist P, Bray GA, Clark JM, et al. Association of the magnitude of weight loss and changes in physical fitness with long-term cardiovascular disease outcomes in overweight or obese people with type 2 diabetes: a post-hoc analysis of the Look AHEAD randomised clinical trial. Lancet Diabetes Endocrinol. 2016;4:913–21.
101. Jakicic JM, Jaramillo SA, Balasubramanyam A, Bancroft B, Curtis JM, Mathews A, Pereira M, Regensteiner JG, Ribisl PM, Look AHEAD Study Group. Effect of a lifestyle intervention on change in cardiorespiratory fitness in adults with type 2 diabetes: results from the Look AHEAD Study. Int J Obes. 2009;33:305–16.

102. Kokkinos P, Faselis C, Myers J, Sui X, Zhang J, Blair SN. Age-specific exercise capacity threshold for mortality risk assessment in male veterans. Circulation. 2014;130:653–8.
103. Jakicic JM, Egan CM, Fabricatore AN, Gaussoin SA, Glasser SP, Hesson LA, Knowler WC, Lang W, et al. Four-year change in cardiorespiratory fitness and influence on glycemic control in adults with type 2 diabetes in a randomized trial: the Look AHEAD Trial. Diabetes Care. 2013;36:1297–303.
104. Kerns JC, Guo J, Fothergill E, Howard L, Knuth ND, Brychta R, Chen KY, Skarulis MC, Walter PJ, Hall KD. Increased physical activity associated with less weight regain six years after "the biggest loser" competition. Obesity (Silver Spring). 2017;25:1838–43.
105. Johansen MY, MacDonald CS, Hansen KB, Karstoft K, Christensen R, Pedersen M, et al. Effect of an intensive lifestyle intervention on glycemic control in patients with type 2 diabetes a randomized clinical trial. JAMA. 2017;318:637–46.
106. Jang HC. Sarcopenia, frailty, and diabetes in older adults. Diabetes Metab J. 2016;40:182–9.
107. Vandervoort AA. Aging of the human neuromuscular system. Muscle Nerve. 2002;25:17–25.
108. Park SW, Goodpaster BH, Strotmeyer ES, et al. Decreased muscle strength and quality in older adults with type 2 diabetes: the health, aging, and body composition study. Diabetes. 2006;55:1813–8.
109. Seok WP, Goodpaster BH, Jung SL, et al. Excessive loss of skeletal muscle mass in older adults with type 2 diabetes. Diabetes Care. 2009;32:1993–7.
110. Womack L, Peters D, Barrett EJ, Kaul S, Price W, Lindner JR. Abnormal skeletal muscle capillary recruitment during exercise in patients with type 2 diabetes mellitus and microvascular complications. J Am Coll Cardiol. 2009;53:2175–83.
111. Hovanec N, Sawant A, Overend TJ, Petrella RJ, Vandervoort AA. Resistance training and older adults with type 2 diabetes mellitus: strength of the evidence. J Aging Res. 2012;2012:284635.
112. Castaneda C, Layne JE, Munoz-Orians L, Gordon PL, Walsmith J, Foldvari M, Roubenoff R, Tucker KL, Nelson ME. A randomized controlled trial of resistance exercise training to improve glycemic control in older adults with type 2 diabetes. Diabetes Care. 2002;25:2335–41.
113. Brooks N, Layne JE, Gordon PL, Roubenoff R, Nelson ME, Castaneda-Sceppa C. Strength training improves muscle quality and insulin sensitivity in Hispanic older adults with type 2 diabetes. Int J Med Sci. 2007;4:19–27.
114. Dunstan DW, Daly RM, Owen N. High-intensity resistance training improves glycemic control in older patients with type 2 diabetes. Diabetes Care. 2002;25:1729–36.
115. Pesta DH, Goncalves RLS, Madiraju AK, Strasser B, Sparks LM. Resistance training to improve type 2 diabetes: working toward a prescription for the future. Nutr Metab. 2017;14:24. https://doi.org/10.1186/s12986-017-0173-7.
116. Sigal RJ, Kenny GP, Boulé NG, Wells GA, Prud'homme D, Fortier M, et al. Effects of aerobic training, resistance training, or both on glycemic control in type 2 diabetes: a randomized trial. Ann Intern Med. 2007;147:357–69.
117. Church TS, Blair SN, Cocreham S, Johannsen N, Johnson W, Kramer K, et al. Effects of aerobic and resistance training on hemoglobin a1c levels in patients with type 2 diabetes: a randomized controlled trial. JAMA. 2010;304:2253–62.
118. American Diabetes Association. 4. Lifestyle management. Diabetes Care. 2017;40(suppl1):s33–43.
119. Aguiar EJ, Morgan PJ, Collins CE, Plotnikoff RC, Callister R. Efficacy of interventions that include diet, aerobic and resistance training components for type 2 diabetes prevention: a systematic review with meta-analysis. Int J Behav Nutr Phys Act. 2014;11:2. https://doi.org/10.1186/1479-5868-11-2.
120. Dempsey PC, Larsen RN, Sethi P, Sacre JW, Straznicky NE, Cohen ND, et al. Benefits for Type 2 diabetes of interrupting prolonged sitting with brief bouts of light walking or simple resistance activities. Diabetes Care. 2016;39:964–72.
121. Winding KM, Munch GW, Iepsen UW, Van Hall G, Pedersen BK, Mortensen SP. The effect of low-volume high-intensity interval training versus endurance training on glycemic control in individuals with type 2 diabetes. Diabetes Obes Metab. 2017;20:1131. https://doi.org/10.1111/dom.13198.
122. Jelleyman C, Yates T, O'Donovan G, Gray LJ, King JA, Khunti J, Davies MJ. The effect of high intensity interval training on glucose regulation and insulin resistance; a meta analysis. Obes Rev. 2015;16:942–61.
123. Stephens NA, Sparks LM. Resistance to the beneficial effects of exercise in type 2 diabetes: are some individuals programmed to fail? J Clin Endocrinol Metab. 2015;100:43.
124. Williams CJ, Williams MG, Eynon N, Ashton KJ, Little JP, Wisloff U, Coombes JS. Genes to predict VO2max trainability: a systematic review. BMC Genomics. 2017;18(Suppl 8):831. https://doi.org/10.1186/s12864-017-4192-6.
125. Sattar N, Preiss D, Murray HM, Welsh P, Buckley BM, de Craen AJ, et al. Statins and risk of incident diabetes: a collaborative meta-analysis of randomised statin trials. Lancet. 2010;375:735–42.
126. Allard NAE, Schirris TJJ, Verheggen RJ, Russel FGM, Rodenburg RJ, Smeitink JAM, et al. Statins affect skeletal muscle performance: evidence for disturbances in energy metabolism. J Clin Endocrinol Metab. 2018;103:75–84.
127. Bahls M, Groß S, Ittermann T, Busch R, Gläser S, Ewert R, et al. Statins are related to impaired exercise capacity in males but not females. PLoS One. 2017;12(6):e0179534.
128. Nylén ES, Faselis C, Kheirbek R, Myers J, Panagiotakos D, Kokkinos P. Statins modulate the mortality risk associated with obesity and cardiorespiratory fitness in diabetics. J Clin Endocrinol Metab. 2013;98:3394–401.

129. Kelley DE, He J, Menshikova EV, Ritov VB. Dysfunction of mitochondria in human skeletal muscle in type 2 diabetes. Diabetes. 2002;51:2944–50.
130. Radice M, Rocca A, Bedon E, Musacchio N, Morabito A, Segalini G. Abnormal response to exercise in middle-aged NIDDM patients with and without autonomic neuropathy. Diabet Med. 1996;13:259–65.
131. Joshi D, Shiwalkar A, Cross MR, Sharma SK, Vachhani A, Dutt C. Continuous, non-invasive measurement of the haemodynamic response to submaximal exercise in patients with diabetes mellitus: evidence of impaired cardiac reserve and peripheral vascular response. Heart. 2010;96:36–41.
132. Mendes R, Sousa N, Reis VM, Themudo-Barata JL. Prevention of exercise-related injuries and adverse events in patients with type 2 diabetes. Postgrad Med J. 2013;89(1058):715–21.
133. Courties A, Sellam J. Osteoarthritis and type 2 diabetes mellitus: what are the links? Diabetes Res Clin Pract. 2016;122:198–206.
134. Mortuza R, Chakrabarti S. Glucose-induced cell signalling in the pathogenesis of diabetic cardiomyopathy. Heart Fail Rev. 2014;19:75–86.
135. Jia G, DeMarco VG, Sowers JR. Insulin resistance and hyperinsulinaemia in diabetic cardiomyopathy. Nat Rev Endocrinol. 2016;12:144–53.
136. Wong CY, O'Moore-Sullivan T, Leano R, Byrne BE, Marwick TH. Alterations of left ventricular myocardial characteristics associated with obesity. Circulation. 2004;110:3081–7.
137. Jewiss D, Ostman C, King N, Smart NA. Clinical outcomes to exercise training in type 1 diabetes: a systematic review and meta-analysis. Diabetes Res Clin Pract. 2017. https://doi.org/10.1016/j.diabres.2017.11.036.
138. Morris JN, Heady JA, Raffle PA, Roberts CG, Parks JW. Coronary heart-disease and physical activity of work. Lancet. 1953;265:1053–7.
139. Hoffman NJ, Parker BL, Chaudhuri R, Fisher-Wellman KH, Kleinert M, et al. Global phosphoproteomic analysis of human skeletal muscle reveals a network of exercise-regulated kinases and AMPK substrates. Cell Metab. 2015;22:922–35.
140. Sparks LM. Exercise training response heterogeneity: physiological and molecular insights. Diabetologia. 2017;60:2329–36.
141. https://commonfund.nih.gov/MolecularTransducers.
142. Ross R, Blair SN, Arena R, Church TS, Després JP, et al., American Heart Association Physical Activity Committee of the Council on Lifestyle and Cardiometabolic Health; Council on Clinical Cardiology; Council on Epidemiology and Prevention; Council on Cardiovascular and Stroke Nursing; Council on Functional Genomics and Translational Biology; Stroke Council. Importance of assessing cardiorespiratory fitness in clinical practice: a case for fitness as a clinical vital sign: a scientific statement from the American Heart Association. Circulation. 2016;134(13):e653–99.
143. Sinharay R, Gong J, Barratt B, Ohman-Strickland P, Ernst S, Kelly F, et al. Respiratory and cardiovascular responses to walking down a traffic-polluted road compared with walking in a traffic-free area in participants aged 60 years and older with chronic lung or heart disease and age-matched healthy controls: a randomised, crossover study. Lancet. 2018;391:339–49.
144. American Diabetes Association. Economic costs of diabetes in the U.S. in 2017. Diabetes Care. 2018. https://doi.org/10.2337/dci18-0007.
145. Myers J, Doom R, King R, Fonda H, Chan K, Kokkinos P, Rehkopf DH. Association between cardiorespiratory fitness and health care costs: the veterans exercise testing study. Mayo Clin Proc. 2018;93(1):48–55. https://doi.org/10.1016/j.mayocp.2017.09.019.
146. Wahl MP, Scalzo RL, Regensteiner JG, Reusch JEB. Mechanisms of aerobic exercise impairment in diabetes: a narrative review. Front Endocrinol. 2018;9:181. https://doi.org/10.3389/fendo.2018.00181.

12 Cardiorespiratory Fitness, Physical Activity, and Metabolic Syndrome

Eric S. Nylén, Shruti M. Gandhi, and Raj Lakshman

Abbreviations

ACC	Acetyl-CoA carboxylase
AHA	American Heart Association
AMPK	Adenosine 5′ monophosphate-activated protein kinase
ATP	Adenosine triphosphate
BP	Blood pressure
CRF	Cardiorespiratory fitness
CVD	Cardiovascular disease
DM2	Type 2 diabetes
DPP	Diabetes Prevention Program
GLUT-4	Glucose transporter 4
HAT	Histone acetyltransferase
HIIT	High-intensity interval training
HTN	Hypertension
IDF	International Diabetes Federation
IL-6	Interleukin-6
MAP	Mitogen-activated protein
MS	Metabolic syndrome
NHANES	National Health and Nutritional Examination Survey
NNT	Numbers needed to treat
P13K	Phosphoinositide 3-kinase
PGC1α	Peroxisome proliferator receptor coactivator 1-alpha
PPAR α	Peroxisome proliferator-activated receptor alpha
PPAR β	Peroxisome proliferator receptor coactivator 1-beta
SIRT1	Sirtuin-1
SREB1c	Sterol regulatory element-binding proteins 1c
TNF-alpha	Tumor necrosis factor-alpha

E. S. Nylén (✉)
Department of Endocrinology, VAMC and George Washington University School of Medicine, Washington, DC, USA
e-mail: Eric.Nylen@va.gov

S. M. Gandhi
Department of Endocrinology, Washington D.C. VA Medical Center, Washington, DC, USA

R. Lakshman
Veterans Affairs Medical Center and George Washington University School of Medicine, Washington, DC, USA

Introduction

Metabolic syndrome (MS) refers to a clustering of physiologic, metabolic, and biochemical factors increasing the risk of cardiovascular disease (CVD) and type 2 diabetes (DM2). This syndrome has undergone diagnostic iterations by several societies, the most recent being the International Diabetes Federation (IDF) in conjunction with the American Heart Association (AHA) which in 2009 proposed a consensus for diagnosis which includes the presence of three of the following: (1) elevated waist circumference (population and country-specific definitions), (2) elevated triglycerides ≥150 mg/dl, (3) decreased

P. Kokkinos, P. Narayan (eds.), *Cardiorespiratory Fitness in Cardiometabolic Diseases*,
https://doi.org/10.1007/978-3-030-04816-7_12

HDL <40 mg/dL in men and <50 mg/dL in women, (4) elevated BP ≥ 130/85 mm Hg, or (5) elevated fasting glucose ≥100 mg/dl [1]. The early origins of an association of metabolic consequences related to lifestyle were proposed in 1923 by Kylin consisting of a syndrome of hypertension (HTN), hyperglycemia, obesity, and hyperuricemia [2]. Himsworth introduced the concept insulin resistance (IR) in 1936 [3] and the role of "androgenic obesity" contributing to diabetes, and CVD was proposed by Vague in 1940 [4]. However, the term as used currently originated in 1988, when Reaven gave the Banting lecture and coined the term Syndrome X, later renamed MS, to describe the role of IR as the driver of atherosclerotic dyslipidemia, DM2, HTN, and obesity [5].

Metabolic syndrome constitutes a considerable healthcare challenge estimated to affect 25% of the population worldwide and continues to rise. According to the National Health and Nutrition Examination Survey (NHANES), the prevalence of MS among US adults aged 18 years or older has increased from approximately 25% during the 1999–2006 period to 34.2% in 2007–2012 period [6]. MS significantly impacts healthcare outcomes and is associated with an approximate increased risk of CVD (twofold), DM2 (fivefold), stroke (two- to fourfold), myocardial infarction (three- to fourfold), and all-cause mortality [7]. It is also associated with increased risk of certain forms of cancer, polycystic ovarian disease, nonalcoholic fatty liver disease, and neurodegeneration. It is important to point out that certain groups tend to have an increased risk of developing MS, such as Caucasian males, African-American women, the elderly, or being of low socioeconomic status. Although we are in the midst of an obesity and diabetes epidemic and MS has received ICD-10 disease status (i.e., E88.81), this diagnosis does not give rise to unique treatment options, it has no unique genetic associations, and it is certainly not without its detractors [8] including those of Reaven [9, 10]. Considering that the incidence of MS has been shown to be inversely proportional to cardiorespiratory fitness (CRF), and that all-cause and CVD mortality are associated with CRF in MS, this chapter will explore these associations [11, 12].

Pathophysiology

Metabolic syndrome is a complex condition with underlying IR and impaired adipose tissue fuel handling at its core. Insulin resistance was recognized as far back as 1936 by Himsworth [3] soon after the introduction of insulin therapy to describe the occasional need for large doses of insulin to control hyperglycemia, but it was more formally defined by Yalow and Berson following the successful measurement of insulin itself as "a state in which a greater than normal amount of insulin is required to elicit a quantitatively normal response" [13], mainly occurring in the adipose, muscle, and liver. The nature of IR is complex and still not fully understood, but it occurs in a spectrum of obesity-related clinical conditions. A 2009 Joint Scientific Statement from the AHA stated that "most persons with the MS have abdominal obesity and IR. Both of the latter conditions appear to contribute to the development of metabolic risk factors, although the mechanisms underlying these contributions are not fully understood" [1].

Normally, insulin binds to its receptor leading to tyrosine phosphorylation of downstream substrates and activation of the phosphoinositide 3-kinase (PI3K) pathway and the mitogen-activated protein (MAP) kinase pathway. The former pathway is affected in IR, while the MAP kinase pathway functions normally. Subnormal PI3K-Akt activity leads to a reduction in endothelial nitric oxide formation and endothelial dysfunction, reduction in glucose transporter 4 (GLUT4) translocation, and decreased skeletal muscle and fat glucose uptake [14]. Concurrently, the persistence of MAP kinase activity results in augmented expression of endothelin-1 and endothelial adhesion molecules with vascular smooth muscle cell mitogenesis which leads to vascular abnormalities and increased atherosclerosis risk.

Glucose utilization during exercise is modulated by the intensity of exercise. Exercise intensities greater than 50% of maximal aerobic capacity (VO_2 max) in most people (75% of VO_2 max in highly trained athletes) favor glucose over free fatty acids (FFA) as the predominant substrate to meet the energy demands of the working muscles. Physical work or exercise disrupts the euglycemic state at rest achieved by the interaction of three hormones: insulin, glucagon, and catecholamines. As glucose demands increase with exercise, blood glucose concentrations decrease. This decreases the release of insulin from islet cells while glucagon increases, resulting in an increase in hepatic glycogen degradation (glycogenolysis). This, along with gluconeogenesis from substrates such as lactate, pyruvate, amino acids, and glycerol, assures adequate blood glucose concentrations (Fig. 12.1). Glucose uptake by the working myocytes is now enhanced by the increased concentrations of catecholamines. Conversely, the energy demands of the working muscles during prolonged exercise of low to moderate intensities, referred to as aerobic, are met predominantly by FFA with glucose and other substrates playing a secondary role.

Regularly performed aerobic exercises of adequate intensity (low to moderate) and volume result in a more efficient use of energy and enhance the capacity of metabolic tissues to switch between substrates in order to meet their metabolic demands (from ATP) depending on nutrient availability and energy demands. The capacity of the organism to adapt fuel oxidation to fuel availability is referred to as metabolic flexibility. The inability to modify fuel oxidation in response to changes in nutrient availability has been implicated in the accumulation of intramyocellular lipid and IR [15]. Reversal of IR by exercise stimulates lipid hydrolysis and oxidation and improves metabolic flexibility [15].

Notable changes with exercise include quantity and quality of mitochondria, enhanced mitochondrial electron transport chain, and fatty acid oxidation enzyme activities within skeletal muscle (see the chapter by Dr. Gidlund). Exercise also increases the number of "slow-twitch" muscle fibers and the development of vascularization via de novo muscle capillaries [16]. On a cellular level, glucose transport is achieved by insulin (via PI3K) and also by muscle contraction or hypoxia (via 5′AMP-activated protein kinase) [17]. Insulin-responsive GLUT4 shows increased mobilization from intracellular stores to the cell surface, resulting in increased glucose uptake and insulin sensitivity (Fig. 12.1). Whole-body utilization of glucose encompasses both mitochondrial glucose oxidation and non-oxidative glycogen synthesis, both of which are reduced in those with IR. Interestingly, non-oxidative glucose disposal appears to be more responsive to exercise training in subjects with early stages of DM2 which may pertain to MS [18].

Additional abnormalities associated with IR include FFA excess as well as low-grade inflammation (i.e., elevated IL-6, CRP, uric acid): the latter is observed in fat, muscle, liver, pancreatic islets, and nutrient-transporting blood [19]. Paradoxically, contracting skeletal muscle during exercise produces IL-6, which in this context has anti-inflammatory properties [20].

Adipocyte fuel malfunction manifests as adipocyte hypertrophy and ectopic lipid deposition in vital organs such as the liver, pancreas, muscle, and heart by means of abnormal transcriptional control. Energy deficit following acute or long-term exercise contributes to increased post-exercise insulin sensitivity which also stimulates a host of transcription factors. Fat synthesis is regulated by lipogenic genes (via sterol regulatory element-binding proteins 1c [SREBP1c]), whereas fat oxidation is regulated by fatty acid oxidation genes (via peroxisome proliferator-activated receptor alpha [PPARα]). Significantly, SREBP1c and PPARα are tightly controlled by peroxisome proliferator-activated receptor beta (PGC1β) and alpha (PGC1α), respectively. Sirtuin-1(SIRT1), the eukaryotic equivalent of SIR2 gene in prokaryotes, is an NAD-dependent deacetylase (histone deacetylase-HDAC) that has been linked to many beneficial effects of cellular processes including IR, glucose homeostasis, fatty acid metabolism, gene silencing, and aging [21]. SIRT1 activates PGC1α by deacetylation, which in concert with PPARα increases fatty acid oxidation. In contrast, histone acetyltransferase (HAT) has just the opposite effects. Thus, SIRT1 and HAT play dynamic roles in regulating the functional forms of SREBP1c and PGC1α.

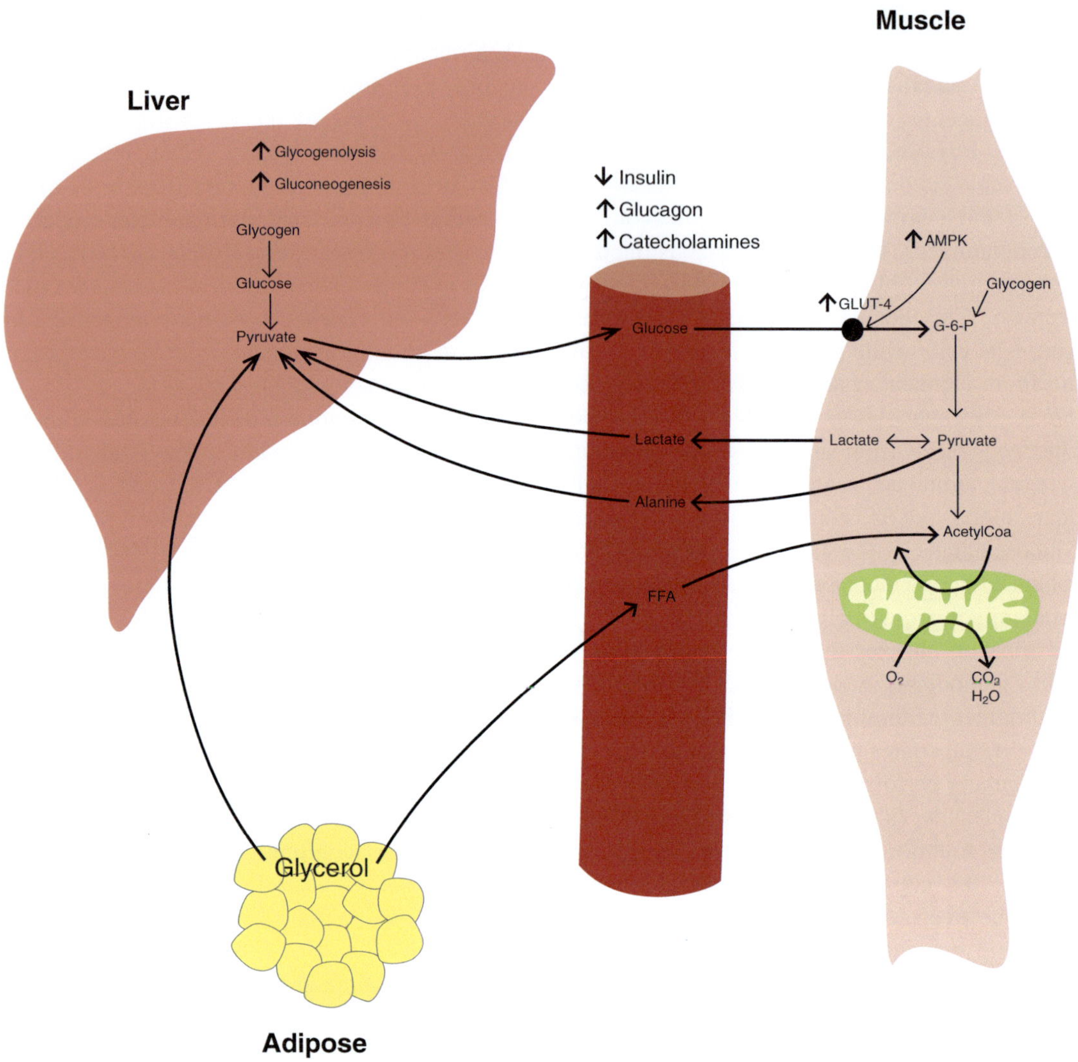

Fig. 12.1 Schematic outline of glucose utilization by muscle during exercise. Important features include the change in insulin, glucagon, and catecholamines as shown which stimulates liver glycogenolysis and gluconeogenesis and adipose lipolysis. There is a lack of glucose-6-phosphatase in muscle, and this compound stays in muscle such that blood levels of glucose cannot be provided from muscle. Increased AMP activates the master metabolic switch AMPKinase, and exercise, independent of insulin, stimulates the insertion of GLUT4 via AMPK. Note that GLUT4 is both insulin and exercise sensitive, and these two pathways are additive. In general, the intensity and duration of exercise determines the source(s) of energy fuels. Fat sources (intramuscular triglycerides and plasma free fatty acids) provides the primary fuel for exercise of low intensity while carbohydrates (muscle glycogen and and blood glucose) provides the fuel at higher intensities. Long-term training often increases fat utilization via greater oxidation of fats from intramuscular sources. Protein such alanine provides a small amount of energy during prolonged exercise

Whereas SIRT1 destabilizes SREBP1c by deacetylation, HAT stabilizes SREBP1c by acetylation. On the other hand, SIRT1 activates PGC1α by deacetylation, while HAT inactivates PGC1α by acetylation. Significantly, high fat activates P38 MAPK by phosphorylation, which inactivates PGC1α or stabilizes SREBP1c by activating HAT. Thus, activation/inactivation of

PGC1β, in concert with SREBP1c, would regulate lipid synthesis, while activation/inactivation of PGC1α, in concert with PPARα, would regulate lipid oxidation. Thus, transcriptional coactivators PGC1α, PGC1β, as well as SREBPs play vital roles in regulating the lipid-oxidizing and lipogenic genes and thereby control the progression of obesity and MS.

Similarly, adenosine 5′ monophosphate-activated protein kinase (AMPK) plays dynamic role, regulating a multitude of critical pathways in lipid metabolism [22]. AMPK is a metabolic, stress-sensing enzyme that is activated by exercise (i.e., a high AMP:ATP ratio) and inhibited (i.e., a low AMP:ATP ratio) by physical inactivity. AMPK is activated by phosphorylation, which then inactivates the key lipogenic enzyme acetyl-CoA carboxylase (ACC), leading to decreased synthesis of malonyl-CoA and long-chain fatty acids and their subsequent esterification to form triacylglycerol. This lipogenic pathway is under tight dietary and hormonal regulation. Thus, exercise and associated energy deprivation shut off fat synthesis, whereas high caloric intake (as in a high-carbohydrate, fat-free diet) induces this pathway. Moreover, one could expect the lipogenic pathway to be blocked with a low malonyl-CoA/long-chain acyl-CoAs ratio, as found during caloric restriction and possibly after exercise, whereas the mitochondrial pathway should be blocked by a high malonyl-CoA/long-chain acyl-CoAs ratio, as encountered during increased caloric intake and a sedentary lifestyle.

Adipocyte fuel malfunction is also indicated by abnormal levels of adipokines that show a strong association with MS, including elevated leptin, plasminogen activator inhibitor-1, retinol-binding protein-4, chemerin, interleukin-1, interleukin-6, interleukin-8, lipopolysaccharide, and fetuin-A, and decreased adiponectin and omentin-1. The strongest influence appears to be changes in adiponectin, adipocyte fatty acid-binding protein, chemerin, and fibroblast growth factor 21 [23]. Another common adipocyte feature of MS is the elevated triglyceride and decreased HDL ratio that can predict CVD comparable to the MS criteria [24].

MS, Physical Activity, and IR

Insulin resistance is strongly suspected to be the pathophysiologic link between the metabolic abnormalities associated with MS [25]. According to Reaven adiposity and physical fitness explain approximately half of the variability in insulin action, with genetic differences likely to account for the other half [26]. Indeed, repeated exercise bouts (exercise-training) have been demonstrated to increase GLUT4 concentrations in populations with MS, and the salutary response may be reflected in increased VO2max and related to the dose of exercise [27]. However, in the absence of weight loss, IR did not change in some studies despite improvements in GLUT4 and mitochondrial parameters [28]. There is also evidence to support that high-intensity interval training (HIIT) or sprint interval training (SIT) may result in greater improvement in insulin sensitivity and pancreatic beta cell function observed with increased CRF [29]. This response is consistent with the concept that exercise-induced adaptations are specific to the demand imposed by exercise, since both HIIT and SIT modes of exercise challenge the anaerobic pathways more so than low to moderate intensity exercise.

Prevention of Metabolic Syndrome

The emergence of new-onset MS is sensitive to lifestyle intervention including exercise and dietary modulations as well as to pharmacological agents that impact glucose status. Lifestyle that includes increases in physical activity appears to be necessary to favorably modify the cluster of the risk factors associated with MS. In the Diabetes Prevention Program (DPP), 53% of the participants had MS. In participants in the lifestyle intervention group that included aerobic exercise 150 min per week and nutritional counseling (participants experienced 7% weight loss), there was a 41% reduction of new onset of MS and 38% reversal of MS [30]. In contrast, treatment with metformin only reduced new cases of MS by 17%. In addition, the progression to DM2 in the exercise-arm of DPP was considerably higher in those with MS compared to baseline subjects with IGT. In comparison, in the ATTICA study, adherence to the Mediterranean diet was associated with a 29% lower risk of all MS components [31]. Similarly, a meta-analysis of 50 studies ($n = 534{,}906$) revealed that adherence to Mediterranean dietary patterns was associated with lower MS prevalence and progression [32]. Finally, in the STOP-NIDDM trial using the anti-hyperglycemic agent acarbose (an alpha-glucosidase inhibitor), 61% had MS at baseline, and the NNT to prevent DM2 was 5.6 compared to 16.5 without baseline MS [33].

Physical Activity, CRF, and MS

Increased physical activity and structured exercise programs have been recognized as a cornerstone in both the prevention and treatment of chronic diseases related to IR and MS. Thus, high levels of PA and/or CRF are associated with reduced prevalence of cardiometabolic risk factors associated with MS including hypertension, hyperlipidemia, inflammation, and IR and lower incident rates of MS itself. The impact of CRF on the risk of MS is also considered a strong metabolic risk factor, independent of obesity [34]. Low CRF is associated with increased MS-related morbidity and mortality regardless of body weight [12, 35]. Thus, poor CRF itself appears to be a feature of MS expression [36, 37].

Two meta-analyses using self-reported PA questionnaires reported lower incidence of MS in subjects with moderate or high levels of leisure-time PA compared to low levels [38, 39]. For example, there was a reduction of 8% in MS risk per ten metabolic equivalent of task (MET) hours/week increment [40]. Likewise, MS risk was 32–53% lower across age groups in those who were fit compared to those that were unfit [41]. Reduced daily PA in healthy young adults was associated with decreased insulin sensitivity and increased abdominal fat [42].

Cardiorespiratory fitness, assessed objectively by standardized exercise protocols, was strongly and inversely associated with MS in both men and women, with the strongest association to lower waist circumference and fasting glucose [43]. Moreover, measured PA by energy expenditure had a stronger association to MS than did measured VO_2 max, especially in those that were considered unfit (by VO2max), who therefore would benefit more from PA than fit subjects [44]. When PA pattern was measured using accelerometry, similar findings showed independent association of various levels of PA to MS prevalence after controlling for fitness [45]. In a study following the development of MS over 4 years, the highest risk group were those who were sedentary and unfit by CRF standards [46]. Engaging in PA >3 h/week vs 1 h/week reduced the risk of MS by 50% independent of BMI and other confounders.

Type of Exercise and MS

Aerobic exercise of individuals with MS improves hemodynamics by reducing diastolic blood pressure, systemic vascular resistances, and the so-called double product (the product of systolic blood pressure and heart rate) [47]. Likewise, resistance training can favorably impact metabolic parameters such as dysglycemia, dyslipidemia, and blood pressure. In a 4-year study, meeting the guidelines for resistance training alone lowered the risk of developing MS by 17%, and performing less than 1 h of resistance exercise/week lowered the risk of MS by 25%. However, larger volumes of resistance training did not yield additional benefits [48]. In a meta- analysis, aerobic exercise and/or combined exercise and resistance training both improved all MS components, but in some studies, the combined approach was less efficacious [49]. Thus, combined aerobic and resistance exercise was no more effective than aerobic exercise alone, but randomized studies reveal an advantage of the combined approach [50]. Resistance exercise alone may or may not change MS status, but it may help reduce systolic blood pressure levels and/or mortality related to stroke or heart disease in MS as shown in other studies [51]. More recently, low-volume (i.e., 51 min/week) high-intensity interval training (HIIT) has been shown to be as effective as high-volume HIIT (i.e., 114 min/week) and traditional moderate intensity exercise (i.e., 150 min/week) in ameliorating MS severity [52]. However, improvements in insulin dynamics as measured by proinsulin were responsive only to higher-volume HIIT [53].

Summary

The MS concept is a clinical construct centered on insulin resistance attributed to Dr. Reaven [54]. It is clearly evident that increased physical activity and CRF have a favorable effect on all MS components and can attenuate the MS epidemic. CRF interacts strongly with MS expression, and a sedentary state and low CRF have been suggested to be included in the definition of MS. Thus, implementation of lifestyle measures to enhance physical fitness can be adapted by clinicians and other healthcare professional to prevent, attenuate, and even reverse the MS rate. In most studies, aerobic exercise appears to be the most efficacious approach to improve dysglycemia, dyslipidemia, and elevated blood pressure. In addition, some studies also show that resistance training has a favorable impact on components of MS. Although not seen in all studies, the combination of aerobic with resistance activity can be additive. Alternative approaches such as HIIT can positively modulate MS although high-intensity exercises may not be easily tolerated by middle-aged and older individuals burdened with comorbidities and can be associated with an increase in the risk of injury and even death. Finally, although measured peak fitness plays an important role vis-à-vis MS, all aspects of physical activity need to be assessed, and the deleterious impact of being sedentary (i.e., minimal muscular contractile inactivity) as an independent contributor to metabolic dysfunction and health risk needs to be recognized [55].

References

1. CDC. https://www.cdc.gov/pcd/issues/2017/16_0287.htm.
2. Alberti KG, Eckel RH, Grundy SM, Zimmet PZ, Cleeman JI, Donato KA, et al. Harmonizing the metabolic syndrome: a joint interim statement of the International Diabetes Federation Task Force on Epidemiology and Prevention; National Heart, Lung, and Blood Institute; American Heart Association; World Heart Federation; International Atherosclerosis Society; and International Association for the Study of Obesity International Diabetes Federation Task Force on Epidemiology and Prevention., National Heart, Lung, and Blood Institute., American Heart Association., World Heart Federation., International Atherosclerosis Society., International Association for the Study of Obesity. Circulation. 2009;120(16):1640–5.
3. Kylin E. Studien über das Hypertonie-Hyperglykämie-Hyperurikämiesyndrom. Zentralblatt für Innere Medizin. 1923;44:105–27. 5–9.
4. Himsworth HP. Diabetes mellitus: its differentiation into insulin-sensitive and insulin-insensitive types. Lancet. 1936;i:127–30.
5. Vague J. The degree of masculine differentiation of obesities. Am J Clin Nutr. 1956;4:20–34.
6. Reaven GM. Banting lecture 1988. Role of insulin resistance in human disease. Diabetes. 1988;37(12):1595–607.
7. Wilson PW, D'Agostino RB, Parise H, Sullivan L, Meigs JB. Metabolic syndrome as a precursor of cardiovascular disease and type 2 diabetes mellitus. Circulation. 2005;112(20):3066–72.
8. Meigs JB. Insulin resistance syndrome? Syndrome X? Multiple metabolic syndrome? A syndrome at all? Factor analysis reveals patterns in the fabric of correlated metabolic risk factors. Am J Epidemiol. 2000;152(10):908–11.
9. Salazar MR, Carbajal HA, Espeche WG, Dulbecco CA, Aizpurúa M, Marillet AG, et al. Relationships among insulin resistance, obesity, diagnosis of the metabolic syndrome and cardio-metabolic risk. Diab Vasc Dis Res. 2011;2:109–16.
10. Reaven GM. The metabolic syndrome: time to get off the merry-go-round? J Intern Med. 2011;269(2):127–36.
11. LaMonte MJ, Barlow CE, Jurca R, Kampert JB, Church TS, Blair SN. Cardiorespiratory fitness is inversely associated with the incidence of metabolic

syndrome: a prospective study of men and women. Circulation. 2005;112:505–12.
12. Katzmarzyk PT, Church TS, Blair SN. Cardiorespiratory fitness attenuates the effects of the metabolic syndrome on all-cause and cardiovascular disease mortality in men. Arch Intern Med. 2004;164:1092–7.
13. Yalow RS, Berson SA. Plasma insulin concentrations in nondiabetic and early diabetic subjects. Determinations by a new sensitive immuno-assay technique. Diabetes. 1960;9:254–60.
14. Sylow L, Kleinert M, Richter EA, Jensen TE. Exercise-stimulated glucose uptake regulation and implications for glycaemic control. Nat Rev Endocrinol. 2017;13:133.
15. Goodpaster BH, Sparks LM. Metabolic flexibility in health and disease. Cell Metab. 2017;25(5):1027–36.
16. Olfert IM, Baum O, Hellsten Y, Egginton S. Advances and challenges in skeletal muscle angiogenesis. Am J Physiol Heart Circ Physiol. 2015;310:H326–36.
17. Goodyear LJ. AMP-activated protein kinase: a critical signaling intermediary for exercise-stimulated glucose transport? Exerc Sport Sci Rev. 2000;28:113–6.
18. Yokoyama H, Mori K, Emoto M, Araki T, Teramura M, Mochizuki K, et al. Non-oxidative glucose disposal is reduced in type 2 diabetes, but can be restored by aerobic exercise. Diabetes Obes Metab. 2008;10:400–7.
19. Wellen KE, Hotamisligil GS. Inflammation, stress, and diabetes. J Clin Invest. 2005;115(5):1111–9.
20. Pedersen BK, Steensberg A, Schjerling P. Exercise and interleukin-6. Curr Opin Hematol. 2001;8:137–41.
21. Reyes-Gordillo K, Shah R, Varatharaialu R, Garige M, Leckey LC, Lakhsman MR. Low-w3 fatty acid and soy protein attenuate alcohol-induced fatty liver and injury by regulating the opposing lipid oxidation lipogenic signaling pathways. Oxidative Med Cell Longev. 2016;2016:1840513.
22. Thirupathi A, de Souza CT. Multi-regulatory network of ROS: the interconnection of ROS, PGC1alpha, and AMPK-SIRT1 during exercise. J Physiol Biochem. 2017;73:487–94.
23. Ebert T, Gebhardt C, Scholz M, Wohland T, Schleinitz D, Fasshauer M, et al. Relationship between 12 adipocytokines and distinct components of the metabolic syndrome. J Clin Endocrinol Metab. 2018;103(3):1015–23. https://doi.org/10.1210/jc.2017-02085.
24. Salazar MR, Carbajal HA, Espeche WG, Alzpurua M, Dulbecco CA, Reaven GM. Comparison of two surrogate estimates of insulin resistance to predict cardiovascular disease in apparently healthy individuals. Nutr Metab Cardiov Dis. 2017;27:366–73.
25. Reaven GM. Insulin resistance: the link between obesity and cardiovascular disease. Med Clin North Am. 2011;95:875–92.
26. Reaven MG. The metabolic syndrome: is this diagnosis necessary? Am J Clin Nutr. 2006;83:1237–47.
27. Bird SR, Hawley, Stuart CA, South MA, Lee ML, et al. Insulin responsiveness in metabolic syndrome after eight weeks of cycle training. Med Sci Sports Exerc. 2013;45:2021–9.
28. Stuart CA, South MA, Lee ML, McCurry MP, Howell ME, Ramsey MW, Stone MH. Insulin responsiveness in metabolic syndrome after eight weeks of cycle training. Med Sci Sports Exerc. 2013;45:2021–9.
29. Ramos JS, Dalleck LC, Borrani F, Fassett RG, Coombes JS. Cardiorespiratory fitness is positively associated with pancreatic beta cell function independent of fatness in individuals with the metabolic syndrome: fitness versus fatness. J Sci Med Sport. 2017;20:45–9.
30. Florez H, Temprosa MG, Orchard TJ, Mather KJ, Marcovina SM, Barrett-Connor E. Metabolic syndrome components and their response to lifestyle and metformin interventions are associated with differences in diabetes risk in persons with impaired glucose tolerance. Diabetes Obes Metab. 2014;16:326–33.
31. Kastorini CM, Panagiotakos DB, Chrysohoou C, Georgousopoulou E, ATTICA Study Group. Metabolic syndrome, adherence to the Mediterranean diet and 10-year cardiovascular disease incidence: the ATTICA study. Atherosclerosis. 2016;246:87–93.
32. Kastorini CM, Milionis J, Esposito K, Giugliano D, Goudevenos JA, Panagiotakos DB. The effect of Mediterranean diet on metabolic syndrome and its components: a meta-analysis of 50 studies and 534,906 individuals. J Am Coll Cardiol. 2011;57:1299–313.
33. Hanefeld M, Karasik A, Koehler C, Westermeier T, Chiasson JL. Metabolic syndrome and its single traits as risk factors for diabetes in people with impaired glucose tolerance: the STOP-NIDDM trial. Diab Vasc Dis Res. 2009;6:32–7.
34. Lätt E, Jurimäe J, Harro J, Loit HM, Mäestu J. Low fitness is associated with metabolic risk independent of central adiposity in a cohort of 18-year olds. Scand J Med Sci Sports. 2018;28:1084–91.
35. Farrell SW, Cheng YJ, Blair SN. Prevalence of the metabolic syndrome across cardiorespiratory fitness levels in women. Obes Res. 2004;12:824–30.
36. Lakka TA, Laaksonen DE, Lakka HM, Männikkö N, Niskanen LK, Rauramaa R, Salonen JT. Sedentary lifestyle, poor cardiorespiratory fitness, and metabolic syndrome. Med Sci Sports Exerc. 2003;35:1279–86.
37. Hassinen M, Lakka TA, Savonen K, Litmanen H, Kiviaho L, Laaksonen DE, Komulainen P, Rauramaa R. Cardiorespiratory fitness as a feature of metabolic syndrome in older men and women. Diabetes Care. 2008;31:1242–7.
38. Huang Y, Liu X. Leisure-time physical activity and the risk of metabolic syndrome: meta-analysis. Eur J Med Res. 2014;19:22. https://doi.org/10.1186/2047-783X-19-22.
39. He D, Xi B, Xue J, Huai P, Zhang M, Li J. Association between leisure time physical activity and metabolic syndrome: a meta-analysis of prospective cohort studies. Endocrine. 2014;46:231–40.
40. Zhang D, Liu X, Liu Y, Sun X, Wang B, Ren Y, et al. Leisure-time physical activity and incident metabolic syndrome: a systematic review and dose-response

meta analysis of cohort studies. Metabolism. 2017;75:36–44. 2017;75:36–44.
41. Ingle L, Mellis M, Brodie D, Sandercock GR. Associations between cardiorespiratory fitness and the metabolic syndrome in British men. Heart. 2017;103:524–8.
42. Olsen RH, Krogh-Madsen R, Thomsen C, Booth FW, Pedersen BK. Metabolic responses to reduced daily steps in healthy non-exercising men. JAMA. 2008;299:1261–3.
43. Earnest CP, Artero CG, Sui X, Church TS, Blair SN. Maximal estimated cardiorespiratory fitness, cardiometabolic risk factors, metabolic syndrome in the aerobics center longitudinal study. Mayo Clin Proc. 2013;88:259–70.
44. Franks PW, Ekelund U, Brage S, Wong M-Y, Wareham NJ. Does the association of habitual activity with the metabolic syndrome differ by level of cardiorespiratory fitness? Diabetes Care. 2004;27:1187–93.
45. Ekblom Ö, Ekblom-Bak E, Rosengren A, Hallsten M, Bergström G, Börjesson M. Cardiorespiratory fitness, sedentary behaviour and physical activity are independently associated with the metabolic syndrome, results from the SCAPIS pilot study. PLoS One. 2015;10(6):e0131586.
46. Laaksonen D, Lakka H-M, Salonen JT, Niskanen LK, Rauramaa R, Lakka TA. Low levels of leisure-time physical activity and cardiorespiratory fitness predict development of the metabolic syndrome. Diabetes Care. 2002;25:1612–8.
47. Mora-Rodriguez R, Fernandez-Elias VE, Morales-Palomo F, Pallares JG, Ramirez-Jimenez M, Ortega JF. Aerobic interval training reduces vascular resistances during submaximal exercise in obese metabolic syndrome individuals. Eur J Appl Physiol. 2017;117:2065–73.
48. Bakker EA, Lee D-C, Sui X, Artero EG, Ruiz JR, Eijsvogels TMH, Lavie CJ, Blair SN. Association of resistance exercise, independent and combined with aerobic exercise, with the incident of metabolic syndrome. Mayo Clin Proc. 2017;92:1214–22.
49. Ostam C, Smart NA, Morcos D, Duller A, Ridley W, Jewiss D. The effects of exercise training on clinical outcomes in patients with the metabolic syndrome; a systematic review and meta analysis. Cardiovasc Diabetol. 2017;16:2–11.
50. Bateman LA, Slentz CA, Willis LH, Shields AT, Piner LW, Bales CW, et al. Comparison of aerobic versus resistance exercise training effects on metabolic syndrome (from the Studies of a Targeted Risk Reduction Intervention Through defined exercise-STRRIDE-AT/RT). Am J Cardiol. 2011;108:838–44.
51. Lemes ÍR, Ferreira PH, Linares SN, Machado AF, Pastre CM, Júnior NJ. Resistance training reduces systolic blood pressure in metabolic syndrome: a systematic review and meta-analysis of randomized controlled trials. Br J Sports Med. 2016;50(23):1438–42.
52. Ramos JS, Dalleck LC, Borrani F, Beetham KS, Wallen MP, Mallard AR, et al. Low-volume high-intensity interval training is sufficient to ameliorate the severity of metabolic syndrome. Metab Syndr Relat Disord. 2017;15:319–28.
53. Ramos JS, Dalleck LC, Borrani F, Mallard AR, Clark B, Keating S, et al. The effect of different volumes of high-intensity interval training on proinsulin in participants with the metabolic syndrome: a randomized trial. Diabetologia. 2016;59:2308–20.
54. Despres JP. The Reaven syndrome: a tribute to a giant. Nature Rev Endocrinol. 2018;14:319–20.
55. Hamilton MT, Hamilton GD, Zderic TW. Sedentary behavior as a mediator of type 2 diabetes. Med Sport Sci. 2014;60:11–26.

Exercise Interventions in Patients with Diabetes and Peripheral Artery Disease

13

Mary M. McDermott

Lower extremity peripheral artery disease (PAD), or atherosclerosis of the arteries supplying the lower extremities, affects approximately 8.5 million people in the United States and more than 200 million people worldwide [1–3]. People with PAD have an increased rate of acute coronary events, stroke, and mortality compared to those without PAD [3, 4]. Insufficient oxygen supply to the lower extremities during walking activity leads to ischemic lower extremity muscle, resulting in pain, tightness, weakness, or other discomfort in lower extremity muscle during walking activity. It is well established that people with PAD have greater functional impairment, more rapid functional decline, and higher rates of mobility loss than those without PAD [5–9].

Diabetes mellitus is a major risk factor for PAD [1–3, 10]. Of five studies that assessed the association of diabetes mellitus with PAD, four reported a significant independent association of diabetes mellitus with increased prevalence of PAD, with odds ratios ranging from 1.9 to 4.0 [11–14]. A fifth study, the Framingham Offspring Study, reported a significant association of diabetes mellitus with PAD that was no longer statistically significant in a multivariable-adjusted model [15]. Diabetes mellitus is associated with a twofold increased risk of intermittent claudication, the most classic symptom of PAD [2]. More severe diabetes mellitus and more long-standing diabetes mellitus are associated with higher risks of PAD [2, 10, 16]. As the prevalence of obesity increases, the prevalence of diabetes mellitus will also increase. Thus, the number of people in the world with PAD and diabetes is likely to grow in the foreseeable future.

Diabetes and Clinically Important Outcomes in PAD Patients

Among patients with PAD, those with diabetes mellitus have more adverse outcomes than those without diabetes mellitus. People with PAD and diabetes mellitus have a threefold higher risk of mortality and a fivefold higher rate of amputation compared to people with PAD who do not have diabetes [2, 17]. They also have greater functional impairment and faster functional decline than those without diabetes [18]. In a cross-sectional study of 460 patients with PAD recruited from several medical centers in Chicago, those with diabetes walked significantly shorter distances in the 6-min walk test (1040 vs. 1168 ft, $P < 0.001$), had slower fast-paced walking velocity (0.83 vs. 0.90 m/s, $P < 0.001$), and had a poorer short physical performance battery score (7.3 vs. 8.6, $P < 0.001$). People with more severe diabetes mellitus, determined by the use

M. M. McDermott (✉)
Northwestern University Feinberg School of Medicine, Department of Medicine, Division of general internal medicine and geriatrics, Chicago, IL, USA
e-mail: mdm608@northwestern.edu

P. Kokkinos, P. Narayan (eds.), *Cardiorespiratory Fitness in Cardiometabolic Diseases*,
https://doi.org/10.1007/978-3-030-04816-7_13

Table 13.1 Characteristics of peripheral artery disease in the setting of diabetes mellitus

Characteristic	Findings compared to people with PAD who do not have diabetes mellitus
Distribution of lower extremity atherosclerosis	People with diabetes mellitus have more distal atherosclerosis than those without diabetes mellitus
Leg symptoms	People with PAD and diabetes mellitus have a higher prevalence of atypical leg symptoms than those without diabetes mellitus
Functional impairment	People with PAD and diabetes mellitus have even greater functional impairment than people with PAD who do not have diabetes mellitus
Endovascular interventions for PAD	People with PAD and diabetes mellitus have poorer outcomes after endovascular revascularization compared to those without diabetes mellitus
Supervised treadmill exercise therapy	People with PAD and diabetes have significant benefits from supervised treadmill exercise. Whether the magnitude of benefit is similar between people with and without diabetes mellitus is unclear
Home-based walking exercise therapy	People with PAD and diabetes benefit from home-based walking exercise

of diabetes medication, performed more poorly on functional testing than those not using diabetes medications [18]. Table 13.1 summarizes some clinically important differences in characteristics of patients with PAD with vs. without diabetes mellitus.

Medical Management of Walking Impairment in PAD

A major treatment goal for PAD is to improve functional performance. Although lower extremity revascularization improves walking performance in PAD, many patients with PAD and diabetes mellitus are not candidates for endovascular revascularization, which is the most common and least invasive form of lower extremity revascularization for PAD. Endovascular revascularization is more effective when performed in the proximal arteries (i.e., the aortoiliac arteries). However, diabetic patients with PAD have more distal and more diffuse atherosclerosis than those with PAD and diabetes mellitus [7]. Therefore, many patients with PAD and diabetes mellitus are not candidates for endovascular revascularization. In addition, few medications have been identified that meaningfully improve walking performance in PAD patients. Just two medications, cilostazol and pentoxifylline, are FDA approved for treating PAD-associated walking impairment [19–23]. Of these two medications, benefits from cilostazol are modest, and recent evidence suggests that pentoxifylline is not much better than placebo for improving walking performance in PAD [19, 20]. Current clinical practice guidelines recommend against pentoxifylline for improving walking performance in patients with PAD [20]. Cilostazol improves treadmill walking performance in people with PAD and intermittent claudication by approximately 25% or approximately 40 m in maximal treadmill walking distance [19–25]. However, side effects from cilostazol are common and include headache, diarrhea, light-headedness, and palpitations. One study reported that as many as 20% of patients who were prescribed cilostazol for PAD-related walking impairment discontinued the drug due to side effects [26].

Supervised Treadmill Exercise for Peripheral Artery Disease

Consistent evidence from randomized clinical trials demonstrates that supervised treadmill exercise significantly and substantially improves pain-free and maximal treadmill walking distance in patients with PAD [27–32]. Supervised treadmill exercise sessions typically take place in a cardiac rehabilitation or hospital setting and consist of walking exercise on a treadmill, supervised by a nurse, exercise physiologist, or other trained personnel with knowledge of exercise treatment in PAD. Supervised exercise is typically conducted 3 days per week for a minimum of 12 weeks. The walking exercise program should be tailored to the individual patient with PAD. Many patients with PAD begin the supervised treadmill exercise program by walking a total of 10–15 min in the initial exercise sessions. Since PAD is associated with pain, weakness, or other disabling leg symptoms during walking exercise, PAD patients typically need to alternate walking exercise with rest periods. Patients should be encouraged to increase walking exercise time each week by about 5 min per session, until a total of 40–50 min of walking exercise is achieved per session (excluding rest periods). Improvement in walking endurance and leg symptoms in response to supervised exercise training does not begin immediately but typically is appreciated by the patient with PAD approximately 4–6 weeks after the start of the exercise program [33, 34]. Maximum improvement in treadmill walking performance occurs approximately 12 weeks after the start of supervised exercise training, while improvement in 6-min walk performance continues during the 3- to 6-month period after the start of supervised exercise [30, 35]. Once a supervised treadmill exercise program is completed, benefits in treadmill walking performance are largely sustained, up to 12 months after completion of the supervised exercise [27]; however benefits in the 6-min walk are not durable after a supervised exercise intervention is completed. The more favorable sustained effect of supervised treadmill exercise on treadmill walking performance vs. 6-min walk performance may be related to a learning effect observed after treadmill exercise on the treadmill walking outcome that is not observed for the 6-min walk outcome [36].

In a meta-analysis of 25 randomized trials of supervised exercise in patients with PAD, supervised treadmill exercise was associated with a 180-m greater increase in maximal treadmill walking distance and a 128-m greater increase in pain-free treadmill walking distance, compared to the control group that did not receive exercise [28]. Supervised treadmill exercise also achieves clinically important improvement in 6-min walk distance in patients with PAD [29–30, 32]. The effects of supervised treadmill exercise on physical activity and quality of life are variable. Supervised treadmill exercise has not been shown consistently to improve physical activity or quality of life [27, 29, 37].

Supervised Treadmill Exercise in Patients with PAD and Diabetes Mellitus

Since diabetes mellitus is a major risk factor for PAD, many PAD participants in randomized clinical trials of supervised exercise have diabetes. In three of the largest randomized trials of supervised exercise in PAD patients, the prevalence of diabetes mellitus was 36–45% [29, 30, 32]. Despite this, relatively few studies have specifically assessed how diabetes mellitus affects responsiveness to supervised treadmill exercise in patients with PAD. A systematic review identified just three studies that had evaluated the impact of diabetes mellitus on improvement in treadmill walking performance in patients with PAD, after a supervised treadmill exercise program [38]. Of the three studies [39–41], two were small randomized trials of 27 and 60 participants, respectively. In post hoc analyses, Gardner et al. reported that PAD participants without diabetes mellitus increased their maximal treadmill walking distance by 57%, compared to 30% in the PAD participants with diabetes mellitus [40]. However, a significant interaction between diabetes mellitus and improvement in maximal treadmill walking distance following supervised exercise was not observed. Allen et al. reported significant improvement in maximal treadmill walking distance among 13 patients with diabetes mellitus and 14 without diabetes mellitus, respectively, but did not statistically compare the degree of improvement in participants with vs. without diabetes mellitus. An observational study from the Netherlands evaluated changes in treadmill walking performance in 775 patients with PAD referred for supervised treadmill exercise, according to presence or absence of diabetes mellitus [41]. Of the 775 PAD patients referred for supervised treadmill exercise, 230 (30%) had diabetes mellitus. At baseline, those with diabetes mellitus had significantly poorer maximal treadmill walking distance than those without diabetes mellitus. Just 440 of the 775 patients with PAD were available for follow-up. There was no difference in the degree of improvement in maximal treadmill walking distance between those with and without diabetes mellitus (270 m vs. 400 m) [41]. The overall conclusion of the review was that there were insufficient data to determine whether diabetes mellitus impairs response to supervised treadmill exercise in patients with PAD [38]. However, it is important to point out that participants with diabetes mellitus in all trials improved their treadmill walking performance following supervised exercise.

In another review of randomized trials of supervised exercise that included greater proportions of patients with PAD and diabetes mellitus, the authors reported that absolute improvement in treadmill walking performance following exercise intervention was poor [42]. However, patients with PAD and diabetes mellitus typically have poorer functional performance and shorter treadmill walking distance at baseline than PAD patients with no diabetes mellitus [18, 41]. Thus, the percent improvement in treadmill walking distance, or the degree of improvement relative to baseline, is a more relevant metric for comparison than absolute improvement in treadmill walking distance. Available evidence suggests that patients with PAD and diabetes mellitus improve their walking performance following supervised treadmill exercise interventions [38–42].

How to Implement a Supervised Treadmill Exercise Program for Patients with PAD and Diabetes Mellitus

Supervised treadmill exercise programs must be tailored for the individual patient. It is ideal to have a treadmill for exercise that can accommodate speeds as low as 0.50 miles per hour, since some patients with PAD, especially those with diabetes mellitus, cannot tolerate high exercise speeds [18]. In addition, some PAD patients with diabetes are unable to complete more than 10–15 min of walking exercise per session in their first week of exercise. Patients with PAD should aim to increase the total number of minutes walking for exercise each session by 5 min per week, until they achieve 40–50 min of walking exercise per session. Patients with PAD should also be instructed to alternate periods of walking exercise with rest during a typical treadmill exercise session. Based on current evidence, PAD patients should be advised to walk to near-maximal leg pain for maximum gains in exercise capacity. There is also some evidence to suggest that patients with PAD who walk at a slow or comfortable pace can still achieve significant gains in walking endurance [28]. Based on current evidence, if a patient with PAD is able to walk for treadmill exercise for 10 min without experiencing ischemic leg symptoms, the workload should be increased, by increasing either the speed or grade of the treadmill [29, 30].

Centers for Medicare and Medicaid Services Coverage for Supervised Exercise in PAD

Until recently, many PAD patients in the United States did not have access to supervised treadmill exercise because of lack of medical insurance coverage. In 2017, the Centers for Medicare and Medicaid Services (CMS) released a decision memorandum, indicating that they would begin providing coverage for supervised exercise for patients with symptomatic PAD [43]. This change in policy by CMS is expected to make supervised treadmill exercise more accessible to many PAD patients.

In order to provide coverage, CMS requires that supervised exercise for PAD must be ordered during a face-to-face physician office visit, during which cardiovascular disease risk factors must be addressed. CMS provides coverage for 12 weeks and 36 sessions of supervised exercise for symptomatic PAD. The supervised exercise must take place in a hospital setting or medical office affiliated with a hospital and must be conducted by qualified personnel with training in basic and advanced cardiac life support and PAD-related

Table 13.2 Elements of supervised exercise required for coverage by the Centers for Medicare and Medicaid Services[a]

Exercise must be prescribed by a physician after a face-to-face meeting with the patient that includes counseling on cardiovascular disease prevention
Prescribed exercise must consist of 12 weeks of exercise sessions that occur three times weekly
After completing 12 weeks of supervised exercise, an additional 36 sessions may be prescribed, with written justification, after the first 12 weeks is completed and may take place over a longer period of time
The exercise sessions must take place in a physician's office or outpatient hospital-affiliated setting
Exercise must be delivered by qualified personnel with training in basic and advance life support and exercise therapy for PAD
Exercise must be supervised by a physician, physician's assistant, or nurse practitioner/clinical nurse specialist

[a]Reprinted with permission from the American College of Cardiology [58].

exercise therapy [43]. A physician must be on-site. After the 12 weeks and 36 sessions of supervised exercise are completed, CMS may provide coverage for an additional 36 sessions of supervised exercise therapy, if a physician can justify the need for the additional sessions. Table 13.2 summarizes characteristics of supervised exercise programs that are covered by CMS.

Home-Based or Unsupervised Walking Exercise in People with PAD and Diabetes Mellitus

For many patients with PAD, participation in supervised treadmill exercise can be difficult even when paid for by medical insurance. In an analysis of 1541 patients with PAD who were eligible to participate in randomized trials of supervised exercise, and therefore had free access to supervised exercise, 69% declined participation, because of inconvenience, lack of interest, or comorbidities that interfered with participation [44]. When supervised exercise is inconvenient or not feasible, home-based or unsupervised exercise may be an effective alternative to supervised treadmill exercise. While home-based exercise was previously considered not an effective therapy for people with PAD, early studies of home-based walking exercise in PAD did not incorporate behavioral change therapies [45–47]. More recent randomized clinical trial evidence demonstrates that when behavioral change methods are incorporated into the intervention, home-based exercise therapy can significantly improve walking endurance in PAD patients [31, 32, 48]. However, close monitoring of the PAD patient is required to ensure ongoing adherence to home-based exercise [49].

Three large clinical trials, published between 2011 and 2014, demonstrated that home-based exercise can improve walking performance in PAD patients [31, 32, 48]. The largest of these three trials was the Group-Oriented Arterial Leg Study (GOALS), which tested the efficacy of a Group-Mediated Cognitive Behavioral (GMCB) intervention to help patients with PAD adhere to a home-based walking exercise program [48]. In the GOALS trial, 192 participants with PAD were randomized to either a GMCB intervention or an attention control group for 6 months [48]. The GMCB intervention used behavioral change methods including self-monitoring, goal setting, group support, and self-efficacy to help people with PAD adhere to a home-based walking exercise program. During the first 6 months of the GOALS intervention, PAD participants in the intervention met in groups once per week at the exercise center with other PAD patients and a coach. The coach led group discussions that fostered group support and focused on specific behaviors necessary for successful behavior change, including goal setting, self-efficacy, self-monitoring, and overcoming obstacles to exercise adherence. PAD participants in the GOALS intervention were instructed to walk for exercise 5 days per week, gradually building up to 40–50 min of walking exercise per session, at a pace that elicited moderate to severe ischemic leg symptoms. Participants were instructed to stop and rest in between bouts of ischemia-inducing walking exercise activity. After 6 months, participants in the GMCB home-based exercise intervention group significantly improved their 6-min walk distance (primary outcome) by 54 m relative to the control group, consistent with a large meaningful improvement [49]. Pain-free treadmill and maximal treadmill walking time also improved significantly compared to the control group [48]. The home-based exercise intervention also significantly improved physical activity levels and participants' perception of walking endurance, measured by the Walking Impairment Questionnaire (WIQ) distance score, compared to the control group. Furthermore, in subgroup analyses, the intervention significantly improved 6-min walk in participants both with and without diabetes mellitus, respectively [48]. Specifically, 6-min walk distance increased by 53 m among participants without diabetes mellitus and by 54 m among participants with diabetes mellitus.

After 6 months of the weekly on-site sessions, participants in the GOALS intervention were transitioned from the weekly group meetings to telephone contact only and received periodic telephone calls from the coach between months 7 and 12. At 12-month follow-up, 6 months after the more intensive on-site study intervention was completed, change in 6-min walk distance compared to baseline remained significantly better in the intervention group compared to the control group, consistent with a durable benefit from the intervention [50].

Findings in the GOALS trial were confirmed in two other randomized trials of home-based exercise in people with PAD [31, 32]. One of these trials randomized 180 participants with PAD and intermittent claudication to one of the three groups: supervised treadmill exercise, home-based walking exercise, and an attention control group for 12 weeks [32]. In the supervised treadmill exercise group, participants performed treadmill walking exercise to maximal ischemic leg pain, 3 days per week, for up to 40 min per session. In the home-based walking exercise group, participants walked for exercise at home 3 days per week, at a self-selected pace, for up to 45 min per session. PAD participants in the home exercise group wore an activity monitor during exercise and returned to the medical center at 1-, 4-, 8-, and 12-week follow-up to meet with a study investigator, review their step count data, and set goals for the next 4 weeks. After 12 weeks, both exercise groups significantly improved their 6-min walk distance, maximum treadmill walking distance, and pain-free treadmill walking distance, relative to the control group. Furthermore, the home-based walking exercise group improved their 6-min walk distance more than the supervised treadmill exercise group. At 12-week follow-up, 6-min walk distance increased by 45 m in the home-based exercise group, by 15 m in the supervised exercise group, and by 45 m in the home-based exercise group. Since corridor walking more closely simulates over ground walking, home-based exercise programs may be more helpful in achieving improved walking in daily life for people with PAD. In summary, home-based walking exercise interventions that include regular visits to the medical center improve walking performance in PAD patients, including those with diabetes mellitus [48]. Table 13.3 summarizes evidence from both supervised and home-based exercise trials regarding benefits of supervised and home-based exercise interventions in PAD participants with and without diabetes mellitus.

In another randomized trial of home-based walking exercise intervention that included only patients with PAD and diabetes mellitus, the findings were somewhat different. Collins et al. randomized 145 participants with PAD and diabetes to a behavioral intervention vs. an attention control group for 6 months [51]. The intervention consisted of an individualized counseling session at baseline, followed by one walking session per week with an instructor and other patients with PAD at an exercise center and 3 days of walking at home each week, for up to 50 min of exercise per session. Participants in the intervention also received bi-weekly telephone calls, in which an instructor reviewed their walking progress and provided feedback. The attention control group received bi-weekly calls from a study investigator during which the participant and study investigator discussed glucose control, blood pressure, and cholesterol levels during the previous month. After 6 months, there were no differences in treadmill walking performance between the home-based walking exercise intervention and the control group. Therefore, in this study of participants with diabetes mellitus and PAD, a

Table 13.3 Studies comparing improvement in walking performance between PAD participants with and without diabetes mellitus

Study	Sample size	Study design	Primary findings	Comments
Supervised treadmill exercise interventions				
Van Pul et al. [41]	$N = 755$ $N = 230$ (30%) with diabetes mellitus	Observational longitudinal analysis of patients referred to supervised treadmill exercise in the Netherlands	At 3-month follow-up, maximal treadmill walking distance increased by 73% in people without diabetes vs. 67% in people with diabetes. At 6-month follow-up, maximal treadmill walking distance increased by 100% and 91%, respectively ($P = 0.48$ for comparison of change between those with and without diabetes)	Follow-up data were available for just 440 of 755 participants
Allen et al. [39]	$N = 27$ $N = 13$ (48%) with diabetes	Randomized trial of supervised exercise in PAD. Data analyzed according to the presence vs. absence of diabetes	At 3-month follow-up, PAD participants with diabetes increased maximal treadmill walking performance by 52%, and those without diabetes increased maximal treadmill walking performance by 29%	Small sample size is a study limitation
Gardner et al. [40]	$N = 60$ $N = 25$ (42%) with diabetes mellitus	Randomized trial of supervised exercise in PAD	At 3-month follow-up, maximal treadmill walking distance increased by 57% (198 m) in participants with diabetes vs. 30% (87 m) in those without diabetes	Small sample size is a study limitation
Home-based walking exercise interventions				
McDermott et al. [48]	$N = 194$ 64 (33%) had diabetes	Randomized clinical trial of home-based exercise using a group-mediated cognitive behavioral intervention	At 6-month follow-up, 6-min walk distance increased by 53 m among participants without diabetes and by 54 m among participants with diabetes mellitus	Improvement in 6-min walk distance is consistent with a large meaningful change
McDermott et al. [49]	$N = 200$ 67 (33.5%) had diabetes	Randomized clinical trial of telephone counseling + wearable device to improve walking ability in PAD	At 9-month follow-up, there was no improvement overall in 6-min walk distance between the intervention and control groups. Results did not differ by the presence vs. absence of diabetes	

home-based exercise intervention did not improve treadmill walking performance more than a control group. Both groups (intervention and control group) improved in this trial, and the 6-min walk test was not measured.

Practical Aspects of Prescribing Home-Based Walking Exercise for Patients with PAD and Diabetes Mellitus

Prior to initiating a new home-based exercise program, it is reasonable for PAD patients with diabetes mellitus to complete a baseline treadmill cardiac stress test to evaluate them for significant coronary ischemia, which may become manifest during walking exercise as leg symptoms improve. A regular treadmill exercise stress test (without imaging) should be sufficient to evaluate most PAD patients for coronary ischemia prior to initiating a new exercise program. PAD patients whose baseline treadmill exercise stress test indicates coronary ischemia should undergo additional evaluation prior to initiating an exercise intervention.

Effective home-based exercise programs for people with PAD have used activity monitors and/or incorporated throughout the intervention principles of behavioral change theory [31, 32, 48]. Behavioral change techniques that have been successful for promoting home-based walking exercise in PAD have included goal setting, building self-efficacy, monitoring progress, and a "coach" to whom the patient feels accountable [31, 32, 48]. Therefore, patients with PAD engaged in home-based exercise should be advised to write down walking exercise goals and record their walking exercise activity each week, and this information should be reviewed periodically by a coach or a clinician who provides regular feedback to the patient. Successful home-based programs have incorporated coach contact with the participant as infrequently as monthly [32]. A home-based exercise intervention for PAD participants that consisted of providing a wearable activity monitor and telephone coaching was not effective [49]. Thus, available evidence suggests that effective home-based exercise programs for PAD may require ongoing contact with a coach, at least during the first 6 months of the intervention [49–52].

Additional Alternative Exercise Strategies for PAD Patients

Relatively few exercise modalities other than walking exercise have been studied for PAD patients. Several randomized trials that implemented upper and lower limb ergometry, or upper and lower extremity cycling, improved walking performance in people with PAD and intermittent claudication [53–55]. Zwierska et al. randomized 104 participants with PAD into an upper limb aerobic ergometry intervention, a lower limb aerobic ergometry intervention, or a non-exercise control group for 6 months [53]. Exercise sessions occurred twice per week and consisted of 2 min of arm or leg cranking ergometry exercise followed by 2 min of rest for a total of ten cycles (20 min of exercise per session). After 6 months of ergometry exercise, the maximal walking distance, measured by a shuttle-walk test, increased by 29% in the upper limb ergometry group and by 31% in the lower limb ergometry group. The improvement in walking endurance following upper limb exercises is unexpected and counterintuitive, as exercise benefits are highly specific to an imposed demand. Improved cardiovascular fitness following upper limb exercise may contribute to improved walking endurance as a result of systemic improvement in endothelial function or if poor cardiorespiratory fitness contributed importantly to the functional impairment, rather than atherosclerotic obstruction of the lower extremity arteries. It is apparent that more studies are needed to define the specific mechanisms involved. These trials have not evaluated benefit specifically in people with PAD and diabetes mellitus.

Resistance Exercise Training for PAD Patients

Lower extremity resistance training has been evaluated in PAD patients in several randomized clinical trials [29, 56, 57]. In the largest of these trials, 156 participants with PAD were randomized to supervised treadmill exercise, supervised resistance training, or a control group for 6 months. At 6-month follow-up, supervised treadmill exercise achieved a statistically significant and clinically meaningful improvement in 6-minute walk performance (+35.9 meters vs. the control group), while supervised lower extremity resistance training did not improve the six-minute walk more than the control group (+12.4 meters). Resistance training has not been separately evaluated in PAD participants with diabetes mellitus, to the author's knowledge.

Conclusions

Diabetes mellitus is common in PAD patients. Patients with PAD and diabetes mellitus have significantly greater impairment in walking endurance and higher rates of mobility loss than those without diabetes mellitus. The distribution of lower extremity atherosclerosis in people with PAD makes these less well suited for endovascular revascularization, which is most beneficial when performed for more proximal lower extremity stenosis.

Patients with peripheral artery disease with and without diabetes mellitus benefit from both supervised and home-based walking exercise. The magnitude of improvement following supervised treadmill exercise may be less for patients with PAD and diabetes mellitus compared to patients with PAD who do not have diabetes mellitus. Nevertheless, evidence supports that exercise interventions are effective in improving walking performance or exercise capacity in PAD patients with and without diabetes mellitus and therefore exercise should be considered as part of the therapeutic strategy of these patients.

References

1. Go AS, Mozaffarian D, Roger VL, Benjamin EJ, Berry JD, Borden WB, et al. Executive summary: heart disease and stroke statistics--2013 update: a report from the American Heart Association. Circulation. 2013;127(1):143–52.
2. Fowkes FG, Rudan D, Rudan I, Aboyans V, Denenberg JO, McDermott MM, et al. Comparison of global estimates of prevalence and risk factors for peripheral artery disease in 2000 and 2010: a systematic review and analysis. Lancet. 2013;382(9901):1329–40.
3. Criqui MH, Aboyans V. Epidemiology of peripheral artery disease. Circ Res. 2015;116:1509–26.
4. Fowkes FG, Murray GD, Butcher I, Heald CL, Lee RJ, Chambless LE, et al. Ankle brachial index combined with Framingham risk score to predict cardiovascular events and mortality: a meta-analysis. JAMA. 2008;300(2):197–208.
5. McDermott MM, Greenland P, Liu K, Guralnik JM, Celic L, Criqui MH, et al. The ankle brachial index is associated with leg function and physical activity: the walking and leg circulation study. Ann Intern Med. 2002;136(12):873–83.
6. McDermott MM, Liu K, Greenland P, Guralnik JM, Criqui MH, Chan C, et al. Functional decline in peripheral arterial disease: associations with the ankle brachial index and leg symptoms. JAMA. 2004;292(4):453–61.
7. McDermott MM, Guralnik JM, Tian L, Liu K, Ferrucci L, Liao Y, et al. Associations of borderline and low normal ankle-brachial index values with functional decline at 5-year follow-up: the WALCS (Walking and Leg Circulation Study). J Am Coll Cardiol. 2009;53:1056–62.
8. McDermott MM, Guralnik JM, Tian L, Ferrucci L, Liu K, Liao Y, et al. Baseline functional performance predicts the rate of mobility loss in persons with peripheral arterial disease. J Am Coll Cardiol. 2007;50:974–82.
9. McDermott MM, Fried L, Simonsick E, Ling S, Guralnik JM. Asymptomatic peripheral arterial disease is independently associated with impaired lower extremity functioning: the women's health and aging study. Circulation. 2000;101(9):1007–12.
10. Joosten MM, Pai JK, Bertoia ML, Rimm EB, Spiegelman D, Mittleman MA, et al. Associations between conventional cardiovascular risk factors and risk of peripheral artery disease in men. JAMA. 2012;308(16):1660–7.
11. Newman AB, Siscovick DS, Manolio TA, Polak J, Fried LP, Borhani NO, et al. Ankle-arm index as a marker of atherosclerosis in the Cardiovascular Health Study. Cardiovascular Heart Study (CHS) Collaborative Research Group. Circulation. 1993;88(3):837–45.
12. Murabito JM, D'Agostino RB, Silbershatz H, Wilson WF. Intermittent claudication. A risk profile from The Framingham Heart Study. Circulation. 1997 Jul;96:44–9.
13. Meijer WT, Grobbee DE, Hunink MG, Hofman A, Hoes AW. Determinants of peripheral arterial disease in the elderly: the Rotterdam study. Arch Intern Med. 2000;160:2934–8.
14. Allison MA, Criqui MH, McClelland RL, Scott JM, McDermott MM, Liu K, et al. The effect of novel cardiovascular risk factors on the ethnic-specific odds for peripheral arterial disease in the Multi-Ethnic Study of Atherosclerosis (MESA). J Am Coll Cardiol. 2006;48:1190–7.
15. Murabito JM, Evans JC, Nieto K, Larson MG, Levy D, Wilson PW. Prevalence and clinical correlates of peripheral arterial disease in Framingham Offspring Study. Am Heart J. 2002;143:961–5.
16. Beks PJ, Mackaay AJ, de Neeling JN, de Vries H, Bouter LM, Heine RJ. Peripheral arterial disease in relation to glycaemic level in an elderly Caucasian population: the Hoorn study. Diabetologia. 1995;38:89–96.
17. Jude EB, Oyibo SO, Chalmers N, Boulton AJ. Peripheral arterial disease in diabetic and nondiabetic patients: a comparison of severity and outcome. Diabetes Care. 2001;24:1433.
18. Dolan NC, Liu K, Criqui MH, Greenland P, Guralnik JM, Chan C, et al. Peripheral artery disease, diabetes, and reduced lower extremity functioning. Diabetes Care. 2002;25:113–20.
19. Girolami B, Bernardi E, Prins MH, Ten Cate JW, Hettiarachchi R, Prandoni P, Girolami A, Buller HR. Treatment of intermittent claudication with physical training, smoking cessation, pentoxifylline, or nafronyl: a meta-analysis. Arch Intern Med. 1999;159:337–45.
20. Gerhard-Herman MD, Gornik HL, Barrett C, Barshes NR, Corriere MA, Drachman DE, et al. 2016 AHA/ACC guideline on the management of patients with lower extremity peripheral artery disease: a report of the American College of

Cardiology/American Heart Association Task Force on Clinical Practice Guidelines. Circulation. 2017;135(120):e726–79.
21. Stevens JW, Simpson E, Harnan S, Squires H, Meng Y, Thomas S, et al. Systematic review of the efficacy of cilostazol, naftidrofuryl oxalate and pentoxifylline for the treatment of intermittent claudication. Br J Surg. 2012;99:1630–8.
22. Dawson DL, Cutler BS, Meissner MH, Strandness DE Jr. Cilostazol has beneficial effects in treatment of intermittent claudication: results from a multicenter, randomized, prospective, double-blind trial. Circulation. 1998;98:678–86.
23. Money SR, Herd JA, Isaacsohn JL, Davidson M, Cutler B, Heckman J, et al. Effect of cilostazol on walking distances in patients with intermittent claudication caused by peripheral vascular disease. J Vasc Surg. 1998;27:267–74.
24. Beebe HG, Dawson DL, Cutler BS, Herd JA, Strandness DE Jr, Bortey EB, et al. A new pharmacological treatment for intermittent claudication: results of a randomized, multicenter trial. Arch Intern Med. 1999;159:2041–50.
25. Bedenis R, Stewart M, Cleanthis M, Robless P, Mikhailidis DP, Stansby G. Cilostazol for intermittent claudication. Cochrane Database Syst Rev. 2014;2014(10):CD003748.
26. Lee C, Nelson PR. Effect of cilostazol prescribed in a pragmatic treatment program for intermittent claudication. Vasc Endovasc Surg. 2014;48:224–9.
27. Murphy TP, Cutlip DE, Regensteiner JG, Mohler ER, Cohen DJ, Reynolds MR, et al. Supervised exercise, stent revascularization, or medical therapy for claudication due to aortoiliac peripheral artery disease: the CLEVER study. J Am Coll Cardiol. 2015;65(10):999–1009.
28. Fakhry F, van de Luijtgaarden KM, Bax L, den Hoed PT, Hunink MG, Rouwet EV, et al. Supervised walking therapy in patients with intermittent claudication. J Vasc Surg. 2012;56:1132–42.
29. McDermott MM, Ades P, Guralnik JM, Dyer A, Ferrucci L, Liu K, et al. Treadmill exercise and resistance training in patients with peripheral arterial disease with and without intermittent claudication: a randomized controlled trial. JAMA. 2009;301(2):165–74.
30. McDermott MM, Ferrucci L, Tian L, Guralnik JM, Lloyd-Jones D, Kibbe MR, et al. Effect of granulocyte-macrophage colony-stimulating factor with or without supervised exercise on walking performance in patients with peripheral artery disease: the PROPEL randomized clinical trial. JAMA. 2017;318(21):2089–98.
31. Gardner AW, Parker DE, Montgomery PS, Scott KJ, Blevins SM. Efficacy of quantified home-based exercise and supervised exercise in patients with intermittent claudication: a randomized controlled trial. Circulation. 2011;123(5):491–8.
32. Gardner AW, Parker DE, Montgomery PS, Blevins SM. Step-monitored home exercise improves ambulation, vascular function, and inflammation in symptomatic patients with peripheral artery disease: a randomized controlled trial. J Am Heart Assoc. 2014;3(5):e001107.
33. McDermott MM. Medical management of functional impairment in peripheral artery disease: a review. Prog Cardiovascular Dis. 2018;60:586–92.
34. McDermott MM. Exercise rehabilitation for peripheral artery disease: a review. J Cardiopulm Rehabil Prev. 2018;38(2):63–9.
35. Gardner AW, Montgomery PS, Parker DE. Optimal exercise program length for patients with claudication. J Vasc Surg. 2012;55(5):1346–54.
36. McDermott MM, Guralnik JM, Criqui MH, Liu K, Kibbe MR, Ferrucci L. Six-minute walk is a better outcome measure than treadmill walking tests in therapeutic trials of patients with peripheral artery disease. Circulation. 2014;130(1):61–8.
37. Gardner AW, Katzel LI, Sorkin JD, Bradham DD, Hochberg MC, Flinn WR, et al. Exercise rehabilitation improves functional outcomes and peripheral circulation in patients with intermittent claudication: a randomized controlled trial. J Am Geriatr Soc. 2001;49(6):755–62.
38. Hageman D, Gommans LN, Scheltinga MR, Teijink JA. Effect of diabetes mellitus on walking distance parameters after supervised exercise therapy for intermittent claudication: a systematic review. Vasc Med. 2017;22:21–7.
39. Allen JD, Stabler T, Kenjale AA, et al. Diabetes status differentiates endothelial function and plasma nitrite response to exercise stress in peripheral arterial disease following supervised training. J Diabet Complications. 2014;28:219–25.
40. Gardner AW, Parker DE, Montgomery PS, et al. Diabetic women are poor responders to exercise rehabilitation in the treatment of claudication. J Vasc Surg. 2014;59:1036–43.
41. van Pul KM, Kruidenier LM, Nicolaï SP, de Bie RA, Nieman FH, Prins MH, et al. Effect of supervised exercise therapy for intermittent claudication in patients with diabetes mellitus. Ann Vasc Surg. 2012;26:957–63.
42. Lyu X, Li S, Peng S, Cai H, Liu G, Ran X. Intensive walking exercise for lower extremity peripheral artery disease: a systematic review and meta-analysis. J Diabetes. 2016;8:363–77.
43. Jensen TS, Chin J, Ashby L, Schafer J, Dolan D. Proposed national coverage determination for supervised exercise therapy (SET) for symptomatic peripheral artery disease (PAD) [Internet]. Baltimore (MD). Centers for Medicare and Medicaid Services. 2017 Mar 2. Available from: https://www.cms.gov/medicare-coverage-database/details/nca-proposed-decision-memo.aspx?NCAId=287. Accessed May 1, 2018.
44. Harwood AE, Smith GE, Cayton T, Broadbent E, Chetter IC. A systematic review for the uptake and adherence rates to supervised exercise programs in patients with intermittent claudication. Ann Vasc Surg. 2016;34:280–9.

45. Regensteiner JG, Meyer TJ, Krupski WC, Cranford LS, Hiatt WR. Hospital vs. home-based exercise rehabilitation for patients with peripheral arterial occlusive disease. Angiology. 1997;48(4):291–300.
46. Savage P, Ricci MA, Lynn M, Gardner A, Knight S, Brochu M, et al. Effects of home versus supervised exercise for patients with intermittent claudication. J Cardpulm Rehabil. 2001;21(3):152–7.
47. Menard JR, Smith HE, Riebe D, Braun CM, Blissmer B, Patterson RB. Long-term results of peripheral arterial disease rehabilitation. J Vasc Surg. 2004;39(6):1186–92.
48. McDermott MM, Liu K, Guralnik JM, Criqui MH, Spring B, Tian L, et al. Home-based walking exercise intervention in peripheral artery disease: a randomized clinical trial. JAMA. 2013;310(1):57–65.
49. McDermott MM, Spring B, Berger JS, Treat-Jacobson D, Conte MS, Creager MA, et al. Effect of a home-based exercise intervention of wearable technology and telephone coaching on walking performance in peripheral artery disease: the HONOR randomized clinical trial. JAMA. 2018;319(16):1665–76.
50. McDermott MM, Guralnik JM, Criqui MH, Ferrucci L, Zhao L, Liu K, et al. Home-based walking exercise in peripheral artery disease: 12-month follow-up of the GOALS randomized trial. J Am Heart Assoc. 2014;3(3):e000711.
51. Collins TC, Lunos S, Carlson T, Henderson K, Lightbourne M, Nelson B, et al. Effects of a home-based walking intervention on mobility and quality of life in people with diabetes and peripheral arterial disease: a randomized controlled trial. Diabetes Care. 2011;34(10):2174–9.
52. McDermott MM, Polonsky T. Home-based exercise: a therapeutic option for peripheral artery disease. Circulation. 2016;134(16):1127–9.
53. Zwierska I, Walker RD, Chosky SA, Male JS, Pockley AG, Saxton JM. Upper vs. lower limb aerobic exercise rehabilitation in patients with symptomatic peripheral arterial disease: a randomized controlled trial. J Vasc Surg. 2005;42(6):1122–30.
54. Tew G, Nawaz S, Zwierska I, Saxton JM. Limb-specific and cross-transfer effects of arm-crank exercise training in patients with symptomatic peripheral arterial disease. Clin Sci (Lond). 2009;117(12):405–13.
55. Bronas UG, Treat-Jacobson D, Leon AS. Comparison of the effect of upper body-ergometry aerobic training vs treadmill training on central cardiorespiratory improvement and walking distance with claudication. J Vasc Surg. 2011;53(6):1557–64.
56. McGuigan MR, Bronks R, Newton RU, Sharman MJ, Graham JC, Cody DV, et al. Resistance training in patients with peripheral arterial disease: effects on myosin isoforms, fiber type distribution, and capillary supply to skeletal muscle. J Gerontol A Biol Sci Med Sci. 2001;56(7):B302–10.
57. Regensteiner JG, Steiner JF, Hiatt WR. Exercise training improves functional status in patients with peripheral arterial disease. J Vasc Surg. 1996;23(1):104–15.
58. McDermott MM. Supervised treadmill exercise therapy for peripheral artery disease. http://www.acc.org. August 3, 2017. http://www.acc.org/latest-in-cardiology/articles/2017/07/12/12/55/supervised. treadmill-exercise-therapy-for-peripheral-artery-disease (last accessed December 9, 2017).

Physical Activity, Cardiorespiratory Fitness, and Obesity

14

Louise de Lannoy and Robert Ross

Introduction

Obesity is an excess accumulation of fat. Overweight and obesity are most commonly defined by increased body mass index (BMI), calculated by dividing weight in kilograms by the square of height in meters. According to the World Health Organization (WHO), overweight is defined as BMI ≥ 25 kg/m^2 and obesity as BMI ≥ 30 kg/m^2 [1]. The prevalence of overweight and obesity is increasing; currently, nearly 40% of adults are overweight, and 13% are obese worldwide [1]. This is a major health concern as obesity has recently been identified as the leading risk factor for noncommunicable diseases [2]. Epidemiological evidence suggests that the decline in physical activity energy expenditure (PAEE), observed in the last few decades, is a major contributor to the rise in overweight and obesity [3]. Following a thorough review on the importance of physical activity (PA) for obesity management, the American College of Sports Medicine [4] published weight loss guidelines that recommend moderate-intensity PA greater than 250 min/week in combination with dietary restriction for adults looking to achieve clinically significant weight loss.

L. de Lannoy · R. Ross (✉)
Queen's University, School of Kinesiology and Health Studies, Kingston, ON, Canada
e-mail: rossr@queensu.ca

In this chapter we will explore the role that PA has in the management of obesity. Specifically, the following topics will be reviewed: (1) the search method utilized; (2) nomenclature related to obesity, PA, and cardiorespiratory fitness (CRF; a physiological trait often considered a surrogate measure of PA); (3) epidemiological and (4) randomized controlled trial (RCT) evidence on the interaction between obesity, PA, and CRF on health outcomes; and finally (5) clinical and public health insights for weight management.

A PubMed search was performed using the following keywords: (obesity OR overweight OR obese) and (exercise OR physical activity) and (cardiorespiratory fitness). The search strategy included the following filters: publication date 1994–2018, humans, English language, and adults >18 years old. Identified studies were included in this chapter based on the following inclusion criteria: (1) Participants were older than 18 years, and (2) analysis of the interaction between at least two of the following variables: body weight or fat mass or waist circumference (WC) or abdominal fat mass, cardiorespiratory fitness, and physical activity or exercise.

Obesity and Health Outcomes

Obesity is associated with a number of cardiometabolic risk factors including hypertension, dyslipidemia, and insulin resistance, as well as

P. Kokkinos, P. Narayan (eds.), *Cardiorespiratory Fitness in Cardiometabolic Diseases*,
https://doi.org/10.1007/978-3-030-04816-7_14

chronic diseases such as type 2 diabetes and nonalcoholic fatty liver disease [5]. Quality of life in this patient population is also frequently reduced as activities of daily living such as getting groceries and cleaning are impaired at a younger age with the onset of obesity [6]. Further, obesity is associated with increased mortality risk due to the presence of multiple comorbid conditions, making surgical interventions and medical treatments more complex [6].

Regional distribution of fat is a key determinant of cardiometabolic risk. Regional accumulation of abdominal subcutaneous (SAT) and visceral adipose tissue (VAT) are major contributors to cardiometabolic dysfunction [7] and are therefore important clinical targets for reducing health risk. SAT and VAT are most accurately measured by computed tomography (CT) or magnetic resonance imaging (MRI); however, given the high cost of imaging technologies, these measures are infrequently used. Surrogate measures such as WC, BMI, and waist-to-hip ratio (WHR) have been validated against objective measures of abdominal adiposity [8–12], where combining WC with BMI produces the most accurate estimate of non-abdominal adipose tissue, SAT, and VAT.

Physical Activity

PA is a behavior, defined as any bodily movement that exerts energy above resting levels. PA can induce a negative energy balance where chronic negative energy balance ultimately leads to a reduction in body weight. Higher amounts of PA performed on a regular basis are associated with a lower risk of developing obesity [13, 14]. Conversely, the decline in occupational PA observed over the last 40 years corresponds closely to actual increases in weight in middle-aged men and women in the workforce over this time period [3]. Thus, a decline in PA, and in particular occupational PA, is a major contributor to the rise in overweight and obesity observed in the last few decades. There is also substantive evidence highlighting the inverse dose-response association between PA and risk of morbidity and mortality [15–17]; thus, engaging in PA is important not only to reduce obesity but to improve long-term health as well.

PA can be unstructured (e.g., occupational, transportation-based, incidental PA) and structured (leisure time moderate-to-vigorous PA; exercise). Common methods to measure PA include questionnaires, pedometers, and accelerometers. Questionnaires are quick to perform and simple to administer and interpret, though are prone to recall bias [18]. For this reason questionnaires may be most useful for broadly categorizing patients as meeting PA guidelines or not [19]. In contrast, pedometers and accelerometers can objectively measure PA and so may be more useful for tracking patient PA behavior over time [19]. In addition, recent advances in accelerometry-based devices have prompted investigation into the 24-h activity cycle and the relationships between sleep, sedentary time, varying intensities of PA (light, moderate, vigorous), and health [20]. Such advances have highlighted the importance of considering the health benefits of all activity intensity domains, as opposed to focusing solely on exercise [20].

Cardiorespiratory Fitness

Cardiorespiratory fitness (CRF) is a physiological characteristic that defines the ability of the respiratory, circulatory, and muscular systems to distribute and use oxygen during continuous physical activity. CRF is inversely associated with overweight and obesity [21], and as outlined in a recent statement paper from the American Heart Association [22], it is also a strong and independent predictor of morbidity and mortality beyond traditional risk factors.

Maximal CRF is assessed directly using standardized exercise protocols (treadmill or cycle ergometer) and expressed as maximal oxygen consumption (VO_2 max) or estimated either from submaximal tests or non-exercise algorithms [22]. PA is the primary modifiable determinant of CRF, where PA leads to an improvement in both central [23] (stroke volume) and peripheral [24] (mitochondrial density and increased vascularization) determinants of CRF. Collectively, these improvements result in increased oxygen delivery and uptake of the exercising muscles, thereby increasing CRF. Thus, CRF is often considered a surrogate measure of PA and an objective measure of the effect of PA on long-term outcomes. However, in longitudinal trials the association between PA and CRF is modest [25, 26]. This is likely due in part to how PA and CRF are assessed. For example, self-report PA questionnaires are often used to assess PA, which are subjective and correlate poorly with direct measures of PA [27], while CRF is typically assessed by a VO_2 max test, which represents a direct and objective assessment of CRF. In addition, there is a strong heritability component in the response of CRF to PA leading to large interindividual differences in CRF improvement following the adoption of PA [28]. Nonetheless, increased PA of adequate intensity, duration, and volume is the primary factor for improving CRF; thus, improvements in CRF generally reflect changes in PA.

Epidemiological Evidence of the Interactions Between CRF, PA, and Obesity

Independent Effects of PA and CRF on Obesity

Both PA and CRF are inversely associated with obesity, where PA is the primary modifiable determinant of CRF. However, CRF is often more strongly associated with obesity [29, 30] and obesity-related metabolic risk [21, 31] than PA. Moreover, these observations are seen when PA is measured through self-report [30, 31] and objectively [21, 29]. A potential explanation for these observations is that CRF is a reflection of both the physiological response to PA as well as genetic predisposition and thus may more accurately reflect the combined effect of intrinsic (genetics, sex) and acquired (PA) factors on health risk. Since PA is the only verified method to improve CRF and is associated with weight loss in a dose-response manner [32], PA should be encouraged to improve CRF, and reduce obesity and obesity-related health risk.

PA and Obesity: Current Guideline Recommendations

Several public health committees [4, 33, 34] recommend PA as an important component of weight loss, weight loss maintenance, and weight gain prevention strategies. Collectively, these committees recommend PA in excess of 250 min per week to promote weight loss and weight loss maintenance and 150–250 min per week of moderate-intensity PA to prevent weight gain [4, 33, 34].

PA and Obesity: Observations on PA Amount

The aforementioned guidelines are based on longitudinal studies that have explored the inverse association between the amount of regular PA performed and obesity. For example, Di Pietro and colleagues [14] examined the association between daily PA and weight change in men with sedentary desk jobs over a 5-year period. The authors reported that daily PA was inversely associated with weight gain in this population [14]. Moreover, the authors proposed that, consistent with the above guidelines, approximately 45–60 min of moderate PA per day was necessary to prevent weight gain [14].

In women, the role of PA amount on weight gain prevention is less straightforward. Consistent with Di Pietro and colleagues, Lee et al. [13] reported that sustaining high amounts (60 min of moderate PA per day) of PA was required to prevent weight gain in women. However, the authors also reported that this association was only observed in women who did not have overweight or obesity at baseline [13]. Therefore, they suggest that for overweight or obese women, increasing PA does not help prevent weight gain, and instead controlling caloric intake may be more important for weight maintenance [13]. However, the discrepancy observed between men and women may be due to an inconsistency in the way in which daily PA levels were measured. For example, occupational PA levels were not measured in the female cohort, whereas occupational

PA was controlled for in the male cohort. As mentioned previously, the decline in occupational PA over the last few decades has substantially contributed to weight gain in adults [3]. Thus, further investigations on the role of PA on weight change are warranted. Incorporating 45–60 min/day of moderate PA within work time hours, by introducing standing/treadmill desks, taking walking breaks, and/or walking meetings, may be a practical strategy to prevent weight gain long term.

PA and Obesity: Observations on PA Intensity

Current weight management recommendations do not address the issue of exercise intensity for weight loss or maintenance [34]. Yet, findings from longitudinal studies indicate a dose-response relationship between intensity of PA and risk of overweight or obesity [35–37]. In older adults, moderate-to-vigorous PA (MVPA; >3 METs, i.e., walking at ≥2.5 mph), but not light PA (LPA; 1.5–<3 METs, i.e., walking at <2.5 mph), is independently associated with lean mass and negatively associated with fat mass [35]. Similarly, in young adults [36], there is a strong association between body fat percentage and moderate PA (MPA; 3–<6 METs), whereas no association is observed between LPA and measures of obesity. Interestingly, in this publication the association between vigorous PA (VPA; ≥6 METs, i.e., very brisk walking at >4.0 mph) and body fat percentage was not as robust as the association with MPA, though very little time was spent in VPA relative to MPA. As energy expenditure (EE) and a subsequent negative energy balance are the primary determinants of change in body weight [4, 38], it is unsurprising that small amounts of VPA, and thus minimal EE, was not strongly associated with body composition.

Collectively, evidence from longitudinal studies suggests that PA intensity above three METs (i.e., walking at ≥2.5 mph) is beneficial for reducing risk of overweight and obesity, though further research is required on PA intensity above 6 METs (i.e., very brisk walking at >4.0 mph). However, accurate assessment of the intensity of PA in longitudinal trials is challenging, as PA intensity, often assessed by self-report, is unreliable [18]. The increase in the use of accelerometry to objectively measure PA in more recent longitudinal trials [39–41] will prove crucial in clarifying the effect of PA intensity on obesity-related health outcomes. For now, the intensity of various activities is available in the 2011 Compendium of Physical Activities [42].

Physical Activity, CRF, and Obesity as Predictors of Morbidity and Mortality

As stated, PA is the primary modifiable determinant of CRF. However, the modest correlation between these two variables leads to important questions regarding the relationship between PA, CRF, and health outcomes. Specifically, is the impact of PA different and independent of the impact of CRF on health? Similarly, do PA and CRF influence disease risk differently? Do they modify risk associated with obesity differently? Finally, which one of the two is more protective?

CRF, Obesity, and Cardiometabolic Risk

It is well established that CRF and adiposity are each independently associated with cardiometabolic risk factors. However, the strength of the association typically depends on the risk factor assessed. For example, while both CRF and BMI are independently associated with impaired fasting glucose [43–45], elevated BMI is more strongly associated with inflammatory markers [46], dyslipidemia [46], and hypertension [47–50]. However, when obesity is classified by visceral and subcutaneous adiposity, CRF is more strongly associated with hypertension and dyslipidemia than is adiposity [51]. This suggests that CRF modifies the relationship between abdominal obesity and cardiometabolic risk and is therefore protective against abdominal obesity-related metabolic risk. This is supported by observations that increasing CRF attenuates the risk of developing hypertension

[50], metabolic syndrome [50, 52], and hypercholesterolemia [50] in individuals who develop or have overweight and/or obesity. Thus, the aforementioned evidence suggests that both a reduction in body fat and improvement in CRF are important for improving cardiometabolic risk.

CRF, Obesity, and Mortality Risk

It is well established that CRF is inversely associated with all-cause mortality, while obesity is positively associated. Furthermore, evidence suggests that when CRF is added to all-cause [52–54] and CVD [52] mortality risk prediction models, the risk associated with increasing obesity is no longer significant (Table 14.1). This observation has been shown whether obesity is estimated by BMI [52], WC [54], or percent body fat [53]. Further, CRF improves all-cause mortality risk assessment when added to a combined BMI and WC risk model [58]. Thus, CRF predicts risk independent of obesity measures, and when included in obesity-related risk models, it improves risk assessment. These observations highlight the benefit of measuring CRF in a clinical setting, as CRF can improve the ability of practitioners to assess health risk of their patients beyond what is currently measured.

PA, Obesity, and Morbidity Risk

There is overwhelming evidence that PA is associated with a reduction in risk factors associated with type 2 diabetes and cardiovascular disease (CVD). In a review by Janiszewski and Ross [59], the authors emphasized that the favorable impact of PA on visceral adiposity, insulin resistance, and hypertension is independent of significant changes in body weight. However, when looking at long-term health outcomes, longitudinal evidence on the association between PA, obesity, and morbidity risk suggests that obesity is a more important determinant of morbidity than PA. For example, when adults are separated by activity level (active or inactive) and change in BMI over a 10-year period, having a BMI greater than 25 (overweight to obese) for a longer duration was the stronger predictor of CVD risk [60]. In the same analysis, the authors reported that being active attenuated but did not eliminate risk of CVD in overweight or obese individuals. Similar observations have been shown with coronary heart disease (CHD) risk, where weight more strongly predicts CHD risk than PA, though PA was associated with an attenuation in risk [56] (Table 14.1). Interestingly, in individuals with CHD, regular PA but not weight loss was associated with a lower risk of all-cause mortality, suggesting that while obesity may be more important than PA for lowering risk of CVD onset, in individuals who already have CHD, adopting or maintaining PA is more important for survival [61]. Thus, both PA and obesity management are important for long-term health, where PA is especially important for long-term survival in clinical populations.

Interactions Between CRF, PA, and Obesity with Risk Assessment

When self-reported PA and CRF are assessed together, CRF is often associated with risk independent of PA [31, 57]. In individuals with obesity, improving CRF reduces the risk of developing a metabolically unhealthy profile, independent of PA [31]. Further, when PA and CRF are assessed in concert with obesity, CRF is inversely associated with risk of developing metabolic syndrome independent of both PA and obesity [57]. However, when PA is measured objectively, it has a threefold stronger inverse association with risk of developing metabolic syndrome than does CRF [62]. While more evidence on objective measures of PA and long-term health outcomes are required, this initial observation reinforces the importance of engaging in regular PA to decrease risk of morbidity.

Interventional Data on PA, CRF, Obesity, and Outcomes

Based on observations from longitudinal trials showing the benefit of adopting PA, lowering obesity, and improving CRF on lowering risk

Table 14.1 Efficacy of PA, CRF, and obesity on reducing morbidity and mortality risk

Article	*N*	Women (%)	Age (years)	Outcome measure	Method of measurement	Risk[a]			
CRF and obesity						**Obesity**	**CRF**	**Obesity adjusted for CRF**	**CRF adjusted for obesity**
Church et al. [53]	2196	0.0%	49.3 (9.5)	All-cause mortality in men with diabetes	BMI Modified Balke protocol on a treadmill	+4% for every 1 unit increase in BMI[i]	−25% for every 1 MET inc[i]	n/s	−26% for every 1 MET inc[i]
Katzmarzyk et al. [52]	19,173	0.0%	43.1 (9.7)	All-cause mortality in men with metabolic syndrome	BMI	Obese: 55%[j]		Obese: n/s[j]	
Sui et al. [54]	2603	19.8%	64.4 (4.8)	All-cause mortality	BMI Modified Balke protocol on a treadmill	Obese: n/s[k]	Fit: −47%[k]	Obese: n/s[k]	Fit: −49%[k]
PA and obesity						**Obesity**	**PA**	**Obesity adjusted for PA**	**PA adjusted for obesity**
Hu et al. [17]	116,564	100.0%	30–55	All-cause mortality	BMI Self-report PA	Obese: +56%[b]	Inactive: +52%[c]		Inactive: +44%[c]
Hu et al. [55]	47,212	52.0%	25–64	All-cause mortality	BMI Self-report PA	*Men* Obese: +24%[d] *Women* Obese: +37%[d]	*Men* Active: −36%[d] *Women* Active: −41%[d]	*Men* Obese: +17%[e] *Women* Obese: +15%[e]	*Men* Active: −26%[e] *Women* Active: −36%[e]
Li et al. [56]	88,393	100%	34–59	Coronary heart disease	BMI Self-report PA	Obese: +207%[f]	Inactive: +58%[g]		Inactive: +43%[g]
Yu et al. [57]	184	100%	61.1 (3.1)	Metabolic syndrome	BMI Self-report PA		Active: −56%[h]		Active: −58%[h]

All values significant at $p < 0.05$ unless otherwise stated

PA physical activity, *CRF* cardiorespiratory fitness, *HR* hazard ratio, *RR* relative risk, *OR* odds ratio

[a]Risk measured as hazard ratio [54, 55], relative risk [17, 31, 52, 53, 56], odds ratio [57]

[b]Adjusted for: age

[c]Adjusted for: age, smoking status, alcohol consumption, parental history of CHD, postmenopausal status and hormone use, BMI (where indicated)

[d]Adjusted for: age, examination year

[e]Adjusted for: age, examination year, education, smoking status, systolic blood pressure, cholesterol, diabetes at baseline, and PA/BMI (where indicated)

[f]Adjusted for: age

[g]Adjusted for: age, smoking status, alcohol consumption, parental history of CVD, postmenopausal status and hormone use, aspirin use, BMI (where indicated)

[h]Adjusted for: age, BMI (where indicated)

[i]Adjusted for: age, examination year, BMI (where indicated)

[j]Adjusted for: age, examination year, smoking status, alcohol consumption, CVD, parental history of CVD, CRF (where indicated)

[k]Adjusted for: age, sex, examination year, smoking status, abnormal ECG, baseline health status (CVD, hypertension, diabetes, hypercholesterolemia), BMI, and CRF (where indicated)

of morbidity and mortality, many randomized controlled trials have been performed to better isolate the effects of PA, CRF, and weight loss on health outcomes. The next sections will discuss evidence from RCTs on the effect of PA on weight management, as well as the combined effect of increasing PA and CRF and lowering obesity on cardiometabolic risk factors.

PA and Weight Loss

It is well established that in a well-controlled, supervised environment, a negative energy balance induced by exercise in the absence of caloric reduction is associated with a substantial reduction in weight and measures of abdominal adiposity [63–66]. These observations are countered by behavioral-based interventions [67] wherein the strategy is to sustain PA for long periods without supervision. In these trials the effect of exercise on weight loss is modest at best [67]. Collectively, these observations show that in a well-controlled environment, exercise is effective at inducing weight loss and reducing abdominal obesity. However, under real-world conditions, encouraging adults to sustain exercise long term is extremely difficult and remains a major public healthcare challenge.

PA and Weight Loss Maintenance

One of the greatest challenges in weight loss interventions is long-term maintenance. Diet-based interventions have been criticized for their lack of long-term effectiveness [68], where up to two-thirds of dieters regain more weight than was lost following completion of diet-only interventions [68, 69]. Interventions that combine exercise with diet are more successful than diet alone in preventing weight regain. In a meta-analysis Franz and colleagues [67] reported that at 12 months diet-only trials, especially very low calorie diet trials, resulted in greater weight recidivism than diet and exercise combined. The amount of PAEE also influences risk of regain; in a 3-year exercise intervention, Jakicic et al. [70] reported that individuals who sustained 10% weight loss or more after 2 years performed substantially more exercise (275 min/week) than those who did not. These observations by Jakicic et al. [70] are consistent with those of Di Pietro et al. [14], Lee et al. [13], and Hu et al. [71] that more than 30 min/day of moderate PA is required to prevent weight gain. These findings are also reflected in obesity management recommendations by the American College of Sports Medicine (ACSM) [4], distinguishing between PA for health benefit and PA for weight loss maintenance. PA in excess of 250 min per week is recommended for weight loss maintenance, but only 150 min is required for health benefit.

PA and Prevention of Weight Gain

There is substantial experimental data to suggest that the body defends more strongly against a negative energy balance than a positive balance [72, 73]; therefore, it may be easier to prevent against weight not yet acquired than to lose existing weight [74, 75]. Given the lack of success many adults experience losing weight and maintaining weight loss, a more achievable strategy to reduce the prevalence of overweight and obesity may be to prevent weight gain. Moreover, data on long-term weight regain shows that individuals whose weight cycles from loss to gain experience a greater reduction in lean mass during weight loss and accumulation of fat mass during weight gain compared to non-weight cyclers [31]. Since weight gain is associated with an increased risk of morbidity and mortality in a dose-response manner [17, 55, 75, 76], limiting weight gain may be more beneficial and realistic for overall health than continual weight loss efforts.

Based on observations of weight gain in the past two decades, Hill and colleagues [74] argue that an energy deficit of 100 kilocalories per day could prevent weight gain in 90% of adults [77]. Consistent with this theory, two short-term pilot studies have shown that a modest decrease in energy intake (100 kcal/day less) combined with a small increase in PA (an additional 2000 steps/day, equivalent to 20 min/day of MPA) was successful in preventing weight gain in families [78, 79]. In fact, a RCT is under way to determine the long-term effectiveness of this approach [80]. Though the findings from this long-term RCT are yet to be published, the success of the above pilot studies combined with the observation that PA level is inversely associated with future weight gain [14, 66] suggests that PA has an important role in preventing weight gain in adults. Therefore, encouraging patients to make small changes in diet (100 kcal less/day) and PA (adopt 20 min of MPA/day in 10 min bouts or more) may be an effective method to prevent weight gain and a pragmatic first step toward reducing obesity.

PA, CRF, and Obesity Reduction in the Absence of Weight Loss

PA is associated with an improvement in CRF and health-related outcomes regardless of weight change [81–84]. PA is also associated with an increase in lean mass and a reduction in visceral adiposity independent of changes in body weight [65, 84]. Collectively, these observations indicate that healthcare professionals should encourage their patients to engage in regular PA for effective obesity and obesity-related risk management and not gauge successful obesity reduction solely through reductions in body weight.

PA, CRF, and Obesity Reduction in Relation to Cardiometabolic Risk Factors

There is substantive epidemiological evidence that physical inactivity, low CRF, and obesity are associated with a poor cardiovascular profile and an increased risk of morbidity and mortality. To better identify the causal relationship between PA, CRF, and obesity on health, several research groups have examined the effect of exercise on CRF and obesity in relation to risk factors of morbidity and mortality. This next section will summarize evidence from RCTs on the interacting and combined effects of PA, CRF, and obesity on dyslipidemia, insulin resistance, and hypertension.

Dyslipidemia

Dyslipidemia is defined by an abnormal lipid profile that includes high blood levels of total cholesterol, low-density lipoprotein (LDL) cholesterol, and/or triglycerides (TG) or low levels of high-density lipoprotein (HDL) cholesterol, and is associated with an increased risk of morbidity and CVD mortality [85]. Moreover, excess adiposity, physical inactivity, and low CRF are associated with a dyslipidemic profile [86–88]. Several RCTs have examined the effects of exercise and weight loss on the lipid profile of inactive overweight and obese individuals. Consistent in the literature is that higher amounts of PAEE are associated with greater improvements in the lipid profile of participants [59, 89–92] (Table 14.2 and Fig. 14.1). A meta-analysis of 25 RCTs including studies from both men and women across a wide age range [107] concluded that moderate-intensity walking and an improvement in CRF were both correlated with improvements in LDL and the total cholesterol (TC)-to-HDL ratio independent of body composition. Important to note in this meta-analysis is that adhering to guideline-type PA was associated with a reduction in the TC-to-HDL ratio such that on average, individuals who became active were more likely to shift out of the high-risk category (10-year risk, 20%) for coronary artery disease [108]. A more recent study found that aerobic, resistance, and combined exercises resulted in similar improvements in the TC-to-HDL ratio in abdominally obese women when similar amounts of PAEE within guideline recommendations were prescribed [93]. Thus, the adoption of PA consistent with current guidelines is sufficient to incur clinically relevant improvements in the lipid profile of high-risk individuals.

Table 14.2 Efficacy of PA vs obesity reduction on improving cardiometabolic risk factors

Article	*N*	Women (%)	Age (years)	PA intervention	Outcome measures: Change in body weight	Outcome measures: Change in cardiometabolic risk factor
Dyslipidemia						
Slentz et al. [89]	240	45.8%	40–65	Amount: 125 min/week Intensity: 65–80% VO_2peak Duration: 24 weeks	Subjects counseled to maintain body weight	LDL: 1.7 (16.0) mg/dl VLDL-TG: −13.7 (52.0) mg/dl HDL: 1.3 (5.5) mg/dl
				Amount: 203 min/week Intensity: 40–55% VO_2peak Duration: 24 weeks		LDL: n/s VLDL-TG: −33.6 (66.0) mg/dl HDL: n/s
				Amount: 207 min/week Intensity: 65–80% VO_2peak Duration: 24 weeks		LDL: n/s VLDL-TG: −17.1 (49.0) mg/dl HDL: 2.7 (6.7) mg/dl
Ades et al. [90]	74	37.8%	64 (9)	Amount: 75–120 min/week Intensity: 65–70% VO_2peak Duration: 20 weeks Group counseled to consume 500 kcal less than predicated maintenance calories	Weight: 3.7 (5.0) kg WC: −5.0 (5.0) cm Body fat: −2.8 (3.0) kg	HDL: n/s Triglycerides: n/s
				Amount: 225–420 min/week Intensity: 50–60% VO_2peak Duration: 20 weeks Group counseled to consume 500 kcal less than predicated maintenance calories	Weight: −8.2 (4.0) kg WC: −7.0(5.0) cm Body fat: −5.9 (4.0) kg	HDL: 3.0 mg/dl Triglycerides: −31.0 mg/dl
Pagels et al. [92]	33	45.5%	25–45	Amount: 210 min/week Intensity: 65–80% VO_2peak Duration: 3 weeks	Weight: −0.7(1.2) kg BMI: −0.2 (0.4) kg/m^2	Total cholesterol: −5.0(8.6) mg/dl LDL: −5.4(8.1) mg/dl
Choo et al. [93]	110	100.0%	18–65	Amount: 180 min/week Intensity: 50–70% heart rate reserve Duration: 36 weeks	Weight: −5.1 kg	TC-to-HDL ratio: −0.62
				Resistance: 180 min/week, 8 exercises, 2 sets of 8–12 repetitions Intensity: 40–50% of maximum strength Duration: 36 weeks	Weight: −7.8 kg	TC-to-HDL ratio: −0.35
				Combination: 90 min/week aerobic, 90 min/week resistance Duration: 36 weeks	Weight: −7.0 kg	TC-to-HDL ratio: −0.82

(continued)

Table 14.2 (continued)

Article	*N*	Women (%)	Age (years)	PA intervention	Outcome measures: Change in body weight	Outcome measures: Change in cardiometabolic risk factor
Insulin resistance						
Hersey et al. [94]	42	50.0%	70–79	Amount: 105–135 min/week Intensity: 75–85% heart rate reserve Duration: 24 weeks	Weight: n/s Percent body fat: −2.0%	Insulin AUC: −16%
				Resistance: 1 set 10 exercises, 8–12 repetitions, 3x/week Intensity: to volitional fatigue Duration: 24 weeks	Weight: n/s Percent body fat: n/s	Insulin AUC: n/s
Perseghin et al. [95]	18	66.7%	19–43	Amount: 180 min/week Intensity: 65% VO_2 max Duration: 6 weeks Offspring of parents with NIDDM	Counseled to maintain weight	Plasma insulin: −2 uU/ml (basal), −9 uU/ml (second phase) Whole body glucose: −2.5 mg/kg*min
Dengel et al. [96]	97	0.00%	50–70	Amount: 120 min/week Intensity: 75–85% HRR Duration: 36 weeks	Weight: n/s	Fasting glucose: n/s Fasting insulin: n/s Glucose AUC: 1069 mg/min*dL Insulin AUC: −2875 uU*min/ml
Wing et al. [97]	154	79%	45.7 (4.4)	Amount: 150 min/week Intensity: 60–85% VO_2peak Duration: 24 weeks Counseled to adhere to 800–1000 kcal/day diet for first 16 weeks, adjusted to 1200–1500 kcal/day thereafter	Weight: −2.1 (4.2) kg BMI: −0.8 (1.5) kg/m^2 WHR: −0.03 (0.05)	HbA1c: n/s Fasting plasma glucose: n/s Fasting insulin: n/s
Rice et al. [98]	29	0.0%	39–47	Amount: 300 min/week Intensity: 85% HRmax Duration: 16 weeks Counseled to reduce EI by 1000 kcal/day	Weight: −11.5(3.9) kg BMI: −3.7 (1.1) kg/m^2 WC: −12.9 (4.0) cm SAT: −2.1 (0.8) L VAT: −1.5 (0.9) L	Fasting glucose: n/s Fasting insulin: −8.4 (6.7) ulU/ml Glucose AUC: n/s Insulin AUC: −582 (244) pmol/l*2 h
				Resistance: 90 min/week, 8–12 repetitions Intensity: to failure Duration: 16 weeks Counseled to reduce EI by 1000 kcal/day	Weight: −13.6 (4.1) kg BMI: −4.3 (1.4) kg/m^2 WC: −11.9 (3.9) cm SAT: −2.8 (0.9) L VAT: −1.2 (0.6) L	Fasting glucose: n/s Fasting insulin: −7.7 (7.1) ulU/ml Glucose AUC: n/s Insulin AUC: −594 (370) pmol/l*2 h

Poehlman et al. [99]	51	100%	18–35	Amount: 180 min/week Intensity: 85% HR max Duration: 24 weeks	Weight: n/s	Insulin sensitivity: 69 mg/min
				Resistance: 3 sets, 9 exercises, 10 repetitions, 3x/week Intensity: 80% of 1RM Duration: 24 weeks	Weight: +2 kg	Insulin sensitivity: n/s
Pratley et al. [100]	17	0.0%	59 (2.0)	Amount: 135–240 min/week Intensity: 80–85% heart rate reserve Duration: 36 weeks	Weight: −1.1 kg Percent body fat: −2.0% WC: −1.7 cm WHR: −1.0%	Insulin AUC: −16%
Ross et al. [64]	52	0.0%	42–46	Exercise-weight loss Amount: 300 min/week Intensity: 80% VO_2peak Duration: 12 weeks	Weight: −7.5 kg BMI: −2.4 kg/m^2 SAT: −4.2 kg VAT: −52 cm^2	Fasting glucose: n/s Fasting insulin: n/s OGTT glucose: −3.4 mg/dl*2 h OGTT insulin: −899 pmol/l*2 h Glucose disposal: −7.2 mg/kg muscle*min
				Exercise-no weight loss: Amount: 300 min/week Intensity: 80% VO_2peak Replace kcal expended from PA Duration: 12 weeks	Weight: n/s BMI: n/s SAT: n/s VAT: −32 cm^2	Fasting glucose: n/s Fasting insulin: n/s OGTT glucose: n/s OGTT insulin: n/s Glucose disposal: n/s
Ross et al. [65]	54	100.0%	41–43	Exercise-weight loss Amount: 300 min/week Intensity: 80% VO_2peak Duration: 14 weeks	Weight: −5.9 kg BMI: 2.4 kg/m^2 WC: 6.5 cm SAT: −1.1 kg VAT: −0.7 kg	Fasting glucose: n/s Fasting insulin: n/s OGTT glucose: n/s OGTT insulin: −430 pM/2 hours Glucose disposal: 6.3 mg/kg muscle*min
				Exercise-no weight loss Amount: 300 min/week Intensity: 80% VO_2peak Replace kcal expended from PA Duration: 14 weeks	Weight: n/s BMI: n/s WC: −3.1 cm SAT: −0.3 kg VAT: −0.4 kg	Fasting glucose: n/s Fasting insulin: n/s OGTT glucose: n/s OGTT insulin: n/s Glucose disposal: n/s
O'Leary et al. [101]	16	68.8%	63 (1)	Amount: 300 min/week Intensity: 85% HRmax Duration: 12 weeks Counseled not to change energy intake	Weight: −3.2 kg VAT: −40 cm^2 SAT: −46 cm^2	Fasting glucose: n/s Fasting insulin: −4.1 uU/ml Glucose AUC: 95 units Insulin AUC: 15,213

(continued)

Table 14.2 (continued)

Article	*N*	Women (%)	Age (years)	PA intervention	Outcome measures: Change in body weight	Outcome measures: Change in cardiometabolic risk factor
Sigal et al. [102]	251	36.3%	39–70	Aerobic Amount: 135 min/week Intensity: 75% HRmax Duration: 22 weeks	Weight: −2.6 kg BMI: −0.8 kg/m^2 WC: −3.0 cm SAT: −17 cm^2	HbA1c: −0.4%
				Resistance: 7 exercises, 3 sets of 7–9 repetitions Intensity: to volitional fatigue Duration: 22 weeks	Weight: n/s BMI: n/s WC: n/s SAT: −18 cm^2	HbA1c: −0.3%
				Combined Full aerobic and resistance regimen Duration: 22 weeks	Weight: −2.6 kg BMI: −0.8 kg/m^2 WC: −4.0 cm SAT: −27 cm^2	HbA1c: −0.9%
Tjonna et al. [103]	32	46.9%	52.3 (3.7)	Amount: 120 min/week Intensity: 90% HRmax Duration: 16 weeks	Weight: −2.3 kg BMI: −0.7 kg/m^2 WC: −5.0 cm	Insulin sensitivity (HOMA): +15%
				Amount: 141 min/week Intensity: 70% HRmax Duration: 16 weeks	Weight: −3.6 kg BMI: −1.2 kg/m^2 WC: −6.0 cm	Insulin sensitivity (HOMA): n/s
Ades et al. [90]	74	37.8%	64 (9)	Amount: 75–120 min/week Intensity: 65–70% VO_2peak Duration: 20 weeks Group counseled to consume 500 kcal less than predicated maintenance calories	Weight: 3.7 (5) kg WC: −5.0 (5) cm Body fat: −2.8 (3) kg	Fasting insulin: −3 uIU/ml Fasting glucose: n/s Glucose disposal: −1.0 mg/FFM*min
				Amount: 225–420 min/week Intensity: 50–60% VO_2peak Duration: 20 weeks Group counseled to consume 500 kcal less than predicated maintenance calories	Weight: −8.2 (4) kg WC: −7.0(5) cm Body fat: −5.9 (4) kg	Fasting insulin: – 6uIU/ml Fasting glucose: −7.0 mg/dl Glucose disposal: −1.8 mg/FFM*min

Davidson et al. [104]	136	58.1%	60–80	Aerobic Amount: 150 min/week Intensity: 60–75% VO_2peak	Weight: −2.77(0.33) kg BMI: −0.96 (0.12) kg/m^2 WC: −5.08 (0.46) cm SAT: −0.40 (0.07) kg VAT: −0.43 (0.08) kg	Fasting insulin: n/s Insulin resistance: −6.51(1.27) M/I
				Resistance: 150 min/week Intensity: 1 set of 9 exercises to volitional fatigue	Weight: −2.31(0.33) kg BMI: −0.84 (0.12) kg/m^2 WC: −4.61 (0.47) cm SAT: −0.40 (0.06) kg VAT: −0.35 (0.05) kg	Fasting insulin: n/s Insulin resistance: −9.22(1.33) M/I
				Combined: 150 min/week Intensity: 60–75% VO_2peak for aerobic, volitional fatigue for resistance Participants counseled to maintain weight	Weight: n/s BMI: n/s WC: −3.18 (0.49) cm SAT: −0.21 (0.07) kg VAT: −0.21 (0.06) kg	Fasting insulin: n/s Insulin resistance: n/s
Ross et al. [63]	300	65.3%	51.4 (8.1)	Amount: 150 min/week Intensity: 50% VO_2peak Duration: 36 weeks	Weight: −3.8 (−5.5, −2.1) kg WC: −3.9 (−5.6, −2.3) cm	2-hour glucose: n/s
				Amount: 200 min/week Intensity: 75% VO_2peak Duration: 36 weeks	Weight: −4.6 (−6.3, −2.9) kg WC: −4.6 (−6.3, −2.9) cm	2-hour glucose: −12.6 (−23.4 to −1.8) mg/dl
				Amount: 300 min/week Intensity: 50% VO_2peak Duration: 36 weeks	Weight: −4.9 (−6.5, −3.3) kg WC: −4.6 (−6.2, −3.0) cm	2-hour glucose: n/s
Hypertension						
Dengel et al. [96]	97	0.00%	50–70	Amount: 120 min/week Intensity: 75–85% HRR Duration: 36 weeks	Weight: n/s	SBP: −6.4(1.3) DBP: −5.2(1.0)
Dengel et al. [105]	17	0.00%	50–70	Amount: 120 min/week Intensity: 75–85% HRR Duration: 24 weeks Restrict diet by 300–500 kcal/day Normotensive vs hypertensive	Weight: −9.1 kg WC: −10.1 cm	SBP: −14(3) mmHg DBP: −10(2) mmHg

(continued)

Table 14.2 (continued)

Article	N	Women (%)	Age (years)	PA intervention	Outcome measures: Change in body weight	Outcome measures: Change in cardiometabolic risk factor
Church et al. [106]	464	100.0%	57.3 (6.4)	Amount: 75 min/week Intensity: 50% VO_2peak Duration: 24 weeks Counseled to replace kcal expended through PA	Weight: n/s WC: 1.9 cm	SBP: n/s DBP: n/s
				Amount: 150 min/week Intensity: 50% VO_2peak Duration: 24 weeks Counseled to replace kcal expended through PA	Weight: n/s WC: 2.9 cm	SBP: n/s DBP: n/s
				Amount: 225 min/week Intensity: 50% VO_2peak Duration: 24 weeks Counseled to replace kcal expended through PA	Weight: n/s WC: 1.4 cm	SBP: −3.3 (1.1) mmHg DBP: n/s
Ades et al. [90]	74	37.8%	64 (9)	Amount: 75–120 min/week Intensity: 65–70% VO_2peak Duration: 20 weeks Group counseled to consume 500 kcal less than predicated maintenance calories	Weight: 3.7 (5.0) kg WC: −5.0 (5.0) cm Body fat: −2.8 (3.0) kg	SBP: −10 mmHg DBP: −4 mmHg
				Amount: 225–420 min/week Intensity: 50–60% VO_2peak Duration: 20 weeks Group counseled to consume 500 kcal less than predicated maintenance calories	Weight: −8.2 (4.0) kg WC: −7.0 (5.0) cm Body fat: −5.9 (4.0) kg	SBP: −8 mmHg DBP: −7 mmHg

All values significant at $p < 0.05$ unless otherwise stated

Insulin Resistance

Insulin resistance is a major metabolic disturbance that drives the onset of both type 2 diabetes and CVD [109]. The primary modifiable determinants of insulin resistance are physical inactivity and abdominal obesity [49, 110]. Several RCTs have explored the interacting and combined effects of PA, CRF, and weight loss on reducing the onset of insulin resistance and improving glucose metabolism (Table 14.2 and Fig. 14.1). The findings from these trials support that a reduction in abdominal adiposity, and not an increase in CRF, predicts improvement in insulin sensitivity in middle-aged and older adults following the adoption of regular aerobic exercise [100, 110, 111]. Similarly, O'Leary et al. [101] observed that while change in insulin resistance was positively associated with visceral adipose tissue (VAT) and negatively associated with CRF following a 12-week aerobic exercise program, the association was stronger with VAT. Further, results from a 2-year diet and exercise intervention in individuals with a family history of diabetes [97] revealed that weight loss, achieved either through diet or exercise, was the strongest negative predictor of type 2 diabetes onset.

There is also evidence that an improvement in insulin sensitivity induced by weight loss may be different in men and women. For example, Ross and colleagues [65] reported that insulin sensitivity improves through exercise-induced but not diet-induced weight loss in women, likely due to a greater reduction in total and abdominal

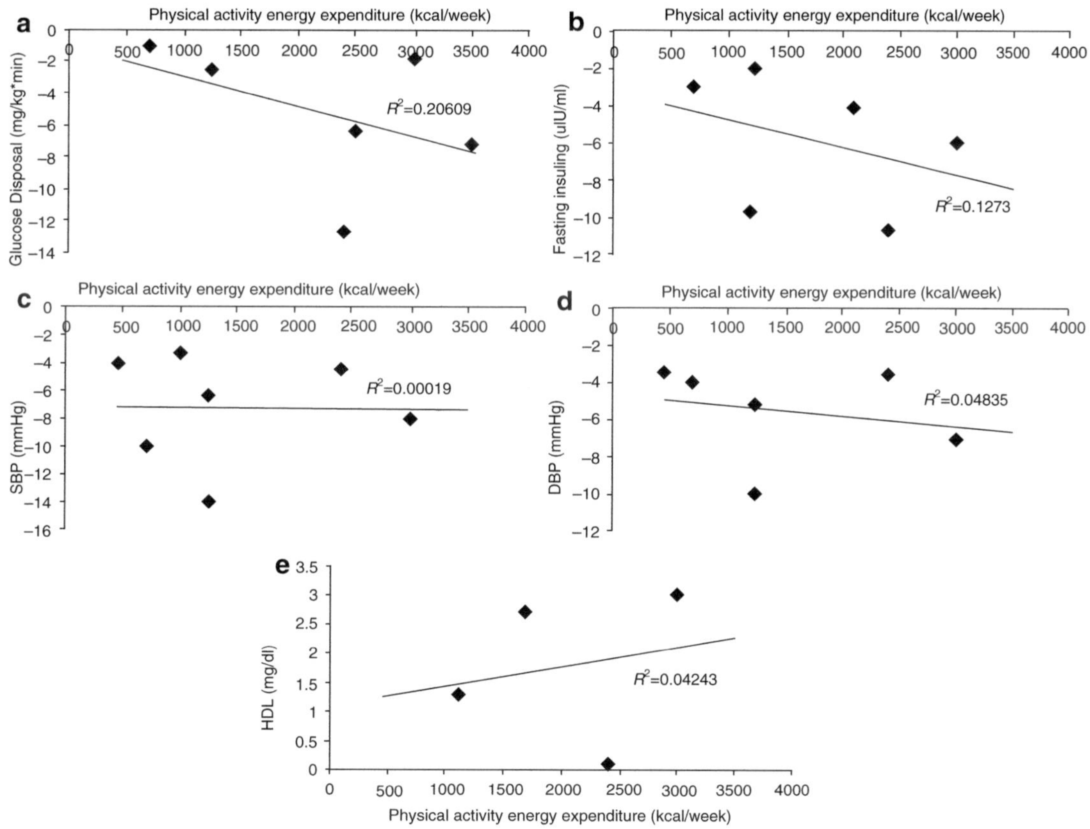

Fig. 14.1 Change in cardiometabolic variables in response to differing amounts of exercise as measured by physical activity energy expenditure. (**a**) Glucose disposal [63–65, 90, 95], (**b**) fasting insulin [63, 90, 95, 101], (**c**) systolic blood pressure (SBP) [63, 90, 91, 96, 105, 106], (**d**) diastolic blood pressure (DBP) [63, 90, 91, 96, 105], and (**e**) high-density lipoprotein (HDL) cholesterol [63, 89, 90]. Data points represent group means from the above-cited randomized controlled trials

adiposity with exercise. In another study, these investigators reported that diet- or exercise-induced weight loss led to similar reductions in VAT and similar improvements in insulin sensitivity in men [64]. However, several studies have shown that in both men and women, the combination of diet and exercise incurs the greatest improvement insulin sensitivity [96, 98, 105, 112]. It is also well established that exercise improves insulin sensitivity acutely in men and women, though this effect dissipates rapidly beyond 48 h [95, 113]. Therefore, regular PA is necessary to sustain the exercise-induced acute benefit, and the combination of diet and regular PA is optimal for long-term benefit in both men and women.

Both aerobic and resistance exercises [63, 94, 98, 99, 102, 104] are associated with improvements in insulin sensitivity, though aerobic exercise is often more effective due to higher EE and subsequent greater fat mass loss. Interestingly, when EE is matched, guideline-type aerobic exercise and a combination of aerobic and resistance exercises result in similar improvements in abdominal adiposity and insulin sensitivity [104, 114]. In contrast, higher-intensity exercise (80–90% of maximum heart rate) is associated with greater improvements in insulin sensitivity, even when PAEE is matched [63, 103, 115]. Thus, reducing abdominal adiposity and engaging in regular PA with emphasis on increasing PA intensity are important targets for improving insulin sensitivity.

Hypertension

Hypertension is a major risk factor for CVD [116], where physical activity [117] and weight loss [50] are considered as effective non-pharmaceutical methods to lower blood pressure. It is important to note that even small reductions in diastolic blood pressure (2 mmHg) may substantially reduce the prevalence of hypertension, risk of CHD, and stroke [118]. In a systematic review of 22 lifestyle-based interventions for weight loss and cardiovascular risk factor reduction in individuals with overweight/obesity, Schwingshackl et al. [119] reported that exercise consistent with current guidelines, combined with a healthful diet ($\leq$ 30% total energy from fat, reduce intake of saturated fats, increased intake of fruit, vegetables, and fiber), resulted in substantive reductions in body weight (~4 kg) and clinically relevant reductions in systolic blood pressure (~2 mmHg). Thus, application of lifestyle-based strategies to lower blood pressure could considerably reduce the prevalence of hypertension-related morbidity (Table 14.2 and Fig. 14.1).

However, it remains unclear whether the exercise-related reduction in blood pressure is independent of weight loss. For example, in a meta-analysis on PA and blood pressure, PA-based interventions were associated with clinically significant reductions in blood pressure (~3.0 mmHg) despite minimal reductions in weight loss (−1.2 kg) [120]. In contrast, Ades et al. [90] found that PAEE and subsequent fat mass loss best predicted an improvement in blood pressure, suggesting that weight loss is the mediating factor between PA and blood pressure reduction. In line with these observations, Church and colleagues [106] reported that when weight was maintained in postmenopausal women, neither PA nor improvements in CRF affected blood pressure. This was true even when PA was prescribed up to 150% of guidelines. Thus, while further research is required to better elucidate the interactions between PA, obesity, and blood pressure, healthy lifestyle behaviors that include adequate PA in combination with a healthful diet are positively associated with improvements in blood pressure.

Recommendations

The preceding evidence suggests that to improve CRF and manage body weight, patients should engage in moderate-intensity PA consistent with current physical activity guidelines (150 min per week at 50% of maximum heart rate, i.e., brisk walking). For weight loss and weight loss maintenance, PA in excess of 250 min per week is recommended [4]. It is also important to note that higher PA intensity and volume is associated with a greater improvements in CRF [63].

However, adoption and maintenance of such large PA volumes are challenging for most people. In addition, poor adherence to weight loss strategies and subsequent weight cycling is associated with greater health risk than weight-stable overweight and obesity [31]. Thus, encouraging patients to first prevent weight gain by incorporating small changes in PA (2000 steps/day increase) and diet (100 kcal/day reduction) may be a more pragmatic and effective first step toward managing the current obesity epidemic.

Public Health/Clinical Significance

One-third of US adults now have obesity [122] where costs associated with overweight, obesity, and comorbidities are in excess of $150 billion USD annually [123]. Epidemiological evidence on PA behaviors strongly suggests that the decline in PA observed in the last few decades is a major contributor to the rise in overweight and obesity, where a higher level of PA [124, 125] and CRF [21, 30, 126–128] is associated with a lower prevalence of obesity across a wide age range. However, PA and CRF are associated with a targeted reduction in waist circumference, VAT, and cardiometabolic risk factors [64, 65, 81–84, 121] even in the absence of weight loss. Collectively, this evidence suggests that while the lowest-risk phenotype includes individuals who are at a normal weight, are active, and have high fitness [129], adopting PA regardless of the effect on weight has important health implications. Further, a singular focus on weight loss as the optimal treatment target may in fact be detrimental to the health of the patient if unsuccessful weight loss leads to discontinued adherence to healthy lifestyle behaviors [75]. Thus, shifting the focus away from weight loss and instead toward the importance of an active lifestyle is a crucial public health message that could substantially reduce the risk of morbidity and mortality in the United States.

References

1. WHO. Obesity and overweight: Fact Sheet 2016 [updated June 2016. Available from: http://www.who.int/mediacentre/factsheets/fs311/en/.
2. Global Burden of Metabolic Risk Factors for Chronic Diseases C, Lu Y, Hajifathalian K, Ezzati M, Woodward M, Rimm EB, et al. Metabolic mediators of the effects of body-mass index, overweight, and obesity on coronary heart disease and stroke: a pooled analysis of 97 prospective cohorts with 1.8 million participants. Lancet. 2014;383(9921):970–83.
3. Church TS, Thomas DM, Tudor-Locke C, Katzmarzyk PT, Earnest CP, Rodarte RQ, et al. Trends over 5 decades in U.S. occupation-related physical activity and their associations with obesity. PLoS One. 2011;6(5):e19657.
4. Donnelly JE, Blair SN, Jakicic JM, Manore MM, Rankin JW, Smith BK, et al. American College of Sports Medicine Position Stand. Appropriate physical activity intervention strategies for weight loss and prevention of weight regain for adults. Med Sci Sports Exerc. 2009;41(2):459–71.
5. Despres JP, Lemieux I. Abdominal obesity and metabolic syndrome. Nature. 2006;444(7121):881–7.
6. Hurt RT, Kulisek C, Buchanan LA, McClave SA. The obesity epidemic: challenges, health initiatives, and implications for gastroenterologists. Gastroenterol Hepatol (N Y). 2010;6(12):780–92.
7. Bjorntorp P. "Portal" adipose tissue as a generator of risk factors for cardiovascular disease and diabetes. Arteriosclerosis. 1990;10(4):493–6.
8. Ross R, Leger L, Morris D, de Guise J, Guardo R. Quantification of adipose tissue by MRI: relationship with anthropometric variables. J Appl Physiol (1985). 1992;72(2):787–95.
9. Janssen I, Heymsfield SB, Allison DB, Kotler DP, Ross R. Body mass index and waist circumference independently contribute to the prediction of nonabdominal, abdominal subcutaneous, and visceral fat. Am J Clin Nutr. 2002;75(4):683–8.
10. Chan DC, Watts GF, Barrett PH, Burke V. Waist circumference, waist-to-hip ratio and body mass index as predictors of adipose tissue compartments in men. QJM. 2003;96(6):441–7.
11. Borruel S, Molto JF, Alpanes M, Fernandez-Duran E, Alvarez-Blasco F, Luque-Ramirez M, et al. Surrogate markers of visceral adiposity in young adults: waist circumference and body mass index are more accurate than waist hip ratio, model of adipose distribution and visceral adiposity index. PLoS One. 2014;9(12):e114112.
12. Nazare JA, Smith J, Borel AL, Aschner P, Barter P, Van Gaal L, et al. Usefulness of measuring both body mass index and waist circumference for the estimation of visceral adiposity and related cardiometabolic risk profile (from the INSPIRE ME IAA study). Am J Cardiol. 2015;115(3):307–15.

13. Lee IM, Djousse L, Sesso HD, Wang L, Buring JE. Physical activity and weight gain prevention. JAMA. 2010;303(12):1173–9.
14. Di Pietro L, Dziura J, Blair SN. Estimated change in physical activity level (PAL) and prediction of 5-year weight change in men: the Aerobics Center Longitudinal Study. Int J Obes Relat Metab Disord. 2004;28(12):1541–7.
15. Strath SJ, Kaminsky LA, Ainsworth BE, Ekelund U, Freedson PS, Gary RA, et al. Guide to the assessment of physical activity: clinical and research applications: a scientific statement from the American Heart Association. Circulation. 2013;128(20):2259–79.
16. Wannamethee SG, Shaper AG, Walker M. Changes in physical activity, mortality, and incidence of coronary heart disease in older men. Lancet. 1998;351(9116):1603–8.
17. Hu FB, Willett WC, Li T, Stampfer MJ, Colditz GA, Manson JE. Adiposity as compared with physical activity in predicting mortality among women. N Engl J Med. 2004;351(26):2694–703.
18. Sylvia LG, Bernstein EE, Hubbard JL, Keating L, Anderson EJ. Practical guide to measuring physical activity. J Acad Nutr Diet. 2014;114(2):199–208.
19. Ainsworth B, Buchholz SW. How to assess physical activity in clinical practice and for scholarly work. J Nurse Pract. 2017;13(1):14–20.
20. Rosenberger ME, Buman MP, Haskell WL, McConnell MV, Carstensen LL. Twenty-four hours of sleep, sedentary behavior, and physical activity with nine wearable devices. Med Sci Sports Exerc. 2016;48(3):457–65.
21. Brock DW, Irving BA, Gower B, Hunter GR. Differences emerge in visceral adipose tissue accumulation after selection for innate cardiovascular fitness. Int J Obes. 2011;35(2):309–12.
22. Ross R, Blair SN, Arena R, Church TS, Despres JP, Franklin BA, et al. Importance of assessing cardiorespiratory fitness in clinical practice: a case for fitness as a clinical vital sign: a scientific statement from the American Heart Association. Circulation. 2016;134(24):e653–e99.
23. Weiner RB, Baggish AL. Exercise-induced cardiac remodelling: the need for assessment of regional myocardial function. J Physiol. 2012;590(Pt 12):2829–30.
24. Saltin B, Nazar K, Costill DL, Stein E, Jansson E, Essen B, et al. The nature of the training response; peripheral and central adaptations of one-legged exercise. Acta Physiol Scand. 1976;96(3):289–305.
25. Myers J, Kaykha A, George S, Abella J, Zaheer N, Lear S, et al. Fitness versus physical activity patterns in predicting mortality in men. Am J Med. 2004;117(12):912–8.
26. Williams PT. Physical fitness and activity as separate heart disease risk factors: a meta-analysis. Med Sci Sports Exerc. 2001;33(5):754–61.
27. Prince SA, Adamo KB, Hamel ME, Hardt J, Connor Gorber S, Tremblay M. A comparison of direct versus self-report measures for assessing physical activity in adults: a systematic review. Int J Behav Nutr Phys Act. 2008;5:56.
28. Bouchard C, An P, Rice T, Skinner JS, Wilmore JH, Gagnon J, et al. Familial aggregation of VO(2max) response to exercise training: results from the HERITAGE Family Study. J Appl Physiol (1985). 1999;87(3):1003–8.
29. Wientzek A, Tormo Diaz MJ, Castano JM, Amiano P, Arriola L, Overvad K, et al. Cross-sectional associations of objectively measured physical activity, cardiorespiratory fitness and anthropometry in European adults. Obesity (Silver Spring). 2014;22(5):E127–34.
30. Lakoski SG, Barlow CE, Farrell SW, Berry JD, Morrow JR Jr, Haskell WL. Impact of body mass index, physical activity, and other clinical factors on cardiorespiratory fitness (from the Cooper Center longitudinal study). Am J Cardiol. 2011;108(1):34–9.
31. Fung MD, Canning KL, Mirdamadi P, Ardern CI, Kuk JL. Lifestyle and weight predictors of a healthy overweight profile over a 20-year follow-up. Obesity (Silver Spring). 2015;23(6):1320–5.
32. Slentz CA, Duscha BD, Johnson JL, Ketchum K, Aiken LB, Samsa GP, et al. Effects of the amount of exercise on body weight, body composition, and measures of central obesity: STRRIDE – a randomized controlled study. Arch Intern Med. 2004;164(1):31–9.
33. Committee PAGA. Physical Activity Guidelines Advisory Committee report. In: Services DoHaH, editor. Washington, DC; 2008.
34. Jensen MD, Ryan DH, Apovian CM, Ard JD, Comuzzie AG, Donato KA, et al. AHA/ACC/TOS guideline for the management of overweight and obesity in adults: a report of the American College of Cardiology/American Heart Association Task Force on Practice Guidelines and The Obesity Society. Circulation. 2013:2013.
35. Bann D, Kuh D, Wills AK, Adams J, Brage S, Cooper R, et al. Physical activity across adulthood in relation to fat and lean body mass in early old age: findings from the Medical Research Council National Survey of Health and Development, 1946–2010. Am J Epidemiol. 2014;179(10):1197–207.
36. Drenowatz C, Prasad VK, Hand GA, Shook RP, Blair SN. Effects of moderate and vigorous physical activity on fitness and body composition. J Behav Med. 2016;39(4):624–32.
37. Bernstein MS, Costanza MC, Morabia A. Association of physical activity intensity levels with overweight and obesity in a population-based sample of adults. Prev Med. 2004;38(1):94–104.
38. Ross R, Janssen I. Physical activity, total and regional obesity: dose-response considerations. Med Sci Sports Exerc. 2001;33(6 Suppl):S521–7; discussion S8–9.
39. Lee IM, Shiroma EJ, Evenson KR, Kamada M, LaCroix AZ, Buring JE. Accelerometer-measured physical activity and sedentary behavior in relation to all-cause mortality: the Women's health study. Circulation. 2018;137(2):203–5.
40. Doherty A, Jackson D, Hammerla N, Plotz T, Olivier P, Granat MH, et al. Large scale population assessment of physical activity using wrist worn

accelerometers: the UK biobank study. PLoS One. 2017;12(2):e0169649.
41. Hooker SP, Hutto B, Zhu W, Blair SN, Colabianchi N, Vena JE, et al. Accelerometer measured sedentary behavior and physical activity in white and black adults: the REGARDS study. J Sci Med Sport. 2016;19(4):336–41.
42. Ainsworth BE, Haskell WL, Herrmann SD, Meckes N, Bassett DR Jr, Tudor-Locke C, et al. 2011 Compendium of Physical Activities: a second update of codes and MET values. Med Sci Sports Exerc. 2011;43(8):1575–81.
43. Lee DC, Sui X, Church TS, Lee IM, Blair SN. Associations of cardiorespiratory fitness and obesity with risks of impaired fasting glucose and type 2 diabetes in men. Diabetes Care. 2009;32(2):257–62.
44. Wei M, Gibbons LW, Mitchell TL, Kampert JB, Lee CD, Blair SN. The association between cardiorespiratory fitness and impaired fasting glucose and type 2 diabetes mellitus in men. Ann Intern Med. 1999;130(2):89–96.
45. Waldburger R, Wilms B, Ernst B, Thurnheer M, Schultes B. Cardio-respiratory fitness is independently associated with cardio-metabolic risk markers in severely obese women. Exp Clin Endocrinol Diabetes. 2014;122(3):190–4.
46. Diaz VA, Player MS, Mainous AG 3rd, Carek PJ, Geesey ME. Competing impact of excess weight versus cardiorespiratory fitness on cardiovascular risk. Am J Cardiol. 2006;98(11):1468–71.
47. Chen J, Das S, Barlow CE, Grundy S, Lakoski SG. Fitness, fatness, and systolic blood pressure: data from the Cooper Center Longitudinal Study. Am Heart J. 2010;160(1):166–70.
48. Huot M, Arsenault BJ, Gaudreault V, Poirier P, Perusse L, Tremblay A, et al. Insulin resistance, low cardiorespiratory fitness, and increased exercise blood pressure: contribution of abdominal obesity. Hypertension. 2011;58(6):1036–42.
49. Lin CY, Chen PC, Kuo HK, Lin LY, Lin JW, Hwang JJ. Effects of obesity, physical activity, and cardiorespiratory fitness on blood pressure, inflammation, and insulin resistance in the National Health and Nutrition Survey 1999–2002. Nutr Metab Cardiovasc Dis. 2010;20(10):713–9.
50. Lee DC, Sui X, Church TS, Lavie CJ, Jackson AS, Blair SN. Changes in fitness and fatness on the development of cardiovascular disease risk factors hypertension, metabolic syndrome, and hypercholesterolemia. J Am Coll Cardiol. 2012;59(7):665–72.
51. Lee S, Kuk JL, Katzmarzyk PT, Blair SN, Church TS, Ross R. Cardiorespiratory fitness attenuates metabolic risk independent of abdominal subcutaneous and visceral fat in men. Diabetes Care. 2005;28(4):895–901.
52. Katzmarzyk PT, Church TS, Janssen I, Ross R, Blair SN. Metabolic syndrome, obesity, and mortality: impact of cardiorespiratory fitness. Diabetes Care. 2005;28(2):391–7.
53. Church TS, Cheng YJ, Earnest CP, Barlow CE, Gibbons LW, Priest EL, et al. Exercise capacity and body composition as predictors of mortality among men with diabetes. Diabetes Care. 2004;27(1):83–8.
54. Sui X, LaMonte MJ, Laditka JN, Hardin JW, Chase N, Hooker SP, et al. Cardiorespiratory fitness and adiposity as mortality predictors in older adults. JAMA. 2007;298(21):2507–16.
55. Hu G, Tuomilehto J, Silventoinen K, Barengo NC, Peltonen M, Jousilahti P. The effects of physical activity and body mass index on cardiovascular, cancer and all-cause mortality among 47 212 middle-aged Finnish men and women. Int J Obes. 2005;29(8):894–902.
56. Li TY, Rana JS, Manson JE, Willett WC, Stampfer MJ, Colditz GA, et al. Obesity as compared with physical activity in predicting risk of coronary heart disease in women. Circulation. 2006;113(4):499–506.
57. Yu R, Yau F, Ho SC, Woo J. Associations of cardiorespiratory fitness, physical activity, and obesity with metabolic syndrome in Hong Kong Chinese midlife women. BMC Public Health. 2013;13:614.
58. Ricketts TA, Sui X, Lavie CJ, Blair SN, Ross R. Addition of cardiorespiratory fitness within an obesity risk classification model identifies men at increased risk of all-cause mortality. Am J Med. 2016;129(5):536.e13–20.
59. Janiszewski PM, Ross R. The utility of physical activity in the management of global cardiometabolic risk. Obesity (Silver Spring). 2009;17(Suppl 3):S3–S14.
60. Dankel SJ, Loenneke JP, Loprinzi PD. The impact of overweight/obesity duration on the association between physical activity and cardiovascular disease risk: an application of the "fat but fit" paradigm. Int J Cardiol. 2015;201:88–9.
61. Moholdt T, Lavie CJ, Nauman J. Sustained physical activity, not weight loss, associated with improved survival in coronary heart disease. J Am Coll Cardiol. 2018;71(10):32–9.
62. Franks PW, Ekelund U, Brage S, Wong MY, Wareham NJ. Does the association of habitual physical activity with the metabolic syndrome differ by level of cardiorespiratory fitness? Diabetes Care. 2004;27(5):1187–93.
63. Ross R, Hudson R, Stotz PJ, Lam M. Effects of exercise amount and intensity on abdominal obesity and glucose tolerance in obese adults: a randomized trial. Ann Intern Med. 2015;162(5):325–34.
64. Ross R, Dagnone D, Jones PJ, Smith H, Paddags A, Hudson R, et al. Reduction in obesity and related comorbid conditions after diet-induced weight loss or exercise-induced weight loss in men. A randomized, controlled trial. Ann Intern Med. 2000;133(2):92–103.
65. Ross R, Janssen I, Dawson J, Kungl AM, Kuk JL, Wong SL, et al. Exercise-induced reduction in obesity and insulin resistance in women: a randomized controlled trial. Obes Res. 2004;12(5):789–98.
66. Swift DL, Johannsen NM, Lavie CJ, Earnest CP, Church TS. The role of exercise and physical activ-

ity in weight loss and maintenance. Prog Cardiovasc Dis. 2014;56(4):441–7.
67. Franz MJ, VanWormer JJ, Crain AL, Boucher JL, Histon T, Caplan W, et al. Weight-loss outcomes: a systematic review and meta-analysis of weight-loss clinical trials with a minimum 1-year follow-up. J Am Diet Assoc. 2007;107(10):1755–67.
68. Mann T, Tomiyama AJ, Westling E, Lew AM, Samuels B, Chatman J. Medicare's search for effective obesity treatments: diets are not the answer. Am Psychol. 2007;62(3):220–33.
69. Wadden TA, Sternberg JA, Letizia KA, Stunkard AJ, Foster GD. Treatment of obesity by very low calorie diet, behavior therapy, and their combination: a five-year perspective. Int J Obes. 1989;13(Suppl 2):39–46.
70. Jakicic JM, Marcus BH, Lang W, Janney C. Effect of exercise on 24-month weight loss maintenance in overweight women. Arch Intern Med. 2008;168(14):1550–9; discussion 9–60.
71. Hu FB, Li TY, Colditz GA, Willett WC, Manson JE. Television watching and other sedentary behaviors in relation to risk of obesity and type 2 diabetes mellitus in women. JAMA. 2003;289(14):1785–91.
72. Jebb SA, Prentice AM, Goldberg GR, Murgatroyd PR, Black AE, Coward WA. Changes in macronutrient balance during over- and underfeeding assessed by 12-d continuous whole-body calorimetry. Am J Clin Nutr. 1996;64(3):259–66.
73. Dulloo AG, Jacquet J. Adaptive reduction in basal metabolic rate in response to food deprivation in humans: a role for feedback signals from fat stores. Am J Clin Nutr. 1998;68(3):599–606.
74. Hill JO, Wyatt HR, Peters JC. Energy balance and obesity. Circulation. 2012;126(1):126–32.
75. Ross R, Blair S, de Lannoy L, Despres JP, Lavie CJ. Changing the endpoints for determining effective obesity management. Prog Cardiovasc Dis. 2015;57(4):330–6.
76. Kumanyika SK, Obarzanek E, Stettler N, Bell R, Field AE, Fortmann SP, et al. Population-based prevention of obesity: the need for comprehensive promotion of healthful eating, physical activity, and energy balance: a scientific statement from American Heart Association Council on Epidemiology and Prevention, Interdisciplinary Committee for Prevention (formerly the expert panel on population and prevention science). Circulation. 2008;118(4):428–64.
77. Hill JO, Wyatt HR, Reed GW, Peters JC. Obesity and the environment: where do we go from here? Science. 2003;299(5608):853–5.
78. Rodearmel SJ, Wyatt HR, Barry MJ, Dong F, Pan D, Israel RG, et al. A family-based approach to preventing excessive weight gain. Obesity (Silver Spring). 2006;14(8):1392–401.
79. Rodearmel SJ, Wyatt HR, Stroebele N, Smith SM, Ogden LG, Hill JO. Small changes in dietary sugar and physical activity as an approach to preventing excessive weight gain: the America on the Move family study. Pediatrics. 2007;120(4):e869–79.
80. Ross R, Hill JO, Latimer A, Day AG. Evaluating a small change approach to preventing long term weight gain in overweight and obese adults - Study rationale, design, and methods. Contemp Clin Trials. 2016;47:275–81.
81. Jakicic JM, Davis KK. Obesity and physical activity. Psychiatr Clin North Am. 2011;34(4):829–40.
82. Clarke J, de Lannoy L, Ross R. Comparison of measures of maximal and submaximal fitness in response to exercise. Med Sci Sports Exerc. 2017;49(4):711–6.
83. Kong Z, Sun S, Liu M, Shi Q. Short-term high-intensity interval training on body composition and blood glucose in overweight and obese young women. J Diabetes Res. 2016;2016:4073618.
84. Ross R, Janiszewski PM. Is weight loss the optimal target for obesity-related cardiovascular disease risk reduction? Can J Cardiol. 2008;24 Suppl D:25D–31D.
85. Expert Panel on Detection E, Treatment of High Blood Cholesterol in A. Executive Summary of the third report of The National Cholesterol Education Program (NCEP) expert panel on Detection, evaluation, and treatment of high blood cholesterol in adults (adult treatment panel III). JAMA. 2001;285(19):2486–97.
86. Ebbert JO, Jensen MD. Fat depots, free fatty acids, and dyslipidemia. Nutrients. 2013;5(2):498–508.
87. Hamburg NM, McMackin CJ, Huang AL, Shenouda SM, Widlansky ME, Schulz E, et al. Physical inactivity rapidly induces insulin resistance and microvascular dysfunction in healthy volunteers. Arterioscler Thromb Vasc Biol. 2007;27(12):2650–6.
88. Sarzynski MA, Schuna JM Jr, Carnethon MR, Jacobs DR Jr, Lewis CE, Quesenberry CP Jr, et al. Association of fitness with incident dyslipidemias over 25 years in the coronary artery risk development in young adults study. Am J Prev Med. 2015;49(5):745–52.
89. Slentz CA, Houmard JA, Johnson JL, Bateman LA, Tanner CJ, McCartney JS, et al. Inactivity, exercise training and detraining, and plasma lipoproteins. STRRIDE: a randomized, controlled study of exercise intensity and amount. J Appl Physiol (1985). 2007;103(2):432–42.
90. Ades PA, Savage PD, Toth MJ, Harvey-Berino J, Schneider DJ, Bunn JY, et al. High-calorie-expenditure exercise: a new approach to cardiac rehabilitation for overweight coronary patients. Circulation. 2009;119(20):2671–8.
91. Proper KI, Hildebrandt VH, Van der Beek AJ, Twisk JW, Van Mechelen W. Effect of individual counseling on physical activity fitness and health: a randomized controlled trial in a workplace setting. Am J Prev Med. 2003;24(3):218–26.
92. Pagels P, Raustorp A, Archer T, Lidman U, Alricsson M. Influence of moderate, daily physical activity on

body composition and blood lipid profile in Swedish adults. J Phys Act Health. 2012;9(6):867–74.
93. Choo J, Lee J, Cho JH, Burke LE, Sekikawa A, SY J. Effects of weight management by exercise modes on markers of subclinical atherosclerosis and cardiometabolic profile among women with abdominal obesity: a randomized controlled trial. BMC Cardiovasc Disord. 2014;14:82.
94. Hersey WC 3rd, Graves JE, Pollock ML, Gingerich R, Shireman RB, Heath GW, et al. Endurance exercise training improves body composition and plasma insulin responses in 70- to 79-year-old men and women. Metabolism. 1994;43(7):847–54.
95. Perseghin G, Price TB, Petersen KF, Roden M, Cline GW, Gerow K, et al. Increased glucose transport-phosphorylation and muscle glycogen synthesis after exercise training in insulin-resistant subjects. N Engl J Med. 1996;335(18):1357–62.
96. Dengel DR, Galecki AT, Hagberg JM, Pratley RE. The independent and combined effects of weight loss and aerobic exercise on blood pressure and oral glucose tolerance in older men. Am J Hypertens. 1998;11(12):1405–12.
97. Wing RR, Venditti E, Jakicic JM, Polley BA, Lang W. Lifestyle intervention in overweight individuals with a family history of diabetes. Diabetes Care. 1998;21(3):350–9.
98. Rice B, Janssen I, Hudson R, Ross R. Effects of aerobic or resistance exercise and/or diet on glucose tolerance and plasma insulin levels in obese men. Diabetes Care. 1999;22(5):684–91.
99. Poehlman ET, Dvorak RV, DeNino WF, Brochu M, Ades PA. Effects of resistance training and endurance training on insulin sensitivity in nonobese, young women: a controlled randomized trial. J Clin Endocrinol Metab. 2000;85(7):2463–8.
100. Pratley RE, Hagberg JM, Dengel DR, Rogus EM, Muller DC, Goldberg AP. Aerobic exercise training-induced reductions in abdominal fat and glucose-stimulated insulin responses in middle-aged and older men. J Am Geriatr Soc. 2000;48(9):1055–61.
101. O'Leary VB, Marchetti CM, Krishnan RK, Stetzer BP, Gonzalez F, Kirwan JP. Exercise-induced reversal of insulin resistance in obese elderly is associated with reduced visceral fat. J Appl Physiol (1985). 2006;100(5):1584–9.
102. Sigal RJ, Kenny GP, Boule NG, Wells GA, Prud'homme D, Fortier M, et al. Effects of aerobic training, resistance training, or both on glycemic control in type 2 diabetes: a randomized trial. Ann Intern Med. 2007;147(6):357–69.
103. Tjonna AE, Lee SJ, Rognmo O, Stolen TO, Bye A, Haram PM, et al. Aerobic interval training versus continuous moderate exercise as a treatment for the metabolic syndrome: a pilot study. Circulation. 2008;118(4):346–54.
104. Davidson LE, Hudson R, Kilpatrick K, Kuk JL, McMillan K, Janiszewski PM, et al. Effects of exercise modality on insulin resistance and functional limitation in older adults: a randomized controlled trial. Arch Intern Med. 2009;169(2):122–31.
105. Dengel DR, Hagberg JM, Pratley RE, Rogus EM, Goldberg AP. Improvements in blood pressure, glucose metabolism, and lipoprotein lipids after aerobic exercise plus weight loss in obese, hypertensive middle-aged men. Metabolism. 1998;47(9):1075–82.
106. Church TS, Earnest CP, Skinner JS, Blair SN. Effects of different doses of physical activity on cardiorespiratory fitness among sedentary, overweight or obese postmenopausal women with elevated blood pressure: a randomized controlled trial. JAMA. 2007;297(19):2081–91.
107. Kelley GA, Kelley KS, Tran ZV. Walking, lipids, and lipoproteins: a meta-analysis of randomized controlled trials. Prev Med. 2004;38(5):651–61.
108. Genest J, Frohlich J, Fodor G, McPherson R, Working Group on H, Other D. Recommendations for the management of dyslipidemia and the prevention of cardiovascular disease: summary of the 2003 update. CMAJ. 2003;169(9):921–4.
109. Bray GA, Bellanger T. Epidemiology, trends, and morbidities of obesity and the metabolic syndrome. Endocrine. 2006;29(1):109–17.
110. Ko G, Davidson LE, Brennan AM, Lam M, Ross R. Abdominal adiposity, not cardiorespiratory fitness, mediates the exercise-induced change in insulin sensitivity in older adults. PLoS One. 2016;11(12):e0167734.
111. Brennan AM, Lam M, Stotz P, Hudson R, Ross R. Exercise-induced improvement in insulin sensitivity is not mediated by change in cardiorespiratory fitness. Diabetes Care. 2014;37(5):e95–7.
112. Mora-Rodriguez R, Ortega JF, Guio de Prada V, Fernandez-Elias VE, Hamouti N, Morales-Palomo F, et al. Effects of simultaneous or sequential weight loss diet and aerobic interval training on metabolic syndrome. Int J Sports Med. 2016;37(4):274–81.
113. Henriksson J. Influence of exercise on insulin sensitivity. J Cardiovasc Risk. 1995;2(4):303–9.
114. Church TS, Blair SN, Cocreham S, Johannsen N, Johnson W, Kramer K, et al. Effects of aerobic and resistance training on hemoglobin A1c levels in patients with type 2 diabetes: a randomized controlled trial. JAMA. 2010;304(20):2253–62.
115. Weston KS, Wisloff U, Coombes JS. High-intensity interval training in patients with lifestyle-induced cardiometabolic disease: a systematic review and meta-analysis. Br J Sports Med. 2014;48(16):1227–34.
116. Weinberger MH. Antihypertensive therapy and lipids. Evidence, mechanisms, and implications. Arch Intern Med. 1985;145(6):1102–5.
117. Faselis C, Doumas M, Pittaras A, Narayan P, Myers J, Tsimploulis A, et al. Exercise capacity and all-cause mortality in male veterans with hypertension aged >/=70 years. Hypertension. 2014;64(1):30–5.

118. Cook NR, Cohen J, Hebert PR, Taylor JO, Hennekens CH. Implications of small reductions in diastolic blood pressure for primary prevention. Arch Intern Med. 1995;155(7):701–9.
119. Schwingshackl L, Dias S, Hoffmann G. Impact of long-term lifestyle programmes on weight loss and cardiovascular risk factors in overweight/obese participants: a systematic review and network meta-analysis. Syst Rev. 2014;3:130.
120. Cornelissen VA, Fagard RH. Effects of endurance training on blood pressure, blood pressure-regulating mechanisms, and cardiovascular risk factors. Hypertension. 2005;46(4):667–75.
121. Hunter GR, Chandler-Laney PC, Brock DW, Lara-Castro C, Fernandez JR, Gower BA. Fat distribution, aerobic fitness, blood lipids, and insulin sensitivity in African-American and European-American women. Obesity (Silver Spring). 2010;18(2):274–81.
122. Ogden CL, Carroll MD, Fryar CD, Flegal KM. Prevalence of obesity among adults and youth: United States, 2011–2014. NCHS Data Brief. 2015;(219):1–8.
123. Hammond RA, Levine R. The economic impact of obesity in the United States. Diabetes Metab Syndr Obes. 2010;3:285–95.
124. Martinez-Gonzalez MA, Martinez JA, Hu FB, Gibney MJ, Kearney J. Physical inactivity, sedentary lifestyle and obesity in the European Union. Int J Obes Relat Metab Disord. 1999;23(11):1192–201.
125. Dwyer T, Hosmer D, Hosmer T, Venn AJ, Blizzard CL, Granger RH, et al. The inverse relationship between number of steps per day and obesity in a population-based sample: the AusDiab study. Int J Obes. 2007;31(5):797–804.
126. Fogelholm M, Malmberg J, Suni J, Santtila M, Kyrolainen H, Mantysaari M. Waist circumference and BMI are independently associated with the variation of cardio-respiratory and neuromuscular fitness in young adult men. Int J Obes. 2006;30(6):962–9.
127. Kim TN, Park MS, Kim YJ, Lee EJ, Kim MK, Kim JM, et al. Association of low muscle mass and combined low muscle mass and visceral obesity with low cardiorespiratory fitness. PLoS One. 2014;9(6):e100118.
128. Lesser IA, Dick TJ, Guenette JA, Hoogbruin A, Mackey DC, Singer J, et al. The association between cardiorespiratory fitness and abdominal adiposity in postmenopausal, physically inactive South Asian women. Prev Med Rep. 2015;2:783–7.
129. Blair SN, Brodney S. Effects of physical inactivity and obesity on morbidity and mortality: current evidence and research issues. Med Sci Sports Exerc. 1999;31(11 Suppl):S646–62.

The Obesity Paradox and Cardiorespiratory Fitness

15

Michelle Phuong Nguyen, Sergey Kachur, and Carl J. Lavie

Abbreviations

AF	Atrial fibrillation
BMI	Body mass index
CHD	Coronary heart disease
CRF	Cardiorespiratory fitness
CVD	Cardiovascular diseases
DM2	Diabetes mellitus
HF	Heart failure
HLD	Hyperlipidemia/dyslipidemia
HTN	Hypertension
LDL-C	Low-density lipoprotein cholesterol
METs	Metabolic equivalent
MetS	Metabolic syndrome
OP	Obesity paradox
PA	Physical activity
VO2	Maximal oxygen uptake
WC	Waist circumference

Introduction

According to the National Health and Nutrition Examination Survey of adults between 2013 and 2014, a third were considered to be overweight as defined by body mass index (BMI 25.0–29.9 kg/m^2) and over a third obese (BMI > 30 kg/m^2). Given long-standing evidence that obesity is a risk factor for numerous diseases, including cardiovascular diseases (CVD), with the trend of increasing BMI over the last 50 years, the obesity epidemic has become a national health concern [1–4].

However, in the last two decades, numerous studies have provided evidence of a paradoxical association between obesity as expressed in BMI and chronic illness, termed the obesity paradox (OP). Specifically, overweight and obese individuals appear to have a substantially lower risk of mortality than similarly matched normal-weight and lean individuals [5–7]. These findings contradict the dogma of obesity as detrimental to public health and mortality, and the concept has spurred significant study.

Unlike obesity, increasing cardiorespiratory fitness (CRF) has been associated with reductions in all-cause and CVD mortality across the full spectrum of BMI [8–15]. Many of the deleterious effects of obesity are attenuated by increased CRF. This is often measured as either maximal oxygen uptake (VO2 max) or levels of physical activity (PA) using metabolic equivalents

M. P. Nguyen
UCF/HCA Graduate Medical Education - Internal Medicine, Ocala Regional Medical Center, Ocala, FL, USA

S. Kachur
Graduate Medical Education, Ocala Regional Medical Center, Ocala, FL, USA

C. J. Lavie (✉)
Department of Cardiology, Ochsner Medical Center, New Orleans, LA, USA
e-mail: clavie@ochsner.org

P. Kokkinos, P. Narayan (eds.), *Cardiorespiratory Fitness in Cardiometabolic Diseases*,
https://doi.org/10.1007/978-3-030-04816-7_15

(METs) [16, 17]. In this review, we discuss the interactions between OP, CRF, and CVD morbidity and mortality.

Effects of Obesity on the Cardiovascular System

Obesity potentiates diseases considered risk factors for coronary heart diseases (CHD), such as metabolic syndrome (MetS), dyslipidemia (HLD), type 2 diabetes mellitus (DM2), and hypertension (HTN). Excess caloric intake contributes to the proliferation of adipose tissue, which has endocrine functions that disrupt normal metabolism and promote inflammation via the action of adipokines [18–20]. These include a number of interleukins (1β, 6), as well as tumor necrosis factor-α, which work with leptin to induce insulin resistance, impair vaso-reactivity, and alter lipid metabolism [21–23].

Increased low-density lipoprotein cholesterol (LDL-C) is also closely associated with excess adiposity through mechanisms such as leptin-associated proprotein convertase subtilisin/kexin type 9 (PCSK9) expression. Excess LDL-C promotes atherosclerosis through subendothelial deposition of LDL-C/apolipoprotein B-containing particles that stimulate macrophage activity, phagocytosis, and foam cell formation, leading to atherosclerosis including CHD [24, 25]. Obesity further contributes to atherosclerosis through its association with small, dense LDL-C and oxidized LDL-C [26]. Both oxidized and dense LDL-C are associated with a higher level of oxidative stress, MetS, smooth muscle proliferation, and higher risks for CHD [27–29].

Obesity is also positively related to HTN, a well-accepted risk factor for CVD. The Framingham Heart Study suggests that weight gain contributes to 78% of blood pressure increases in males and 65% in females [30]. The postulated mechanisms for this effect include impairment of renal-pressure natriuresis via three proposed mechanisms: physical renal compression, adipose tissue-derived angiotensinogen activating the renin-angiotensin-aldosterone system and mineralocorticoid receptors, and leptin-mediated stimulation of renal sympathetic nerve activity [31–33] (Fig. 15.1).

These factors tie in closely with obesity's effects on cardiac remodeling and associated heart failure (HF) (Fig. 15.2). One mechanism is through increased total blood volume and cardiac output associated with adiposity, resulting in increases in left ventricular stroke volume, ultimately contributing to concentric ventricular remodeling and HF [34]. The

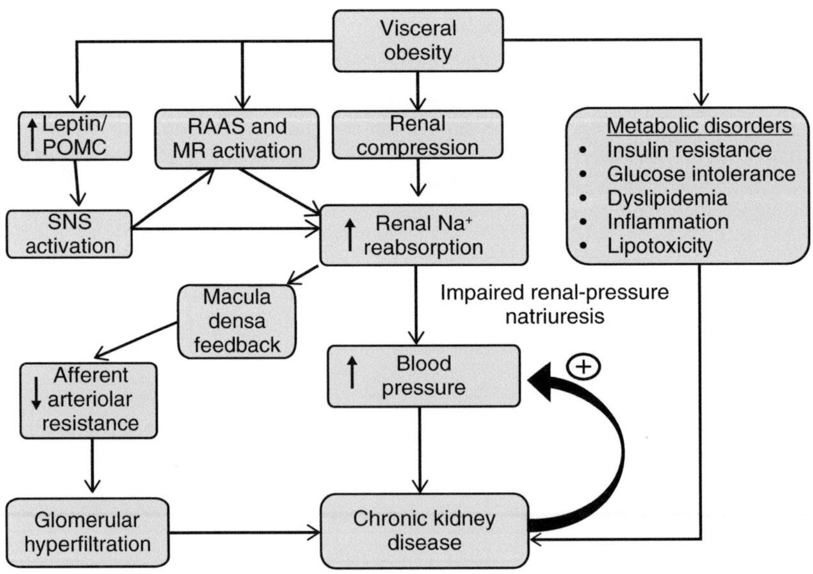

Fig. 15.1 Obesity-induced hypertension and renal injury. SNS sympathetic nervous system, RAAS renin-angiotensin-aldosterone system, MR mineralocorticoid receptor, POMC proopiomelanocortin, neurons. (Modified from Hall et al. [33])

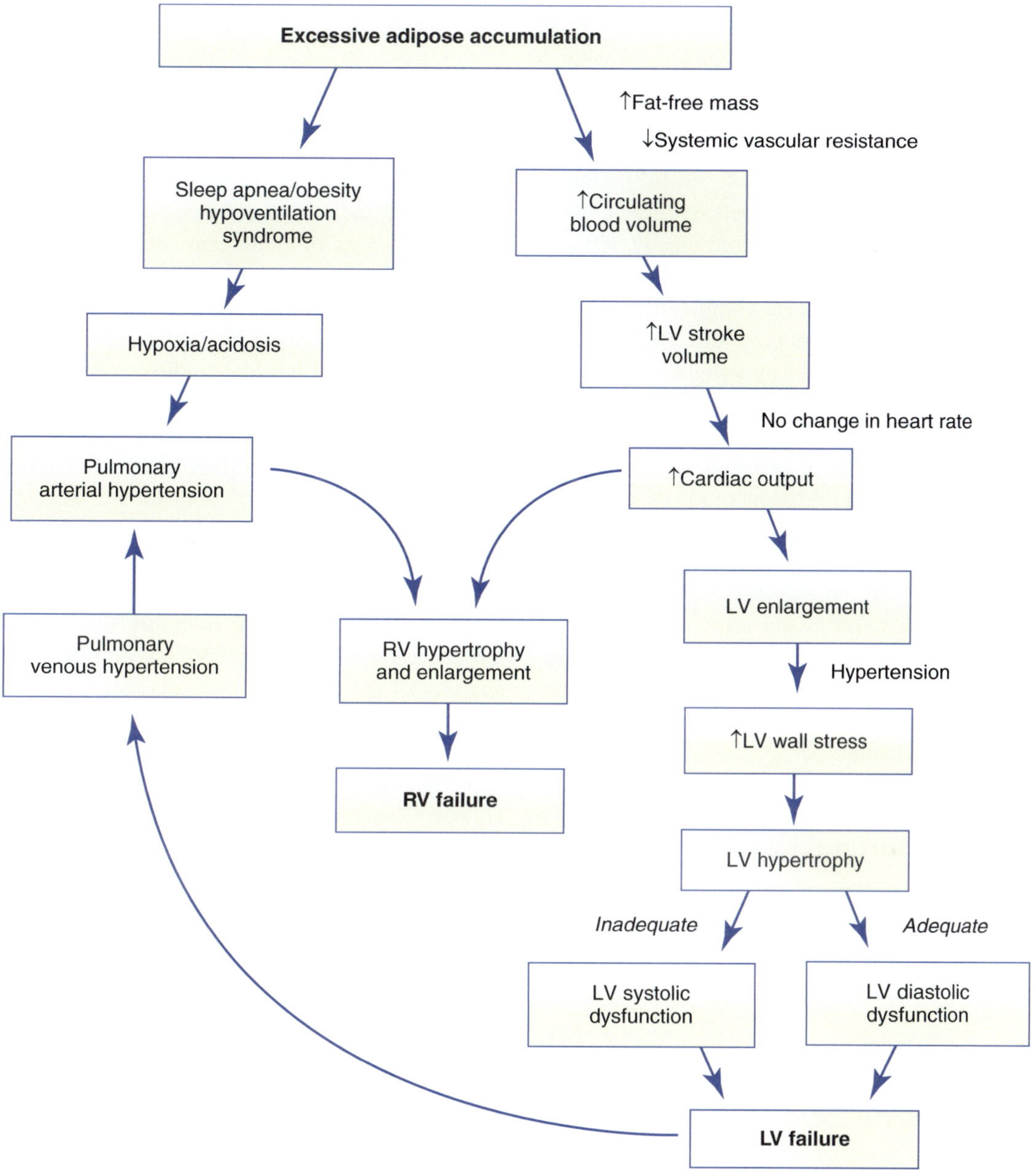

Fig. 15.2 Pathophysiology of obesity cardiomyopathy. This diagram shows the consequences of excessive adipose tissue accumulation, resulting in LV and RV failure. LV left ventricle, RV right ventricle. (Modified from Lavie et al. [53])

Framingham Heart Study of 5881 subjects showed that every 1 kg/m^2 increase in BMI resulted in a 5% increased risk of HF in males and 7% in females during a 14-year follow-up [35]. Similarly, in a study of normotensive, morbidly obese subjects, obesity was the strongest predictor of HF [36].

Excess adipose tissue likewise contributes to maladaptations and alterations of the cardiac structure and function that promote atrial fibrillation (AF) [33, 37–39]. Changes in left ventricular morphology have been associated with bimodal increases in AF reflecting both dilated and hypertrophied variants of dysfunctional ventricular morphology [40]. There also appears to be an independent association of left atrial remodeling with higher BMI which is also associated with increases in AF risk [40, 41]. These mechanisms help explain findings that every 1 unit increase in BMI elevates AF risk by 4–5% [42]. Gender may also play a role in incidence of AF in obese people. In a Danish study examining 47,589 subjects, an increase in BMI correlated with a greater incidence of AF in males compared to females [43]. Additionally, we have already discussed that obesity potentiates hypertension, which is another risk factor for AF [44].

Although weight gain has significant associations with an increased risk for a spectrum of CV diseases, the relationship is dynamic. AF studies have shown that weight loss results in decreased duration and burden of AF and long-term weight loss reduces its recurrence [45–47]. On the other hand, many retrospective studies suggest that weight loss (especially unintentional) in HF is associated with poor outcomes [48, 49]. This will be discussed in more detail later in the chapter.

Data Supporting the Obesity Paradox

Over the last two decades, numerous studies have found mortality benefits in obese patients with chronic disease compared to their leaner counterparts. In 22,576 subjects with HTN and CHD, overweight and obese subjects had lower rates of all-cause mortality than normal-weight subjects [50]. When data on patients with CHD was pooled into a meta-analysis of 89 studies, overweight and obese subjects were found to have lower risks of short-term (<6 months) and long-term (≥6 months) mortality [51]. Likewise, low BMI and HF were associated with a higher incidence of hospital readmissions and mortality [52, 53]. In one of the first studies on the OP in HF by Horwich et al., the best HF prognosis was found in overweight subjects, followed by obese subjects, whereas the worst prognosis was found in underweight subjects, followed by subjects with normal BMI (Fig. 15.3) [54]. Similarly, in a meta-analysis by Oreopoulous et al., patients with HF who were overweight and obese had lower CVD and all-cause mortality than counterparts with normal BMI [55]. A retrospective analysis of the CHARM trial supports this relationship by finding that individuals who were underweight or had normal BMI had higher mortality than overweight and obese subjects [56]. However, several studies have demonstrated a U-shaped curve between BMI and HF morbidity/mortality, suggesting loss of protective effects of the OP in morbidly obese people [57, 58].

The OP in AF is somewhat more surprising. AF was found to be a significant independent risk

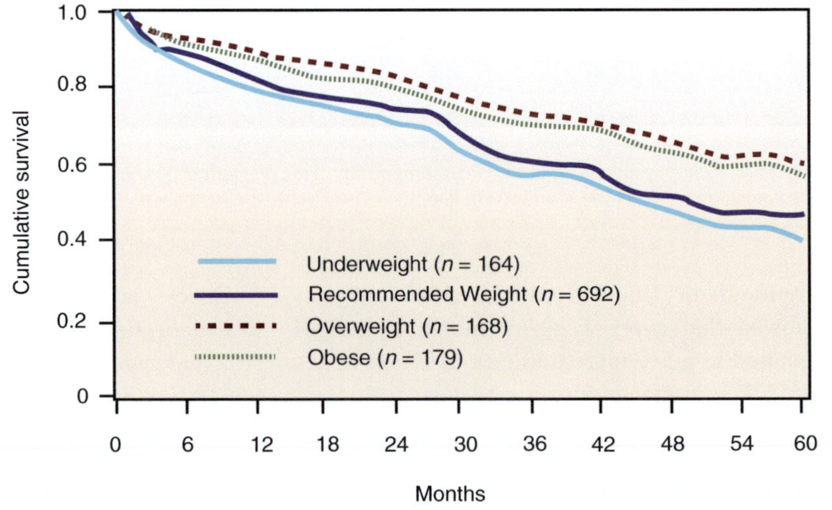

Fig. 15.3 Obesity and survival in heart failure. Highest survival was found in overweight and obesity groups, respectively. Lowest survival was found in underweight and recommended weight. (Modified from Lavie CJ, et al., *JACC* 2009;53(21):1925–32)

factor for death in the original Framingham cohort of 5209 subjects and numerous other studies [59, 60]. Given that both advancing age and increasing obesity have been found to be risk factors for developing AF, a plausible conclusion would be that increasing obesity leading to an increasing burden of AF would be associated with higher mortality [42, 43]. However, there has been significant evidence for the OP in the AF population [61, 62]. In two post hoc analyses from the Atrial Fibrillation Follow-up Investigation of Rhythm Management (AFFIRM), overweight status and obesity were associated with lower risk of all-cause mortality compared to normal-weight subjects with AF [63]. Similarly overweight AF subjects enrolled in Chinese hospitals had a higher survival rate compared to normal and underweight counterparts [64]. Additionally, the apixaban for reduction in stroke and other thromboembolic events in atrial fibrillation (ARISTOTLE) trial by Sandhu et al. showed higher BMI and waist circumference (WC) were associated with a favorable prognosis [65].

In addition to CVD, the OP has been documented in numerous other disease states, including those with chronic kidney disease, the critically ill, and surgical patients: non-bariatric general surgery, coronary bypass, both open and catheter-directed valve replacement, and colorectal surgical patients [66–68]. Notable exceptions to this include renal transplant patients (poorer survival and graft survival than ideal-body-weight patients) and aortoiliac bypass patients (metabolic syndrome rather than obesity was a significant predictor of reintervention) [69, 70].

Proposed Mechanisms of the Obesity Paradox in CVD

The OP is a phenomenon that highlights protective mechanisms for overweight to mildly obese people with chronic disease. The mechanisms of the OP are not clearly understood, but several have been proposed (Table 15.1). One effect related to the OP is that higher lean muscle mass rather than fat mass is associated with improved CRF in those with higher BMI [71, 72]. Coutinho and colleagues attempted to evaluate the hypothesis of an OP due to lean mass versus fat mass by stratifying 15,547 CHD patients by a combination of BMI and WC. In this analysis individuals with BMI of ≤22 and WC ≥101 cm had a significantly higher mortality than both individuals of similar BMI and lower WC and individuals with higher BMI and variable WC [73]. De Schutter and colleagues examined 47,866 patients who were stratified based on BMI and lean mass, noting that when body fat was examined in the setting of lean mass, it was a poor predictor of mortality in all but underweight patients [74]. Thus, although the OP by BMI is evident in the CHD population, positive associations are more consistent in those with higher lean mass than higher body fat (or associated central obesity).

Table 15.1 Mechanisms of the obesity paradox

Additional metabolic reserves allow for more prolonged catabolic states
Better nutritional status
Tolerating higher doses of cardioprotective medications
Increased body mass leads to increased muscle mass/strength and increased CRF
Earlier presentation/screening associated with lead time bias
Increased sequestration of cytokines
Exclusion of cachectic/frail individuals with high mortality

HF is characterized by a catabolic state, especially in its later stages, thus a strong possibility exists that normal-weight patients are captured in a downward trend of BMI characteristic of end-stage disease. This is a plausible explanation since weight loss exceeding 5% of starting body weight was found to be a significant predictor of mortality in HF [48, 49]. However, Khalid and colleagues studied this hypothesis in 1487 patients enrolled in the Atherosclerosis Risk in Communities study by comparing pre-HF BMI to outcomes over a 10-year span and found that the overweight and obese appeared to have better survival than patients with normal BMI [75]. Additionally, Ahmad et al. studied patients from ages 45–55 through 95 years old and found that obesity does lengthen life-span during a HF disease state, but overall longevity is shorter for the obese than nonobese [76]. It is plausible then that most studies identify an obesity survival paradox in HF due to a bias toward studying diseased (rather than disease-free) populations.

Given that inflammatory stress is posited to play a significant role in AF, the cytokine sequestration hypothesis (i.e. the presence of tumor necrosis-α receptors in adipose tissue) may play a significant role in reducing AF-associated morbidity [77]. Another explanation for the OP in AF is that higher levels of BMI are associated with higher levels of CRF (due to increased lean mass), which may confer mortality benefits [71, 72]. Interestingly the relationship between CRF and AF has been shown to be an inverse one above levels of moderate PA/CRF, which will be discussed more later in this chapter [78, 79].

Effects of Cardiorespiratory Fitness

CRF is a measurement of the ability of the circulatory and respiratory systems to supply oxygen during sustained PA which can be measured with exertional metrics, such as the estimated METs or through maximal VO2 consumption [80]. Assessing CRF has become an important cornerstone of studying the OP, because of the dynamic interactions between levels of CRF and mortality benefits derived from excess BMI.

As discussed elsewhere in the text, CRF counters CVD risk factors, such as hyperglycemia, HTN, and HLD. In a study of 29,854 men who underwent the Balke maximal exercise treadmill test, it was estimated that a 1-MET increase in CRF conferred a 20% decrease in CHD risk [81]. Barlow and colleagues evaluated CRF associations with mortality and CVD events and found that a 1-unit MET increase in baseline CRF was associated with 11% and 18% reductions in all-cause and CVD mortality, respectively [82]. In HF patients, a 1-MET increase in CRF was associated with a 16% risk reduction of HF, and patients with exercise capacity of 6–12 METS had an 81% reduction of HF compared to patients with a capacity of <6 METs (Fig. 15.4) [83]. These effects have translated into both lower hospitalization and mortality rates and have resulted in the FDA approval of cardiac rehabilitation for a HF indication [84–86].

Higher CRF is associated with lower incidence of AF to a point. In a retrospective study using data from the Henry Ford Exercise Testing Project, there was an inverse relationship between CRF and incidence of AF, especially for obese patients compared to nonobese patients [79]. More specifically, there was a 7%

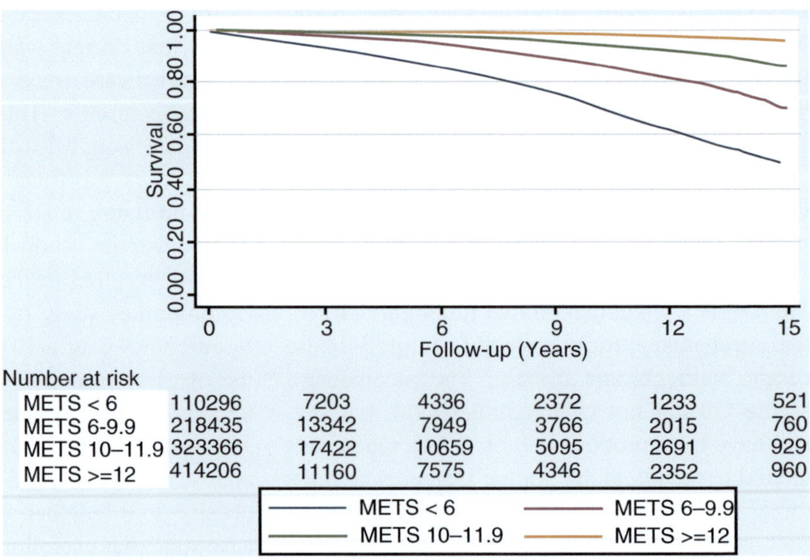

Fig. 15.4 Survival stratified by CRF groups. Kaplan-Meier survival curves of HF incidence according to CRF categories. A graded decrease in survival with decreasing functional capacity is illustrated ($P < 0.001$). (Modified from Kupsky et al. [83])

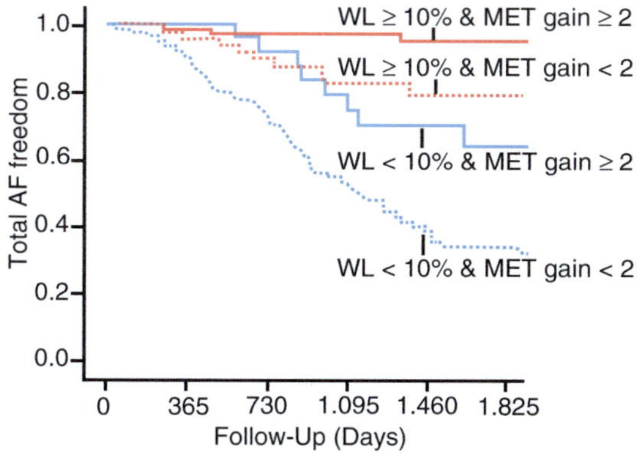

Fig. 15.5 Atrial fibrillation stratified by weight loss and CRF. Kaplan-Meier curve for AF incidence. The lowest burden of AF was found in the category with the greatest weight loss (WT) and CRF (MET). (Modified from Pathak et al. [87])

lower risk of AF for every 1-MET increase in CRF. In the CARDIO-FIT Study, weight loss and increases in CRF had a synergistic effect on reduction of AF recurrence (Fig. 15.5) [87]. Among obese subjects, an increase in CRF of 1 MET alone would result in a 20% reduction in occurrence of arrhythmias. Improving PA has been shown to reduce the risk factors of AF such as autonomic dysfunction, elevated blood pressure, insulin resistance, poor arterial function, and inflammation [88–90]. However, some data suggest intensive, sustained physical training is associated with increasing risk of AF, especially in elite endurance athletes [91, 92]. This would indicate that CRF can be protective for AF with light-to-moderate exercise, but the benefits plateau at higher levels of PA, especially endurance exercise [78].

In discussing weight loss with respect to the OP, data has shown marked differences between intentional (usually fat losses) versus unintentional weight loss. In the National Health Interview Survey, intentional weight loss lowered mortality rate by 24% (HR 0.76; 95% confidence interval, 0.60–0.97). In contrast, unintentional weight loss was associated with a 31% higher mortality rate (HR 1.31; 95% confidence interval, 1.01–1.70) [93]. In a comparison between the Tecumseh Health prospective study and Framingham study, weight loss (LM) and fat loss (BF) were isolated; weight loss increased HR by 29–39%, while fat loss reduced HR by 15–17% [94]. In the HUNT study, weight gain was associated with improved mortality, whereas weight loss was only associated with higher mortality risk in normal-weight individuals [95]. In the setting of cardiac rehabilitation (CR), weight loss was associated with lower rate of CVD regardless of baseline BMI (HR = 0.62; $P = 0.018$) [96]. Given the variability in data surrounding weight loss, the difficulty of distinguishing "healthy" from "unhealthy" weight loss, and the strong support for the OP in chronic disease, at this time weight loss is not a recommended method of improving outcomes.

Interactions of CRF, Obesity, and the OP

Those with low PA often have more abdominal obesity and higher CVD risk. Although increasing PA attenuates the CVD risk associated with obesity, leanness does not seem to ameliorate the adverse effects of being sedentary [97–99]. Thus, both CRF and obesity have been found to be independent modifiers of CVD and mortality [15, 100, 101].

In some studies body composition appears to play a minimal role when stratified by CRF. In the Aerobic Center Longitudinal Study, in patients with CHD, there were no significant differences in CVD and mortality risk among categories of BMI, WC, and % BF. This mirrors findings in a separate cohort of individuals with CVD where obesity did not have significant effects on mortality [14, 102]. Likewise, in the HUNT study, only those overweight and obese subjects who did not adhere to recommended PA had reduced all-cause and CVD mortality [103]. However, a systematic review by Fogelholm concluded that people with high BMI and CRF had lower risk of all-cause and CVD mortality compared to people with normal BMI with poor CRF [104]. McAuley and colleagues also found that body composition had mortality effects; overweight-obese men with moderate CRF had similar mortality risk compared to high CRF normal-weight

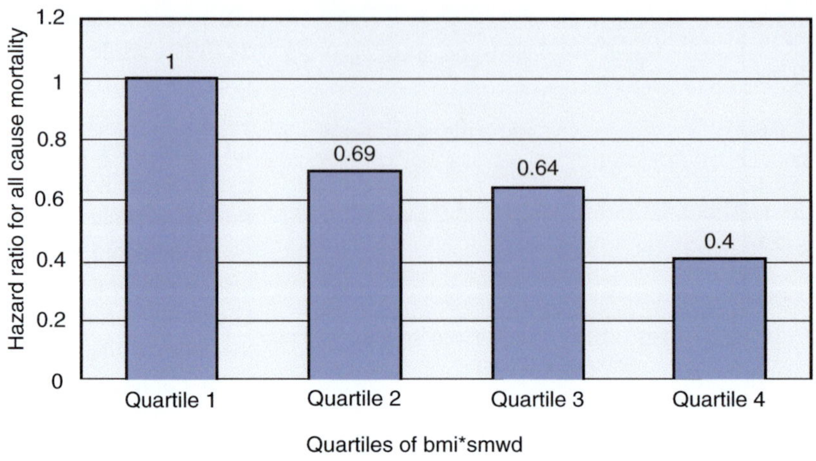

Fig. 15.6 Impact of BMI and 6-min walk distance product on mortality. Adjusted hazard ratio for all-cause mortality according to the product of BMI and physical capacity assessed by the SMWD test. SMWD, six-minute walk distance. (Modified from Zafrir et al. [106])

men [105]. Zafrir et al. examined the product of BMI and CRF (as measured by the 6-min walk distance test) and found that there was a stepwise decrease in mortality by viewing BMI and CRF as a combined metric (Fig. 15.6) [106].

Other data shows an independent effect of body composition on mortality when stratified by CRF. Goel and colleagues investigated CHD patients from the Mayo Clinic cardiac rehabilitation program and found that differences in mortality were bimodal, stratifying into just two groups of low and high risk. The low-risk cluster contained individuals with high CRF regardless of body composition and the low CRF obese, while the high-risk cluster contained all other low CRF individuals, indicating that obesity was associated with comparable mortality benefits to CRF [107]. Additionally, in the previously referenced study by McAuley, subgroup analyses suggested that being overweight and having moderate CRF were equivalent to being normal-weight and having high CRF [105].

However, other data shows significant interactions between BMI and CRF with respect to mortality benefits. Kokkinos et al. explored the BMI-mortality risk association in 18,033 male veterans and found that lower BMI was associated with higher mortality risks in the low-fit and moderately fit categories, but not in the high-fit categories (METs > 11.1) [108]. In several studies of HF patients, the OP has been observed in unfit patients with advanced HF [109, 110]; it was noted that BMI 18.5–24.9 was associated with decreased survival in the low CRF group, while survival was highest in the high CRF group regardless of BMI [110]. Lastly, PA and exercise training have been shown to reduce adiposity and increase CRF while improving prognosis in both HF and CHD populations, which suggests that lean mass displaces fat mass in physically active individuals [95, 111, 112]. As of now, data supports the OP in populations with low to moderate CRF, whereas in the high CRF population, the OP is more of a lean paradox [113, 114].

Conclusions

Obesity is associated with many risk factors for CVD, such as MetS, HLD, glucose intolerance, and HTN. Among individuals with CVD, many studies have found a favorable association between improved survival and having a BMI in the overweight to mildly obese range when compared to normal-weight or lean groups. In exploring the mechanisms of pathology associated with obesity and the data behind the OP in CVD, it is evident that there are significant benefits to excess body weight in the CVD population. However, these benefits diminish with increasing CRF reserves.

Matthew Budoff has recently discussed the utility of CRF as gauge of biological age [115]. Given existing data that obesity is detrimental to life-span for younger patients and that the OP has not been demonstrated in individuals with high CRF, it is reasonable to encourage PA that increases CRF in all populations throughout the life-span, with the aspiration of improving health through higher CRF regardless of BMI [76, 116]. Therefore, we recommend exercise training and PA to improve CRF to attenuate risk factors of CVD in individuals who are overweight or obese.

References

1. Flegal KM, Kruszon-Moran D, Carroll MD, Fryar CD, Ogden CL. Trends in obesity among adults in the United States, 2005 to 2014. JAMA. 2016;315(21):2284–91.
2. Ogden CL, Carroll MD, Lawman HG, Fryar CD, Kruszon-Moran D, Kit BK, et al. Trends in obesity prevalence among children and adolescents in the United States, 1988–1994 through 2013–2014. JAMA. 2016;315(21):2292–9.
3. Fryar CD, Carroll MD, Ogden CL. Prevalence of overweight, obesity, and extreme obesity among adults aged 20 and over: United States, 1960–1962 through 2013–2014 [Internet]. Atlanta: Centers for Disease Control; 2016. p. 6. (National Center for Health Statistics). Available from: https://www.cdc.gov/nchs/data/hestat/obesity_adult_13_14/obesity_adult_13_14.pdf.
4. Fryar CD, Carroll MD, Ogden CL. Prevalence of overweight and obesity among children and adolescents aged 2–19 years: United States, 1963–1965 through 2013–2014 [Internet]. Atlanta: Centers for Disease Control; 2016. p. 6. (National Center for Health Statistics). Available from: https://www.cdc.gov/nchs/data/hestat/obesity_child_13_14/obesity_child_13_14.pdf.
5. Lavie CJ, De Schutter A, Parto P, Jahangir E, Kokkinos P, Ortega FB, et al. Obesity and prevalence of cardiovascular diseases and prognosis—the obesity paradox updated. Prog Cardiovasc Dis. 2016;58(5):537–47.
6. Lavie CJ, Sharma A, Alpert MA, De Schutter A, Lopez-Jimenez F, Milani RV, et al. Update on obesity and obesity paradox in heart failure. Prog Cardiovasc Dis. 2016;58(4):393–400.
7. Oktay AA, Lavie CJ, Kokkinos PF, Parto P, Pandey A, Ventura HO. The interaction of cardiorespiratory fitness with obesity and the obesity paradox in cardiovascular disease. Prog Cardiovasc Dis. 2017;60(1):30–44.
8. Blair SN, Kohl HW, Paffenbarger RS, Clark DG, Cooper KH, Gibbons LW. Physical fitness and all-cause mortality. A prospective study of healthy men and women. JAMA. 1989;262(17):2395–401.
9. Gulati M, Black HR, Shaw LJ, Arnsdorf MF, Merz CNB, Lauer MS, et al. The prognostic value of a nomogram for exercise capacity in women. N Engl J Med. 2005;353(5):468–75.
10. Kokkinos P, Myers J, Kokkinos JP, Pittaras A, Narayan P, Manolis A, et al. Exercise capacity and mortality in black and white men. Circulation. 2008;117(5):614–22.
11. Mora S, Redberg RF, Cui Y, Whiteman MK, Flaws JA, Sharrett AR, et al. Ability of exercise testing to predict cardiovascular and all-cause death in asymptomatic women: a 20-year follow-up of the lipid research clinics prevalence study. JAMA. 2003;290(12):1600–7.
12. Myers J, Prakash M, Froelicher V, Do D, Partington S, Atwood JE. Exercise capacity and mortality among men referred for exercise testing. N Engl J Med. 2002;346(11):793–801.
13. Physical fitness as a predictor of mortality among healthy, middle-aged Norwegian men. NEJM [Internet]. 2017 [cited 2017 Oct 30]. Available from: http://www.nejm.org.ezproxy.net.ucf.edu/doi/full/10.1056/NEJM199302253280803.
14. Lee CD, Blair SN, Jackson AS. Cardiorespiratory fitness, body composition, and all-cause and cardiovascular disease mortality in men. Am J Clin Nutr. 1999;69(3):373–80.
15. Sui X, LaMonte MJ, Laditka JN, Hardin JW, Chase N, Hooker SP, et al. Cardiorespiratory fitness and adiposity as mortality predictors in older adults. JAMA. 2007;298(21):2507–16.
16. Aadahl M, Kjaer M, Jørgensen T. Associations between overall physical activity level and cardiovascular risk factors in an adult population. Eur J Epidemiol. 2007;22(6):369–78.
17. Kavanagh T, Mertens DJ, Hamm LF, Beyene J, Kennedy J, Corey P, et al. Peak oxygen intake and cardiac mortality in women referred for cardiac rehabilitation. J Am Coll Cardiol. 2003;42(12):2139–43.
18. Kachur S, Lavie CJ, de Schutter A, Milani RV, Ventura HO. Obesity and cardiovascular diseases. Minerva Med. 2017;108(3):212–28.
19. Redinger RN. The pathophysiology of obesity and its clinical manifestations. Gastroenterol Hepatol. 2007;3(11):856–63.
20. Coppack SW. Pro-inflammatory cytokines and adipose tissue. Proc Nutr Soc. 2001;60(3):349–56.
21. Lumeng CN, Bodzin JL, Saltiel AR. Obesity induces a phenotypic switch in adipose tissue macrophage polarization. J Clin Invest. 2007;117(1):175–84.
22. Li P, Wang L, Liu C. Overweightness, obesity and arterial stiffness in healthy subjects: a systematic review and meta-analysis of literature studies. Postgrad Med. 2017;129(2):224–30.
23. Despres JP, Krauss RM. Obesity and lipoprotein metabolism. In: Handbook of obesity: etiology and pathophysiology. 2nd ed. New York: Marcel Dekker; 2004. p. 845–71.
24. Tabas I, Williams KJ, Boren J. Subendothelial lipoprotein retention as the initiating process in

atherosclerosis: update and therapeutic implications. Circulation. 2007;116(16):1832–44.
25. Du Y, Li S, Cui C-J, Zhang Y, Yang S-H, Li J-J. Leptin decreases the expression of low-density lipoprotein receptor via PCSK9 pathway: linking dyslipidemia with obesity. J Transl Med [Internet]. 2016 [cited 2016 Dec 8];14(1). Available from: http://translational-medicine.biomedcentral.com/articles/10.1186/s12967-016-1032-4.
26. Kulanuwat S, Tungtrongchitr R, Billington D, Davies IG. Prevalence of plasma small dense LDL is increased in obesity in a Thai population. Lipids Health Dis [Internet]. 2015 [cited 2016 Dec 21];14(1). Available from: http://lipidworld.biomedcentral.com/articles/10.1186/s12944-015-0034-1.
27. Norris AL, Steinberger J, Steffen LM, Metzig AM, Schwarzenberg SJ, Kelly AS. Circulating oxidized LDL and inflammation in extreme pediatric obesity. Obesity. 2011;19(7):1415–9.
28. Holvoet P, Kritchevsky SB, Tracy RP, Mertens A, Rubin SM, Butler J, et al. The metabolic syndrome, circulating oxidized LDL, and risk of myocardial infarction in well-functioning elderly people in the health, aging, and body composition cohort. Diabetes. 2004;53(4):1068–73.
29. Holvoet P, Mertens A, Verhamme P, Bogaerts K, Beyens G, Verhaeghe R, et al. Circulating oxidized LDL is a useful marker for identifying patients with coronary artery disease. Arterioscler Thromb Vasc Biol. 2001;21(5):844–8.
30. Garrison RJ, Kannel WB, Stokes J, Castelli WP. Incidence and precursors of hypertension in young adults: the Framingham offspring study. Prev Med. 1987;16(2):235–51.
31. Bell BB, Rahmouni K. Leptin as a mediator of obesity-induced hypertension. Curr Obes Rep. 2016;5(4):397–404.
32. Taddei S, Virdis A, Mattei P, Favilla S, Salvetti A. Angiotensin II and sympathetic activity in sodium-restricted essential hypertension. Hypertension. 1995;25(4):595–601.
33. Hall JE, do Carmo JM, da Silva AA, Wang Z, Hall ME. Obesity-induced hypertension: interaction of neurohumoral and renal mechanisms. Circ Res. 2015;116(6):991–1006.
34. Ho JE, Lyass A, Lee DS, Vasan RS, Kannel WB, Larson MG, et al. Predictors of new-onset heart failure clinical perspective: differences in preserved versus reduced ejection fraction. Circ Heart Fail. 2013;6(2):279–86.
35. Kenchaiah S, Evans JC, Levy D, Wilson PWF, Benjamin EJ, Larson MG, et al. Obesity and the risk of heart failure. N Engl J Med. 2002;347(5):305–13.
36. Alpert MA, Terry BE, Mulekar M, Cohen MV, Massey CV, Fan TM, et al. Cardiac morphology and left ventricular function in normotensive morbidly obese patients with and without congestive heart failure, and effect of weight loss. Am J Cardiol. 1997;80(6):736–40.
37. Bastien M, Poirier P, Lemieux I, Després J-P. Overview of epidemiology and contribution of obesity to cardiovascular disease. Prog Cardiovasc Dis. 2014;56(4):369–81.
38. Poirier P, Martin J, Marceau P, Biron S, Marceau S. Impact of bariatric surgery on cardiac structure, function and clinical manifestations in morbid obesity. Expert Rev Cardiovasc Ther. 2004;2(2):193–201.
39. Knuiman M, Briffa T, Divitini M, Chew D, Eikelboom J, McQuillan B, et al. A cohort study examination of established and emerging risk factors for atrial fibrillation: the Busselton Health Study. Eur J Epidemiol. 2014;29(3):181–90.
40. Bekwelem W, Misialek JR, Konety S, Solomon SD, Soliman EZ, Loehr LR, et al. Echocardiographic measures of cardiac structure and function are associated with risk of atrial fibrillation in blacks: the Atherosclerosis Risk in Communities (ARIC) study. PLoS One. 2014;9(10):e110111.
41. Sasson Z, Rasooly Y, Gupta R, Rasooly I. Left atrial enlargement in healthy obese: prevalence and relation to left ventricular mass and diastolic function. Can J Cardiol. 1996;12(3):257–63.
42. Wang TJ. Obesity and the risk of new-onset atrial fibrillation. JAMA. 2004;292(20):2471.
43. Frost L, Hune LJ, Vestergaard P. Overweight and obesity as risk factors for atrial fibrillation or flutter: the Danish Diet, Cancer, and Health Study. Am J Med. 2005;118(5):489–95.
44. O'Neal WT, Soliman EZ, Qureshi W, Alonso A, Heckbert SR, Herrington D. Sustained pre-hypertensive blood pressure and incident atrial fibrillation: the multi-ethnic study of atherosclerosis. J Am Soc Hypertens JASH. 2015;9(3):191–6.
45. Abed HS, Wittert GA, Leong DP, Shirazi MG, Bahrami B, Middeldorp ME, et al. Effect of weight reduction and cardiometabolic risk factor management on symptom burden and severity in patients with atrial fibrillation: a randomized clinical trial. JAMA. 2013;310(19):2050–60.
46. Pathak RK, Middeldorp ME, Meredith M, Mehta AB, Mahajan R, Wong CX, et al. Long-term effect of goal-directed weight management in an atrial fibrillation cohort: a Long-Term Follow-Up Study (LEGACY). J Am Coll Cardiol. 2015;65(20):2159–69.
47. Lavie CJ, Pandey A, Lau DH, Alpert MA, Sanders P. Obesity and atrial fibrillation prevalence, pathogenesis, and prognosis. J Am Coll Cardiol. 2017;70(16):2022–35.
48. Pocock SJ, McMurray JJV, Dobson J, Yusuf S, Granger CB, Michelson EL, et al. Weight loss and mortality risk in patients with chronic heart failure in the candesartan in heart failure: assessment of reduction in mortality and morbidity (CHARM) programme. Eur Heart J. 2008;29(21):2641–50.
49. Zamora E, Díez-López C, Lupón J, de Antonio M, Domingo M, Santesmases J, et al. Weight loss in obese patients with heart failure. J Am Heart Assoc. 2016;5(3):e002468.

50. Uretsky S, Messerli FH, Bangalore S, Champion A, Cooper-Dehoff R, Zhou Q, et al. Obesity paradox in patients with hypertension and coronary artery disease. Am J Med. 2007;120(10):863–70.
51. Wang ZJ, Zhou YJ, Galper BZ, Gao F, Yeh RW, Mauri L. Association of body mass index with mortality and cardiovascular events for patients with coronary artery disease: a systematic review and meta-analysis. Heart. 2015;101(20):1631–8.
52. Khaled S, Matahen R. Obesity paradox in heart failure patients – female gender characteristics-KAMC-single center experience. Egypt Heart J. 2017;69(3):209–13.
53. Lavie CJ, Alpert MA, Arena R, Mehra MR, Milani RV, Ventura HO. Impact of obesity and the obesity paradox on prevalence and prognosis in heart failure. JACC Heart Fail. 2013;1(2):93–102.
54. Horwich TB, Fonarow GC, Hamilton MA, MacLellan WR, Woo MA, Tillisch JH. The relationship between obesity and mortality in patients with heart failure. J Am Coll Cardiol. 2001;38(3):789–95.
55. Oreopoulos A, Padwal R, Kalantar-Zadeh K, Fonarow GC, Norris CM, McAlister FA. Body mass index and mortality in heart failure: a meta-analysis. Am Heart J. 2008;156(1):13–22.
56. Kenchaiah S, Pocock SJ, Wang D, Finn PV, Zornoff LAM, Skali H, et al. Body mass index and prognosis in patients with chronic heart failure: insights from the candesartan in heart failure: assessment of reduction in mortality and morbidity (CHARM) program. Circulation. 2007;116(6):627–36.
57. Sharma A, Lavie CJ, Borer JS, Vallakati A, Goel S, Lopez-Jimenez F, et al. Meta-analysis of the relation of body mass index to all-cause and cardiovascular mortality and hospitalization in patients with chronic heart failure. Am J Cardiol. 2015;115(10):1428–34.
58. Vest AR, Wu Y, Hachamovitch R, Young JB, Cho L. The heart failure overweight/obesity survival paradox: the missing sex link. JACC Heart Fail. 2015;3(11):917–26.
59. Benjamin EJ, Wolf PA, D'Agostino RB, Silbershatz H, Kannel WB, Levy D. Impact of atrial fibrillation on the risk of death: the Framingham Heart Study. Circulation. 1998;98(10):946–52.
60. González-Cambeiro MC, Abu-Assi E, Raposeiras-Roubín S, Rodríguez-Mañero M, Otero-Raviña F, R González-Juanatey J, et al. Exploring the obesity paradox in atrial fibrillation. AFBAR (Atrial Fibrillation Barbanza Area) Registry Results. J Atr Fibrillation. 2014;6(5):991.
61. Stewart S, Hart CL, Hole DJ, McMurray JJV. A population-based study of the long-term risks associated with atrial fibrillation: 20-year follow-up of the Renfrew/Paisley study. Am J Med. 2002;113(5):359–64.
62. Vidaillet H, Granada JF, Chyou PO, Maassen K, Ortiz M, Pulido JN, et al. A population-based study of mortality among patients with atrial fibrillation or flutter. Am J Med. 2002;113(5):365–70.
63. Badheka AO, Rathod A, Kizilbash MA, Garg N, Mohamad T, Afonso L, et al. Influence of obesity on outcomes in atrial fibrillation: yet another obesity paradox. Am J Med. 2010;123(7):646–51.
64. Wang J, Yang Y, Zhu J, Zhang H, Shao X, Tian L, et al. Overweight is associated with improved survival and outcomes in patients with atrial fibrillation. Clin Res Cardiol. 2014;103(7):533–42.
65. Sandhu RK, Ezekowitz J, Andersson U, Alexander JH, Granger CB, Halvorsen S, et al. The 'obesity paradox' in atrial fibrillation: observations from the ARISTOTLE (Apixaban for Reduction in Stroke and Other Thromboembolic Events in Atrial Fibrillation) trial. Eur Heart J. 2016;37(38):2869–78.
66. Camilleri B, Bridson JM, Sharma A, Halawa A. From chronic kidney disease to kidney transplantation: the impact of obesity and its treatment modalities. Transplant Rev. 2016;30(4):203–11.
67. Mariscalco G, Wozniak MJ, Dawson AG, Serraino GF, Porter R, Nath M, et al. Body mass index and mortality among adults undergoing cardiac surgery clinical perspective: a nationwide study with a systematic review and meta-analysis. Circulation. 2017;135(9):850–63.
68. Lv W, Li S, Liao Y, Zhao Z, Che G, Chen M, et al. The "obesity paradox" does exist in patients undergoing transcatheter aortic valve implantation for aortic stenosis: a systematic review and meta-analysis. Interact Cardiovasc Thorac Surg. 2017;25(4):633–42.
69. Tanaka A, Perlick A, Miller CC, Sandhu HK, Afaq S, Safi HJ, et al. Metabolic syndrome but not obesity adversely affects outcomes after open aortoiliac bypass surgery. Ann Vasc Surg. 2018;46:155–61.
70. Meier-Kriesche H-U, Arndorfer JA, Kaplan B. The impact of body mass index on renal transplant outcomes: a significant independent risk factor for graft failure and patient death. Transplantation. 2002;73(1):70–4.
71. Wannamethee SG, Shaper AG, Whincup PH, Lennon L, Papacosta O, Sattar N. The obesity paradox in men with coronary heart disease and heart failure: the role of muscle mass and leptin. Int J Cardiol. 2014;171(1):49–55.
72. Zavin A, Daniels K, Arena R, Allsup K, Lazzari A, Joseph J, et al. Adiposity facilitates increased strength capacity in heart failure patients with reduced ejection fraction. Int J Cardiol. 2013;167(6):2468–71.
73. Coutinho T, Goel D, Correa de Sa RE, Carter DO, Hodge C, Kragelund AM, et al. Combining body mass index with measures of central obesity in the assessment of mortality in subjects with coronary disease: role of 'normal weight central obesity'. J Am Coll Cardiol. 2013;61(5):553–60.
74. De Schutter A, Lavie CJ, Kachur S, Patel DA, Milani RV. Body composition and mortality in a large cohort with preserved ejection fraction: untangling the obesity paradox. Mayo Clin Proc. 2014;89(8):1072–9.
75. Khalid U, Ather S, Bavishi C, Chan W, Loehr LR, Wruck LM, et al. Pre-morbid body mass index

and mortality after incident heart failure: the ARIC Study. J Am Coll Cardiol. 2014;64(25):2743–9.
76. Ahmad FS, Ning H, Rich JD, Yancy CW, Lloyd-Jones DM, Wilkins JT. Hypertension, obesity, diabetes, and heart failure–free survival. JACC Heart Fail. 2016;4(12):911–9.
77. Mohamed-Ali V, Goodrick S, Bulmer K, Holly JM, Yudkin JS, Coppack SW. Production of soluble tumor necrosis factor receptors by human subcutaneous adipose tissue in vivo. Am J Phys. 1999;277(6 Pt 1):E971–5.
78. Khan H, Kella D, Rauramaa R, Savonen K, Lloyd MS, Laukkanen JA. Cardiorespiratory fitness and atrial fibrillation: a population-based follow-up study. Heart Rhythm. 2015;12(7):1424–30.
79. Qureshi WT, Alirhayim Z, Blaha MJ, Juraschek SP, Keteyian SJ, Brawner CA, et al. Cardiorespiratory fitness and risk of incident atrial fibrillation: results from the Henry Ford ExercIse Testing (FIT) Project. Circulation. 2015;131(21):1827–34. https://doi.org/10.1161/CIRCULATIONAHA.114.014833.
80. Caspersen CJ, Powell KE, Christenson GM. Physical activity, exercise, and physical fitness: definitions and distinctions for health-related research. Public Health Rep Wash DC 1974. 1985;100(2):126–31.
81. Gander JC, Sui X, Hébert JR, Hazlett LJ, Cai B, Lavie CJ, et al. Association of cardiorespiratory fitness with coronary heart disease in asymptomatic men. Mayo Clin Proc. 2015;90(10):1372–9.
82. Barlow CE, DeFina LF, Radford NB, Berry JD, Cooper KH, Haskell WL, et al. Cardiorespiratory fitness and long-term survival in "low-risk" adults. J Am Heart Assoc Cardiovasc Cerebrovasc Dis [Internet]. 2012 [cited 2017 Oct 31];1(4). Available from: https://www.ncbi.nlm.nih.gov/pmc/articles/PMC3487345/.
83. Kupsky DF, Ahmed AM, Sakr S, Qureshi WT, Brawner CA, Blaha MJ, et al. Cardiorespiratory fitness and incident heart failure: The Henry Ford Exercise Testing (FIT) Project. Am Heart J. 2017;185(Suppl C):35–42.
84. Pandey A, Patel M, Gao A, Willis BL, Das SR, Leonard D, et al. Changes in mid-life fitness predicts heart failure risk at a later age independent of interval development of cardiac and noncardiac risk factors: the Cooper Center Longitudinal Study. Am Heart J. 2015;169(2):290–297.e1.
85. Farrell SW, Finley CE, Radford NB, Haskell WL. Cardiorespiratory fitness, body mass index, and heart failure mortality in MenClinical perspective: Cooper Center Longitudinal Study. Circ Heart Fail. 2013;6(5):898–905.
86. O'Connor CM, Whellan DJ, Lee KL, Keteyian SJ, Cooper LS, Ellis SJ, et al. Efficacy and safety of exercise training in patients with chronic heart failure: HF-ACTION randomized controlled trial. JAMA. 2009;301(14):1439.
87. Pathak RK, Elliott A, Middeldorp ME, Meredith M, Mehta AB, Mahajan R, et al. Impact of CARDIOrespiratory FITness on arrhythmia recurrence in obese individuals with atrial fibrillation: the CARDIO-FIT Study. J Am Coll Cardiol. 2015;66(9):985–96.
88. Soares-Miranda L, Sattelmair J, Chaves P, Duncan G, Siscovick DS, Stein PK, et al. Physical activity and heart rate variability in older adults: the Cardiovascular Health Study. Circulation. 2014;129(21):2100–10.
89. Cornelissen VA, Smart NA. Exercise training for blood pressure: a systematic review and meta-analysis. J Am Heart Assoc Cardiovasc Cerebrovasc Dis [Internet]. 2013 [cited 2017 Oct 31];2(1). Available from: https://www.ncbi.nlm.nih.gov/pmc/articles/PMC3603230/.
90. Tinken TM, Thijssen DHJ, Black MA, Cable NT, Green DJ. Time course of change in vasodilator function and capacity in response to exercise training in humans. J Physiol. 2008;586(Pt 20):5003–12.
91. Myrstad M, Nystad W, Graff-Iversen S, Thelle DS, Stigum H, Aarønæs M, et al. Effect of years of endurance exercise on risk of atrial fibrillation and atrial flutter. Am J Cardiol. 2014;114(8):1229–33.
92. Guasch E, Nattel S. CrossTalk proposal: prolonged intense exercise training does lead to myocardial damage. J Physiol. 2013;591(Pt 20):4939–41.
93. Gregg EW, Gerzoff RB, Thompson TJ, Williamson DF. Intentional weight loss and death in overweight and obese U.S. adults 35 years of age and older. Ann Intern Med. 2003;138(5):383–9.
94. Allison DB, Zannolli R, Faith MS, Heo M, Pietrobelli A, VanItallie TB, et al. Weight loss increases and fat loss decreases all-cause mortality rate: results from two independent cohort studies. Int J Obes Relat Metab Disord. 1999;23(6):603–11.
95. Moholdt T, Lavie CJ, Nauman J. Sustained physical activity, not weight loss, associated with improved survival in coronary heart disease. J Am Coll Cardiol. 2018;71(10):1094–101.
96. Sierra-Johnson J, Romero-Corral A, Somers VK, Lopez-Jimenez F, Thomas RJ, Squires RW, et al. Prognostic importance of weight loss in patients with coronary heart disease regardless of initial body mass index. Eur J Cardiovasc Prev Rehabil. 2008;15(3):336–40.
97. Arsenault BJ, Rana JS, Lemieux I, Després J-P, Kastelein JJP, Boekholdt SM, et al. Physical inactivity, abdominal obesity and risk of coronary heart disease in apparently healthy men and women. Int J Obes. 2009;34(2):340–7.
98. Kaminsky LA, Arena R, Beckie TM, Brubaker PH, Church TS, Forman DE, et al. The importance of cardiorespiratory fitness in the United States: the need for a National Registry: a policy statement from the American Heart Association. Circulation. 2013;127(5):652–62.
99. Li TY, Rana JS, Manson JE, Willett WC, Stampfer MJ, Colditz GA, et al. Obesity as compared with physical activity in predicting risk of coronary heart disease in women. Circulation. 2006;113(4):499–506.

100. Katzmarzyk PT, Church TS, Blair SN. Cardiorespiratory fitness attenuates the effects of the metabolic syndrome on all-cause and cardiovascular disease mortality in men. Arch Intern Med. 2004;164(10):1092–7.
101. Sui X, Laditka JN, Hardin JW, Blair SN. Estimated functional capacity predicts mortality in older adults. J Am Geriatr Soc. 2007;55(12):1940–7.
102. McAuley PA, Artero EG, Sui X, Lee D, Church TS, Lavie CJ, et al. The obesity paradox, cardiorespiratory fitness, and coronary heart disease. Mayo Clin Proc. 2012;87(5):443–51.
103. Moholdt T, Lavie CJ, Nauman J. Interaction of physical activity and body mass index on mortality in coronary heart disease: data from the Nord-Trøndelag Health Study. Am J Med. 2017;130(8):949–57.
104. Fogelholm M. Physical activity, fitness and fatness: relations to mortality, morbidity and disease risk factors. A systematic review. Obes Rev. 2010;11(3):202–21.
105. McAuley PA, Kokkinos PF, Oliveira RB, Emerson BT, Myers JN. Obesity paradox and cardiorespiratory fitness in 12,417 male veterans aged 40 to 70 years. Mayo Clin Proc. 2010;85(2):115–21.
106. Zafrir B, Salman N, Amir O. Joint impact of body mass index and physical capacity on mortality in patients with systolic heart failure. Am J Cardiol. 2014;113(7):1217–21.
107. Goel K, Thomas RJ, Squires RW, Coutinho T, Trejo-Gutierrez JF, Somers VK, et al. Combined effect of cardiorespiratory fitness and adiposity on mortality in patients with coronary artery disease. Am Heart J. 2011;161(3):590–7.
108. Kokkinos P, Faselis C, Myers J, Pittaras A, Sui X, Zhang J, et al. Cardiorespiratory fitness and the paradoxical BMI-mortality risk association in male veterans. Mayo Clin Proc. 2014;89(6):754–62.
109. Clark AL, Fonarow GC, Horwich TB. Impact of cardiorespiratory fitness on the obesity paradox in patients with systolic heart failure. Am J Cardiol. 2015;115(2):209–13.
110. Lavie CJ, De Schutter A, Alpert MA, Mehra MR, Milani RV, Ventura HO. Obesity paradox, cachexia, frailty, and heart failure. Heart Fail Clin. 2014;10(2):319–26.
111. Vissers D, Hens W, Taeymans J, Baeyens J-P, Poortmans J, Gaal LV. The effect of exercise on visceral adipose tissue in overweight adults: a systematic review and meta-analysis. PLoS One. 2013;8(2):e56415.
112. Bekfani T, Pellicori P, Morris DA, Ebner N, Valentova M, Steinbeck L, et al. Sarcopenia in patients with heart failure with preserved ejection fraction: impact on muscle strength, exercise capacity and quality of life. Int J Cardiol. 2016;222(Suppl C):41–6.
113. Lavie CJ, De Schutter A, Patel DA, Romero-Corral A, Artham SM, Milani RV. Body composition and survival in stable coronary heart disease: impact of lean mass index and body fat in the "obesity paradox". J Am Coll Cardiol. 2012;60(15):1374–80.
114. Lavie CJ, De Schutter A, Patel D, Artham SM, Milani RV. Body composition and coronary heart disease mortality—an obesity or a lean paradox? Mayo Clin Proc. 2011;86(9):857–64.
115. Budoff MJ. Exercise capacity and biological age. Heart. 2016;102(6):415.
116. Lavie CJ, Kokkinos P, Ortega FB. Survival of the fittest—promoting fitness throughout the life span. Mayo Clin Proc. 2017;92(12):1743–5.

Physical Activity, Exercise, and Lipids and Lipoproteins

16

J. Larry Durstine, Elizabeth Anderson, Ryan R. Porter, and Xuewen Wang

Abbreviations

Apo	Apolipoprotein
BMI	Body mass index
CAD	Coronary artery disease
CETP	Cholesteryl ester transfer protein
CVD	Cardiovascular disease
HDL	High-density lipoprotein
HDL-C	High-density lipoprotein cholesterol
HDL-P	Total HDL particles
HL	Hepatic lipase
HLP	Large HDL-P
HMP	Medium HDL-P
HSP	Small HDL-P
HZ	HDL particle size
IDL	Intermediate-density lipoprotein
IDL-P	Intermediate-density lipoprotein particles
Kcal	Kilocalories
LCAT	Lecithin/cholesterol acyltransferase
LDL	Low-density lipoprotein
LDL-C	Low-density lipoprotein cholesterol
LDL-P	Total LDL particles
LLP	Large LDL-P
LPL	Lipoprotein lipase
LSP	Small LDL-P
LZ	LDL particle size
NMR	Nuclear magnetic resonance
PA	Physical activity
TG	Triglyceride
VLCP	Large VLDL-P plus chylomicron particles
VLDL	Very low-density lipoprotein
VLDLCP	VLDL-P plus chylomicron particles
VLDL-P	VLDL particles
VLZ	VLDL particle size
VMP	Medium VLDL-P
VSP	Small VLDL-P

Introduction

Existing evidence overwhelmingly supports that physical activity (PA) and exercise have a positive effect on improving overall health. These positive PA and exercise effects are important for the prevention and treatment of adverse health conditions such as coronary artery disease (CAD), cardiovascular disease (CVD), and stroke by reducing disease risk factors such as high blood pressure and elevated blood lipids [1]. Various blood lipids exist and are necessary for normal body functioning [2]. Nevertheless, when blood lipids like cholesterol and triglyceride levels are abnormally elevated, risk for CVD is increased. Hyperlipidemia and dyslipidemia are

J. L. Durstine (✉) · E. Anderson · R. R. Porter
X. Wang
Department of Exercise Science, Norman J. Arnold School of Public Health, University of South Carolina, Columbia, SC, USA
e-mail: ldurstin@mailbox.sc.edu

P. Kokkinos, P. Narayan (eds.), *Cardiorespiratory Fitness in Cardiometabolic Diseases*,
https://doi.org/10.1007/978-3-030-04816-7_16

Table 16.1 Lipid definitions [139]

Term	Definition
Apolipoprotein	The protein portion of the lipoprotein that combines with lipids, forming a lipid-protein particle (see Table 16.4)
Cholesterol	A common steroid found in food and in the body, consumed in the diet and synthesized in the liver, and contribute to forming cell membranes, bile, and sex hormones
Dyslipidemia	Elevated blood lipid concentrations based on a combination of genetic, environmental, and other pathological factors
Hypercholesterolemia	Elevated blood cholesterol concentrations
Hyperlipidemia	Chronically elevated blood triglyceride and cholesterol as a result of lifestyle
Hyperlipoproteinemia	Elevated lipoprotein concentrations possibly related to other underlying diseases
Hypertriglyceridemia	Elevated triglyceride concentrations
Lipoprotein	The combining of lipids such as cholesterol and triglycerides with soluble proteins, making the lipids capable of transportation to body tissues through the plasma
Postprandial lipidemia	A dramatic rise in triglyceride-rich lipoproteins after eating a fat-rich meal. Several lines of evidence exist suggesting that postprandial lipemia increases the risk of atherogenesis
Triglyceride	A group of three fatty acids connected to glycerol. Fatty acids are consumed in the diet, synthesized in the liver, used as energy, or stored in body tissues as fat – not soluble in an aqueous solution

Information modified from: Durstine and Moore [139]

terms used to describe abnormal blood triglyceride and cholesterol profiles, but numerous other terms such as dyslipoproteinemia also exist. These terms with broad definitions are presented in Table 16.1.

The first classic exercise study evaluating blood lipids was published by Holloszy et al. [3]. Their work provided two basic premises regarding blood lipids that are still constant today: total blood cholesterol does not usually change with exercise unless body weight is changed or dietary intake is changed [4], and blood triglyceride levels are usually lower following exercise training [3]. Since the publishing of this important study, a plethora of exercise studies examining lipid and lipoprotein metabolism have been published. Though more knowledge is yet to be learned, we now have a much clearer understanding of lipid and lipoprotein function, the regulation for their formation, lipid and lipoprotein transportation both extracellularly by the blood to tissue cells and intracellular movement, and greater details pertaining to abnormal lipid and lipoprotein profile and disease risk. Now after more than 50 years of scientific examination, many factors are known to exist affecting the regulation of lipid and lipoprotein metabolism with lifestyle interventions such as diet, PA, and exercise. A list of some of these factors is found in Table 16.2. Much of our expanded knowledge surrounding lipoprotein metabolism has come from understanding the different genetic and environmental factors influencing the lipoprotein metabolic pathways and ultimately lipoprotein composition. Environmental factors include gender; age; body composition and body fat distribution; dietary intake including fat, cholesterol, carbohydrates, fiber, and alcohol; cigarette smoking; medication use (see Table 16.3); change in body weight; PA; regular participation in exercise; and a single exercise session. The intent of this chapter is to provide an appraisal of the existing knowledge concerning blood lipids and lipoproteins related to PA, regularly practiced exercise, and a single exercise session.

Pathophysiology

Lipoprotein Composition and Metabolic Pathways

Blood lipoproteins are part of a complex system for moving exogenous and endogenous lipids from the intestine and liver to systemic tissues. Because lipids are not soluble in water, lipids must combine with proteins (apolipoprotein – apo) (see Table 16.4) to form lipid-protein parti-

Table 16.2 Factors affecting blood lipids and lipoproteins

Factors	Explanation
Age	Lipid profiles tend to alter as we age and are likely a reflection in the change in blood hormone levels [82, 140]
Body fat distribution	The distribution of body fat is related to adverse changes in serum lipids and lipoproteins rather than the amount: abdominal obesity results in increases of triglycerides [141, 142]
Cigarette smoking	Smoking is associated with low HDL-C levels and higher triglyceride concentrations [143]
Considerations for women	Include the type of oral contraceptives used and the subjects' day in the menstrual cycle [9, 144]
Diet	If an experimental protocol involves several exercise treatments and/or lasts for an extended period, dietary composition must be held constant as part of the experimental design [9, 81, 145]
Fasting state	Postprandial vs fasting status influences triglyceride values but not cholesterol [146]. A fasting lipid panel is preferred [137]
Medications	See Table 16.3 on medications
Plasma volume changes	Plasma volume can contract during an exercise session or expand in the days after exercise. An appropriate estimate of this change would incorporate measurement of both hemoglobin and hematocrit and/or measurement of total plasma proteins [9, 147]
Pre-exercise lipid concentrations	If pre-exercise lipid concentrations are high or low for change to occur, persons with initially high HDL-C or low total cholesterol concentrations may have to complete a larger volume of work [9]
Time of day variation	Lipid concentrations will vary throughout the day. The time of the day that the blood samples are collected (morning, afternoon, etc.) needs to be consistent throughout the study [146]
Timing of follow-up blood collection	Single exercise session – changes that occur in lipoprotein metabolism may develop within the 72-h postexercise period, not necessarily during exertion Exercise training – blood collection should be at least 48 h after the last exercise session [9]
Training state	An inactive person may require a smaller absolute volume of exercise to elicit change than an active person [9, 94]
Use of alcohol	High alcohol intake has a greater impact on overweight individuals by increasing triglyceride, VLDL, and chylomicron levels. Usually when triglycerides are elevated, HDL-C is lower. However, alcohol may in this case cause an increase in HDL-C [148, 149]
Weight change	Weight change will affect triglyceride, LDL-C, and total cholesterol concentrations [4]
Exercise volume (kcals, MET-minutes)	The volume of work or exercise completed should be quantified so that various activities may be compared in either kcals or Met-minutes [9, 52, 150]

cles referred to as lipoproteins. These particles have defined dimensions, are spherical in shape and water-soluble, and contain phospholipid, triglyceride, both free and esterified cholesterol, and various apolipoproteins. Four basic lipoprotein categories exist and are identified based on each lipoproteins' gravitational density properties. All lipoprotein classes such as HDL-C are divided into HDL_2-C and HDL_3-C (see Table 16.5). Chylomicron is the least dense lipoprotein, is very large in size, is comprised mostly of lipid (triglyceride), is mostly produced during food digestion, to a lesser degree is produced by the liver, and is important for the transport of triglyceride to systemic tissues. Very low-density lipoprotein (VLDL) also provides for the transport of triglyceride to systemic tissue and is formed mostly in the liver and, to a lesser extent, in the gut during digestion. Low-density lipoprotein (LDL) is the catabolized remains of VLDL, is created by the action of hepatic lipase (HL) [5], is found in the endothelial lining of the liver and lipoprotein lipase (LPL) [6], is found in the endothelial lining of peripheral blood capillary wall, and is the primary transport mechanism for cholesterol to systemic tissue. High-density lipoprotein (HDL) is created in the breakdown of other lipoproteins and by absorption during digestion in the small intestine. With the actions of the enzymes cholesteryl ester transfer protein

Table 16.3 Drug interactions with lipids and lipoproteins [96, 151]

Class of drug	Effect on lipids and lipoproteins
Lipid altering drugs and supplements[a]	
Bile acid sequestrants	Decreases total cholesterol
Cholesterol absorption inhibitor	Inhibits cholesterol absorption in the small intestine
HMG-CoA reductase inhibitors	Inhibits cholesterol synthesis, increases LDL receptors
Fibric acid derivatives	Activates LPL, decreases VLDL and triglycerides, and increases HDL
Nicotinic acid	Increases HDL, decreases VLDL synthesis
Fish oils	Decreases triglycerides
Common drugs and supplements given for other health conditions[b]	
Anticonvulsants	Variable effects on LDL and HDL
Antipsychotics	Increase triglyceride
Beta-blockers[c]	Increase triglyceride and decrease HDL
Immunosuppressive drugs	Increases triglyceride, LDL, and HDL
Corticosteroids	Variable effects, but tends to increase LDL and triglyceride
Growth hormone	Increases LDL, might slightly increase HDL
Retinoids	Increases triglyceride and LDL
Anabolic steroids	Increases LDL, decreases HDL
Protease inhibitors	Increases triglyceride and LDL
Estrogen	Decreases LDL but increases both triglyceride and HDL

[a]Modified from Moore et al. [96]
[b]Modified from Herink and Ito [151]
[c]Varies based on individual drug dose

Table 16.4 Major human apolipoproteins [46, 152]

Apolipoprotein	Major function	CAD risk factor
A-I	LCAT activator	Inversely related with CAD risk
A-II	LCAT inhibitor and/or activator of heparin releaseable hepatic triglyceride hydrolase	Not associated with CAD risk
B-48	Required for synthesis of chylomicron	Directly associated with CAD risk
B-100	LDL receptor-binding site	Directly associated with CAD risk
(a)	Similar characteristics between apo(a) and plasminogen, thus may have a prothrombolytic role by interfering with function of plasminogen, possible acute phase reactant to tissue damage	Directly associated with CAD risk
C-I	LCAT activator	Not associated with CAD risk
C-II	LPL activator	Not associated with CAD risk
C-III	LPL inhibitor, several forms depending on content of sialic acids	Not associated with CAD risk
D	Core lipid transfer protein, possibly identical to the cholesteryl ester transfer protein	Not associated with CAD risk
E	Remnant receptor binding, present in excess in the beta-VLDL of patients with type III hyperlipoproteinemia and exclusively with HDL-C	Not associated with CAD risk
H	Cofactor in phospholipid binding, involved in lipoprotein metabolism, possible LPL activator, plays a role in immune clearance of foreign particles by macrophages, and inhibits certain aspects of platelet activity	Unclear as to CAD risk

VLDL very low-density lipoprotein, *IDL* intermediate-density lipoprotein, *LDL* low-density lipoprotein, *HDL* high-density lipoprotein, *CAD* coronary artery disease, *LCAT* lecithin:cholesterol acyltransferase, *LPL* lipoprotein lipase
Reprinted with permission Durstine et al. [46]
Crook and Apolipoprotein [152]

(CETP) and lecithin:cholesterol acyltransferase (LCAT), HDL is involved in the reverse transport process of returning excessive amounts of cholesterol and triglyceride back to the liver for breakdown and excretion [7].

In the past, differential centrifugation density gradient technology was used for the specific classification of all lipoproteins to include chylomicrons, VLDL, intermediate-density lipoprotein (IDL), LDL, and HDL (see Table 16.5). With the advancement of technology for blood analysis techniques, nuclear magnetic resonance (NMR) spectroscopy methods are now available allowing for the analysis of lipoprotein concentrations based on particle size. Using NMR methodology, lipoprotein particles are segregated into the following: VLDL particles (VLDL-P) plus chylomicron particles (VLDLCP); large VLDL-P plus chylomicron particles (VLCP); small and medium VLDL-P (VSP and VMP, respectively); IDL particles (IDL-P); total LDL particles (LDL-P); small and large LDL-P (LSP and LLP, respectively); total HDL particle (HDL-P); and small, medium, and large HDL-P (HSP, HMP, and HLP, respectively). NMR spectroscopy also analyzes average VLDL, LDL, and HDL particle sizes (VLZ, LZ, and HZ, respectively) [8].

Lipids have different important biological uses in the body. Triglyceride is a fat or lipid formed as glycerol, combines with three fatty acids in the liver or through intestinal absorption during digestion, and is used for energy. Excessive amounts are stored intramuscularly or in adipose tissue. Cholesterol is also a fat or lipid, is synthesized by all animal cells, is an essential structural component of cell membranes, and is necessary in the biosynthesis of steroid hormones, bile acid, and vitamin D [9].

Table 16.5 Characteristics of plasma lipids and lipoproteins [46]

		Composition						
				Percentage of total lipid				
Lipid/ Lipoprotein	Source	Protein%	Total lipid %	TG	Chol	Phosp	Free Chol	Apolipoprotein
Chylomicron	Intestine	1–2	98–99	88	8	3	1	Major: A-IV, B-48, B-100, H Minor: A-I, A-II, C-I, C-II, C-III, E
VLDL	Major: liverMinor: intestine	7–10	90–93	56	20	15	8	Major: B-100, C-III, E, G Minor: A-I, A-II, B-48, C-II, D
IDL	Major: VLDLMinor: chylomicron	11	89	29	26	34	9	Major: B-100 Minor: B-48
LDL	Major: VLDLMinor: chylomicron	21	79	13	28	48	10	Major: B-100 Minor: C-I, C-II, (a)
HDL_2	Major: HDL_3	33	67	16	43	31	10	Major: A-1, A-II, D, E, F Minor: A-IV, C-I, C-II, C-III
HDL_3	Major: liver and intestine Minor VLDL and Chylomicron Remnants	57	43	13	46	29	6	Major: A-1, A-II, D, E, F Minor: A-IV, C-I, C-II, C-III
Chol	Liver and diet		100			70–75	25–30	
TG	Diet and liver		100	100				

VLDL very low-density lipoprotein, *IDL* intermediate-density lipoprotein, *LDL* low-density lipoprotein, *HDL* high-density lipoprotein, *Chol* cholesterol, *TG* triglyceride, *Phosp* phospholipid
Modified from Durstine et al. [46]

For movement to various body tissues, triglyceride is wrapped into the core of the large chylomicron and VLDL and is circulated to systemic tissues by the cardiovascular and lymphatic systems. Chylomicron and VLDL interact with HL [5] found in the liver endothelial walls and LPL [6] found in the systemic endothelial walls. Both HL and LPL hydrolyze the triglyceride core of chylomicron and VLDL. Free fatty acids and glycerol are released during the HL and LPL hydrolysis process, are taken up by the tissue, utilized as fuel (beta oxidation), or stored as fat intramuscularly or in adipose tissue. The remaining remnant, IDL, is either catabolized in the liver by HL or in the peripheral vascular system by LPL to become LDL. The resulting LDL particle is the primary transported mechanism for cholesterol systemically. LDL binds to LDL receptors found on the surface of all cells. Once taken-up by the LDL receptor, LDL is internalized into the cell. When the cell no longer needs cholesterol, a negative feedback system reduces cellular LDL receptor synthesis, suppressing LDL receptors on the outside of the cell preventing additional cellular uptake of LDL [10].

Excessive cholesterol is removed by the reverse cholesterol process and excreted as bile [7, 9]. The most notable pathway for cholesterol elimination from the body uses nascent HDL particles secreted by the liver, enriched with free cholesterol and phospholipid derived from LPL-mediated chylomicron, and VLDL catabolism. Free cholesterol is esterified and moved into the core of the HDL_3 by the action of LCAT with apo A-I as a cofactor and provides a constant cholesterol supply to maintain a chemical gradient for a continuous LCAT reaction. As the HDL_3 core expands, the particle transforms into HDL_2. As this series of reactions are taking place, two other separate groups of metabolic reactions are occurring. In the first group of reactions, the enzyme CETP [11] facilitates an exchange for the newly obtained HDL_2 cholesteryl ester with triglyceride obtained from triglyceride-rich lipoprotein remnants, and the remaining lipid-depleted lipoprotein remnant is moved to the liver for removal. Another group of reactions facilitated by HL removes triglyceride and cholesterol from the HDL_2 particle that previously gained triglyceride by CETP action, resulting in a smaller denser HDL_3 particle that returns to the circulation providing substrate to continue this process. Finally, two other cholesterol removal pathways exist. The first pathway is the direct HDL_2 withdrawal from circulating blood by liver cells through the combined action of phospholipase and HL. Another pathway is the hepatic apo E receptor-mediated removal of an HDL_2 cholesteryl ester. In this reaction cholesteryl ester-rich HDL_2 particles containing apo E are withdrawn from circulating blood by hepatic LDL receptor-mediated endocytosis.

Lipoprotein Oxidation

Lipoprotein oxidation is both detrimental and beneficial [12]. Excessive LDL circulating through the cardiovascular system, if not metabolized by the liver, is oxidized [13]. Oxidation occurs when LDL reacts with free radicals, causing the protein portion of the LDL to undergo changes, resulting in an altered radical-mediated damaged protein containing free radical by-products (uncharged particles that are typically highly reactive and short-lived). Oxidation is a nonenzymatic process altering the amino acids and their cross-linking bonds, changing the composition and structure of apolipoprotein B (apo B), the major protein associated with LDL. Oxidized LDL will facilitate further lipid degradation and/or peroxidation of the lipid core. The modified surface of an oxidized LDL is now recognized by leukocytes, triggering an immune system reaction that causes an inflammatory response [14, 15]. Monocytes and macrophages are now attracted to the site and engulf the damaged LDL [13]. The oxidized LDL causes a chemical reaction inside the macrophage, causing foam cell formation and potentiating long-term damage and adhesion to blood vessel walls which initiates endothelial plaque formation [14, 16–18]. Long-term damage and plaque buildup are reportedly due to various factors including diets high in saturated fats [19] and/or a sedentary lifestyle [20], leading to lasting problematic health conditions such as atherosclerosis, stroke, CAD, and peripheral artery disease.

HDL oxidation also occurs and is both beneficial and detrimental. While LDL oxidation is usually associated with adverse health consequences, HDL oxidation is usually associated with positive health outcomes [12]. One positive benefit of HDL oxidation is that macrophages do not recognize oxidized HDL, thus reducing foam cell formation. Unlike oxidized LDL, oxidized HDL can leave the intima and return to the liver, be metabolized, and be excreted [14]. Oxidized HDL does not undergo apolipoprotein proteolysis like oxidized LDL [13]. The effectiveness of oxidized HDL when compared to their unoxidized counterparts remains unclear. Some existing evidence supports oxidized HDL as having a diminished capacity to accept cholesterol from cells [21]. On the other hand, oxidized HDL promotes cholesterol efflux from macrophages more effectively than normal HDL depending on the type of radical and oxidant used [12] which is beneficial because increased efflux capacity is inversely related to CHD [22].

HDL, in addition to being a positive component for reverse cholesterol transport, offers added protection against atherosclerosis. HDL has been proposed to interfere with LDL oxidation by absorbing free radicals. If this interference with LDL oxidation effect is true, this explanation can help to elucidate why HDL is a major carrier of lipid peroxides [14]. Thus, elevated HDL not only removes excess cholesterol but is effective in the clearance of lipid peroxides, allowing for a more effective protection against atherosclerosis [17, 18, 23].

Epidemiological Evidence for the Scope of the Disease (Prevalence and Incidence)

According to the Center for Disease Control and Prevention and the American Heart Association, 95 million adults 20 years of age and older living in the United States (US) (13% women and 11% men of total population) have total serum cholesterol levels above 200 mg/dL [24, 25]. Approximately 29 million or 12% of the adults in the USA require cholesterol-lowering medication because their blood cholesterol levels are greater than 240 mg/dL [24, 26]. Non-Hispanic blacks represent a lower percentage of adults with high total cholesterol (9%) than non-Hispanic whites (13%) and all Hispanic adults (13%). However, 6% of US adults are unaware of their high cholesterol levels [24]. At the same time, 70% of US adults had their cholesterol levels checked within the last 5 years [24]. Most notable is that at least 10% of patients having office-based physician visits had their blood cholesterol measurements completed when more than 20% of the patients had in their medical record an indication of hyperlipidemia and needed follow-up measurements [26].

As the incidence of adolescent chronic diseases is increasing in the USA, the number of adolescents (12–19 years of age) having abnormal cholesterol levels is 20%. The percentage of adolescents having elevated total cholesterol and are normal weight is 14%; those adolescents that are overweight with high total cholesterol is 22%; and those adolescents who are obese and have high total cholesterol is 43% [24].

On a positive note, the prevalence of elevated cholesterol in the USA has been decreasing. The percentage of US adults 20 years and older with elevated total cholesterol has decreased from 18% in 2000 to 11% in 2014, and this trend appears to be worldwide. The decline in total cholesterol levels in adults is associated with the increased usage of cholesterol-lowering medications rather than lifestyle improvements [24]. At the same time, the prevalence of elevated total cholesterol in US youth has also declined from 11% between the ages of 6 and 19 years in 1988–1994 to 8% in 2007–2010. However, according to the American Academy of Pediatrics, less than 1% of children are eligible for cholesterol-lowering medications [24].

As the need for lipid-lowering medication is considered, 78 million or 37% of the US adults 20 years of age and older had LDL-C levels high enough for medication in 2012 [25] and represents one in three Americans having elevated LDL-C levels [27]. Fortunately, the prevalence of elevated

LDL-C in the USA has also decreased in adults from 59% in 1976 to1980 to 27% in 2007 to 2010 with the mean LDL-C levels at 113 mg/dL in 2011 to 2014. The prevalence of elevated LDL-C is higher in men (31%) than in women (24%) [24].

Limited data is available for LDL-C levels in youth. Adolescents LDL-C levels are higher in girls when compared to boys. In 2014 elevated LDL-C concentrations were prevalent in 8% of girls while elevated in only 6% of boys between the ages of 12–19 years. The overall mean LDL-C levels in adolescents are 88 mg/dL. Only slight mean LDL-C level variations were found between racial and ethnic groups [24]:

- Non-Hispanic whites 87 mg/dL for boys and 89 mg/dL for girls
- Non-Hispanic blacks 86 mg/dL for boys and 91 mg/dL for girls
- Hispanic youth 86 mg/dL for boys and 88 mg/dL for girls
- Non-Hispanic Asians 85 mg/dL for boys and 97 mg/dL for girls

The mean HDL-C level in adults during 2011 to 2014 was 53 mg/dL. Unfortunately, the percentage of adults having low HDL-C levels (lower than 40 mg/dL) was 17% of the US adults in 2012 [24]. Fortunately, the percentage of adults having low HDL-C has decreased by 20% since 2010. The prevalence of low HDL-C levels varies by gender with men having a higher prevalence of low HDL-C compared to women. When comparing race/ethnicity, blacks have the lowest prevalence of low HDL-C levels. Among US adults 20 years of age and older, low HDL-C levels for [24]:

- Non-Hispanic whites were 17% (25% of men and 9% of women).
- Non-Hispanic blacks were 13% (19.1% of men and 7.8% of women).
- Non-Hispanic Asians were 14% (24.5% of men and 5.1% of women).
- Hispanic adults were 22% (32.6% of men and 11.3% of women).

During the time from 2011 to 2014, children between 6 and 11 years of age had a mean HDL-C level of 54. mg/dL. Adolescents between ages of 12–19 years had a mean HDL-C level of 51 mg/dL. The prevalence of low HDL-C among adolescents during that time was 19% for males and 13% for females [24].

Approximately 24% of adults 20 years of age and older in the USA have elevated triglyceride levels (≥150 mg/dL) with a mean triglyceride level of 104 mg/dL. Mean triglyceride levels were higher in men (112 mg/dL) than in women (96 mg/dL) with non-Hispanic black men and women having the lowest mean triglyceride levels when compared to the other racial/ethnic populations between 2011 and 2014 [24].

Among adolescents, mean triglyceride levels were 79 mg/dL in 2014 with boys having higher mean triglyceride levels compared to girls. Non-Hispanic blacks had lower mean levels of triglycerides compared to the other racial/ethnic groups. The prevalence of high triglycerides in adolescents was 9% in boys and 6% in girls [24].

Although US adults are making progress in decreasing the prevalence of dyslipidemia because of increased medication usage, other lipid-lowering interventions including lifestyle modifications should still be considered as first-line intervention before starting medications [1]. If an improved diet, increased PA and exercise were regularly practiced, society would decrease the need for medications while experiencing improved health benefits and quality of life [24].

Epidemiologic Association Between Disease and Fitness

Blood lipid and lipoprotein levels are associated with risk for CVD in individuals irrespective of age, race, nationality, or gender [24, 28–32]. In 2015, worldwide deaths associated with ischemic heart disease totaled 8.76 million (World Health Organization, 2017). In 2012, the cost associated with CVD and stroke was an estimated $316.1 billion [24]. By 2030, 40% of the US population is projected to have some form of CVD resulting in a $918 billion annual cost [24].

Though elevated blood lipids and lipoproteins are associated with increased risk for chronic disease, lipids and lipoproteins are essential for proper body function. Lipoproteins are transporters of triglyceride and cholesterol and are utilized for multiple essential processes within the body [2]. Only when blood lipid and lipoproteins reach abnormal levels do lipids and lipoproteins become associated with elevated risk for chronic disease [28, 33]. Changeable behaviors such as PA, exercise, diet, and sleep are known modifiers of blood lipid and lipoproteins [9, 34–38], thereby changing CVD risk without the necessity for pharmacological intervention.

Until recently, CVD risk was determined by utilizing only blood markers such as triglyceride, total cholesterol, HDL-C, and LDL-C (see Table 16.6). With the development of the new NMR technology, lipoprotein concentration and particle size provide greater detail allowing for greater precision in understanding the relationship between disease risk and the various lipoproteins and their subfractions [8, 39]. As a reminder, the new NMR methodology provides various lipoprotein particles including very low-density lipoprotein particles (VLDL-P) and chylomicron particles (VLDLCP); large VLDL-P and chylomicron particles (VLCP); small and medium VLDL-P (VSP and VMP, respectively); intermediate-density lipoprotein (IDL) particles (IDL-P); total LDL particles (LDL-P); small and large LDL-P (LSP and LLP, respectively); total HDL particle (HDL-P); and small, medium, and large HDL-P (HSP, HMP, and HLP, respectively) [8].

Present scientific investigations have established that CVD risk is increased with elevated LDL-C and decreased HDL-C levels. In addition, lipoprotein particle function also provides added information in determining CVD pathophysiology. Investigations examining lipoprotein subfractions and their function have concluded that elevated concentrations of LSP and HSP are better atherogenic indicators than their larger counterparts [40–43]. Smaller mean LZ and HZ are also associated with greater CVD risk compared to larger mean LZ and HZ [44, 45]. Since the NMR technology used to analyze lipoprotein concentrations is relatively new, detailed investigation of how to most effectively modulate lipids and lipoproteins via lifestyle is still needed.

As is well established by observational and clinical trials, increased PA and regularly practiced exercise contribute to favorable blood lipid and lipoprotein profiles by decreasing blood triglyceride

Table 16.6 LDL cholesterol goals and cut points for therapeutic lifestyle changes (TLC) and drug therapy in different risk categories [153]

Risk category	LDL goal	LDL level at which to initiate therapeutic lifestyle changes	LDL level at which to consider drug therapy
CHD or CHD risk equivalents (10-year risk >20%)	<100 mg/dL	100 mg/dL	130 mg/dL (100–129 mg/dL: Drug optional)[a]
2+ risk factors (10-year risk ≤20%)	<130 mg/dL	130 mg/dL	10-year risk 10–20%: 130 mg/dL
			10-year risk <10: 160 mg/dL
0–1 Risk factor[b]	<160 mg/dL	160 mg/dL	190 mg/dL (160–189 mg/dL: LDL-lowering drug optional) [see Reference 137]

[a]Almost all people with 0–1 risk factor have a 10-year <10%; thus, 10-year risk assessment in people with 0–1 risk factor is not necessary

[b]Some authorities recommend the use of LDL-lowering drugs in this category if an LDL cholesterol <100 mg/dL cannot be achieved by therapeutic lifestyle changes. Others prefer the use of drugs that primarily modify triglycerides and HDL, e.g., nicotinic acid or fibrate. Clinical judgment also may call for deferring drug therapy in this subcategory.

Reprinted with permission National Cholesterol Education Program. National Heart, Lung, and Blood Institute, National Institutes of Health. NIH Publication No. 01-3670, May 2001. https://www.nhlbi.nih.gov/files/docs/guidelines/atp3xsum.pdf

Also found in Expert Panel on Detection, Evaluation, and Treatment of High Blood Cholesterol in Adults [153]

concentration and increasing blood HDL-C levels [9, 46]. With the arrival of NMR spectroscopy, the effect of exercise on multiple lipoprotein subfractions is now well established [47–51]. A recent meta-analysis by Sarzynski et al. [39] concluded that exercise training significantly decreased large VLDL-P, SLP, and HMP concentrations as well as mean VLZ. In addition, exercise training significantly increased LLP and HLP concentrations and increased mean LZ.

Cleary, PA and exercise training have positively impacted the lipoprotein profile, but the lipoprotein particles being significantly affected by PA and exercise vary from study to study. One possible explanation for these inconsistent results is the wide variety of exercise training protocols utilized across studies. Not yet thoroughly investigated is the precise PA or exercise volume or dose that will influence different lipoprotein subfractions. The volume, amount, or dose does make a difference when examining the impact of PA and exercise on blood lipids and lipoproteins [49, 52, 53]. Kraus et al. [49] demonstrated that a high exercise dose or volume impacted 10 of 11 lipoprotein outcomes compared to a lower dose exercise of similar intensity. Exercise volume or dose has yet to be investigated in respect to NMR spectroscopy-based lipoprotein separation. Prior to lipoprotein subfraction analysis, multiple cross-sectional studies demonstrated greater amounts of exercise, resulting in greater decreases in triglyceride and total cholesterol/HDL-C ratio by increasing HDL-C concentration [52, 54–60]. Though these studies demonstrate that lipoprotein cholesterol respond differently to different exercise volumes, no published data is available concerning the effect of exercise volume on lipoprotein subfractions separated using NMR spectroscopy.

Weight loss by dietary caloric restriction is commonly utilized as a method to decrease CVD risk [61]. Caloric restriction generally decreases CVD risk by decreasing blood cholesterol and LDL-C and/or elevating HDL-C [62–64]. A prevalence of LSP and HSP particles are associated with overweight and obesity [43]. Weight loss by means of caloric restriction and alternate-day fasting demonstrated decreased LDL-C and decreased proportion of LSP among total LDL-P, as well as an increase in LZ particles [65–68].

Like caloric restriction and exercise, evidence exists that sleep duration also affects blood lipid and lipoprotein profiles. As a modifiable lifestyle behavior, sleep has only been studied in relation to lipoprotein particles and CVD for the past decade. Thus, our understanding of the relationship is limited. Population-based studies have concluded that sleep duration is associated with blood triglyceride, total cholesterol, HDL-C, and LDL-C levels [34, 69]. These studies demonstrate the existence of optimal sleep duration of 6–8 h. Consistent patterns of sleeping less than 6 h or more than 8 h are associated with blood lipid and lipoprotein levels associated with elevated CVD risk [34]. Only one human study has utilized NMR to analyze the effect of short-term (5 days) sleep deprivation on lipoprotein subfractions and reported a decreased concentration of small, medium, LLP, and VSP. No significant concentration change in small, medium, or HLP were found [70]. Presently, no studies exist that utilize NMR spectroscopy to analyze the effect of experimental chronic sleep restriction on lipoprotein subfractions.

Interventional Evidence

Impact of Aerobic Exercise on the Blood Lipid Profile

Aerobic exercise has been the focus of most scientific investigations involving the effects of PA and exercise on the blood lipid and lipoprotein profile, and much of the evidence has linked higher levels of aerobic PA and exercise to lower CVD rates and other chronic diseases [1]. Well-designed investigations evaluating fitness and other lifestyles have eliminated or controlled for confounding factors such as diet composition, gender including women's phase of their menstrual cycle, age, body fat distribution, alcohol use, cigarette smoking, medication use, and regular participation of exercise (see Table 16.2). A summary of the results from these studies concerning the impact of exercise training on blood lipids and lipoproteins is presented in Table 16.7. The literature is rather clear

Table 16.7 Lipids and lipoprotein changes associated with exercise [46]

Lipid/lipoprotein	Single exercise session	Exercise training
Triglyceride	Decreases of 14–50% Approximate mean change 20%	Decrease of 4–40% Approximate mean change 24%
Cholesterol	No change[a]	No change[b]
LDL-C	No change	No change
Small dense LDL-C particles	Literature unclear	Can increase LDL particle size, usually associated with triglyceride lowering
Lp(a)	No change	No change
HDL-C	Increase of 4–18% Approximate mean change 10%	Increase of 4–18% Approximate mean change 8%

[a]No change unless the exercise session is prolonged (see text)
[b]No change if bodyweight and diet do not change (see text)
Reprinted with permission Durstine et al. [36]

regarding the following two points. First, blood triglyceride levels are usually reduced after exercise training. Second, unless diet is changed or body weight is reduced after exercise training, total cholesterol levels do not change.

Triglycerides

Endurance exercise is almost always associated with reduced triglyceride levels. Holloszy et al. [3] in a classic study from 1964 compared two groups of sedentary middle-aged male subjects. One group performed organized endurance exercises (i.e., distance running 2–4 miles and endurance calisthenics) with an exercise trainer, while another group performed a less organized and unsupervised exercise program. After 6 months of aerobic exercise training, triglyceride levels did drop significantly from 208 ± 127 to 125 ± 78 mg/dL or by 40% in the organized/supervised group. An added important observation was that triglyceride reductions started to occur within 2–3 h following the exercise session and last up to 2 days. This study was the first to demonstrate that serum triglyceride levels are lowered with exercise training and is maintained when aerobic exercise is regularly performed [3].

The extent of triglyceride reductions usually produced with regular endurance exercise training is dependent upon the pretraining concentrations and the exercise volume completed throughout the training program. Blood triglyceride reductions ranging from 4% to 40% have been reported (see Table 16.7) [9, 52]. Serum triglyceride levels are reduced primarily by increasing LPL content and activity. This increase in LPL activity is responsible for increasing triglyceride hydrolysis in both active and sedentary populations [71]. Therefore, most individuals gain health benefits from regular aerobic exercise training by reducing their blood triglyceride levels.

Plaisance et al. [72] observed the effects of aerobic exercise in combination with extended-release niacin usage on postprandial triglyceride levels in men with the metabolic syndrome. Subjects underwent each of four different interventions: control, only a high-fat meal (100 g fat); exercise, 1 h before consuming the high-fat meal, subjects completed an aerobic exercise session by expending 500 kcal of treadmill running; niacin, completed 6 weeks of niacin therapy before consuming the high-fat meal; and niacin plus exercise, after completing 6 weeks of niacin therapy and 1 h before consuming the high-fat meal, subjects completed an aerobic exercise session by expending 500 kcal doing treadmill running. Exercise alone reduced postprandial triglyceride concentrations without affecting fasting triglycerides. In contrast, extended-release niacin alone reduced fasting triglycerides but had little effect on postprandial triglyceride levels. The intervention having the greatest effect on triglyceride levels was the exercise plus niacin therapy. These results demonstrate the importance of including an aerobic exercise program with pharmacological therapy in men with metabolic syndrome [72].

Cholesterol

Historically, existing evidence does not support that aerobic exercise alone reduces blood cholesterol concentrations [73]. Rather, endurance exercise does not change blood total cholesterol levels unless body weight is decreased. Holloszy et al. reported serum total cholesterol levels did not change after exercise training [3]. This same finding has been reported time after time (see Table 16.7) [4, 9, 35]. Although total cholesterol is not changed with exercise training, regular exercise does positively affect lipid and lipoprotein profiles. For example, increasing PA and exercise have become a regular recommendation for individuals with hypercholesterolemia [74].

HDL-Cholesterol

Aerobic exercise training will increase blood HDL-C concentrations but not always [9, 52, 75]. Existing evidence supports an inverse relationship between blood HDL-C and triglyceride levels. In a classic study from 1978, Schaefer et al. [76] evaluated a large group of patients with hypolipoproteinemia. Subjects having high fasting concentrations of triglycerides and/or chylomicrons had significantly lower HDL-C levels when compared to normal controls. As triglyceride levels decrease after exercise training, HDL-C concentrations increase, implying that endurance exercise has a positive effect on HDL-C levels.

Aerobic exercise is associated with elevated HDL-C concentrations in men with low HDL-C levels, high triglyceride levels, and abdominal adiposity. As part of the HERITAGE Family Study, male subjects completed cycle ergometer exercise at 75% of maximal oxygen consumption (VO_2max) for 50 min, three times per week for 21 weeks. Men with higher waist circumference and blood triglyceride levels at baseline showed the most improvement in their blood HDL-C levels [77]. Nonetheless, not all individuals in this study or other exercise studies had this beneficial HDL-C response. In fact, considerable interindividual variability, or heterogeneity of responsiveness, to regular exercise participation exists regarding changes in both cardiorespiratory fitness and cardiometabolic risk factors [78–80]. Thus, some subjects' HDL-C levels will have little or no response to exercise regardless of the exercise volume completed. This individual variability in response to exercise is consequent to the interaction of the individual's genotype, familial factors, and environment. The lack of beneficial cardiometabolic risk factor responses to exercise is not yet well understood.

LDL-Cholesterol

When considering the effects of aerobic exercise on LDL-C concentrations, many studies report no exercise effect unless associated with body weight or body fat percentage change or an altered diet [9, 35, 73]. Stefanick et al. [81] evaluated the effects of exercise or the National Cholesterol Education Program (NCEP) diet in women and men who have blood lipid and lipoprotein levels that place them at a high risk for CAD. Diet and exercise alone did not alter LDL-C. Rather, diet and exercise combined lowered body weight and LDL-C.

Kraus et al. [49] developed the STRRIDE project to evaluate the exercise volume and the exercise intensity needed to effect lipids, lipoproteins, and lipoprotein subfractions, while body weight was maintained at baseline value. Subjects were randomly assigned to one of four different groups: high-amount-high-intensity group, low-amount-high-intensity group, low-amount-moderate-intensity group, or a non-exercise control group for a 34-week training period. The high-amount-high-intensity group expended the caloric equivalent of exercising about 20 miles per week at 65–80% of peak oxygen consumption (VO_2peak) expending 23 kcals per kilogram per week. The low-amount-high-intensity group expended the caloric equivalent of exercising 12 miles per week at 65–80% of VO_2peak. The low-amount-moderate-intensity group expended the caloric equivalent of walking 12 miles per week at 40–55% of VO_2peak. Subject body weight remained constant throughout the study period. The concentrations of small LDL-C and LDL particles decreased, while the size of the LDL particles increased only in the high-amount-high-intensity group [49].

VLDL-Cholesterol

VLDL-C is normally reduced with regular aerobic exercise training based on the many observations that endurance athletes have lower VLDL-C concentrations than sedentary controls [9, 35, 73].

Postprandial Lipemia

Postprandial lipemia is characterized by exaggerated levels of triglycerides in the blood that fails to return to baseline levels within 8–10 h after consumption of high volume of dietary fat [82]. Postprandial lipemia is lower in the hours after completing aerobic exercise of sufficient volume [72, 83, 84] but is increased when exercise is withdrawn for several days [85]. Together, these data suggest that the beneficial influence of exercise on blood lipids and lipoprotein levels is an acute phenomenon that is lost rather quickly after cessation of exercise, even in the most highly trained individuals. Exercise must be repeated regularly to maintain this benefit.

Oxidized Lipoproteins

Tiainen et al. [17] randomized 161 sedentary women from Southern Finland into a control group and an intervention group that completed 6 months of aerobic exercise. Exercise consisted of 50-min aerobic exercise sessions 4 days a week with heart rate maintained at 65–80% maximal heart rate. After intervention, a five-percentage increase in oxidized HDL-C level was achieved by the intervention group compared to a two-percentage decrease in oxidized HDL-C level by the control group. A six-percentage point decrease in blood triglyceride levels in the intervention group was also observed [17].

Valimaki et al. [23] evaluated oxidative stress and lipid oxidation product removal in middle-distance and marathon runners from Southern Finland following a single exercise session. Subjects performed two non-exhaustive treadmill exercise sessions: a 40-min intermittent session (alternating 2-min runs with 2-min rests at a velocity corresponding to 100% $\dot{V}O_{2max}$) and a second 40-min continuous session (at a velocity corresponding to 80% $\dot{V}O_{2max}$). No significant change was seen in oxidized LDL during exercise, but a four-percentage decrease after the intermittent run was observed as well as a 16% decrease after the continuous run. Also, a 26% increase in oxidized HDL was reported for the intermittent run, and 25% for the continuous run was found. Based on these data, continuous exercise and intermittent exercise both decrease oxidized LDL and increase oxidized HDL [23].

Evidence does exist supporting the hypothesis that aerobic exercise training improves resistance to LDL-C oxidation. Medlow et al. placed male subjects into four different groups: young participants (18–25 years), aged participants (50–65 years), and randomly assigning subjects to either an experimental or control group – total of four groups. Subjects assigned to the exercise groups participated in 12 weeks of moderate-intensity exercise training (55–65% $\dot{V}O_{2max}$) and expended 1600 kcals each week. The control group maintained their normal daily lifestyle for 12 weeks. Lipoprotein resistance to oxidation was assessed by measuring the half time ($T½_{max}$) necessary for oxidation to begin. The most notable result was the change in the aged exercising group where $T½_{max}$ increased for the large less dense LDL subfraction was found. Though additional investigations are needed in this area, resistance to oxidation occurs to the large less dense LDL subfraction after moderate-intensity exercise intervention meaning that large LDL is less likely to be oxidized in older populations [86].

Exercise Intensity Versus Exercise Volume

Exercise volume has a greater influence on blood lipids than exercise intensity. For instance, higher HDL-C and lower triglycerides are almost always reported when exercise of greater volume is completed [49, 53]. Even though some evidence suggests an improved blood lipid and lipoprotein profile with higher exercise intensity [58–60, 87], exercise volume has the greatest influence on the blood lipid profile [52].

Crouse et al. [74] evaluated hypercholesterolemic men after a 24-week exercise training program which included 3 days a week of a cycle ergometer exercise training protocol. Subjects were randomized to either a group that trained at 50% VO_{2max} (moderate intensity) or a group that trained at 80% VO_{2max} (high intensity). Both exercise intensity groups improved in aerobic capacity and had significant weight loss and lower percentage body fat measurements after exercise training. Despite different exercise intensities, no differences in the blood lipid and lipoprotein levels were found between groups [74].

Kraus et al. [49] in the STRRIDE project found that high volume exercise completed at 65–80% of VO_2peak, expending the caloric equivalent of exercising about 20 miles per week, and maintained body weight throughout the 34-week study period did not change blood cholesterol or LDL-C levels, but the concentration of small LDL-C decreased. While the size of the LDL particles did become larger, the concentration of LDL particles also decreased. This study further supports the concept that the exercise volume has a greater impact on blood lipid and lipoprotein profiles than does exercise intensity [49].

Effects of Resistance Exercise on the Blood Lipid and Lipoprotein Profile

Resistance exercise training has not received as much attention historically as aerobic exercise when examining blood lipids and lipoprotein profiles. Gordon et al. [73] and Eckel et al. [1] state that resistance training does have an impact on the blood lipid and lipoprotein profile. Nevertheless, earlier reviews report different observations [9, 35, 46, 88]. These inconsistencies are most likely due to variations in energy expenditure and/or lack of incorporating non-exercise control groups into the study design [35, 73]. Resistance exercise has little effect on blood triglyceride levels unless triglyceride levels are elevated. Durstine and Haskell [9] and Franklin et al. [35] reviewed the literature and reported blood cholesterol, VLDL-C, and/or LDL-C which did not change with regular resistance training participation [9, 35]. However, recent reports contradict these earlier reports [1, 89]. Few early studies have presented findings for a reduced LDL-C after resistance training because it did not consider body weight or body fat change [73]. Though few studies report elevated blood HDL-C after resistance training, the consensus is that HDL-C usually does not changed after resistance training [1, 9, 35].

Wooten et al. [90] reported that resistance training reduced LDL-C and total cholesterol. Obese postmenopausal women were randomized into either a resistance exercise training group or a control group. After 12 weeks of supervised resistance exercise training incorporating ten whole body exercises, the resistance exercise trained group had reductions in total cholesterol (16%), LDL-C (23%) and non-HDL-C (20%). No changes were observed in HDL-C, body weight, BMI, or percentage body fat [90]. This resistance training study was well designed and gave consideration for variables such as plasma volume shift (see Table 16.2).

James et al. [91] randomized older men into either an active control or resistance exercise group. After 1 year, the resistance intervention group did not change body weight, but did increase lean body mass and muscle strength, while fat mass decreased. Reductions in blood cholesterol, LDL-C, and non-HDL-C concentrations were reported when compared to the active nonresistance exercise control group. No changes in blood chylomicron, triglyceride, or HDL-C levels were found. These data are consistent with the summary developed for the 2013 guidelines on lifestyle management to reduce cardiovascular risk [1].

A Single Exercise Session and the Blood Lipid and Lipoprotein Profile

Studies designed to evaluate lipid and lipoprotein metabolism after a single exercise session must consider the factors found in Table 16.2. If these confounding factors are not given proper consideration, the results presented are difficult to interpret. When evaluating a single exercise session, exercise or work volume completed must be quantified (i.e., kcals or MET-minutes), pre-exercise lipid concentrations must be measured, subjects' state of training, and plasma volume shifts must be considered. Other factors include the timing of follow-up periods for blood sample collections; diet before, during, and after the exercise training; and special consideration for women regarding oral contraceptive use and timing of the menstrual cycle [9, 46, 92]. Understanding the mechanisms causing change during a single exercise session provides better insight into the health benefits of PA and exercise.

Triglyceride concentrations are generally lower immediately after and/or in the days following a single exercise session if the session is long enough and requires large enough volume of energy expenditure [53]. Cholesterol levels are not likely to change after a single exercise session; however, some evidence exist suggesting a small change in blood cholesterol if the exercise is prolonged and large amounts of energy expended [52, 53]. VLDL-C levels are reduced after exercise, and LDL-C is likely reduced if exercise is prolonged and a large amount of energy is expended [9, 53, 92].

Because physically active persons typically exercise on consecutive days, Wagganer et al. [93] recruited obese, sedentary, male and female subjects to complete three separate protocols to understand the impact of consecutive exercise days on blood lipid and lipoprotein levels. The first protocol had subjects complete one treadmill exercise at 60% VO_{2max} for 90 min. The second protocol had subjects complete the same treadmill exercise at 60% VO_{2max} for 90 min on three consecutive days. A control protocol requiring two fasted blood samples 6 days apart with no exercise during these 6 days was completed. Average energy expenditure for each exercise session was 847 ± 61 kcal. HDL-C levels increased during the three-consecutive-exercise-day protocol when compared to the 1-day protocol. Unexpectedly, LDL-C concentrations were lower following the one-exercise-day protocol with the greatest change observed 48 h postexercise. However, this LDL-C finding is somewhat unique since the past studies have not reported a reduced LDL-C following a single exercise session unless high kcal expenditure or associated weight loss was achieved. The three-consecutive-exercise-day protocol observed a continuous decrease in triglyceride level with blood triglyceride 29% below baseline 24 h after exercise, and a 13% reduction remained 72 h after the third consecutive exercise day. Individuals with the highest baseline triglyceride level had the greatest triglyceride reduction. No blood cholesterol change was observed by either protocol. Three consecutive days of exercise training positively impacted blood lipid and lipoprotein profiles more than one single exercise session [93]. The changes after three consecutive days of exercise are similar to those reported for regular exercise participation [9, 52].

Kantor et al. [94] evaluated cycle ergometer exercise response in subjects working at 80% maximum heart for 1 h in untrained and for 2 h in trained men. Untrained men did not experience a change in HDL-C, while trained men did increased their blood HDL-C levels and decreased blood triglyceride levels immediately after the exercise which remained lower for 48 h after exercise. Blood LDL-C and cholesterol levels decreased in both groups but returned to pre-exercise levels 48 h after exercise [94]. Though not reported in this study but is deserving of comment, trained men exercising for 2 h at 80% of their maximal heart rate completed more work and are likely responsible for causing greater exercise change. Based on completing greater exercise or work volume, trained subjects who responded differently to a single exercise session provide further support for the importance of knowing the exercise volume completed [94].

Whether a single exercise session or regular exercise participation is considered, blood cholesterol and LDL-C are unlikely to change. HDL-C levels can increase approximately average of 8% after a single exercise session and 10% after regular exercise participation. Blood triglyceride levels decrease after a single exercise session and after regular exercise participation (see Table 16.7) [46, 52]. In light of these beneficial changes, the impact of a single exercise session is temporary or transient and lasts for a short period of 24–72 h. To maintain these health improvements, regular exercise should take place at least on nonconsecutive days if not most days of the week [9, 95, 96].

Another consideration is the exercise intensity impact on blood lipid and lipoprotein profiles. Davis et al. [97] exercised active men having high HDL-C levels at two different exercise intensities: a high-intensity exercise session at 75% VO_{2max} for 60 min and a low-intensity exercise session at 50% VO_{2max} for 90 min. Total caloric expenditure of 950 kcals was held constant for each of the two different exercise intensities. After correcting for plasma volume shifts, no change in any blood lipid and lipoprotein levels was reported. The data from this study suggest that exercise intensity is not a criterion for blood lipid profile change and perhaps a minimum threshold of physical exertion is necessary in order to achieve blood lipid and lipoprotein modification [97].

Building on the work of Davis et al. [97], Ferguson et al. [53] determined whether thresholds of energy expenditure exist for blood lipid and lipoprotein change to take place. This study incorporated four different exercise energy expenditures (800, 1100, 1300, or 1500 kcal of energy expenditure), and all exercise sessions were completed at 70% VO_2max. Twenty-four hours following the 800-kcal-exercise session, triglyceride levels decreased by 26%, and VLDL-C decreased by 22%, but these changes returned to baseline 48 h postexercise. Twenty-four hours after the 1100-kcal-exercise session, triglyceride levels decreased by 30%, VLDL-C decreased by 15%, HDL-C increased by 15%, and LPL activity increased by 33%. However, none of these changes persisted 48 h after exercise. Twenty-four hours after the 1300-kcal-exercise session, triglyceride levels decreased by 28%, VLDL-C levels decreased by 15%, HDL-C increased by 15%, and LPL activity increased by 31%. Twenty-four hours after the 1500-kcal-exercise session was completed, triglyceride levels decreased by 36%, VLDL-C and LDL-C levels decreased by 25%, HDL-C levels had increased by 29% with noticeable increases in HDL-C and the subfractions HDL_2-C while HDL_3-C decreased, and LPL activity increased by 49%. After 48 h, all the noted changes from the 1500-kcal-exercise session remained. This study was the first investigation to show that different energy expenditure thresholds or different exercise volume thresholds are necessary for changes to occur in blood lipids and lipoproteins levels [53].

The impact of a single resistance exercise session on blood lipid and lipoprotein levels has not received as much attention as has aerobic exercise [88]. Two recent studies are considered here. Lira et al. [98] evaluated the effects of four different resistance exercise workloads on blood lipids and lipoproteins. Subjects were randomly assigned to complete four different resistance exercises ranging from low exercise intensity to high exercise intensity. The results indicate that low and moderate exercise intensities promote greater changes in blood lipid and lipoprotein profiles than did the higher resistance exercise intensities. A strong point of this study was the quantification of total exercise volume between the different exercise intensities being held constant. Nonetheless, weaknesses of this study were that confounding factors (see Table 16.2) especially plasma volume change were not considered. Because exercise will cause plasma volume shifts and this study did not correct for this factor, interpretations of the data from this study are difficult [98].

Wooten et al. [90] completed an exercise training study incorporating a pre-exercise and postexercise training single exercise session evaluation. This experimental design has not often been used but is a very good design characteristic. In addition, most of the confounding factors pointed out in Table 16.2 were incorporated into the study design including a correction for plasma volume shift. Their exercise group exhibited improvements in muscular strength, but no change in BMI, body mass, or body composition post-training. Blood cholesterol, LDL-C, and non-HDL-C were lowered in the exercise group compared to the control group following 12 weeks of resistance training. These data are consistent with the summary and recommendations developed for the 2013 guidelines on lifestyle management to reduce cardiovascular risk [1].

Mechanisms of Exercise-Induced Change

PA, regularly practiced exercise, and a single exercise session alter blood lipid and lipoprotein levels, lipid transport process, and lipoprotein metabolism. In the last 25 years, the mechanisms responsible for these modifications are better understood but not completely. Diet composition, sleep, adiposity, weight loss, plasma volume change, hormone, and enzyme activity are factors that work singularly or in combination with PA and exercise to alter the rate of synthesis, clearance of lipid and lipoproteins, and lipid transportation. Unquestionably, exercise changes blood triglyceride levels by modifying LPL, HL, LCAT, and CEPT action, and these changes result in chylomicron and VLDL breakdown while enhancing reverse cholesterol transport [99]. In response to routine PA, exercise participation, and a single exercise session, the altered lipoprotein enzyme activity, especially in the enzyme LPL, has provided valuable insight regarding mechanisms responsible for the change in lipoprotein metabolism, composition, and lipid transport.

Lipoprotein Lipase

LPL is responsible for the delipidation of chylomicron and VLDL molecules and promotes the clearance of fatty acids and glycerol from the vascular compartment for either storage or use as substrate in energy metabolism. Cross-sectional studies report that endurance-trained runners at rest have higher heparin releasable LPL activity than less active controls [100, 101] but not always [102]. After completing endurance exercise training, inactive men have higher adipose tissue and post-heparin LPL activity than before training [103, 104]. Peltonen et al. [103] observed an increase in LPL activity after the first week of training and suggested that this increased LPL activity after only 1 week of exercise training is perhaps a response to a single exercise session.

Depletion of intramuscular triglyceride stores during exercise promotes secretion and/or synthesis of LPL by capillary endothelial cells. Sedentary and trained subjects performing a single prolonged endurance cycling exercise session [94] had higher post-heparin LPL activity. Running a marathon increased post-heparin LPL activity and the clearance of an ingested triglyceride emulsion [105]. Higher post-heparin LPL activity is not evident until 4–18 h after exercise. Augmented LPL activity increased chylomicron and VLDL hydrolysis and reduced blood triglyceride levels [53, 94, 106]. Increased catabolism of chylomicrons, VLDL, and their remnants works with HDL_3 in a series of reactions to add cholesterol and triglyceride and grow HDL_3 into HDL_2 [101]. This process of enlarging HDL mass occurs in the vascular compartment of the muscle [106] and adipose tissue [107] following endurance exercise. After 8 weeks of one-leg cycle training, Kiens and Lithell [106] reported increased arterial-venous HDL_2-C concentrations across trained skeletal muscle, but not across non-trained muscle from the same individual. Resting muscle biopsies taken before and after 8 weeks of exercise training showed an increase in resting muscle LPL activity after exercise training. This LPL activity change was not seen immediately after exercise in either muscle group. Rather, muscle LPL activity was higher 4 h after exercise in only trained muscle [106]. These data support that lipoprotein profile changes induced by endurance training are, in part, explained by altered skeletal muscle LPL activity after a single exercise session. Williams et al. [107] proposed that LPL activity is greatest in adipose tissue, and thus, chylomicron and VLDL catabolism occurs in adipose tissue more than in muscle tissue. Endurance training that induces weight loss and causes the depletion of adipocyte triglyceride stores will increase adipocyte LPL activity affecting blood lipoprotein levels [107]. Regardless of which tissue has the more prominent role, both the muscle and adipose tissue are sites for endurance training-induced LPL activity modifications that cause lipoprotein change.

Increased LPL activity can increase HDL synthesis and is often given much of the credit for the elevated HDL mass after endurance exercise. Yet, present knowledge supports the concept that exercise training prolongs HDL apolipoprotein survival. The rate of HDL protein synthesis is similar for competitive runners and sedentary subjects [108] with no change in HDL protein synthesis rate after endurance training [104]. However, the survival time of HDL protein was 27% longer in physically active men [108]. Furthermore, endurance training increased the half-life of apolipoprotein A-I and A-II in formerly inactive men [104], and LPL activity and fat clearance were associated with the increased HDL survival, while post-heparin LPL activity was not [104]. Increased HDL mass found with endurance training is likely a result of both increased synthesis and protein survival.

Hepatic Lipase

HL bound to the endothelial surface of hepatic tissue is involved primarily in reverse cholesterol transport. Cross-sectional studies observe that HL activity is not different between active and inactive groups [101] or is lower in active groups [109]. HL is reduced in middle-aged men after endurance training [103, 104] and after 1 year of weight loss by exercise and/or dieting [110]. HL activity is not affected by a single endurance exercise session [94, 111] or resistive exercise [112]. HDL-C and HL are inversely related in active students [113] and negatively correlated with HDL_2-C but positively correlated with HDL_3-C [114]. Because HL acts in the process of transforming HDL_2 to HDL_3 and because HL activity is either lower or not changed in response to a single exercise session, higher HDL_2 concentrations and lower HDL_3 reported after endurance exercise training are expected.

Lecithin:Cholesterol Acyltransferase

LCAT resides on the surface of lipoprotein particles and catalyzes the transfer of plasma fatty acids from lecithin to cholesterol. Once esterified, cholesterol moves into the hydrophobic core of the preferred substrate HDL_3 creating a gradient favoring the net movement of cholesterol from cell membranes onto the lipoprotein surface [115]. Higher LCAT activity is reported for endurance-trained athletes [116–118], after endurance training of young men [117] and middle-aged men [119], and is thought to contribute to increased synthesis of HDL_2-C. LCAT activity is correlated with HDL-C ($r = 0.49$, $p < 0.01$) [117]. Thomas et al. [120], however, found LCAT activity not to change in men after an 11-week interval training program. Williams et al. [115] observed no LCAT mass change after 1 year of exercise-induced weight loss program. Thompson et al. [121] withdrew routine exercise for 6 weeks from physically active men who were expending about 1000 kcals per week and found no change in LCAT activity. The discrepancy between studies is not apparent but might be related to the exercise training volume completed. Marniemi et al. [117] had athletes complete 10 h per week of aerobic activity, while young military cadets completed 20 h per week of combat and aerobic training. LCAT activity was correlated with VO_{2max} ($r = 0.399, p < 0.01$), whereas Williams et al. [115] reported on subjects exercising 13 km per week and found that VO_{2max} was not related to LCAT activity ($r = 0.23$). If LCAT activity is modified after endurance training, a threshold above 13 km per week is probably needed.

A single endurance exercise session increased LCAT activity [122, 123], but not always [124, 125]. Wallace et al. [126] observed increased LCAT activity in young weight lifters after a 90-min high volume weight lifting session in contrast to a 90-min low volume weight lifting session. These data provide support for the positive impact that PA and exercise have on LCAT activity causing blood lipid and lipoprotein to change. For change, an energy expenditure threshold must be reached.

CETP

CETP promotes the transfer of cholesteryl ester to chylomicron and VLDL remnants in exchange for triglyceride. Once accepted by these lipoproteins, this cholesterol undergoes hepatic degradation or becomes a source for tissue utilization. Little information is available regarding a CEPT exercise training effect, but higher CEPT activity was observed in endurance-trained athletes [116]. Finally, CEPT activity is inversely correlated with lipoprotein ratios (total cholesterol/HDL-C) and is a reflection for reduced CAD risk. Information from these studies provides insight into possible explanations regarding the previous exercise training observations of blood lipid and lipoprotein profiles after exercise training. For example, increased CEPT activity could explain enhanced reverse cholesterol transport despite a coinciding decrease or no change in HDL-C concentration [127].

Clinical/Public Health Relevance

PA and regular exercise participation is recommended for all persons by the 2008 US Department of Health and Human Services Physical Activity Guidelines for Americans [128] and supported by position statements from the ACSM [96, 129–131]. A summary of these exercise guideline recommendations is presented in Table 16.8. These same recommendations are followed for persons having dyslipidemia but no other comorbidities. Most persons starting a PA or exercise program will start at low functional levels and progress at a rate that has been individualized to meet their functional abilities. An important first long-term goal is to exercise 150 min of moderate intensity or 75–150 min of vigorous-intensity physical activity per week or a combination of moderate to vigorous PA. An additional long-term goal of up to 300 min of PA or regular exercise participation may be considered and would provide optimal PA and exercise health benefits if participants can complete this volume of exercise [128]; many individuals may not. Persons with dyslipidemia having other comorbidities should follow the exercise recommendations for their condition(s) (i.e., CAD, stroke, or diabetes) [96, 132]. Even so, all healthy individuals and individuals having other health conditions should receive proper exercise prescriptions and encouragement to complete as much daily PA and regular exercise as their functional capabilities allow.

Investigations evaluating the impact of PA and regular exercise participation on blood lipid and lipoprotein levels support a PA or exercise threshold of 8–10 miles or an expenditure of 1000 kcals

Table 16.8 Exercise prescription [96]

Modes	Goals	Intensity/frequency/duration	Time to goal
Aerobic Large muscle activities	Decrease total cholesterol and triglyceride concentrations Increase endurance and work capacity Increase daily caloric expenditure Decrease adiposity	40–80% peak work rate 40–80% heart rate reserve >5 days/week 20–60 min/session or intermittent sessions (e.g., 2–3 sessions/day of 10–30 min	4 months (fitness) 9–12 months (lipids)
Strength Free weights, machines	Increase muscle strength and endurance	60–80% 1RM 2–4 sets of 8–12 reps 2–3 days/week	4–6 months
Flexibility Upper and lower body ROM activities	Decrease risk of injury	Static stretches: hold for 10–30 s 2–3 days/week	4–6 months

Progression - To optimize the impact of physical activity and exercise, weekly energy expenditure must eventually grow to be greater than 2000 Kcals of energy spent each week or more than 250 or more minutes of physical activity and exercise each week

Reprinted with permission from Moore et al. [96]

of activity each week for improved blood HDL-C levels [133, 134]. An important consideration is for blood lipid, and lipoprotein modifications related to health benefits should rely more on the total PA or exercise volume completed than on the exercise intensity [49, 52, 97]. Though resistance training has limited impact on improving the blood lipid and lipoprotein profile, blood cholesterol and LDL-C levels are somewhat lower after resistance training programs lasting longer than 12 weeks. Regardless, resistance exercise training does have many other health benefits and must be part of any individuals' exercise programming (see Table 16.8).

Various lifestyle management guidelines exist [1, 135, 136] for managing dyslipidemias that support PA and regular exercise participating in conjunction with a proper diet and weight loss. These statements support exercise and diet as first interventions. Medications are used when lifestyle management is not successful [137]. An important consideration is gaining an understanding for the interactive effect of exercise and diet on lipoprotein metabolism and the interactions between exercise and various classes of lipid medications now in use (see Table 16.3). Though few studies of such medication interactions have been completed or published, the optimal medical and exercise management of patients will in part depend on understanding these interactions.

Aerobic exercise has been the focus of most scientific investigations involving the impact of exercise on the blood lipid and lipoprotein profile, and much of the evidence has linked higher levels of aerobic exercise to lower CVD rates. Blood triglyceride levels typically decrease, while blood HDL-C levels increase. Blood cholesterol and LDL-C levels remain unchanged unless associated with weight loss. The main goal for PA and exercise programming is to expend calories. Inactive individuals starting a PA and regular exercise participation should expect improved lipid and lipoprotein measurements after several months of PA and regular exercise programming.

Favorable changes in blood lipids and lipoproteins are optimized when:

- PA and exercise are performed regularly – preferably 5 or more days per week.
- PA and exercise are performed at a moderate intensity to vigorous levels (40% to 80% heart rate reserve).
- Developing an exercise program that progressively moves the individual to 150 min of moderate-intensity exercise or 75 min of vigorous-intensity exercise.
- When 250 min of moderate-intensity exercise or more than 2000 calories are expended each week, optimal impact on blood lipid and lipoprotein levels occur.
- Resistance exercise is incorporated into a training regimen (2–3 days per week).
- Overall calorie and fat intake are reduced.
- Body weight is reduced.

Special PA and Exercise Considerations

If no comorbidities exist, patients with dyslipidemia can follow the American College of Sports Medicine Guidelines for healthy adults. However, modifications in the exercise prescription are needed if other chronic diseases are present such as CAD, diabetes, obesity, or hypertension (ACSM Guidelines and chronic disease recommendation) [96, 132].

Medications and special considerations for PA exercise programming include:

- HMG CoA reductase inhibitors – the most common reported side effect with these medications is muscle discomfort and damage which cause a limited ability to perform exercise. In these cases, always contact your physician. Rhabdomyolysis may occur in rare cases.
- Bile acid sequestrants – major side effects include constipation, bloating, and flatulence, resulting in discomfort during PA and exercise.
- Other medication usage and interaction during exercise should always be considered (see Table 16.3).
- Obesity may limit choices for exercise training.

Conclusions

Scientific investigations report lower blood triglyceride levels because of PA and regular exercise participation for men and women. Blood cholesterol is not changed unless body weight is reduced or dietary intake is changed. Although the triglyceride portion of VLDL is reduced after exercise, the prominent changes in lipoprotein composition after PA and exercise are the increased blood HDL-C and HDL_2-C levels. LDL-C changes from PA and regular exercise are minor without a reduction in adiposity or dietary fat and cholesterol intake. Evidence strongly supports that concentrations of small LDL-C and LDL particles will decrease, while the size of the LDL particles will increase when an exercise program of a high volume completed at moderate to vigorous intensity with a caloric energy equivalence of exercising about 20 miles per week. The consensus is that HDL-C usually does not change after resistance training since few studies report elevated blood HDL-C after a resistance training program. Resistance exercise reductions in blood cholesterol, LDL-C, and non-HDL-C concentrations are reported, while no changes in blood chylomicron and triglyceride levels are found.

The mechanisms responsible for blood lipids and lipoproteins after exercise are related to increased LPL and LCAT enzyme activity. These enzymes enhance the breakdown of the large lipoproteins, promote lipid uptake by tissue, and facilitate reverse cholesterol transport. The process for the removal of cholesterol from HDL is better understood and is related to altered CETP and HL enzyme activity and/or an increased hepatic apo E receptor-mediated pathway. The described exercise-induced responses and adaptations occur in both men and women of all ages and are associated with reduced CAD risk. Thus, abundant evidence is available to support a reduced disease risk by increasing PA and regular exercise participation.

With the introduction of NMR spectroscopy methodology, lipoprotein particles are now segregated into chylomicron particles and VLDL particles; large VLDL-P and chylomicron particles; small and medium VLDL-P; IDL particles; total LDL particles; small and large LDL-P; total HDL particles; and small, medium, and large HDL-P. NMR spectroscopy also allows for analyses of the average VLDL, LDL, and HDL particle sizes. This new methodology provides for the analysis of blood lipoprotein levels in a variety of new ways and adds new clinical perspectives for blood lipid and lipoprotein analysis after PA, regular exercise participation, and a single exercise session. The information gained from this new methodology will afford new insight for clinical management of dyslipidemic persons and a better understanding for the beneficial cardiovascular reduction in CAD morbidity and mortality. Much is already known about the exercise training-induced blood lipid and lipoprotein modifications as well as the lipoprotein enzyme changes, but much is still to learn, and this work should continue with future research focus on the molecular basis for these changes.

Although lifestyle management should always be considered as the first therapeutic method used in dyslipidemia intervention, the primary means for blood lipid and lipoprotein change is likely pharmacological intervention. Health care professionals will and always should consider dietary change, weight loss, and increased PA and exercise as adjunctive therapies. Few randomized controlled studies have been completed evaluating the effects of pharmacological interventions, PA, and exercise on individuals with dyslipidemia. Consequently, the impact of PA and regular exercise on these persons may be substantially different from the PA and exercise effects in persons free of dyslipidemia. Intervention programs emphasizing reductions in dietary fat and cholesterol result in reduced blood cholesterol and LDL-C levels when accompanied with exercise programming. Blood HDL-C levels will either stay the same or increase. Without exercise, a less consistent reduction in blood triglyceride level occurs, while HDL-C tends to decrease.

Finally, knowing the interactive effect of exercise and diet on lipoprotein metabolism is important for proper patient medical management, but knowing the interactions between exercise and various classes of current lipid medications is equally as important. Few studies of such interactions have been published. The optimal medical management of dyslipidemic persons will in part depend on understanding these interactions.

Recommendations Key Points/ Future Directions

In the last 50 years of scientific investigation, major advancements in understanding CVD disease and the association with blood lipid and lipoprotein levels have been achieved. Nonetheless, some major literature limitations currently exist concerning the effects of PA and exercise on blood lipid and lipoprotein levels including the lack of complete quantification of the proper dose response for specific populations, incorporation of confounding factors found in Table 16.2 into experimental study design, complete information for understanding PA, and exercise impact on lipid and lipoprotein oxidation and lipoprotein functionality. In the past, numerous studies have assessed the effects of resistance exercise on blood lipid and lipoprotein levels; however, our ability at that time for systematic quantification of resistance exercise was lacking. But because new methodology exists for quantifying resistance exercise, future resistance exercise studies need to better quantify energy expenditure when evaluating blood lipid and lipoprotein after PA and exercise.

With the introduction of NMR spectroscopy, an entirely different continuum in lipid and lipoprotein science was opened. For example, utilization of NMR spectroscopy provides a new means for completing CVD investigations in gaining new insight into blood lipids and lipoproteins and their subfractions and involvement in oxidation and lipoprotein functionality. NMR spectroscopy may now be used to assess the impact of PA and exercise and determine the precise exercise volume necessary for changing blood lipids, lipoproteins, and lipoprotein subfractions. This methodology also is useful in determining the effects of sleep deprivation on the various lipoprotein subfractions. An interesting new area for future research is the examination of exercise-induced HDL functionality changes and risk of CVD [138].

Regarding lipoprotein oxidation and the work of Medlow et al. [86], the impact of exercise on oxidation time is an important area for future investigations. Understanding the possible mechanisms that alter the oxidized LDL and HDL has implications for reducing atherosclerosis development.

From a clinical practice perspective, understanding the effectiveness for bringing about behavioral change in current clinical practices is important for reducing overall population disease risk [1, 135].

Key Points

- Elevated blood lipid and lipoprotein levels are well-known risk factors for CVD, and overwhelming evidence exists supporting the effects of PA and exercise to improve blood lipid and lipoprotein levels.
- PA and exercise recommendations for adults with dyslipidemia without other comorbidities include at least 30 min per day or 150 min per week of moderate-intensity exercise or 75–150 min of vigorous-intensity exercise per week and even up to 300 min per week (Table 16.8) to optimize blood lipid and lipoprotein levels if individuals are able to exercise this much.
- PA and exercise are also recommended for adults with dyslipidemia but having comorbidities such as CVD, CAD, stroke, diabetes, or other complications. In these cases, the exercise recommendations for the specific condition(s) should be considered when developing an individualized exercise program.
- Current evidence strongly supports longer duration aerobic exercise or greater exercise volume over high-intensity exercise when developing exercise programming.
- For optimal blood lipid and lipoprotein levels, combining exercise and a healthier diet gives the best results.
- Present evidence suggests that resistance exercise can reduce blood cholesterol, LDL-C,

and non-HDL-C levels, providing other health benefits. Thus, when recommending an individualized exercise program, resistance exercise should be part in any individuals' exercise recommendation.

References

1. Eckel RH, Jakicic JM, Ard JD, de Jesus JM, Houston-Miller N, Hubbard VS, et al. 2013 AHA/ACC guideline on lifestyle management to reduce cardiovascular risk: a report of the American College of Cardiology/American Heart Association Task Force on practice guidelines. Circulation. 2014;129(25 Suppl 2):S76–99. https://doi.org/10.1161/01.cir.0000437740.48606.d1.
2. Ginsberg HN. Lipoprotein physiology. Endocrinol Metab Clin N Am. 1998;27(3):503–19. https://doi.org/10.1016/S0889-8529(05)70023-2.
3. Jo H, Js S, Toro G, Tk C. Effects of a six month program of endurance exercise on the serum lipids of middle-aged man. JACC. 1965;14:753–60. https://doi.org/10.1016/0002-9149(64)90004-9.
4. Olefsky J, Reaven G, Farquhar J. Effects of weight reduction on obesity studies of lipid and carbohydrate metabolism in normal and hyperlipoproteinemic subjects. J Clin Invest. 1974;53(1):64–76. https://doi.org/10.1172/JCI107560.
5. Connelly PW. The role of hepatic lipase in lipoprotein metabolism. Clin Chim Acta. 1999;286(1–2):243–55. https://doi.org/10.1016/S0009-8981(99)00105-9.
6. Goldberg IJ. Lipoprotein lipase and lipolysis: central roles in lipoprotein metabolism and atherogenesis. J Lipid Res. 1996;37(4):693–707.
7. Lewis GF. New insights into the regulation of HDL metabolism and reverse cholesterol transport. Circ Res. 2005;96(12):1221–32. https://doi.org/10.1161/01.RES.0000170946.56981.5c.
8. Jeyarajah EJ, Cromwell WC, Otvos JD. Lipoprotein particle analysis by nuclear magnetic resonance spectroscopy. Clin Lab Med. 2006;26(4):847–70. https://doi.org/10.1016/j.cll.2006.07.006.
9. Durstine JL, Haskell WL. Effects of exercise training on plasma lipids and lipoproteins. Exerc Sport Sci Rev. 1994;22:477–521.
10. Brown MS, Goldstein JL. How LDL receptors influence cholesterol and atherosclerosis. Sci Am Nature. 1984;251(5):58–69.
11. Barter P. CETP and atherosclerosis. Arterioscler Thromb Vasc Biol. 2000;20(9):2029–31. https://doi.org/10.1161/01.ATV.20.9.2029.
12. Bergt C, Oram J, Heinecke J. Oxidized HDL. Arterioscler Thromb Vasc Biol. 2003;23(9):1488–90. https://doi.org/10.1161/01.ATV.0000090570.99836.9C.
13. Parthasarathy S, Raghavamenon A, Garelnabi M, Santanam N. Oxidized low-density lipoprotein. Methods Mol Biol. 2010;610:403–17. https://doi.org/10.1007/978-1-60327-029-8_24.
14. Cobbold C, Sherratt J, Maxwell S. Lipoprotein oxidation and its significance for atherosclerosis: a mathematical approach. B Math Biol. 2002;64(1):65–95. https://doi.org/10.1006/bulm.2001.0267.
15. Shapiro MD, Fazio S. From lipids to inflammation: new approaches to reducing atherosclerotic risk. Circ Res. 2016;118(4):732–49. https://doi.org/10.1161/CIRCRESAHA.115.306471.
16. Jacobson TA, Ito MK, Maki KC, Orringer CE, Bays HE, Jones PH, et al. National lipid association recommendations for patient-centered management of dyslipidemia: Part 1--full report. J Clin Lipidol. 2015;9(2):129–69. https://doi.org/10.1016/j.jacl.2015.02.003.
17. Tiainen S, Luoto R, Ahotupa M, Raitanen J, Vasankari T. 6-mo aerobic exercise intervention enhances the lipid peroxide transport function of HDL. Free Rad Res. 2016;50:1279–85. https://doi.org/10.1080/10715762.2016.1252040.
18. Ahotupa M, Suomela J-P, Vuorimaa T, Vasankari T. Lipoprotein-specific transport of circulating lipid peroxides. Ann Med. 2010;42(7):521–9. https://doi.org/10.3109/07853890.2010.510932.
19. Bier D. Saturated fats and cardiovascular disease: interpretations not as simple as they once were. Crit Rev Food Sci Nutr. 2015;56(12):1943–6. https://doi.org/10.1080/10408398.2014.998332.
20. Garber CE, Blissmer B, Deschenes MR, Franklin BA, Lamonte MJ, Lee I-MM, et al. American College of Sports Medicine position stand: quantity and quality of exercise for developing and maintaining cardiorespiratory, musculoskeletal, and neuromotor fitness in apparently healthy adults: guidance for prescribing exercise. Med Sci Sports Exerc. 2011;43(7):1334–59. https://doi.org/10.1249/MSS.0b013e318213fefb.
21. Francis G. High density lipoprotein oxidation: in vitro susceptibility and potential in vivo consequences. Biochim Biophys Acta. 2000;1483(2):217–35. https://doi.org/10.1016/S1388-1981(99)00181-X.
22. Rohatgi A, Khera A, Berry J, Givens E, Ayers C, Wedin K, et al. HDL cholesterol efflux capacity and incident cardiovascular events. N Engl J Med. 2014;371(25):2383–93. https://doi.org/10.1056/NEJMoa1409065.
23. Välimäki IA, Vuorimaa T, Ahotupa M, Vasankari T. Effect of continuous and intermittent exercises on oxidised hdl and ldl lipids in runners. Int J Sports Med. 2016;37(14):1103–9. https://doi.org/10.1055/s-0042-114703.
24. Benjamin E, Blaha M, Chiuve S, Cushman M, Das S, Deo R, et al. Heart disease and stroke statistics—2017 update: a report from the American Heart Association. Circulation. 2017;135(10):e146–603. https://doi.org/10.1161/CIR.0000000000000485.

25. Center for Disease Control and Prevention. High cholesterol facts. 2017. https://www.cdc.gov/cholesterol/facts.htm
26. Center for Disease Control and Prevention. Cholesterol. 2017. https://www.cdc.gov/nchs/fastats/cholesterol.htm
27. Center for Disease Control and Prevention. Cholesterol fact sheet. 2015. https://www.cdc.gov/dhdsp/data_statistics/fact_sheets/fs_cholesterol.htm
28. Austin M, Hokanson J, Edwards K. Hypertriglyceridemia as a cardiovascular risk factor. Am J Cardiol. 1998;81(4):7B–12B. https://doi.org/10.1016/S0002-9149(98)00031-9.
29. Austin MA, Hokanson JE. Epidemiology of triglycerides, small dense low-density lipoprotein, and lipoprotein(a) as risk factors for coronary heart disease. Med Clin N Am. 1994;78(1):99–115. https://doi.org/10.1016/S0025-7125(16)30178-X.
30. Cullen P. Evidence that triglycerides are an independent coronary heart disease risk factor. Am J Cardiol. 2000;86(9):943–9. https://doi.org/10.1016/S0002-9149(00)01127-9.
31. Durstine JL. Gender differences in lipids and lipoproteins after cardiac rehabilitation. J Cardpulm Rehabil. 2004;24(4):257–8.
32. Mykkänen L, Kuusisto J, Haffner SM, Laakso M, Austin MA. LDL size and risk of coronary heart disease in elderly men and women. Arterioscler Thromb Vasc Biol. 1999;19(11):2742–8. https://doi.org/10.1161/01.ATV.19.11.2742.
33. Brewer HB. Hypertriglyceridemia: changes in the plasma lipoproteins associated with an increased risk of cardiovascular disease. Am J Cardiol. 1999;83(9):3–12. https://doi.org/10.1016/S0002-9149(99)00308-2.
34. Bjorvatn B, Sagen I, Øyane N, Waage S, Fetveit A, Pallesen S, et al. The association between sleep duration, body mass index and metabolic measures in the Hordaland Health Study. J Sleep Res. 2007;16(1):66–76. https://doi.org/10.1111/j.1365-2869.2007.00569.x.
35. Franklin BA, Durstine JL, Roberts CK, Barnard RJ. Impact of diet and exercise on lipid management in the modern era. Best Pract Res Clin Endocrinol Metab. 2014;28(3):405–21. https://doi.org/10.1016/j.beem.2014.01.005.
36. Haskell WL. The influence of exercise training on plasma lipids and lipoproteins in health and disease. Acta Med Scand Suppl. 1986;711:25–37. https://doi.org/10.1111/j.0954-6820.1986.tb08929.x.
37. Keys A. Coronary Heart Disease, serum cholesterol, and the diet. Acta Med Scand. 1980;207(3):153–60. https://doi.org/10.1111/j.0954-6820.1980.tb09697.x.
38. Wirth A, Diehm C, Kohlmeier M, Heuck CC, Metabolism V-I. Effect of prolonged exercise on serum lipids and lipoproteins. Metabolism. 1983;32(7):669–72. https://doi.org/10.1016/0026-0495(83)90122-1.
39. Sarzynski M, Burton J, Rankinen T, Blair S, Church T, Després J-P, et al. The effects of exercise on the lipoprotein subclass profile: a meta-analysis of 10 interventions. Atherosclerosis. 2015;243(2):364–72. https://doi.org/10.1016/j.atherosclerosis.2015.10.018.
40. Asztalos B, Cupples L, Demissie S, Horvath K, Cox C, Batista M, et al. High-density lipoprotein subpopulation profile and coronary heart disease prevalence in male participants of the Framingham offspring study. Arterioscler Thromb Vasc Biol. 2004;24(11):2181–7. https://doi.org/10.1161/01.ATV.0000146325.93749.a8.
41. Cheung MC, Brown BG, Wolf AC, Albers JJ. Altered particle size distribution of apolipoprotein A-I-containing lipoproteins in subjects with coronary artery disease. J Lipid Res. 1991;32(3):383–94.
42. Krauss R. Lipoprotein subfractions and cardiovascular disease risk. Curr Opin Lipidol. 2010;21(4):305–11. https://doi.org/10.1097/MOL.0b013e32833b7756.
43. Després J-P. Cardiovascular disease under the influence of excess visceral fat. Critical Pathways Cardiol. 2007;6(2):51. https://doi.org/10.1097/HPC.0b013e318057d4c9.
44. Harchaoui K, Steeg W, Stroes E, Kuivenhoven J, Otvos J, Wareham N, et al. Value of low-density lipoprotein particle number and size as predictors of coronary artery disease in apparently healthy men and women : the EPIC-Norfolk prospective population study. J Am Coll Cardiol. 2007;49(5):547–53. https://doi.org/10.1016/j.jacc.2006.09.043.
45. Lamarche B, Tchernof A, Moorjani S, Cantin B, Dagenais GR, Lupien PJ, et al. Small, dense low-density lipoprotein particles as a predictor of the risk of ischemic heart disease in men: prospective results from the Quebec cardiovascular study. Circulation. 1997;95(1):69–75. https://doi.org/10.1161/01.CIR.95.1.69.
46. Durstine JL, Grandjean PW, Cox CA, Thompson PD. Lipids, lipoproteins, and exercise. J Cardpulm Rehabil. 2002;22(6):385–98.
47. Brown A, Setji T, Sanders L, Lowry K, Otvos J, Kraus W, et al. Effects of exercise on lipoprotein particles in women with polycystic ovary syndrome. Med Sci Sports Exerc. 2009;41(3):497. https://doi.org/10.1249/MSS.0b013e31818c6c0c.
48. Halverstadt A, Phares D, Wilund K, Goldberg A, Hagberg J. Endurance exercise training raises high-density lipoprotein cholesterol and lowers small low-density lipoprotein and very low-density lipoprotein independent of body fat phenotypes in older men and women. Metabolism. 2007;56(4):444–50. https://doi.org/10.1016/j.metabol.2006.10.019.
49. Kraus WE, Houmard JA, Duscha BD, Knetzger KJ, Wharton MB, McCartney JS, et al. Effects of the amount and intensity of exercise on plasma lipoproteins. N Engl J Med. 2002;347(19):1483–92. https://doi.org/10.1056/NEJMoa020194.

50. Seip R, Otvos J, Bilbie C, Tsongalis G, Miles M, Zoeller R, et al. The effect of apolipoprotein E genotype on serum lipoprotein particle response to exercise. Atherosclerosis. 2006;188(1):126–33. https://doi.org/10.1016/j.atherosclerosis.2005.06.050.
51. Shadid S, LaForge R, Otvos J, Jensen M. Treatment of obesity with diet/exercise versus pioglitazone has distinct effects on lipoprotein particle size. Atherosclerosis. 2006;188(2):370–6. https://doi.org/10.1016/j.atherosclerosis.2005.10.038.
52. Durstine JL, Grandjean PW, Davis PG, Ferguson MA, Alderson NL, DuBose KD. Blood lipid and lipoprotein adaptations to exercise: a quantitative analysis. Sports Med. 2001;31(15):1033–62. https://doi.org/10.2165/00007256-200131150-00002.
53. Ferguson MA, Alderson NL, Trost SG, Essig DA, Burke JR, Durstine JL. Effects of four different single exercise sessions on lipids, lipoproteins, and lipoprotein lipase. J Appl Physiol. 1998;85(3):1169–74. https://doi.org/10.1152/jappl.1998.85.3.1169.
54. Drygas W, Jegler A, Kunski H. Study on threshold dose of physical activity in coronary heart disease prevention. Part i. relationship between leisure time physical activity and coronary risk factors. Int J Sports Med. 1988;09(04):275–8. https://doi.org/10.1055/s-2007-1025021.
55. Drygas W, Kostka T, Jegier A, Kuński H. Long-term effects of different physical activity levels on coronary heart disease risk factors in middle-aged men. Int J Sports Med. 2000;21(4):235–41. https://doi.org/10.1055/s-2000-309.
56. Kokkinos PF, Holland JC, Narayan P, Colleran JA, Dotson CO, Papademetriou V. Miles run per week and high-density lipoprotein cholesterol levels in healthy, middle-aged men. A dose-response relationship. Arch Intern Med. 1995;155(4):415–20. https://doi.org/10.1001/archinte.1995.00430040091011.
57. Lakka TA, Salonen JT. Physical activity and serum lipids: a cross-sectional population study in eastern Finnish men. Am J Epidemiol. 1992;136(7):806–18. https://doi.org/10.1093/aje/136.7.806.
58. Williams PT. Relationship of distance run per week to coronary heart disease risk factors in 8283 male runners: the National Runners' health study. Arch Intern Med. 1997;157(2):191–8. https://doi.org/10.1001/archinte.1997.00440230063008.
59. Williams PT. High-density lipoprotein cholesterol and other risk factors for coronary heart disease in female runners. N Engl J Med. 1996;334(20):1298–303. https://doi.org/10.1056/NEJM199605163342004.
60. Williams PT. Relationships of heart disease risk factors to exercise quantity and intensity. Arch Intern Med. 1998;158(3):237–45. https://doi.org/10.1001/archinte.158.3.237.
61. Siri-Tarino P, Krauss R. Diet, lipids, and cardiovascular disease. Curr Opin Lipidol. 2016;27(4):323–8. https://doi.org/10.1097/MOL.0000000000000310.
62. Fontana L, Meyer T, Klein S, Holloszy J. Long-term calorie restriction is highly effective in reducing the risk for atherosclerosis in humans. P Natl Acad Sci USA. 2004;101(17):6659–63. https://doi.org/10.1073/pnas.0308291101.
63. Katzel LI, Bleecker ER, Colman EG, Rogus EM, Sorkin JD, Goldberg AP. Effects of weight loss vs aerobic exercise training on risk factors for coronary disease in healthy, obese, middle-aged and older men. A randomized controlled trial. JAMA. 1995;274(24):1915–21. https://doi.org/10.1001/jama.1995.03530240025035.
64. Verdery RB, Walford RL. Changes in plasma lipids and lipoproteins in humans during a 2-year period of dietary restriction in biosphere 2. Arch Intern Med. 1998;158(8):900–6. https://doi.org/10.1001/archinte.158.8.900.
65. Bhutani S, Klempel M, Kroeger C, Trepanowski J, Varady K. Alternate day fasting and endurance exercise combine to reduce body weight and favorably alter plasma lipids in obese humans. Obesity. 2013;21(7):1370–9. https://doi.org/10.1002/oby.20353.
66. Tzotzas T, Evangelou P, Kiortsis D. Obesity, weight loss and conditional cardiovascular risk factors. Obes Rev. 2011;12(5):e282–9. https://doi.org/10.1111/j.1467-789X.2010.00807.x.
67. Varady KA, Hellerstein MK. Alternate-day fasting and chronic disease prevention: a review of human and animal trials. Am J Clin Nutr. 2007;86(1):7–13. https://doi.org/10.1093/ajcn/86.1.7.
68. Varady K, Bhutani S, Klempel M, Kroeger C. Comparison of effects of diet versus exercise weight loss regimens on LDL and HDL particle size in obese adults. Lipids Health Dis. 2011;10(1):1–5. https://doi.org/10.1186/1476-511X-10-119.
69. Kaneita Y, Uchiyama M, Yoshiike N, Ohida T. Associations of usual sleep duration with serum lipid and lipoprotein levels. Sleep. 2008;31(5):645–52. https://doi.org/10.1093/sleep/31.5.645.
70. Aho V, Ollila H, Kronholm E, Bondia-Pons I, Soininen P, Kangas A, et al. Prolonged sleep restriction induces changes in pathways involved in cholesterol metabolism and inflammatory responses. Sci Reports. 2016;6(1):24828. https://doi.org/10.1038/srep24828.
71. Plaisance EP, Grandjean PW, Mahurin AJ. Independent and combined effects of aerobic exercise and pharmacological strategies on serum triglyceride concentrations: a qualitative review. Phys Sportsmed. 2009;37(1):11–9. https://doi.org/10.3810/psm.2009.04.1678.
72. Plaisance EP, Mestek ML, Mahurin AJ, Taylor JK, Moncada-Jimenez J, Grandjean PW. Postprandial triglyceride responses to aerobic exercise and extended-release niacin. Am J Clin Nutr. 2008;88(1):30–7. https://doi.org/10.1093/ajcn/88.1.30.
73. Gordon B, Chen S, Durstine JL. The effects of exercise training on the traditional lipid profile and

beyond. Curr Sports Med Rep. 2014;13(4):253–9. https://doi.org/10.1249/JSR.0000000000000073.
74. Crouse SF, O'Brien BC, Grandjean PW, Lowe RC, Rohack JJ, Green JS, et al. Training intensity, blood lipids, and apolipoproteins in men with high cholesterol. J Appl Physiol. 1997;82(1):270–7. https://doi.org/10.1152/jappl.1997.82.1.270.
75. Blazek A, Rutsky J, Osei K, Maiseyeu A, Rajagopalan S. Exercise-mediated changes in high-density lipoprotein: impact on form and function. Am Heart J. 2013;166(3):392–400. https://doi.org/10.1016/j.ahj.2013.05.021.
76. Schaefer EJ, Levy RI, Anderson DW, Danner RN, Brewer HB, Blackwelder WC. Plasma-triglycerides in regulation of H.D.L.-cholesterol levels. Lancet. 1978;2(8086):391–3. https://doi.org/10.1016/S0140-6736(78)91863-9.
77. Couillard C, Despres J-P, Lamarche B, Bergeron J, Gagnon J, Leon AS, et al. Effects of endurance exercise training on plasma HDL cholesterol levels depend on levels of triglycerides : evidence from men of the health, risk factors, exercise training and genetics (HERITAGE) Family Study. Arterioscler Thromb Vasc Biol. 2001;21(7):1226–32. https://doi.org/10.1161/hq0701.092137.
78. Bouchard C, Rankinen T. Individual differences in response to regular physical activity. Med Sci Sports Exerc. 2001;33(6 Suppl):S446–51.; discussion S452–3. https://doi.org/10.1097/00005768-200106001-00013.
79. Bouchard C, Blair S, Church T, Earnest C, Hagberg J, Häkkinen K, et al. Adverse metabolic response to regular exercise: is it a rare or common occurrence? PLoS One. 2012;7(5):e37887. https://doi.org/10.1371/journal.pone.0037887.
80. Leon AS, Gaskill SE, Rice T, Bergeron J, Gagnon J, Rao DC, et al. Variability in the response of HDL cholesterol to exercise training in the HERITAGE family study. Int J Sports Med. 2002;23(1):1–9. https://doi.org/10.1055/s-2002-19270.
81. Stefanick ML, Mackey S, Sheehan M, Ellsworth N. Effects of diet and exercise in men and postmenopausal women with low levels of HDL cholesterol and high levels of LDL cholesterol. N Engl J Med. 1998;339:12–20. https://doi.org/10.1056/NEJM199807023390103.
82. Kolovou G, Bilianou H, Marvaki A, Mikhailidis D. Aging men and lipids. Am J Mens Health. 2010;5(2):152–65. https://doi.org/10.1177/1557988310370360.
83. MacEneaney O, Harrison M, O'Gorman D, Pankratieva E, O'Connor P, Moyna N. Effect of prior exercise on postprandial lipemia and markers of inflammation and endothelial activation in normal weight and overweight adolescent boys. Eur J Appl Physiol. 2009;106(5):721–9. https://doi.org/10.1007/s00421-009-1073-y.
84. Mestek M, Plaisance E, Ratcliff L, Taylor J, Wee S-O, Grandjean P. Aerobic exercise and postprandial lipemia in men with the metabolic syndrome. Med Sci Sports Exerc. 2008;40(12):2105. https://doi.org/10.1249/MSS.0b013e3181822ebd.
85. Hardman AE, Lawrence JE, Herd SL. Postprandial lipemia in endurance-trained people during a short interruption to training. J Appl Physiol. 1998;84(6):1895–901. https://doi.org/10.1152/jappl.1998.84.6.1895.
86. Medlow P, McEneny J, Murphy M, Trinick T, Duly E, Davison G. Exercise training protects the LDL I subfraction from oxidation susceptibility in an aged human population. Atherosclerosis. 2015;239(2):516–22. https://doi.org/10.1016/j.atherosclerosis.2015.02.012.
87. Kokkinos PF, Holland JC, Pittaras AE, Narayan P, Dotson CO, Papademetriou V. Cardiorespiratory fitness and coronary heart disease risk factor association in women. J Am Coll Cardiol. 1995;26(2):358–64. https://doi.org/10.1016/0735-1097(95)80007-4.
88. Kokkinos PF, Hurley BF. Strength training and lipoprotein-lipid profiles. A critical analysis and recommendations for further study. Sports Med. 1990;9(5):266–72.
89. Kelley G, Kelley K. Impact of progressive resistance training on lipids and lipoproteins in adults: a meta-analysis of randomized controlled trials. Prev Med. 2009;48(1):9–19. https://doi.org/10.1016/j.ypmed.2008.10.010.
90. Wooten JS, Phillips MD, Mitchell JB, Patrizi R, Pleasant RN, Hein RM, et al. Resistance exercise and lipoproteins in postmenopausal women. Int J Sports Med. 2010;32(01):7–13. https://doi.org/10.1055/s-0030-1268008.
91. James A, Whiteford J, Ackland T, Dhaliwal S, Woodhouse J, Prince R, et al. Effects of a 1-year randomised controlled trial of resistance training on blood lipid profile and chylomicron concentration in older men. Eur J Appl Physiol. 2016;116(11–12):2113–23. https://doi.org/10.1007/s00421-016-3465-0.
92. Durstine JL, Thompson PD. Exercise in the treatment of lipid disorders. Cardiol Clin. 2001;19(3):471–88. https://doi.org/10.1016/S0733-8651(05)70230-7.
93. Wagganer J, Robison C, Ackerman T, Davis P. Effects of exercise accumulation on plasma lipids and lipoproteins. Appl Physiol Nutr Metab. 2015;40(5):441–7. https://doi.org/10.1139/apnm-2014-0321.
94. Kantor MA, Cullinane EM, Sady SP, Herbert PN, Thompson PD. Exercise acutely increases high density lipoprotein-cholesterol and lipoprotein lipase activity in trained and untrained men. Metab Clin Exp. 1987;36(2):188–92. https://doi.org/10.1016/0026-0495(87)90016-3.
95. Thompson PD, Crouse SF, Goodpaster B, Kelley D, Moyna N, Pescatello L. The acute versus the chronic response to exercise. Med Sci Sports Exerc. 2001;33(6 Suppl):S438–45.; discussion S452–3. https://doi.org/10.1097/00005768-200106001-00012.
96. Moore G, Durstine JL, Painter P. ACSM's exercise management for persons with chronic diseases and

disabilities. 4th ed. Champaign: Human Kinetics; 2016.
97. Davis PG, Bartoli WP, Durstine JL. Effects of acute exercise intensity on plasma lipids and apolipoproteins in trained runners. J Appl Physiol. 1992;72(3):914–9. https://doi.org/10.1152/jappl.1992.72.3.914.
98. Lira FS, Yamashita AS, Uchida MC, Zanchi NE, Gualano B, Martins E, et al. Low and moderate, rather than high intensity strength exercise induces benefit regarding plasma lipid profile. Diabetol Metab Syndr. 2010;2:31. https://doi.org/10.1186/1758-5996-2-31.
99. Gorski J, Oscai LB, Palmer WK. Hepatic lipid metabolism in exercise and training. Med Sci Sports Exerc. 1990;22(2):213–21.
100. Nikkilä EA, Taskinen MR, Rehunen S, Harkonen M. Lipoprotein lipase activity in adipose tissue and skeletal muscle of runners: relation to serum lipoproteins. Metabolism. 1978;27(11):1661–71. https://doi.org/10.1016/0026-0495(78)90288-3.
101. Thompson PD, Cullinane EM, Sady SP, Flynn MM, Chenevert CB, Herbert PN. High density lipoprotein metabolism in endurance athletes and sedentary men. Circulation. 1991;84:140–52. https://doi.org/10.1161/01.CIR.84.1.140.
102. Sady SP, Cullinane EM, Saritelli A, Bernier DN, Thompson PD. Elevated high-density lipoprotein cholesterol in endurance athletes is related to enhanced plasma triglyceride clearance. Metabolism. 1988;37(6):568–72. https://doi.org/10.1016/0026-0495(88)90173-4.
103. Peltonen P, Marniemi J, Hietanen E, Vuori I, Ehnholm C. Changes in serum lipids, lipoproteins, and heparin releasable lipolytic enzymes during moderate physical training in man: a longitudinal study. Metabolism. 1981;30(5):518–26. https://doi.org/10.1016/0026-0495(81)90190-6.
104. Thompson PD, Cullinane EM, Sady SP, Flynn MM, Bernier DN, Kantor MA, et al. Modest changes in high-density lipoprotein concentration and metabolism with prolonged exercise training. Circulation. 1988;78:25–34. https://doi.org/10.1161/01.CIR.78.1.25.
105. Sady SP, Thompson PD, Cullinane EM, Kantor MA, Domagala E, Herbert PN. Prolonged exercise augments plasma triglyceride clearance. JAMA. 1986;256(18):2552–5. https://doi.org/10.1001/jama.1986.03380180114030.
106. Kiens B, Lithell H. Lipoprotein metabolism influenced by training-induced changes in human skeletal muscle. J Clin Invest. 1989;83(2):558–64. https://doi.org/10.1172/JCI113918.
107. Williams PT, Krauss RM, Vranizan KM, Circulation P. Changes in lipoprotein subfractions during diet-induced and exercise-induced weight loss in moderately overweight men. Circulation. 1990;81:1293–304. https://doi.org/10.1161/01.CIR.81.4.1293.
108. Herbert PN, Bernier DN, Cullinane EM, Edelstein L, Kantor MA, Thompson PD. High-density lipoprotein metabolism in runners and sedentary men. JAMA. 1984;252(8):1034–7. https://doi.org/10.1001/jama.1984.03350080036023.
109. Marniemi J, Peltonen P, Vuori I, Hietanen E. Lipoprotein lipase of human postheparin plasma and adipose tissue in relation to physical training. Acta Physiol. 1980;110:131–5. https://doi.org/10.1111/j.1748-1716.1980.tb06642.x.
110. Stefanick ML, Terry RB, Haskell WL, Wood P. Relationships of changes in postheparin hepatic and lipoprotein lipase activity to HDL-cholesterol changes following weight loss achieved by dieting versus exercise. Cardiovasc Dis. 1987; https://doi.org/10.1007/978-1-4684-5296-9_7.
111. Kantor MA, Cullinane EM, Herbert PN, Thompson PD. Acute increase in lipoprotein lipase following prolonged exercise. Metabolism. 1984;33(5):454–7. https://doi.org/10.1016/0026-0495(84)90147-1.
112. Shoup EE, Durstine JL, Davis JM, Pate RR, Baroli WP. Effects of a single exercise session of resistance exercise on plasma lipoproteins and postheparin lipase activity. *Unpublished data.*
113. Kuusi T, Nikkilä EA, Saarinen P, Varha P, Laitinen LA. Plasma high density lipoproteins HDL2, HDL3 and postheparin plasma lipases in relation to parameters of physical fitness. Atherosclerosis. 1982;41(2–3):209–19. https://doi.org/10.1016/0021-9150(82)90186-1.
114. Taskinen MR, Nikkilä EA. High density lipoprotein subfractions in relation to lipoprotein lipase activity of tissues in man--evidence for reciprocal regulation of HDL2 and HDL3 levels by lipoprotein lipase. Clin Chim Acta. 1981;112(3):325–32. https://doi.org/10.1016/0009-8981(81)90455-1.
115. Williams PT, Albers JJ, Krauss RM, Wood P. Associations of lecithin: cholesterol acyltransferase (LCAT) mass concentrations with exercise, weight loss, and plasma lipoprotein subfraction concentrations in men. Atherosclerosis. 1990;82(1–2):53–8. https://doi.org/10.1016/0021-9150(90)90143-7.
116. Gupta AK, Ross EA, Myers JN, Kashyap ML. Increased reverse cholesterol transport in athletes. Metabolism. 1993;42(6):684–90. https://doi.org/10.1016/0026-0495(93)90233-E.
117. Marniemi J, Dahlström S, Kvist M, SeppAnen A, Hietanen E. Dependence of serum lipid and lecithin: cholesterol acyltransferase levels on physical training in young men. Eur J Appl Physio and Occup Physio. 1982;49(1):25–35. https://doi.org/10.1007/BF00428960.
118. Tsopanakis C, Kotsarellis D, Tsopanakis A. Plasma lecithin: cholesterol acyltransferase activity in elite athletes from selected sports. Eur J Appl Physio and Occup Physio. 1988;58(3):262–5. https://doi.org/10.1007/BF00417260.
119. Marniemi J, Hietanen E. Regulation of Serum Lipids by Physical Exercise. Boca Raton: CRC Press; 1982.
120. Thomas TR, Adeniran SB, Iltis PW, Aquiar CA, Albers JJ. Effects of interval and continuous running

on HDL-cholesterol, apoproteins A-1 and B, and LCAT. Can J Appl Sport Sci. 1985;10(1):52–9.
121. Thompson CE, Thomas TR, Araujo J, Albers JJ, Decedue CJ. Response of HDL cholesterol, apoprotein AI, and LCAT to exercise withdrawal. Atherosclerosis. 1985;54(1):65–73. https://doi.org/10.1016/0021-9150(85)90154-6.
122. Dufaux B, Order U, Muller R, Hollmann W. Delayed effects of prolonged exercise on serum lipoproteins. Metabolism. 1986;35(2):105–9. https://doi.org/10.1016/0026-0495(86)90108-3.
123. Frey I, Baumstark MW, Berg A, Keul J. Influence of acute maximal exercise on lecithin: cholesterol acyltransferase activity in healthy adults of differing aerobic performance. Eur J Appl Physio Occup Physiol. 1991;62(1):31–5. https://doi.org/10.1007/BF00635630.
124. Berger GMB, Griffiths MP. Acute effects of moderate exercise on plasma lipoprotein parameters. Inter J Sports Med. 1987;8(5):336–41. https://doi.org/10.1055/s-2008-1025680.
125. Griffin BA, Skinner ER, Maughan RJ. The acute effect of prolonged walking and dietary changes on plasma lipoprotein concentrations and high-density lipoprotein subfractions. Metabolism. 1988;37(6):535–41. https://doi.org/10.1016/0026-0495(88)90168-0.
126. Wallace MB, Moffatt RJ, Haymes EM, Green NR. Acute effects of resistance exercise on parameters of lipoprotein metabolism. Med Sci Sports Exerc. 1991;23(2):199–204.
127. Seip RL, Moulin P, Cocke T, Tall A, Kohrt WM, Mankowitz K, et al. Exercise training decreases plasma cholesteryl ester transfer protein. Arterioscler Thromb Vasc Biol. 1993;13:1359–67. https://doi.org/10.1161/01.ATV.13.9.1359.
128. Services USDoHH. Physical activity guidelines for Americans. ODPHP Publication No. 2008;U0036:2008.
129. Haskell WL, Lee IM, Pate RR, Powell KE, Blair SN, Franklin BA, et al. Physical activity and public health: updated recommendation for adults from the American College of Sports Medicine and the American Heart Association. Circulation. 2007;116(9):1081–93. https://doi.org/10.1161/CIRCULATION.107.185649.
130. Chodzko-Zajko WJ, Proctor DN, Singh MA, Minson CT, Nigg CR, Salem GJ, et al. Exercise and physical activity for older adults. Med Sci Sports Exerc. 2009;41:1510–30. https://doi.org/10.1249/MSS.0b013e3181a0c95c.
131. Nelson ME, Rejeski WJ, Blair SN, Duncan PW, Judge JO, King AC, et al. Physical activity and public health in older adults: recommendation from the American College of Sports Medicine and the American Heart Association. Circulation. 2007;116(9):1094–105. https://doi.org/10.1161/CIRCULATIONAHA.107.185650.
132. Riebe D. ACSM's Exercise Testing and Prescription. 10th ed. Philadelphia: Wolters Kluwer; 2017.
133. Williams PT, Krauss RM, Wood PD, Lindgren FT, Giotas C, Vranizan KM. Lipoprotein subfractions of runners and sedentary men. Metabolism. 1986;35(1):45–52. https://doi.org/10.1016/0026-0495(86)90094-6.
134. Wood PD, Haskell WL, Blair SN, Williams PT, Krauss RM, Lindgren FT, et al. Increased exercise level and plasma lipoprotein concentrations: a one-year, randomized, controlled study in sedentary, middle-aged men. Metabolism. 1983;32(1):31–9. https://doi.org/10.1016/0026-0495(83)90152-X.
135. Artinian NT, Fletcher GF, Mozaffarian D, Kris-Etherton P, Van Horn L, Lichtenstein AH, et al. Interventions to promote physical activity and dietary lifestyle changes for cardiovascular risk factor reduction in adults: a scientific statement from the American Heart Association. Circulation. 2010;122(4):406–41. https://doi.org/10.1161/CIR.0b013e3181e8edf1.
136. Fletcher B, Berra K, Ades P, Braun LT, Burke LE, Durstine JL, et al. Managing abnormal blood lipids: a collaborative approach. Circulation. 2005;112(20):3184–209. https://doi.org/10.1161/CIRCULATIONAHA.105.169180.
137. Stone NJ, Robinson JG, Lichtenstein AH, Bairey Merz CN, Blum CB, Eckel RH, et al. 2013 ACC/AHA guideline on the treatment of blood cholesterol to reduce atherosclerotic cardiovascular risk in adults: A report of the American College of Cardiology/American Heart Association Task Force on Practice Guidelines. J Am Coll Cardiol. 2014;63(25 Pt B):2889–934. https://doi.org/10.1016/j.jacc.2013.11.002.
138. Sarzynski MA, Ruiz-Ramie JJ, Barber JL, Slentz CA, Apolzan JW, McGarrah RW, et al. Effects of increasing exercise intensity and dose on multiple measures of HDL (High-Density Lipoprotein) function. Arterioscler Thromb Vasc Biol. 2018;38(4):943–52. https://doi.org/10.1161/ATVBAHA.117.310307.
139. Durstine JL, Moore GE. ACSM's Exercise Management for Persons with Chronic Diseases and Disabilities. 2nd ed. Champaign: Human Kinetics; 2003.
140. Auro K, Joensuu A, Fischer K, Kettunen J, Salo P, Mattsson H, et al. A metabolic view on menopause and ageing. Nat Commun. 2014;5:4708. https://doi.org/10.1038/ncomms5708.
141. Després JP, Moorjani S, Lupien PJ, Tremblay A, Nadeau A, Bouchard C. Regional distribution of body fat, plasma lipoproteins, and cardiovascular disease. Arteriosclerosis. 1990;10(4):497–511. https://doi.org/10.1161/01.ATV.10.4.497.
142. Walton C, Lees B, Crook D, Worthington M, Godsland IF, Stevenson JC. Body fat distribution, rather than overall adiposity, influences serum lipids and lipoproteins in healthy men independently of age. Amer J Med Sci. 1995;99(5):459–64. https://doi.org/10.1016/S0002-9343(99)80220-4.
143. Gepner AD, Piper ME, Johnson HM, Fiore MC, Baker TB, Stein JH. Effects of smoking and smok-

ing cessation on lipids and lipoproteins: outcomes from a randomized clinical trial. Am Heart J. 2011;161(1):145–51. https://doi.org/10.1016/j.ahj.2010.09.023.
144. Schijf CP, Mooren MJ, Doesburg WH, Thomas CM, Rolland R. Differences in serum lipids, lipoproteins, sex hormone binding globulin and testosterone between the follicular and the luteal phase of the menstrual cycle. Acta Endocrinol. 1993;129(2):130–3. https://doi.org/10.1530/acta.0.1290130.
145. Ribeiro SM, Luz Sdos S, Aquino Rde C. The role of nutrition and physical activity in cholesterol and aging. Clin Geriatr Med. 2015;31(3):401–16. https://doi.org/10.1016/j.cger.2015.04.010.
146. Langsted A, Freiberg JJ, Nordestgaard BG. Fasting and nonfasting lipid levels: influence of normal food intake on lipids, lipoproteins, apolipoproteins, and cardiovascular risk prediction. Circulation. 2008;118(20):2047–56. https://doi.org/10.1161/CIRCULATIONAHA.108.804146.
147. Dill DB, Costill DL. Calculation of percentage changes in volumes of blood, plasma, and red cells in dehydration. J Appl Physiol. 1974;37(2):247–8. https://doi.org/10.1152/jappl.1974.37.2.247.
148. Crouse JR, Grundy SM. Effects of alcohol on plasma lipoproteins and cholesterol and triglyceride metabolism in man. J Lipid Res. 1984;25:486–96.
149. Klop B, Rego A, Cabezas M. Alcohol and plasma triglycerides. Curr Opin Lipidol. 2013;24(4):321–6. https://doi.org/10.1097/MOL.0b013e3283606845.
150. Ainsworth R, Haskell WL, Herrmann SD, Meckes N, Ssett DR, Tudor-Locke C, et al. 2011 Compendium of physical activities. Med Sci Sports Exerc. 2011;43(8):1575–81. https://doi.org/10.1249/MSS.0b013e31821ece12.
151. Herink M, Ito MK. Medication induced changes in lipid and lipoproteins. Endotext [Internet] 2015; https://www.ncbi.nlm.nih.gov/books/NBK326739/
152. Crook MA, Apolipoprotein H. Its relevance to cardiovascular disease. Atherosclerosis. 2010;209(1):32–4. https://doi.org/10.1016/j.atherosclerosis.2009.11.022.
153. Expert Panel on Detection, Evaluation, and Treatment of High Blood Cholesterol in Adults. Executive summary of the Third Report of the National Cholesterol Education Program (NCEP) expert panel on detection, evaluation, and treatment of high blood cholesterol in adults. JAMA. 2001;285(19):2486–97. https://doi.org/10.1001/jama.285.19.2486.

Physical Activity, Fitness, and Coronary Heart Disease

17

Michael J. LaMonte

Introduction

Coronary heart disease (CHD) mortality among US adults has decreased substantially in recent decades, resulting in 341,745 fewer CHD deaths between 1980 and 2000 [1]. Despite this encouraging trend, CHD remains a major force of morbidity and mortality worldwide and accounts for excessive healthcare in both high- and low-income countries [2]. In 2011–2014, an estimated 16.5 million US adults had existing CHD, of which the age-standardized prevalence is higher in men (7.4%) than women (5.3%) and demonstrates considerable race-ethnic variation [3]. In 2015, cardiovascular disease was the number one cause of death among US adults, with 366,801 (43.8%) deaths due to CHD [3]. About 35% of those who experience an acute CHD event will die from it, and for about 40–55% of women and men who die suddenly from CHD, there was no prior symptom or knowledge of underlying atherosclerotic disease [3]. The proportion of CHD deaths in 2015 was higher in men (57.1%) than women (42.9%). Fatality remains low at younger ages (e.g., <40 years), but rises exponentially until about age 80 with men experiencing higher mortality than women until about age 70. Myocardial infarction ($12 million) and CHD ($nine million) are two of the ten most expensive conditions treated in US hospitals [3]. The estimated total cost of CHD in the United States in 2013 was $204 billion, and this is projected to increase more than 100% by 2030 [3]. Clearly the population burden of CHD is large and will continue to grow in parallel with population aging over the next several decades [4].

CHD has a lengthy induction and incubation period during which biological risk factors interact with genetic and environmental influences to initiate and promote endothelial cell dysfunction, atherosclerotic plaque development, arterial stenosis, and thrombosis [5]. Major clinical manifestations of CHD include angina, myocardial infarction, and sudden death. Prevention of clinical CHD events is typically achieved by reducing the development of new atherosclerotic lesions, stabilizing or limiting progression of existing lesions, and promoting enhanced fibrinolysis and reduced platelet aggregation. The objective is to maintain balance between myocardial oxygen supply and demand under a range of physiologic conditions and perturbations. Major modifiable CHD risk factors account for a large proportion (i.e., >75%) of the variation in clinical CHD between populations [6]. Only a small proportion of individuals will express clinical CHD because of genetic predisposition to these antecedent factors [7]. For most individuals the principal determinant

M. J. LaMonte (✉)
Department of Epidemiology and Environmental Health, University at Buffalo – SUNY, School of Public Health, Buffalo, NY, USA
e-mail: mlamonte@buffalo.edu

P. Kokkinos, P. Narayan (eds.), *Cardiorespiratory Fitness in Cardiometabolic Diseases*,
https://doi.org/10.1007/978-3-030-04816-7_17

is their lifestyle, the modification of which offers tremendous opportunity for controlling CHD in the community [8]. The lifestyle factors that likely benefit CHD prevention and control the most are smoking cessation; reduced dietary saturated fats, cholesterol, sodium, and refined sugars; and increased physical activity [9]. Because regular physical activity has far-reaching beneficial effects on major CHD risk factors, inflammation, oxidative stress, hemostasis, and cardiac structure and function, it has substantial implications to CHD prevention and management.

In this chapter, current evidence will be summarized with respect to benefits of physical activity and cardiorespiratory fitness on CHD. More thorough reviews have been published elsewhere [10–12]. To illustrate key points, individual studies frequently cited in consensus statements and systematic reviews will be discussed. Relevant biological mechanisms that may explain associations between activity, fitness, and CHD will be briefly reviewed.

Physical Activity Terminology

Physical activity refers to a behavior, specifically body movement, that occurs from skeletal muscle contraction resulting in increased energy expenditure above resting metabolic rate [13]. Physical fitness is a set of physiological attributes (e.g., cardiorespiratory fitness, body composition, muscular strength and endurance, flexibility, agility, balance) that may be enhanced through exercise training or through regular participation in PA [13]. The component of physical fitness that most often has been related with CHD outcomes is *cardiorespiratory fitness*, which reflects the body's ability to circulate and utilize oxygen during heavy dynamic physical activities. Determinants of cardiorespiratory fitness include age, sex, health status, and genetics; however, the principal modifiable determinant is habitual physical activity level [13]. In most individuals, and particularly among those who are sedentary, increases in PA result in increases in cardiorespiratory fitness, whereas it declines soon after cessation of physical activity. Thus, cardiorespiratory fitness can be used as a surrogate measure of recent physical activity patterns.

Healthy adults are encouraged to achieve a minimum of 150 min per week of moderate-intensity (3–6 METs) physical activity or at least 75 min per week of vigorous-intensity (>6 METs) activity [13]. The targeted minimum volume of PA is about 8 MET-h/week (≈1000 kcal/week) above routine activities of daily living and can be achieved through a combination of moderate- and vigorous-intensity activities. Recent clinical trial data indicate that recommended levels of moderate-intensity physical activity are a sufficient stimulus to improve cardiorespiratory fitness [14] and that adherence is greater for moderate- compared with high-intensity physical activity programs [15]. An example that fulfils the guideline-recommended energy expenditure for health-related benefits might be 30 min of brisk walking (moderate intensity) on 3 days, plus 20 min of jogging (vigorous intensity) on another 1 day of the week. Given that brisk walking (3.5 mph (5.6 km/h) on level ground) is a 3.8 MET activity and that jogging (10 min/mile (9.6 km/h) on level ground) is a 10 MET activity, the weekly volume of combined moderate-intensity (30 min × 3.8 METs × 3 days = 342 MET-min) and vigorous-intensity (20 min × 10 METs × 1 day = 200 MET-min) physical activity would be 542 MET-min per week, or 9 MET-h per week. In the recent Advisory Committee Report for the 2008 Physical Activity Guidelines for Americans [11], the health outcome with the clearest and strongest evidence supporting benefit at guideline-recommended physical activity levels was CHD incidence and mortality. There currently is no gold standard classification currently exists to classify "recommended cardiorespiratory fitness level." However, many observational epidemiologic studies have demonstrated substantially lower CHD risk (e.g., 35–50% lower risk) among adults in the middle two fifths of the age- and sex-standardized distribution of achieved maximal metabolic equivalents (METs) during incremental exercise ergometry testing, as compared to those in the lowest fifth of the distribution [10, 11]. The MET values that separate the lowest and middle two fifths of cardiorespiratory fitness distributions are about 7–10 METs in men and 6–8 METs in women, ages 20–70 years [16, 17].

Epidemiologic Studies on CHD: *Primary Prevention*

Physical Activity: Men

The field of physical activity epidemiology is rooted in seminal studies demonstrating lower CHD rates in men who were more physically active in their jobs. Prospective cohort studies conducted by Professor Jeremy Morris (1910–2009) in British civil servants (c., 1950); by Professor Ralph Paffenbarger, Jr. (1922–2007) in San Francisco longshoremen (c., 1970); and by Professor Henry Taylor (1919–1983) in US railroad employees (c., 1960) showed that men with higher levels of *occupational physical activity* (e.g., double-deck bus conductors, dockworkers, railroad switchmen) experienced rates of CHD mortality that were about 50% lower than those seen in their less active coworkers (e.g., bus drivers, desk clerks) [18–20]. Figure 17.1 summarizes these findings.

Because classifying physical activity levels by occupational duties provides a crude assessment of overall daily physical activity exposure and because widespread reductions in occupational energy expenditure were occurring throughout the twentieth century, Professors Morris and Paffenbarger expanded their research to include examination of self-reported *leisure-time physical activity* in relation to CHD. Morris' findings in male British civil servants [21] and Paffenbarger's in male Harvard alumni [22] consistently showed higher levels of leisure-time activity were associated with significantly lower CHD mortality. Morris reported a threshold of activity intensity of about 31.5 kJ/min (7.5 kcal/min; high end of moderate absolute intensity by contemporary standards) for at least 20 min on at least 2 days per week to obtain about a 62% reduction in CHD risk. In the landmark report by Paffenbarger on 16,936 male Harvard alumni ages 35–74 at baseline who were followed for 8 years (215 CHD deaths), age-adjusted CHD mortality rates across incremental groups of leisure-time activity-related energy expenditure

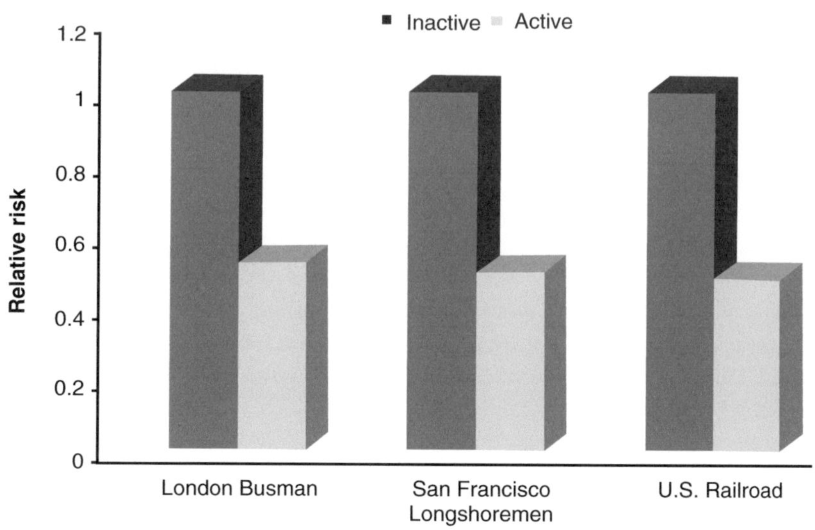

Fig. 17.1 Relative risks of CHD mortality according to occupational physical activity level in three prospective epidemiologic cohort studies on London busmen [18], San Francisco longshoremen [19], and US railroad employees [20]. Inactive men had job classifications of clerks or desk workers and were the referent group. Active men were London double-deck bus conductors, San Francisco dockworkers, and US railroad switchmen. Relative risks were adjusted for age, smoking, systolic blood pressure, and relative weight

(<500, 500–1999, ≥2000 kcal/week in vigorous sports play, stair climbing, brisk walking) were 25.7, 21.2, and 16.4 per 10,000 man-years (trend $P = 0.002$). After adjustment for history of parental CHD, smoking, weight status, and hypertension, the risk of CHD death was 33% lower ($P < 0.001$) among men who expended ≥2000 kcal/week compared to those with less than this amount of activity. Suggestion in both studies that vigorous-intensity activity may be the principal component of overall leisure-time activity that confers CHD benefits focused on ensuing research (and scientific debate) on the relative roles of physical activity intensity and energy expenditure as determinants of CHD morbidity and mortality, and this debate continues today [23].

Several additional studies have been published following the above seminal work, the majority of which have demonstrated that reduced CHD risk is associated with higher amounts of physical activity in men [10, 11]. Table 17.1 provides a summary of findings from selected well-established large prospective epidemiologic cohort studies on physical activity and the risk of primary CHD events [24–32].

Physical Activity: Women

Because early epidemiologic studies on the cardiovascular benefit of physical activity were conducted in men, it was unclear whether similar findings should be expected in women. An initial report from the Framingham Heart Study included 2311 women ages 35–64 years who completed a physical activity questionnaire in 1955–1956 and then were followed for 14 years during which 52 CHD deaths occurred [33]. No association was seen between self-reported levels of physical activity and mortality risk. In this study, activity was quantified using questionnaire items and associated energy costs originally developed and validated in men. Thus, one possible explanation for the null finding may have been due to misclassification of energy costs in women. However, in a later study with longer follow-up on these women, physical activity was found to be significantly related to lower CHD mortality [34]. The authors attributed the difference in findings to greater statistical power in their later analyses.

In another study, 6620 Canadian women ≥30 years of age completed an extensive baseline questionnaire to quantify usual daily physical activity during the past year and were followed 7 years during which 109 women experienced fatal CHD [35]. Age-adjusted odds ratios for CHD death were 1.0 (referent), 0.61, 0.84, and 0.63 (all nonsignificant) across incremental fourths of leisure-time physical activity. Further investigation revealed that of the 8.2 kcal/kg/day average daily total physical activity energy expenditure, only 1.2 kcal/kg/day (15%) was spent in sport and leisure activities, whereas 7.0 kcal/kg/day (85%) was spent in non-leisure activities (e.g., house and family care, commuting). When *non-leisure-time physical activity* was analyzed separately, a significant inverse association was seen with CHD death (OR: 1.00 (referent), 0.71, 0.57, 0.49; $P < 0.05$, each). The data from the Framingham and Canadian studies illustrate an important methodological issue, the influence that physical activity assessment methods can have in studies of health risks in women [36]. The use of assessment methods that are less ideal for measuring physical activity in women may partly explain why a significant inverse association between physical activity and CHD morbidity and mortality is less consistently observed in women than men and, when observed, why the effect sizes tend to be smaller in women than in men [10, 11].

Two of the largest and most comprehensive investigations on physical activity and CHD risk in women have been led by Professor JoAnn Manson in the US Nurses' Health Study [37] and Women's Health Initiative [38]. In each study, more than 70,000 women ages 40–79 years had usual leisure and recreational physical activity levels assessed at baseline using questionnaires relevant to women's lives and were then followed for primary CHD events during an average of 3–8 years. In both studies, multivariable analyses showed that compared with women in the lowest physical activity quintile, CHD risk was 12%,

Table 17.1 Summary of selected results on physical activity and the incidence of primary CHD events as reported in well-established prospective epidemiologic cohort studies

Study	Physical activity assessment	Endpoint follow-up (cases)	Main results	
Men				
Framingham Heart Study: Community-based cohort of 1909 men, ages 35–64, free of known CVD	Questionnaire; occupational, leisure/sports; Physical Activity Index (PAI) score	Fatal and nonfatal CHD 14 years (100 deaths; 351 events)	RR per 1 SD unit increment PAI	
			CHD death	0.18 ($P < 0.05$)
			CHD incidence	0.19 ($P < 0.05$)
Adventist Health Study [24]: Low-risk study population of 10,376 men, age ≥ 25, free of known CVD	Questionnaire; occupational, vigorous exercise; low, medium, high	Fatal and nonfatal CHD 6 years (136 deaths; 122 events)	CHD death	*RR (95% CI)*
			Low	1.00 (referent)
			Med	0.75 (0.46, 1.22)
			High	0.60 (0.39, 0.93)
			CHD incidence	
			Low	1.00 (referent)
			Med	1.50 (0.90, 2.50)
			High	0.90 (0.55, 1.49)
Honolulu Heart Study (Hakim 1999): 2678 physically capable elderly men, ages 71–93, free of known CVD	Questionnaire; walking (miles/day); <0.25, 0.25–1.5, >1.5	Combined fatal and nonfatal CHD 2–4 years (119)	*Miles/day*	*RR (95% CI)*
			>1.5	1.00 (referent)
			0.25–1.5	2.10 (1.20, 3.60)
			<0.255	2.30 (1.30, 4.10)
			P-trend	0.002
Health Professionals Study (Tanasescu 2002) 44,452 US male health professionals, ages 40–75; free of known CVD	Questionnaire; leisure-time; cumulative total activity and walking activity; MET-h/week updated every 2 years	Combined fatal and nonfatal CHD Not specified (1700)	*MET-h/week*	*RR (95% CI)*
			Total physical activity	
			0–6.32	1.00 (referent)
			6.33–14.49	0.93 (0.80, 1.06)
			14.50–25.08	0.90 (0.78, 1.05)
			25.09–41.98	0.87 (0.71, 1.01)
			≥41.99	0.74 (0.63, 0.87)
			P-trend	<0.001
			Walking	
			0–1.19	1.00 (referent)
			1.20–3.49	1.00 (0.83, 1.21)
			3.50–6.99	0.90 (0.74, 1.10)
			7.00–14.74	1.02 (0.84, 1.23)
			≥14.75	0.82 (0.67, 1.00)
			P-trend	0.04
			Walking speed (mph)	
			<2	1.00 (referent)
			2–3	0.74 (0.60, 0.91)
			3–4	0.60 (0.45, 0.79)
			≥4	0.50 (0.31, 0.84)
			P-trend	<0.001

(continued)

Table 17.1 (continued)

Study	Physical activity assessment	Endpoint follow-up (cases)	Main results	
EPIC-nested biomarker case-control study (Boekholdt 2006): 1869 men (663 cases; 1206 controls), mean age 65, free of CVD at baseline	Questionnaire; occupational, leisure-time; inactive, moderately inactive (ModIn), moderately active (ModAc), active	Combined fatal and nonfatal CHD 6 years (663)		*RR (95% CI)*
			Inactive	1.00 (referent)
			ModIn	0.74 (0.55, 0.98)
			ModAc	0.74 (0.54, 1.00)
			Active	0.68 (0.49, 0.93)
			P-trend	0.02
Finn-MONICA Study (Hu 2007): Community-based cohort of 19,707 men, ages 25–64, free of known CVD	Questionnaire; occupational, leisure-time; low, moderate, high	Combined fatal and nonfatal CHD 10 years (1141)	*Occupational*	*RR (95% CI)*
			Low	1.00 (referent)
			Moderate	0.64 (0.54, 0.76)
			High	0.73 (0.64, 0.83)
			P-trend	<0.001
			Leisure-time	
			Low	1.00 (referent)
			Moderate	0.96 (0.85, 1.09)
			High	0.64 (0.51, 0.82)
			P-trend	0.001
ARIC Study (Bell 2013): Community-based cohort of 3707 black and 10,018 white adults (*combined men and women), ages 45–64, without known CVD	Questionnaire; occupational, leisure/sports; minutes/week in moderate-to-vigorous activity: 0 (poor), 1–149 (intermediate), ≥150 (recommended)	Combined fatal and nonfatal CHD 21 years maximum (blacks 465; whites 971)		*RR* (95% CI)*
			Blacks	
			Poor	1.00 (referent)
			Intermediate	0.59 (0.47, 0.75)
			Recommended	0.66 (0.50, 0.86)
			P-trend	<0.001
			Whites	
			Poor	1.00 (referent)
			Intermediate	0.76 (0.65, 0.90)
			Recommended	0.68 (0.58, 0.80)
			P-trend	<0.001
			*Includes adjustment for sex	
Women				
Adventist Health Study (Fraser 1992): Low-risk study population of 17,282 women, age ≥ 25, free of known CVD	Questionnaire; occupational, vigorous exercise; low, medium, high	Fatal and nonfatal CHD 6 years (166 deaths; 81 events)	CHD death	*RR (95% CI)*
			Low	1.00 referent
			Med	0.61 (0.37, 0.98)
			High	0.41 (0.26, 0.64)
			CHD incidence	
			Low	1.00 referent
			Med	0.87 (0.43, 1.75)
			High	0.97 (0.55, 1.71)

Women's Health Study (Lee 2001): 39,372 US female health professionals, age ≥ 45, free of known CVD	Questionnaire; leisure-time and walking; Kcal/week	Combined fatal and nonfatal MI, coronary revascularization 5 years (244)		*RR (95% CI)*
			Total activity	
			<200	1.00 (referent)
			200–599	0.79 (0.56, 1.12)
			600–1499	0.55 (0.37, 0.82)
			≥1500	0.75 (0.50, 1.12)
			P-trend	0.03
			Walking (min/week)	
			0	1.00 (referent)
			1–59	0.86 (0.57, 1.29)
			60–90	0.49 (0.28, 0.86)
			≥90	0.48 (0.29, 0.78)
			P-trend	<0.001
			Walking pace (mph)	
			0	1.00 (referent)
			<2	0.56 (0.32, 0.97)
			2–2.9	0.71 (0.47, 1.05)
			≥3	0.52 (0.30, 0.90)
				0.02
EPIC-nested biomarker case-control study (Boekholdt 2006): 1064 women (368 cases; 696 controls), mean age 66, free of CVD at baseline	Questionnaire; occupational, leisure-time; inactive, moderately inactive (ModIn), moderately active (ModAc), active	Combined fatal and nonfatal CHD 6 years (368)	*RR (95% CI)*	
			Inactive	1.00 (referent)
			ModIn	0.81 (0.57, 1.15)
			ModAc	0.62 (0.40, 0.96)
			Active	0.51 (0.30, 0.87)
			P-trend	0.003
Finn-MONICA Study (Hu 2007): Community-based cohort of 21,346 women, ages 25–64, free of known CVD	Questionnaire; occupational, leisure-time; low, moderate, high	Combined fatal and nonfatal CHD 10 years (392)	*Occupational*	*RR (95% CI)*
			Low	1.00 (referent)
			Moderate	0.45 (0.35, 0.59)
			High	0.50 (0.38, 0.65)
			P-trend	<0.001
			Leisure-time	
			Low	1.00 (referent)
			Moderate	0.71 (0.58, 0.88)
			High	0.51 (0.32, 0.81)
			P-trend	0.001
Swedish Mammography Study (Akesson 2007): 24,444 postmenopausal women, mean age 59, free of known CVD	Questionnaire; walking/bicycling (min/d), exercise (h/week)	Combined fatal and nonfatal MI 6.2 years (308)		*RR (95% CI)*
			Walk/bike	
			≥40 min/week	1.00 (referent)
			<40	1.15 (0.90, 1.47)
			Exercise	
			≥1 h/week	1.00 (referent)
			<1	1.40 (1.10, 1.47)

(continued)

Table 17.1 (continued)

Study	Physical activity assessment	Endpoint follow-up (cases)	Main results	
Nurse's Health Study II (Chomistek 2016): 97,230 US female nurses, ages 27–44, free of CVD	Questionnaire; leisure-time; MET-h/week; updated every 2 years	Combined fatal and nonfatal CHD 20 years (544)		*RR (95% CI)*
			Total activity	
			<1	1.00 (referent)
			1.0–5.9	0.96 (0.76, 1.21)
			6.0–14.9	0.80 (0.63, 1.03)
			15.0–29.9	0.63 (0.47, 0.83)
			≥30	0.75 (0.57, 0.99)
			P-trend	0.01
			Vigorous activity*	
			0	1.00 (referent)
			0.1–2.9	1.16 (0.89, 1.51)
			3.0–7.4	0.99 (0.75, 1.31)
			7.5–14.9	0.89 (0.63, 1.27)
			≥15	0.77 (0.57, 1.03)
			P-trend	0.04
			Moderate activity*	
			0	1.00 (referent)
			0.1–2.9	0.65 (0.49, 0.87)
			3.0–7.4	0.68 (0.54, 0.87)
			7.5–14.9	0.59 (0.44, 0.80)
			≥15	0.67 (0.51, 0.87)
			P-trend	0.01
			*Mutually adjusted for each intensity	

In each study, the point and interval estimates of association were adjusted for age and several other risk predictors; the most fully adjusted associations reported in the original studies are provided in the table

Abbreviations: *CVD* cardiovascular disease, *CHD* coronary heart disease, *MI* myocardial infarction, *RR* relative risk,*CI* confidence interval, *SD* standard deviation, *MET* metabolic equivalent, a unit of physical activity intensity, *MET-h/week* a unit of physical activity energy expenditure computed as the product of duration (h/week) and intensity (MET) for a given physical activity task, *EPIC* European Prospective Investigation into Cancer and Nutrition study, *MONICA* Multinational Monitoring of Trends and Determinants in Cardiovascular Disease Project, *ARIC* Atherosclerosis Risk in Communities, *Kcal* kilocalorie

19%, 22–26%, and 28–34% lower in women in the upper four quintiles, respectively (trend $P \leq 0.002$). Significant inverse associations also were seen when women were categorized by race-ethnicity, smoking status, body mass index, and history of premature parental coronary disease. Perhaps the most provocative finding was that similar CHD risk reduction was seen in walking activity and in vigorous physical activities when energy expenditure was held constant. For example, the multivariable risk of CHD was, on average, 14% and 6% lower ($P < 0.05$ each) for each 5 MET-h increment of energy expenditure in walking and vigorous activity, respectively [37]. This finding suggests that physical activity energy expenditure, not intensity, is more relevant to CHD prevention, which is consistent with current public health guidelines [11, 13].

Cardiorespiratory Fitness: Men and Women

Compared with studies on physical activity and CHD, far fewer studies have been published in which an objective measure of cardiorespiratory fitness (henceforth *fitness*) has been obtained in a defined cohort of adults, without known clinical CVD at the time of fitness assessment, who then are followed up prospectively for the occurrence of incident CHD events [10, 11]. One of the first such studies was completed in 2779 men in Los Angeles (CA), ages 55 and younger, who were employed in law enforcement and firefighting and who completed submaximal cycle ergometry testing to quantify their cardiorespiratory fitness [39]. During a mean follow-up of nearly 5 years, there were 36 myocardial infarctions documented. In analysis controlling for age and major CHD risk factors, men whose fitness level was below the cohort median experienced a twofold higher relative risk ($P < 0.05$) of myocardial infarction compared to men above the median value. The magnitude of association seen for low fitness (RR = 2.2) was comparable to that seen for established CHD risk factors hypercholesterolemia (RR = 2.5), cigarette smoking (RR = 2.8), and high systolic blood pressure (RR = 1.8). Interestingly, the relative risk of CHD was more than sixfold higher in men with low fitness who also had two or more existing CHD risk factors. In the previously described US Railroad Study, initially CVD-free men completed a single-stage submaximal treadmill test to assess their fitness level, which was based on the exercise heart rate response to a standardized work rate (5 min at 5% grade and 3.0 mph) [40]. Lower heart rates, which reflect greater fitness levels, were associated with reduced CHD mortality risks. After adjustments for smoking, serum cholesterol, and systolic blood pressure, the relative risks (95% CI) for CHD mortality across four groups of incrementally higher exercise heart rates were 1.00 (referent), 1.06 (0.98, 1.16), 1.13 (1.04, 1.23), and 1.20 (1.10, 1.26).

Soon after publication of the above studies, a seminal paper was published by Professor Steven Blair, in which more than 10,000 men and 3000 women, ages 20–88 years, completed maximal treadmill exercise tests as part of an elective preventive medical examination at the Cooper Clinic in Dallas, TX, and then were followed 8 years for mortality outcomes [41]. While the numbers of CHD deaths were insufficient to be analyzed separately, rates of total CVD mortality declined steeply across fitness groups defined as the lowest fifth, the middle two fifths, and the upper two fifths of age- and sex-specific maximal treadmill times. Among men, age-adjusted CVD rates (per 10,000 person-years) were 24.6, 7.8, and 3.1 and for women were 7.4, 2.9, and 0.8. A subsequent report from this study on a 10-year follow-up for nonfatal CHD among 20,728 men and 5909 women documented 1222 and 97 events in men and women, respectively [17]. Study results are shown in Fig. 17.2.

Steep inverse gradients in age- and examination year-adjusted incidence rates of nonfatal CHD were observed across incremental fitness levels in both men (trend, $P < 0.001$) and women (trends, $P = 0.004$). Among men, a statistically significant inverse trend in the multivariable-adjusted relative risks for nonfatal CHD was seen (RR = 1.00, 0.89, 0.76; $P = 0.001$), whereas, among women, the inverse trend was observed but did not reach statistical significance

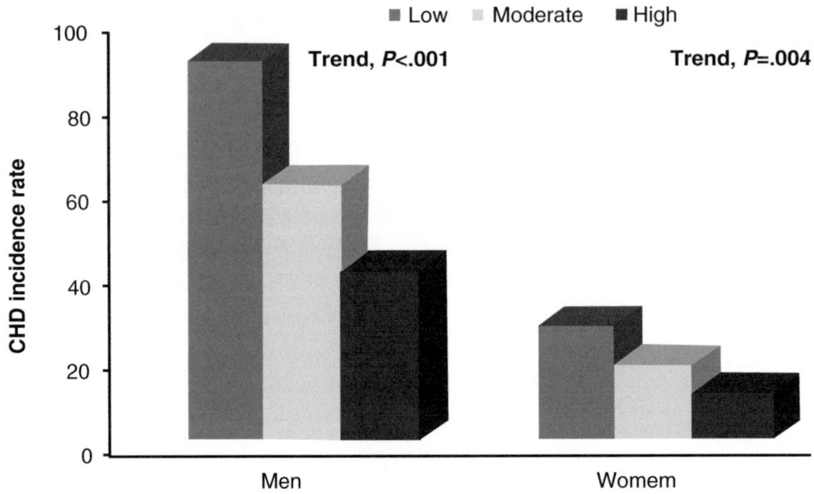

Fig. 17.2 Age- and examination year-adjusted rates (per 10,000 person-years) of CHD (MI, revascularization, cardiac death) according to categories of cardiorespiratory fitness in 20,728 men (1222 events) and 5909 women (97 events) followed 10 years in the Aerobics Center Longitudinal Study. Low, moderate, and high fitness categories were defined as the lower 20%, middle 40%, and upper 40% of the sex- and age-standardized distribution of maximal treadmill exercise test time

(RR = 1.00, 0.93, 0.82; $P = 0.49$), perhaps because of the limited number of CHD events analyzed. Similar to the above study on Los Angeles public servants, in this study, the age- and examination year-adjusted rates of CHD were inversely associated with fitness levels in men and women ($P < 0.05$, each) with especially high CHD risk based on the presence of two or more risk factors at baseline. Similar findings of lower multivariable-adjusted risks of CHD associated with greater levels of fitness determined by maximal treadmill exercise test duration in women and men have been reported in the Mayo ClinicOlmsted County Study [42], Framingham Heart Study [43], and St. James Women Take Heart Project [44].

The apparent benefit on CHD risk associated with higher fitness levels in the above discussed studies is based on estimated cardiorespiratory fitness, either using a physiologic response or work rate achieved during submaximal exercise [39, 40] or extrapolating from maximal exercise time or the final achieved work rate [17, 45]. While providing a reasonable distribution of estimated fitness for use in population health studies, these approaches are prone to misclassification of true cardiorespiratory fitness, defined as the maximal oxygen uptake [13]. Direct measurement of maximal oxygen uptake requires expensive laboratory instrumentation and is more burdensome to participants; thus, it has been included sparsely in large epidemiologic follow-up studies. However, this measurement was included as part of the Kuopio Ischemic Heart Disease Study which followed a cohort of Finnish men, ages 42–60 years without known CVD, for nonfatal myocardial infarction [46] and CHD death [47]. Cardiorespiratory fitness was measured using maximal cycle ergometry and indirect calorimetry analysis of expired air. After extensive adjustments for CVD predictors, each 1-MET (3.5 mL oxygen uptake/kg/min) increment in fitness was associated with a statistically significant ($P < 0.05$) reduced risk of MI (RR = 0.93) and CHD death (RR = 0.82). The inverse association between fitness and CHD mortality persisted when analyses were restricted to men who smoked, were obese, and had hypertension and dyslipidemia. In 1083 asymptomatic adults, ages 46–63 years in the Baltimore Longitudinal Study of Aging, 76 CHD events were documented during 8 years of follow-up [48]. Each 1-MET increment in measured oxygen uptake was associated with a significantly lower CHD risk (RR = 0.92;

$P < 0.001$), following adjustments for age, sex, and major CHD risk factors. Results from the Kuopio Ischemic Heart Disease Study and Baltimore Longitudinal Study of Aging, showing lower CHD risks in adults with higher levels of directly measured cardiorespiratory fitness, enhance confidence in the earlier described epidemiologic studies in which fitness was indirectly estimated.

Physical Activity or Fitness Benefit in High-Risk Groups

CHD risk is elevated in adults with existing conditions, such as diabetes, hypertension, metabolic syndrome, and obesity [49]. These comorbidities can affect the initiation and progression of atherosclerosis as well as potentially contribute to clinical event precipitation [50]. A role for physical activity or fitness in preventing primary CHD in these high-risk population subgroups is becoming established [51–55]. Among women in the Nurses' Health Study [52] with history of diabetes diagnosis, significantly lower multivariable-adjusted CHD risk was seen across incremental quintiles of self-reported physical activity (RR = 1.00 (referent), 1.07, 0.86, 0.61, 0.49, trend $P = 0.003$). Age-adjusted rates of CHD were lower in adults with metabolic syndrome who reported higher physical activity as compared with their less active peers (men, 11.5% vs 21.8%, $P < 0.001$; women, 5.3% vs 12.4%, $P < 0.001$) in the EPIC study [51]. Among adults with hypertension diagnosis, multivariable-adjusted relative risks for CHD comparing the lowest and highest categories of cardiorespiratory fitness were 0.71 ($P < 0.05$) in men and 0.47 ($P = 0.09$) in women [53]. And, in the Women's Health Study [55], CHD risks associated with being overweight or obese were attenuated, though not eliminated, by higher levels of total recreational physical activity as well as walking. For example, compared to active women with normal body weight, relative risks were 1.87 and 2.53 for obese women who were active and inactive, respectively ($P < 0.05$, each). These observational study results reinforce the importance of lifestyle modification as part of managing individual-level CHD risk [49].

Change in Activity or Fitness and CHD Risk

The studies reviewed thus far had a simple prospective epidemiological design where a single baseline measure of physical activity or fitness was related to CHD outcomes in follow-up. A perplexing issue for such studies is whether study participants changed their health habits during follow-up. That is, individuals eating a high-fat diet at baseline can improve their dietary habits at some point during the observation period, whereas others could initiate unhealthy dietary intakes. The same is true for other lifestyle habits such as physical activity and fitness. Those active or fit at the start of the study might reduce their activity levels early or later in the follow-up period and thus might be misclassified on their activity patterns or fitness levels for much of the observational period. This could introduce a biased or "imprecise" measure of association between the exposure and outcome variables of interest. Misclassification bias can reduce the likelihood of showing the true magnitude or significance of an association between the exposure and CHD outcome if such an association does in fact exist. As the field of physical activity epidemiology evolved, it became apparent that a more complete evaluation of the causal hypothesis for physical inactivity or low fitness and CHD incidence would be achieved by evaluating the association of changes in physical activity or fitness and subsequent CHD occurrence.

In the previously described Nurses' Health Study [37], women reported their physical activity levels in 1980 and then again in 1986. Women, who were physically inactive in 1980, were then classified on their activity levels according to the 1986 survey and followed thereafter for occurrence of CHD events. Compared to women who were inactive at both time points, the multivariable relative risks of CHD in those whose physical activity had increased placing them into incremental quartiles were 0.85, 0.79, 0.67, and

0.71 (trend, $P = 0.03$). In the Copenhagen City Heart Study [56], 4487 men and 5956 women, ages 20–93 years, self-reported their physical activity at baseline in 1976–1978 and again in 1981–1983 and then were followed through 2008 for incidence of CHD. Although significant differences in CHD risk factors such as blood pressure and total cholesterol were not seen in relation to patterns of physical activity changes, women and men who were active at baseline and became less active by the second assessment interval had statistically significant higher multivariable-adjusted CHD risks. Similarly, middle-aged men in the British Regional Heart Study who reported increases in physical activity levels across two assessments separated by 12–14 years had significantly lower rates of myocardial infarction and CHD death compared to those with persistent inactivity [57]. Fewer data are available for the association of fitness changes with CHD risk. Blair and colleagues [58] reported significant improvements in CHD risk factors among men whose maximal treadmill exercise duration increased between two tests separated by about 2 years. A subsequent report from this study showed that men with low fitness at the first test and improved fitness at the second test have a 52% ($P < 0.05$) lower multivariable-adjusted relative risk of CVD mortality compared to their peers with low fitness at both tests [59]. The CHD benefit of changing from lower to higher fitness seen in the above and other studies that defined fitness based on indirect assessments has been confirmed in the Baltimore Longitudinal Study of Aging [60] where, as previously described, fitness was determined by directly measuring maximal oxygen uptake. While not as rigorous as experimental data from a randomized controlled trial, the epidemiological findings reported among these studies on the risks of CHD subsequent to change in self-reported physical activity or measured fitness provide important additional evidence for a causal association between these exposures and primary CHD occurrence.

One might argue that any propensity for increasing physical activity and fitness may well reflect genetic prowess in those able to make and sustain such changes and subsequently realize CHD benefit. Quantifying the extent to which the association between physical activity and fitness with CHD is explained by genetics is relevant when allocating limited public health resources for the development of targeted strategies to intervene on modifiable risk factors as a means of controlling the population burden of CHD morbidity and mortality. Exposure-outcome associations largely accounted for by genetic selection likely would not be a cost-effective widespread target for improving population health but instead may be more feasible in population subgroups with specific genetic composition. Recent findings in the Swedish Twin Registry study [61] begin to address this issue as related to physical activity and CVD mortality. Physical activity questionnaires were completed in 1972 by 13,109 twin pairs (40% monozygotic twin pairs), who then were followed for mortality through 2004 (1800 deaths). As expected, in the overall study population, CVD mortality risk was 66% and 45% lower among women and men, respectively, in the high- compared with low-activity groups. When analyses were conducted on physical activity discordant monozygotic twin pairs, the twin with higher physical activity had a 32% lower risk ($P < 0.05$) of CVD mortality compared with their less active co-twin. Similar mortality risk reduction in high- compared with low-activity groups was seen when monozygotic twin pairs were analyzed separately according to sex. Associations between activity and mortality were weaker and not significant among dizygotic twins. The significant protective association between physical activity and mortality observed in monozygotic twins tempers arguments that the association is accounted for principally by genetic selection and supports the hypothesis that the association is one of causality. In another epidemiologic cohort study, the Women's Genome Health Study [62], genes pertaining to cardiorespiratory fitness did not modify the significant inverse association observed between self-reported physical activity and CHD incidence. This finding provides some evidence against the argument that the CHD benefit associated with physical activity habits predominantly reflects a broader effect conferred through fitness pathways. It is important to recognize that complex multifactorial webs of causation underlay most etiological pathways linking lifestyle and other exposures with CHD morbidity and mortality, and genetic components likely are involved in several aspects therein, although these effects may be difficult to assess at present. Ongoing progress in the technological capacity for refined examination of complex gene-gene and gene-environment interactions and the emerging field of epigenetics will no doubt lead to better understanding of the role genetics has in the established health benefits associated with physical activity and fitness.

Epidemiologic Studies on CHD: *Secondary Prevention*

Numerous prospective epidemiologic cohort studies have documented better prognosis associated with higher physical activity or fitness levels in adults with established clinical CHD [10, 11, 63]. Results have shown that levels of activity and fitness prior to [64–67] and following [64, 65, 67–74] primary CHD events are associated with better outcomes in these patients. These studies are summarized in Table 17.2. Prognostic benefit of higher physical activity or fitness is seen in both women and men with established CHD. Fitness, whether estimated from achieved maximal work rate during ergometry testing or directly measured maximal oxygen uptake, is one of the strongest prognostic factors among demographic, medical, and clinical parameters evaluated [64, 68, 70–74]. Even in those with reduced left ventricular ejection fraction (<40%), achieving higher fitness levels (≥4 vs <4 METs) during symptom-limited cycle ergometry was associated with significantly lower age-adjusted 5-year mortality (5% vs 29%, $P < 0.05$) [68]. Among adults with stable CHD who had clinical depression, a major complication of myocardial infarction and other CHD sequelae, low levels of self-reported physical activity as well as measured fitness eliminated the adverse association between depression and secondary CVD events [74]. In this study, when simultaneously adjusted for the presence of depression and other CVD risk predictors, physical inactivity remained a strong determinant of recurrent CVD events (RR = 1.44, $P < 0.05$).

Experimental Studies on CHD Prevention

Primary Prevention

Several studies using experimental designs have demonstrated favorable changes in CHD risk factors, including resting and exercise heart rate and blood pressure; fasting and postprandial blood lipid and glucose concentrations; hemostatic, inflammatory, and stress-response biomarkers; body fat distribution; and physical fitness parameters in adults who increased their physical activity or fitness levels as a result of exercise training. A detailed review of this evidence is beyond the scope of this chapter. Readers are referred elsewhere to published reviews of these findings [10, 11, 13, 75–77]. The LookAhead trial is a recent randomized primary prevention trial conducted among adults who, at enrollment, were overweight or obese and had clinically diagnosed type 2 diabetes in which physical activity was part of a multicomponent intervention [78]. A total of 5145 participants were randomized to either intensive lifestyle intervention (physical activity, dietary restriction, stress management) targeting a modest 10% loss of enrollment body weight or usual care diabetes education and followed for a maximum of 13.5 years. Significant weight loss and improvements in systolic blood pressure, LDL and HDL cholesterol concentrations, glycemic control, and cardiorespiratory fitness were observed in the intervention compared with control group. However, rates (per 100 person-years) of the primary outcome (CVD death, nonfatal MI, stroke, angina) were not different between intervention and control groups (1.83 vs 1.92, $P = 0.51$) nor were rates of a secondary CHD endpoint (fatal and nonfatal MI; intervention, 0.71, vs control, 0.84; $P = 0.11$). Because this trial did not focus exclusively on physical activity or excise training as the sole

Table 17.2 Summary of selected results on physical activity or cardiorespiratory fitness and the incidence of secondary CHD events in adults with established clinical cardiovascular disease

Study	Physical activity or fitness assessment	Endpoint follow-up (cases)	Main results	
Outpatient Cardiac Rehab [64]: 2146 adults (84% men), mean age 60, with prior revascularization, completed 12 weeks of exercise-based C-Rehab	*Fitness*: symptom-limited upright cycle ergometry test (protocol not specified); peak watts (W) achieved Pre- and post-rehabilitation fitness	All-cause and CVD mortality Median 33 months (74 total deaths)	*RR (95% CI)*	
			Fitness <105 W	
			At entry	
			All-cause	2.38 (1.40, 4.06)
			CVD	3.53 (1.80, 6.96)
			At completion	
			All-cause	2.34 (1.23, 4.43)
			CVD	not reported
KAROLA study [65]: 1038 adults (85% men), ages 30–70, with stable CHD	*Physical activity*: questionnaire; leisure-time; frequency of activity (episodes per month); assessed 1, 3, 6, 8, and 10 years after completion of C-Rehab	Fatal and nonfatal CVD 8 years (81 deaths; 112 nonfatal)	*RR (95% CI)*	
			Year 1 activity	
			CVD mortality	
			Daily	1.73 (0.83, 3.60)
			5–6/week	1.19 (0.52, 2.71)
			2–4/week	1.00 (referent)
			1–4/month	1.30 (0.60, 2.85)
			Rarely/never	3.80 (1.84, 7.86)
			Nonfatal CVD	
			Daily	0.71 (0.33, 1.52)
			5–6/week	1.75 (0.99, 3.09)
			2–4/week	1.00 (referent)
			1–4/month	1.63 (0.94, 2.85)
			Rarely/never	1.37 (0.62, 3.01)
			Time-varying activity	
			CVD mortality	
			Daily	2.36 (1.05, 5.34)
			5–6/week	1.23 (0.43, 3.51)
			2–4/week	1.00 (referent)
			1–4/month	1.48 (0.66, 3.32)
			Rarely/never	3.30 (1.61, 3.78)
			Nonfatal CVD	
			Daily	1.21 (0.54, 2.71)
			5–6/week	2.56 (1.26, 5.20)
			2–4/week	1.00 (referent)
			1–4/month	1.30 (0.72, 2.34)
			Rarely/never	2.51 (1.38, 4.56)

Italian AMI Study [66]: 180 adults (69% men), ≥70 years, with vascularized AMI	*Physical activity*: questionnaire; administered about 10-day follow revascularization; tertiles	CHD mortality 30-day, 1-year (53; 86)	*RR (95% CI)*	
			Tertile 3 vs 1	
			30-day death	0.15 (0.04, 0.50)
			1-year death	0.22 (0.07, 0.71)
Corpus Christi Heart Study [67]: 406 adults (70% men), mean age 58, with a primary AMI	*Physical activity*: questionnaire; frequency and intensity of activities asked prior to and following MI	Reinfarction, all-cause mortality 7 years (150 events, 106 deaths)	*RR (95% CI)*	
			Reinfarction	
			Active, both	0.40 (0.24, 0.66)
			Increased	0.22 (0.09, 0.50)
			Decreased	0.93 (0.59, 1.42)
			Sedentary, both	1.00 (referent)
			All-cause mortality	
			Active, both	0.21 (0.10, 0.44)
			Increased	0.11 (0.03, 0.46)
			Decreased	0.49 (0.26, 0.90)
			Sedentary, both	1.00 (referent)
Women's Health Initiative [69]: 856 postmenopausal women, ages 50–79, with a primary AMI	*Physical activity*: questionnaire; duration and intensity of usual activity asked prior to and following MI; MET-Min/week	CVD mortality 7.2 years (120)	*RR (95% CI)*	
			Total activity	
			Maintain low	1.00 (referent)
			Decreased	0.82 (0.44, 1.55)
			Increased	0.59 (0.30, 1.15)
			Maintain high	0.41 (0.24, 0.71)
			Walking:	
			Maintain low	1.00 (referent)
			Decreased	0.77 (0.39, 1.51)
			Increased	0.39 (0.12, 1.22)
			Maintain high	0.57 (0.29, 1.12)

(continued)

Table 17.2 (continued)

Study	Physical activity or fitness assessment	Endpoint follow-up (cases)	Main results	
PAAMI-2 database [68]: 330 adults (74% men), mean age 59, vascularized for acute STEMI	*Fitness*: symptom-limited cycle ergometry test 6 weeks after MI; peak watts achieved, expressed as METs	All-cause mortality 2- and 5-year (13, 28 deaths)	*RR (95% CI)*	
			2-year	
			≥4 METs	1.00 (referent)
			<4 METs	2.70 (0.85, 9.09)
			5-year:	
			≥4 METs	1.00 (referent)
			<4 METs	4.54 (1.77, 11.6)
			Age-adjusted 5-year mortality	
			LVEF <40%	
			≥4 METs	5% (P < 0.05)
			<4 METs	29%
			LVEF ≥40%	
			≥4 METs	3% (P < 0.05)
			<4 METs	20%
Toronto Cardiac Rehabilitation Study [70, 71]: 12,169 men (mean age 55) and 2380 women (mean age 59) with primary CHD (MI or revascularization)	*Fitness*: symptom-limited cycle ergometry test (16 watts/min); maximal oxygen uptake (ml/kg/min) measured by indirect calorimetry	All-cause and CHD mortality Men: 7.9 years (2352, 1336 deaths) Women: 6.1 years (209, 95 deaths)	*RR (95% CI)*	
			Men	
			All-cause death	
			<15 ml/kg/min	1.00 (referent)
			15–22	0.66 (0.59, 0.73)
			>22	0.48 (0.42, 0.55)
			CHD death	
			<15 ml/kg/min	1.00 (referent)
			15–22	0.62 (0.54, 0.71)
			>22	0.39 (0.33, 0.47)
			Women	
			All-cause death:	
			<13 ml/kg/min	1.00 (referent)
			≥13	0.71 (0.53, 0.95)
			CHD death	
			<13 ml/kg/min	1.00 (referent)
			≥13	0.50 (0.38, 0.80)

Henry Ford Heart Institute Cohort [72]: 2812 adults (72% men), mean age 61; with primary CHD (MI, revascularization) entering cardiac rehabilitation	*Fitness*: symptom-limited treadmill ergometry test (Balke protocol); maximal oxygen uptake (ml/kg/min) measured by indirect calorimetry	All-cause and CVD mortality 4.9 years (men, 200, 77 deaths; women, 80, 26 deaths)	*RR (95% CI)*	
			Per 1 ml/kg/min	
			Men	
			All-cause	0.83 (0.80, 0.86)
			CVD	0.84 (0.79, 0.89)
			Women	
			All-cause	0.86 (0.80, 0.93)
			CVD	0.87 (0.76, 0.98)
Palo Alto VA Hospital Cohort [73]: 3679 men, mean age 61, with a history of CVD	*Fitness*: symptom-limited treadmill ergometry test (ramp protocol); achieved METs estimated from test duration	All-cause mortality 6.2 years (968)	*RR (95% CI)*	
			Age-adjusted	
			≥10.7 METs	1.0 (referent)
			8.3–10.6	1.7 (1.4, 2.2)
			6.5–8.2	2.3 (1.7, 2.8)
			5.0–6.4	3.0 (2.4, 3.7)
			1.0–4.9	4.2 (3.3, 5.2)
			Multivariable-adjusted	
			Per 1 MET	0.91 (0.88, 0.94)
Heart and Soul Study [74]: 1017 adults (83% men), mean age 68, with history of stable CHD	*Physical activity*: questionnaire; leisure and sports; frequency (episodes per month)	Total CVD incidence 4.8 years (341 events)	*RR (95% CI)*	
			Active	1.00 (referent)
			Inactive	1.44 (1.14, 1.82)

In each study, the point and interval estimates of association were adjusted for age and several other risk predictors; the most fully adjusted associations reported in the original studies are provided in the table

Abbreviations: *CVD* cardiovascular disease, *CHD* coronary heart disease, *MI* myocardial infarction, *AMI* acute MI, *STEMI* ST elevation MI, *C-Rehab* cardiac rehabilitation, *RR* relative risk, *CI* confidence interval, *LVEF* left ventricular ejection fraction, *MET* metabolic equivalent, a unit of physical activity intensity, *MET-h/week* a unit of physical activity energy expenditure computed as the product of duration (hours/week) and intensity (MET) for a given physical activity task intervention modality, it is not possible to rule out that such an intervention, if of sufficient activity dose and adherence, could be efficacious for primary CHD prevention. However, to date, there has not been a published large randomized controlled trial evaluating the effect of physical activity on the incidence of primary CHD events. Results of an ongoing NHLBI-funded large pragmatic community-based trial, the Women's Health Initiative Strong and Healthy (WHISH) trial [79], to increase physical activity and reduce sedentary time among older postmenopausal women, will provide desperately needed and important scientific understanding in this area.

Secondary Prevention

More evidence is available from experimental studies on the effect that increasing physical activity and fitness have on the prevention of secondary outcomes in adults with established CHD. One of the first such large-scale studies was the National Exercise and Heart Disease Program [80], a 3-year multicenter randomized trial in the United States, in which 351 and 319 men, ages 30–64 years who had acute myocardial infarction 2–36 months prior to enrollment, were randomized to an exercise or control group, respectively. Overall, trial outcomes were more favorable in the exercise compared with control group. The cumulative 3-year rate of all-cause mortality and recurrent myocardial infarction favored the intervention group (4.6% vs 7.3%; 5.3% vs 7.0%), although rate differences did not achieve statistical significance. A recent meta-analysis [81] on the efficacy of exercise-based cardiac rehabilitation for secondary event prevention (16 randomized controlled trials, 14,486 participants, median follow-up 12 months) demonstrated significantly lower CVD mortality (weighted summary RR = 0.74, 95% CI: 0.64, 0.86) and hospitalization (weighted summary RR = 0.82, 95% CI: 0.70, 0.96) associated with physical activity intervention. These findings generally concur with the observational findings shown in Table 17.2. Additional trial results suggest that increasing physical activity is associated with reduced healthcare costs and improved clinical outcomes as compared with percutaneous revascularization in patients with stable CHD [82, 83].

Biologic Mechanisms for CHD Risk Reduction

Existing evidence supports a causal association between physical inactivity and CHD [10, 11, 84]. A key aspect that enhances such a conclusion is the numerous biologic mechanisms that have been demonstrated between physical activity or fitness and CHD. It is beyond the scope of this chapter to provide a detailed comprehensive review of these data. Figure 17.3 illustrates several of these possible mechanisms, grouped into four primary elements, including factors improving *skeletal muscle* substrate utilization and contractile function, factors improving *myocardial* structure and function, factors that prevent or control onset and progression of *atherosclerosis*, and factors related to improved *neurohormonal control* over perturbations in cardiac function as well as intermediary metabolic pathways. Importantly, physical activity appears to reduce both subclinical [85] and clinically evident [86] atherosclerosis. Other potential mechanisms that could link physical activity with a favorable impact on CHD are improved myocardial electrical stability [87], myocardial ischemic preconditioning [88], improved central cardiac components of cardiorespiratory fitness (maximal oxygen uptake) [86], less myocardial ectopic fat deposition [89], as well as telomere lengthening [90] and microRNA responses [91] that may have cardiometabolic benefit particularly with aging. A principal effect desired for CHD risk reduction is to maintain or restore the balance between myocardial oxygen supply and demand. Clinical trials have demonstrated improvements of myocardial perfusion following exercise training in patients with stable CHD, likely owing to regression of atheromatous plaques within the coronary circulation [86], enhanced coronary endothelial function [92, 93], promotion of coronary collateralization [94], and reduced coronary

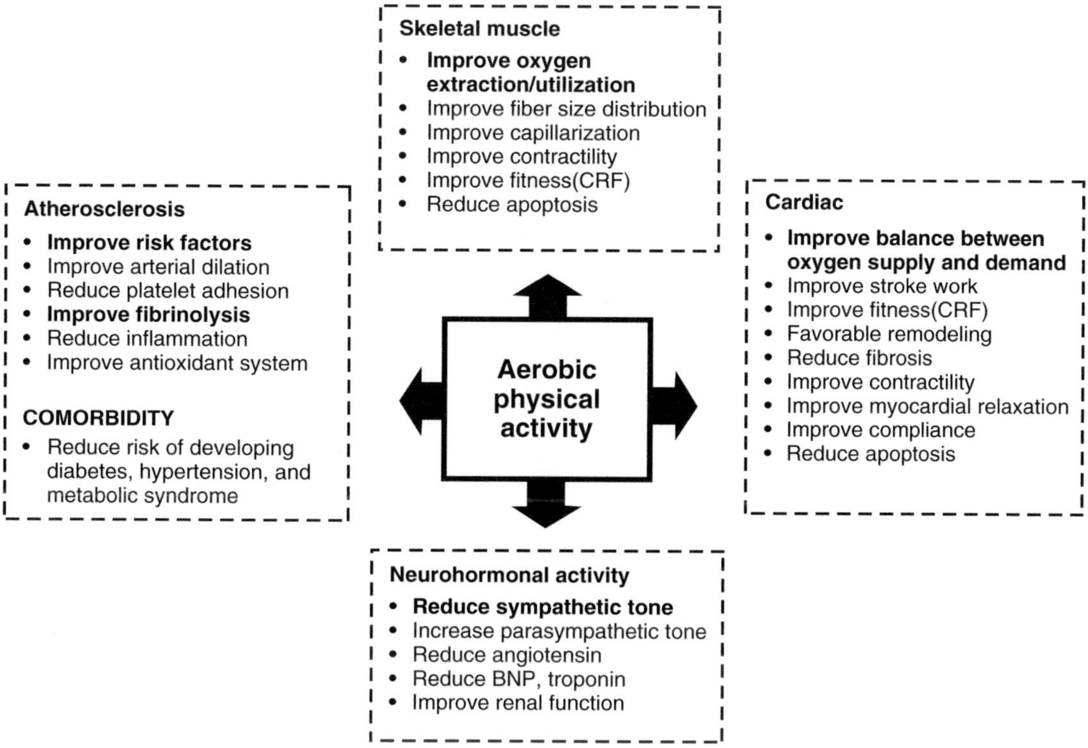

Fig. 17.3 Potential mechanisms through which physical activity reduces CHD risk. Bold elements are likely a major pathway

inflammation [83]. Other elements presented in Fig. 17.3 likely have a direct or indirect influence on either oxygen supply, demand, or both.

Clinical and Public Health Significance

The ongoing accumulation of scientific evidence supports a role, quite likely causal in nature, for physical inactivity and low fitness in the etiology and clinical manifestations of CHD. Compelling evidence derives from large, well-designed prospective observational cohort studies, the results of which tend to show strong inverse associations between self-reported physical activity and measured fitness with the incidence of primary CHD and with secondary event occurrence in those who already have clinical CHD. The apparent CHD benefit associated with physical activity and fitness is consistently observed in studies of diverse populations, using different approaches to the assessment of activity and fitness, and across varying lengths of follow-up for endpoint events. Indeed, the seminal 1996 US Surgeon General Report on Physical Activity and Health [10] concluded:

> The epidemiologic literature supports an inverse causal association between level of physical activity or fitness and CHD. The association is moderate in magnitude, consistent across studies that differed substantially in methods and population, and biologically plausible. Dose-response has been observed in most studies examining more than two levels of exposure. Although controlled trials have not been conducted for CHD, morbidity or mortality controlled trials have shown that increasing physical activity can improve physiologic risk factors and subclinical measures for CHD. From this large body of consistent scientific evidence it is reasonable to conclude physical activity is causally related to CHD.

The biological mechanisms that could explain a causal link between physical activity and CHD continue to evolve, and many more likely will be identified and existing mechanistic theories refined as technologic advances continue in both basic and applied scientific settings, including the potential understanding about targeted preventive and therapeutic applications that might come through precision medicine endeavors. Use of objective measures of physical activity, such as accelerometers, will likely result in less misclassification of activity exposures, which in turn should enhance precision of associations with CHD risk factors and clinical endpoints [95, 96]. Exercise-induced cardiac benefits in adults with stable CHD appear to have a cost advantage over conventional clinical intervention [82]. Taken together, future discovery and improved research methods will expand and refine the paradigm of CHD prevention and management; the downstream consequence ideally will further decline in population CHD rates as seen over the past 25 or so years [2].

However, the important public health and clinical question pertains neither to more comprehensive elucidation of mechanisms nor to whether an association between physical activity and CHD exists independent of these pathways. The more important question is whether the population burden of CHD will decrease if individuals who are physically inactive and have low fitness increase their activity habits and fitness levels, even by relatively small amounts [97]. It is clear that small changes in other modifiable risk factors [98] confer potential for large reductions in the incidence of CHD and other atherosclerotic cardiovascular diseases. Community changes in behavioral factors associated with CHD [99], including physical activity [100], are possible. Guideline recommendations for improving the cardiovascular health of communities continue to emphasize the utility of modifiable lifestyle behavior targets in order to realize these goals [101, 102]. To this point, however, experts argue that more guidelines are not the answer to the public health problem. Instead, widespread efforts to change the US way of living are needed so that the abundance of proven effective CVD guidelines has a chance at being implemented, adopted, and successful in making small but meaningful changes in cardiovascular health measures within communities [103, 104]. Because the population prevalence of physical inactivity is high and its association with CHD is of a moderate-to-strong magnitude [11], the fraction of CHD morbidity attributable to physical inactivity could be as high as 37% [105], which is comparable to or exceeds that for other major modifiable CHD risk factors such as diabetes, hypertension, poor dietary intake, and obesity.

Conclusion

The population burden to CHD remains large in the United States and abroad. Approaches to CHD primary and secondary prevention have led to recent declines in CHD mortality rates; however, the absolute numbers of CHD cases in the community are substantial and will increase with population aging. Healthcare costs will parallel this increasing trend in the coming decades. The review in this chapter demonstrates the role that physical activity and fitness have in both primary and secondary CHD prevention. Evidence will continue to accumulate from studies with improved designs, including genotypic variation in physical activity behavior and the response of CHD risk factors therein, and better measures of activity and fitness in larger and more diverse cohorts. There were 366,801 CHD deaths in 2015 [3]. Assuming the population attributable fraction of CHD is 37% [105] and assuming a causal association between inactivity and CHD, 135,716 CHD deaths in 2015 could have been averted had no one been exposed to inactivity. While such estimates are theoretical, they do provide a realistic context about the contribution physical inactivity makes to the population burden of CHD. Because improvements in physical activity tend to favorably influence blood lipids, blood pressure, insulin sensitivity, and hemostatic factors as well as cardiorespiratory fitness, next to quitting smoking, increasing and maintaining one's physical activity level at recommended levels is one of the least expensive and most beneficial approaches to achieving cardiometabolic health and reducing CHD risk available to the public.

References

1. Ford ES, Ajani UA, Croft JB, Critchley JA, Labarthe DR, Kottke TE, et al. Explaining the decrease in U.S. deaths from coronary disease, 1980-2000. N Engl J Med. 2007;356(23):2388–98.
2. Herrington W, Lacey B, Sherliker P, Armitage J, Lewington S. Epidemiology of atherosclerosis and the potential to reduce the global burden of atherothrombotic disease. Circ Res. 2016;118(4):535–46.
3. Benjamin EJ, Virani SS, Callaway CW, Chamberlain AM, Chang AR, Cheng S, et al. Heart disease and stroke statistics-2018 update: a report from the American Heart Association. Circulation. 2018;137(12):e67–e492.
4. Jones DS, Greene JA. The decline and rise of coronary heart disease: understanding public health catastrophism. Am J Public Health. 2013;103(7):1207–18.
5. Libby P, Theroux P. Pathophysiology of coronary artery disease. Circulation. 2005;111(25):3481–8.
6. Greenland P, Knoll MD, Stamler J, Neaton JD, Dyer AR, Garside DB, et al. Major risk factors as antecedents of fatal and nonfatal coronary heart disease events. JAMA. 2003;290(7):891–7.
7. Hopkins PN, Williams RR. Human genetics and coronary heart disease: a public health perspective. Annu Rev Nutr. 1989;9:303–45.
8. Stampfer MJ, Hu FB, Manson JE, Rimm EB, Willett WC. Primary prevention of coronary heart disease in women through diet and lifestyle. N Engl J Med. 2000;343(1):16–22.
9. Mozaffarian D, Afshin A, Benowitz NL, Bittner V, Daniels SR, Franch HA, et al. Population approaches to improve diet, physical activity, and smoking habits: a scientific statement from the American Heart Association. Circulation. 2012;126(12):1514–63.
10. U.S. Department of Health and Human Services. Physical activity and health: a report of the Surgeon General. Atlanta: U.S. Department of Health and Human Services, Centers for Disease Control and Prevention, National Center for Chronic Disease Prevention and Health Promotion; 1996.
11. Physical Activity Guidelines Advisory Committee. Physical Activity Guidelines Advisory Committee report, 2008. Washington, DC: U.S. Department of Health and Human Services; 2008.
12. Sattelmair J, Pertman J, Ding EL, Kohl HW 3rd, Haskell W, Lee IM. Dose response between physical activity and risk of coronary heart disease: a meta-analysis. Circulation. 2011;124(7):789–95.
13. Garber CE, Blissmer B, Deschenes MR, Franklin BA, Lamonte MJ, Lee IM, et al. American College of Sports Medicine position stand. Quantity and quality of exercise for developing and maintaining cardiorespiratory, musculoskeletal, and neuromotor fitness in apparently healthy adults: guidance for prescribing exercise. Med Sci Sports Exerc. 2011;43(7):1334–59.
14. Church TS, Earnest CP, Skinner JS, Blair SN. Effects of different doses of physical activity on cardiorespiratory fitness among sedentary, overweight or obese postmenopausal women with elevated blood pressure: a randomized controlled trial. JAMA. 2007;297(19):2081–91.
15. Perri MG, Anton SD, Durning PE, Ketterson TU, Sydeman SJ, Berlant NE, et al. Adherence to exercise prescriptions: effects of prescribing moderate versus higher levels of intensity and frequency. Health Psychol. 2002;21(5):452–8.
16. Kokkinos P, Myers J, Franklin B, Narayan P, Lavie CJ, Faselis C. Cardiorespiratory fitness and health outcomes: a call to standardize fitness categories. Mayo Clin Proc. 2018;93(3):333–6.
17. Sui X, LaMonte MJ, Blair SN. Cardiorespiratory fitness as a predictor of nonfatal cardiovascular events in asymptomatic women and men. Am J Epidemiol. 2007;165(12):1413–23.
18. Morris JN, Heady JA, Raffle PA, Roberts CG, Parks JW. Coronary heart-disease and physical activity of work. Lancet. 1953;265(6796):1111–20; concl.
19. Paffenbarger RS, Hale WE. Work activity and coronary heart mortality. N Engl J Med. 1975;292(11):545–50.
20. Taylor HL, Blackburn H, Keys A, Parlin RW, Vasquez C, Puchner T. Coronary heart disease in seven countries. IV. Five-year follow-up of employees of selected U.S. railroad companies. Circulation. 1970;41(4 Suppl):I20–39.
21. Morris JN, Everitt MG, Pollard R, Chave SP, Semmence AM. Vigorous exercise in leisure-time: protection against coronary heart disease. Lancet. 1980;2(8206):1207–10.
22. Paffenbarger RS Jr, Hyde RT, Wing AL, Steinmetz CH. A natural history of athleticism and cardiovascular health. JAMA. 1984;252(4):491–5.
23. Swain DP, Franklin BA. Comparison of cardioprotective benefits of vigorous versus moderate intensity aerobic exercise. Am J Cardiol. 2006;97(1):141–7.
24. Fraser GE, Strahan TM, Sabate J, Beeson WL, Kissinger D. Effects of traditional coronary risk factors on rates of incident coronary events in a low-risk population. The Adventist Health Study. Circulation. 1992;86:406–13.
25. Hakim AA, Curb JD, Petrovitch H, Rodriguez BL, Yano K, Ross GW, White LR, Abbott RD. Effects of walking on coronary heart disease in elderly men. The Honolulu Heart Program. Circulation. 1999;100:9–13.
26. Tanasescu M, Leitzmann MF, Rimm EB, Willett WC, Stamfer MJ, Hu FB. Exercise type and intensity in relation to coronary heart disease in men. JAMA. 2002;288:1994–2000.
27. Boekholdt SM, Sandhu MS, Day NE, Luben R, Bingham SA, Peters RJG, Wareham NJ, Khaw KT. Physical activity, C-reactive protein levels and the risk of future coronary artery disease in apparently healthy men and women: the EPIC-Norfolk prospective population study. Eur J Cardiovasc Prev Rehabil. 2006;13:970–6.
28. Hu G, Tuomilehto J, Borodulin K, Jousilahti P. The joint associations of occupational, commuting, and leisure-time physical activity, and the Framingham risk score on the 10-year risk of coronary heart disease. Eur Heart J. 2007;28:492–8.

29. Bell EJ, Lutsey PL, Windham BG, Folsom AR. Physical activity and cardiovascular disease in African Americans in Atherosclerosis Risk in Communities. Med Sci Sports Exerc. 2013;45:901–7.
30. Lee IM, Rexrode KM, Cook NR, Manson JM, Buring JE. Physical activity and coronary heart disease in women. JAMA. 2001;285:1447–54.
31. Akesson A, Weismayer C, Newby PK, Wolk A. Combined effect of low-risk dietary and lifestyle behaviors in primary prevention of myocardial infarction in women. Arch Intern Med. 2007;167:2122–7.
32. Chomistek AK, Henschel B, Eliassen AH, Mukamal KJ, Rimm EB. Frequency, type, and volume of leisure-time physical activity and risk of coronary heart disease in young women. Circulation. 2016;134:290–9.
33. Kannel WB, Sorlie P. Some health benefits of physical activity. The Framingham Study. Arch Intern Med. 1979;139(8):857–61.
34. Sherman SE, D'Agostino RB, Cobb JL, Kannel WB. Physical activity and mortality in women in the Framingham Heart Study. Am Heart J. 1994;128(5):879–84.
35. Weller I, Corey P. The impact of excluding non-leisure energy expenditure on the relation between physical activity and mortality in women. Epidemiology. 1998;9(6):632–5.
36. LaMonte MJ, Ainsworth BE. Quantifying energy expenditure and physical activity in the context of dose response. Med Sci Sports Exerc. 2001;33(6 Suppl):S370–8.
37. Manson JE, Hu FB, Rich-Edwards JW, Colditz GA, Stampfer MJ, Willett WC, et al. A prospective study of walking as compared with vigorous exercise in the prevention of coronary heart disease in women. N Engl J Med. 1999;341(9):650–8.
38. Manson JE, Greenland P, LaCroix AZ, Stefanick ML, Mouton CP, Oberman A, et al. Walking compared with vigorous exercise for the prevention of cardiovascular events in women. N Engl J Med. 2002;347:716–25.
39. Peters RK, Cady LD Jr, Bischoff DP, Bernstein L, Pike MC. Physical fitness and subsequent myocardial infarction in healthy workers. JAMA. 1983;249(22):3052–6.
40. Slattery ML, Jacobs DR Jr. Physical fitness and cardiovascular disease mortality. The US Railroad Study. Am J Epidemiol. 1988;127(3):571–80.
41. Blair SN, Kampert JB, Kohl HW 3rd, Barlow CE, Macera CA, Paffenbarger RS Jr, et al. Influences of cardiorespiratory fitness and other precursors on cardiovascular disease and all-cause mortality in men and women. JAMA. 1996;276(3):205–10.
42. Roger VL, Jacobsen SJ, Pellikka PA, Miller TD, Bailey KR, Gersh BJ. Prognostic value of treadmill exercise testing: a population-based study in Olmsted County, Minnesota. Circulation. 1998;98(25):2836–41.
43. Balady GJ, Larson MG, Vasan RS, Leip EP, O'Donnell CJ, Levy D. Usefulness of exercise testing in the prediction of coronary disease risk among asymptomatic persons as a function of the Framingham risk score. Circulation. 2004;110(14):1920–5.
44. Gulati M, Pandey DK, Arnsdorf MF, Lauderdale DS, Thisted RA, Wicklund RH, et al. Exercise capacity and the risk of death in women: the St James Women Take Heart Project. Circulation. 2003;108(13):1554–9.
45. Blair SN, Kohl HW 3rd, Paffenbarger RS Jr, Clark DG, Cooper KH, Gibbons LW. Physical fitness and all-cause mortality. A prospective study of healthy men and women. JAMA. 1989;262(17):2395–401.
46. Khan H, Jaffar N, Rauramaa R, Kurl S, Savonen K, Laukkanen JA. Cardiorespiratory fitness and nonfatal cardiovascular events: a population-based follow-up study. Am Heart J. 2017;184:55–61.
47. Laukkanen JA, Kurl S, Salonen R, Rauramaa R, Salonen JT. The predictive value of cardiorespiratory fitness for cardiovascular events in men with various risk profiles: a prospective population-based cohort study. Eur Heart J. 2004;25(16):1428–37.
48. Rywik TM, O'Connor FC, Gittings NS, Wright JG, Khan AA, Fleg JL. Role of nondiagnostic exercise-induced ST-segment abnormalities in predicting future coronary events in asymptomatic volunteers. Circulation. 2002;106(22):2787–92.
49. Grundy SM. Primary prevention of coronary heart disease: integrating risk assessment with intervention. Circulation. 1999;100(9):988–98.
50. Hopkins PN, Williams RR. Identification and relative weight of cardiovascular risk factors. Cardiol Clin. 1986;4(1):3–31.
51. Broekhuizen LN, Boekholdt SM, Arsenault BJ, Despres JP, Stroes ES, Kastelein JJ, et al. Physical activity, metabolic syndrome, and coronary risk: the EPIC-Norfolk prospective population study. Eur J Cardiovasc Prev Rehabil. 2011;18(2):209–17.
52. Hu FB, Stampfer MJ, Solomon C, Liu S, Colditz GA, Speizer FE, et al. Physical activity and risk for cardiovascular events in diabetic women. Ann Intern Med. 2001;134(2):96–105.
53. Sui X, LaMonte MJ, Blair SN. Cardiorespiratory fitness and risk of nonfatal cardiovascular disease in women and men with hypertension. Am J Hypertens. 2007;20(6):608–15.
54. Sui X, LaMonte MJ, Laditka JN, Hardin JW, Chase N, Hooker SP, et al. Cardiorespiratory fitness and adiposity as mortality predictors in older adults. JAMA. 2007;298(21):2507–16.
55. Weinstein AR, Sesso HD, Lee IM, Rexrode KM, Cook NR, Manson JE, et al. The joint effects of physical activity and body mass index on coronary heart disease risk in women. Arch Intern Med. 2008;168(8):884–90.
56. Petersen CB, Gronbaek M, Helge JW, Thygesen LC, Schnohr P, Tolstrup JS. Changes in physical activity in leisure time and the risk of myocardial infarction, ischemic heart disease, and all-cause mortality. Eur J Epidemiol. 2012;27(2):91–9.
57. Wannamethee SG, Shaper AG, Walker M. Changes in physical activity, mortality, and incidence of coronary heart disease in older men. Lancet. 1998;351(9116):1603–8.

58. Blair SN, Cooper KH, Gibbons LW, Gettman LR, Lewis S, Goodyear N. Changes in coronary heart disease risk factors associated with increased treadmill time in 753 men. Am J Epidemiol. 1983;118(3):352–9.
59. Blair SN, Kohl HW 3rd, Barlow CE, Paffenbarger RS Jr, Gibbons LW, Macera CA. Changes in physical fitness and all-cause mortality. A prospective study of healthy and unhealthy men. JAMA. 1995;273(14):1093–8.
60. Talbot LA, Morrell CH, Metter EJ, Fleg JL. Comparison of cardiorespiratory fitness versus leisure time physical activity as predictors of coronary events in men aged < or = 65 years and > 65 years. Am J Cardiol. 2002;89(10):1187–92.
61. Carlsson S, Andersson T, Lichtenstein P, Michaelsson K, Ahlbom A. Physical activity and mortality: is the association explained by genetic selection? Am J Epidemiol. 2007;166(3):255–9.
62. Chomistek AK, Chasman DI, Cook NR, Rimm EB, Lee IM. Physical activity, genes for physical fitness, and risk of coronary heart disease. Med Sci Sports Exerc. 2013;45(4):691–7.
63. Thompson PD, Buchner D, Pina IL, Balady GJ, Williams MA, Marcus BH, et al. Exercise and physical activity in the prevention and treatment of atherosclerotic cardiovascular disease: a statement from the Council on Clinical Cardiology (Subcommittee on Exercise, Rehabilitation, and Prevention) and the Council on Nutrition, Physical Activity, and Metabolism (Subcommittee on Physical Activity). Circulation. 2003;107(24):3109–16.
64. Di Valentino M, Maeder MT, Jaggi S, Schumann J, Sommerfeld K, Piazzalonga S, et al. Prognostic value of cycle exercise testing prior to and after outpatient cardiac rehabilitation. Int J Cardiol. 2010;140(1):34–41.
65. Mons U, Hahmann H, Brenner H. A reverse J-shaped association of leisure time physical activity with prognosis in patients with stable coronary heart disease: evidence from a large cohort with repeated measurements. Heart. 2014;100(13):1043–9.
66. Rengo G, Galasso G, Piscione F, Golino L, Fortunato F, Zincarelli C, et al. An active lifestyle improves outcome of primary angioplasty in elderly patients with acute myocardial infarction. Am Heart J. 2007;154(2):352–60.
67. Steffen-Batey L, Nichaman MZ, Goff DC Jr, Frankowski RF, Hanis CL, Ramsey DJ, et al. Change in level of physical activity and risk of all-cause mortality or reinfarction: the Corpus Christi Heart Project. Circulation. 2000;102(18):2204–9.
68. Dutcher JR, Kahn J, Grines C, Franklin B. Comparison of left ventricular ejection fraction and exercise capacity as predictors of two- and five-year mortality following acute myocardial infarction. Am J Cardiol. 2007;99(4):436–41.
69. Gorczyca AM, Eaton CB, LaMonte MJ, Manson JE, Johnston JD, Bidulescu A, et al. Change in physical activity and sitting time after myocardial infarction and mortality among postmenopausal women in the Women's Health Initiative-Observational Study. J Am Heart Assoc. 2017;6(5):e005354.
70. Kavanagh T, Mertens DJ, Hamm LF, Beyene J, Kennedy J, Corey P, et al. Prediction of long-term prognosis in 12 169 men referred for cardiac rehabilitation. Circulation. 2002;106(6):666–71.
71. Kavanagh T, Mertens DJ, Hamm LF, Beyene J, Kennedy J, Corey P, et al. Peak oxygen intake and cardiac mortality in women referred for cardiac rehabilitation. J Am Coll Cardiol. 2003;42(12): 2139–43.
72. Keteyian SJ, Brawner CA, Savage PD, Ehrman JK, Schairer J, Divine G, et al. Peak aerobic capacity predicts prognosis in patients with coronary heart disease. Am Heart J. 2008;156(2):292–300.
73. Myers J, Prakash M, Froelicher V, Do D, Partington S, Atwood JE. Exercise capacity and mortality among men referred for exercise testing. N Engl J Med. 2002;346(11):793–801.
74. Whooley MA, de Jonge P, Vittinghoff E, Otte C, Moos R, Carney RM, et al. Depressive symptoms, health behaviors, and risk of cardiovascular events in patients with coronary heart disease. JAMA. 2008;300(20):2379–88.
75. Bouchard C, Shephard RJ, Stephens T, editors. Physical activity, fitness, and health: international proceedings and consensus statement. Champaign: Human Kinetics; 1994.
76. Kasapis C, Thompson PD. The effects of physical activity on serum C-reactive protein and inflammatory markers: a systematic review. J Am Coll Cardiol. 2005;45(10):1563–9.
77. Kesaniemi YK, Danforth E Jr, Jensen MD, Kopelman PG, Lefebvre P, Reeder BA. Dose-response issues concerning physical activity and health: an evidence-based symposium. Med Sci Sports Exerc. 2001;33(6 Suppl):S351–8.
78. Wing RR, Bolin P, Brancati FL, Bray GA, Clark JM, et al. Cardiovascular effects of intensive lifestyle intervention in type 2 diabetes. N Engl J Med. 2013;369(2):145–54.
79. ClinicalTrials.gov. Women's Health Initiative Strong and Healthy study (WHISH). Identifier: NCT02425345. 2018. https://clinicaltrials.gov/ct2/show/NCT02425345. Accessed 6 April 2018.
80. Shaw LW. Effects of a prescribed supervised exercise program on mortality and cardiovascular morbidity in patients after myocardial infarction. The National Exercise and Heart Disease Project. Am J Cardiol. 1981;48(1):39–46.
81. Anderson L, Oldridge N, Thompson DR, Zwisler AD, Rees K, Martin N, et al. Exercise-based cardiac rehabilitation for coronary heart disease: cochrane systematic review and meta-analysis. J Am Coll Cardiol. 2016;67(1):1–12.
82. Hambrecht R, Walther C, Mobius-Winkler S, Gielen S, Linke A, Conradi K, et al. Percutaneous coronary angioplasty compared with exercise training in patients with stable coronary artery disease: a randomized trial. Circulation. 2004;109(11):1371–8.

83. Walther C, Mobius-Winkler S, Linke A, Bruegel M, Thiery J, Schuler G, et al. Regular exercise training compared with percutaneous intervention leads to a reduction of inflammatory markers and cardiovascular events in patients with coronary artery disease. Eur J Cardiovasc Prev Rehabil. 2008;15(1):107–12.
84. Powell KE, Thompson PD, Caspersen CJ, Kendrick JS. Physical activity and the incidence of coronary heart disease. Annu Rev Public Health. 1987;8:253–87.
85. Wildman RP, Schott LL, Brockwell S, Kuller LH, Sutton-Tyrrell K. A dietary and exercise intervention slows menopause-associated progression of subclinical atherosclerosis as measured by intima-media thickness of the carotid arteries. J Am Coll Cardiol. 2004;44(3):579–85.
86. Hambrecht R, Niebauer J, Marburger C, Grunze M, Kalberer B, Hauer K, et al. Various intensities of leisure time physical activity in patients with coronary artery disease: effects on cardiorespiratory fitness and progression of coronary atherosclerotic lesions. J Am Coll Cardiol. 1993;22(2):468–77.
87. Dor-Haim H, Lotan C, Horowitz M, Swissa M. Intensive exercise training improves cardiac electrical stability in myocardial-infarcted rats. J Am Heart Assoc. 2017;6(7):e005989.
88. Thijssen DHJ, Redington A, George KP, Hopman MTE, Jones H. Association of exercise preconditioning with immediate cardioprotection: a review. JAMA Cardiol. 2018;3(2):169–76.
89. Rabkin SW, Campbell H. Comparison of reducing epicardial fat by exercise, diet or bariatric surgery weight loss strategies: a systematic review and meta-analysis. Obes Rev. 2015;16(5):406–15.
90. Shadyab AH, LaMonte MJ, Kooperberg C, Reiner AP, Carty CL, Manini TM, et al. Association of accelerometer-measured physical activity with leukocyte telomere length among older women. J Gerontol. 2017;72(11):1532–7.
91. McCarthy JJ. microRNA and skeletal muscle function: novel potential roles in exercise, diseases, and aging. Front Physiol. 2014;5:290.
92. Hambrecht R, Adams V, Erbs S, Linke A, Krankel N, Shu Y, et al. Regular physical activity improves endothelial function in patients with coronary artery disease by increasing phosphorylation of endothelial nitric oxide synthase. Circulation. 2003;107(25):3152–8.
93. Hambrecht R, Wolf A, Gielen S, Linke A, Hofer J, Erbs S, et al. Effect of exercise on coronary endothelial function in patients with coronary artery disease. N Engl J Med. 2000;342(7):454–60.
94. Mobius-Winkler S, Uhlemann M, Adams V, Sandri M, Erbs S, Lenk K, et al. Coronary collateral growth induced by physical exercise: results of the impact of intensive exercise training on coronary collateral circulation in patients with stable coronary artery disease (EXCITE) trial. Circulation. 2016;133(15):1438–48. discussion 48
95. LaMonte MJ, Buchner DM, Rillamas-Sun E, Di C, Evenson KR, Bellettiere J, et al. Accelerometer-measured physical activity and mortality in women aged 63 to 99. J Am Geriatr Soc. 2017;66:886–94.
96. LaMonte MJ, Lewis CE, Buchner DM, Evenson KR, Rillamas-Sun E, Di C, et al. Both light intensity and moderate-to-vigorous physical activity measured by accelerometry are favorably associated with cardiometabolic risk factors in older women: the objective physical activity and cardiovascular health (OPACH) study. J Am Heart Assoc. 2017;6(10):e007064.
97. Rose G. Sick individuals and sick populations. Int J Epidemiol. 1985;14(1):32–8.
98. Cook NR, Cohen J, Hebert PR, Taylor JO, Hennekens CH. Implications of small reductions in diastolic blood pressure for primary prevention. Arch Intern Med. 1995;155(7):701–9.
99. Pennant M, Davenport C, Bayliss S, Greenheld W, Marshall T, Hyde C. Community programs for the prevention of cardiovascular disease: a systematic review. Am J Epidemiol. 2010;172(5):501–16.
100. Eaton CB, Lapane KL, Garber CE, Gans KM, Lasater TM, Carleton RA. Effects of a community-based intervention on physical activity: the Pawtucket Heart Health Program. Am J Public Health. 1999;89(11):1741–4.
101. Lloyd-Jones DM, Hong Y, Labarthe D, Mozaffarian D, Appel LJ, Van Horn L, et al. Defining and setting national goals for cardiovascular health promotion and disease reduction: the American Heart Association's strategic impact goal through 2020 and beyond. Circulation. 2010;121(4):586–613.
102. Pearson TA, Palaniappan LP, Artinian NT, Carnethon MR, Criqui MH, Daniels SR, et al. American Heart Association guide for improving cardiovascular health at the community level, 2013 update: a scientific statement for public health practitioners, healthcare providers, and health policy makers. Circulation. 2013;127(16):1730–53.
103. Ford ES, Capewell S. Coronary heart disease mortality among young adults in the U.S. from 1980 through 2002: concealed leveling of mortality rates. J Am Coll Cardiol. 2007;50(22):2128–32.
104. Greenland P. Cardiovascular guideline skepticism vs lifestyle realism? JAMA. 2018;319(2):117–8.
105. Anand SS, Islam S, Rosengren A, Franzosi MG, Steyn K, Yusufali AH, et al. Risk factors for myocardial infarction in women and men: insights from the INTERHEART study. Eur Heart J. 2008;29(7):932–40.

Physical Activity and Cardiorespiratory Fitness in Heart Failure

18

Jonathan Myers and Peter Kokkinos

Introduction

Historically, recommendations for physical activity in patients with heart failure (HF) have evolved differently than other chronic conditions. Prior to the 1980s, patients with HF were discouraged from participating in exercise programs due to concerns regarding safety and the potential for harm to an already damaged myocardium [1, 2]. However, studies performed over the last three decades have provided extensive insights into both the health outcome benefits of exercise training and the physiological mechanisms underlying these benefits. Studies on the outcome benefits of exercise-based rehabilitation, including mortality and hospitalization, have been consistent and convincing, and these studies recently led to the US Centers for Medicare and Medicaid Services approval for coverage of cardiac rehabilitation for patients with HF with reduced ejection fraction (HFrEF). The landmark HF-ACTION trial [3], among others, has had a major impact on our understanding of the effects of exercise training on health outcomes in patients with HF. This knowledge has provided insight not only into the benefits of exercise training in HF but has also provided a clearer understanding of the dose-response relationship between the volume of exercise performed and clinical outcomes as well as the cost-effectiveness of training in HF. Systematic reviews and meta-analyses have provided strong evidence that exercise-based rehabilitation is associated with clinically significant reductions in hospitalizations and improvements in health-related quality of life among patients with HF. This chapter will provide an overview of evidence related to exercise training in HF, including the impact of cardiorespiratory fitness (CRF) in HF, the epidemiologic sequelae of rehabilitation programs, mechanisms underlying benefits of training in HF, public health implications, and recommendations for future research.

J. Myers (✉)
Department of Cardiology, VA Palo Alto Health Care System/Stanford University, Palo Alto, CA, USA

P. Kokkinos (✉)
Veterans Affairs Medical Center, Department of Cardiology, Washington, DC, USA

Georgetown University School of Medicine, Washington, DC, USA

Department of Kinesiology and Health, Rutgers University, New Brunswick, NJ, USA

George Washington University School of Medicine and Health Sciences, Washington, DC, USA

University of South Carolina, Department of Exercise Science, Arnold School of Public Health, Columbia, SC, USA
e-mail: peter.kokkinos@va.gov

P. Kokkinos, P. Narayan (eds.), *Cardiorespiratory Fitness in Cardiometabolic Diseases*,
https://doi.org/10.1007/978-3-030-04816-7_18

Epidemiologic Perspective on Cardiorespiratory Fitness in Heart Failure

The measurement of CRF has probably had a greater clinical impact in patients with HF than any other condition. The application of direct measures of fitness using cardiopulmonary exercise testing (CPX) during the last 25 years in patients with HF has evolved as an important metric for stratifying risk in HF guidelines [4–6]. Directly measured maximal oxygen uptake, typically expressed as peak VO_2 normalized for body weight (ml O_2•kg^{-1}•min^{-1}), is generally considered to be the measurement that defines the limits of the cardiopulmonary system [7]. Peak VO_2 and other cardiopulmonary exercise test responses have been widely applied in recent years to estimate risk in patients with HF [4–6]. In 1991, Mancini and colleagues published an influential study on the value of peak VO_2 for estimating risk in patients with advanced HF [8]. In a sample of 114 candidates for transplantation, they observed that patients achieving a peak $VO_2 \leq 14$ ml O_2•kg^{-1}•min^{-1} had an extremely poor prognosis (survival rates of 47% and 32% at 1 and 2 years, respectively), while those achieving >14 ml O_2•kg^{-1}•min^{-1} had survival rates similar to patients who received a transplant (94% and 84% at 1 and 2 years, respectively). This study was significant in that it provided a springboard for numerous subsequent studies that further defined the role of cardiopulmonary exercise testing (CRF in particular) in the management of patients with HF. During the 1990s, peak VO_2 became recognized as a reliable prognostic marker, particularly for the timing of cardiac transplantation in advanced HF caused by systolic dysfunction [8–14]. Over the last two decades, numerous editions of HF guidelines and scientific statements have incorporated CRF, expressed as peak VO_2, as part of risk stratification strategies in patients with HF [4, 6, 15, 16]. Because of the many studies documenting its prognostic utility, exercise capacity measured using CPX techniques has become the benchmark for both primary and intermediary outcomes in clinical trials undergoing evaluation by regulatory agencies in HF [4, 6, 15, 16].

Exercise Intervention in Heart Failure

Prior to the 1990s, patients with left ventricular dysfunction were thought to be poor candidates for exercise programs. This was out of concern for safety and the general thinking that they were unable to benefit from training. This has been dispelled, however, by numerous studies that have been published over the last three decades [2]. Today it is recognized that patients with CHF derive considerable benefits from regular exercise. This is important for patients with HF in particular because while the incidence of cardiovascular disease in general has declined in recent decades, there has been an increase in the incidence of HF. This increase is due to the better survival after a myocardial infarction, improvements in therapy (i.e., thrombolytics, ACE inhibitors, beta-blockers, resynchronization therapy), and aging of the population. Therefore, many more patients with HF are available as candidates for rehabilitation programs. As a result of the many studies showing physiologic, quality of life, and outcome benefits of rehabilitation programs for patients with HF, the Centers for Medicare and Medicaid Services (CMS) recently approved coverage for rehabilitation for patients with HFrEF. Although the referral rate of patients with HF to rehabilitation programs remains poor [17–19], CMS reimbursement will undoubtedly bring many more of these patients to rehabilitation programs going forward.

Concerns regarding the effects of training on the hearts of patients with reduced ventricular function after an infarction were intensified in 1988 with the publication of a study from a Canadian group. Judgutt and coworkers [20] studied 13 patients with anterior Q-wave MIs using echocardiography before and after the supervised low-level exercise training. They found that patients with evidence of greater left ventricular asynergy (akinesis or dykinesis) at baseline had more detrimental ventricular shape distortion, with expansion and thinning of their left ventricle after exercise training. This was thought to be secondary to remodeling of an incompletely healed infarct zone. These provocative observations were supported by several animal studies published in the early 1990s, some of which demonstrated severe global left ventricular dilation, left ventricular shape distortion, and scar thinning after periods of training [21–23]. Indeed, while cardiac rehabilitation burgeoned as a therapeutic modality among patients with CAD, guidelines recommended continued bed rest or limited activity for patients with HF in the 1970s and into the 1980s [24–27].

However, subsequent controlled trials among humans did not confirm the concept that exercise training led to further myocardial damage [28–35]. Giannuzzi and colleagues [26] completed a multicenter controlled trial of exercise training in Italy. After 1 year, patients in both the trained and control groups whose ejection fractions were ≤40% demonstrated some degree of additional global and regional dilation. Importantly, however, training had no effect on this response, and there was no effect in either group among patients with ejection fractions >40%. These investigators also completed a larger randomized trial in patients with left ventricular dysfunction after a myocardial infarction [30]. After 6 months, patients in the control group demonstrated increases in both end-systolic and end-diastolic volumes and a worsening in both wall motion abnormalities and regional dilation relative to patients in the exercise group. The latter study was the first to suggest that an exercise program may actually attenuate abnormal remodeling in patients with reduced ventricular function. Novel data from Switzerland in the 1990s employing magnetic resonance imaging (MRI) confirmed that exercise training in patients with reduced left ventricular function following an MI was effective in improving exercise capacity [28] and did not cause further myocardial damage (i.e., wall thinning, infarct expansion, changes in ejection fraction, or increases in ventricular volumes). Longer-term studies confirmed that there were no adverse changes in myocardial remodeling measured using MRI [31], and numerous subsequent studies from the United States and Europe have documented that training does not lead to further myocardial damage in patients with HF [32–36]. Exercise training is now recognized as a useful adjunct to medical therapy in these patients, widely recommended by national and international guidelines on HF [37–40].

Mechanisms of Benefit with Exercise Training in Heart Failure

Studies suggest that the major physiologic benefit from training in CHF occurs in the skeletal muscle rather than in the heart itself [35, 37–41]. Extensive analyses have been performed on the effects of training on central hemodynamics, peripheral blood flow, myocardial remodeling after an MI using echocardiographic and MRI techniques, and skeletal muscle metabolism [28–44]. These studies are nearly universal in their demonstration that training has beneficial effects on these systems. In addition, the rather extensive experience with training in CHF patients now available in the literature has been associated with improved morbidity and mortality (discussed below). Numerous studies have demonstrated improvements in symptoms, and the majority of studies have documented improvements in quality of life [37, 38, 42–46].

Potential mechanisms by which exercise training may improve exercise capacity and improve outcomes in HF are outlined in Table 18.1. Importantly, the extent to which one or a combination of these mechanisms may affect an individual patient's exercise tolerance varies considerably. Peak oxygen consumption (VO_2) is strongly related to prognosis in patients with HF, and exercise training generally improves peak VO_2 in the range of 10–25% [37, 38]. However, even small changes in peak VO_2 are associated with significantly improved outcomes [47]. Numerous central and peripheral factors influence peak VO_2, but increases in peak VO_2 and related benefits from training are fundamentally related to the combination of an improvement in peak cardiac output, improved vascular reactivity, better utilization of oxygen through metabolic changes in the skeletal muscle, and more efficient ventilation. These mechanisms are outlined in the following.

Table 18.1 Potential mechanisms by which exercise training improves outcomes

System	Response to training	Effect on outcomes
Cardiac function	Increased cardiac output Increase or no change in contractility Increased peak VO_2 Improved ventilatory efficiency	Increased exercise capacity Improved quality of life Reduced mortality Reduced hospitalizations
Regional blood flow	Increased vasodilatory capacity Improved endothelial function Improved redistribution of flow	Increased exercise capacity
Skeletal muscle	Increased aerobic enzymes Increased mitochondrial volume and density Increased capillary density Decreased muscle receptor sensitivity	Increased exercise capacity Improved physical function Reduced ventilatory response Reduced mortality
Autonomic nervous system	Decrease in plasma norepinephrine Increased heart rate variability Reduced chemo- and ergoreceptor sensitivity Reduced ventilatory response	Reduced cardiac rhythm disturbances Reduced or no change in mortality

Central Adaptations As mentioned above, a general consensus exists that the benefits of exercise training in patients with HF are due largely to adaptations in the peripheral vasculature and skeletal muscle rather than the heart itself [37, 38, 48, 49]. Although the focus of these studies has been on patients with HFrEF, this also appears to be the case among patients with HF with preserved EF (HFpEF) [49, 50]. This consensus evolved in part due to the recognition that EF is poorly correlated with exercise capacity [37, 38, 41]. However, while the preponderance of studies has reported that EF and other measures of contractility show minimal change following training, a number of studies have reported significant improvements in these indices [34, 51–53]. The majority of studies have focused on resting EF, and less is known regarding indices of contractility during exercise. Because of the difficulty measuring cardiac output directly, it has not been widely reported, but studies using thermodilution techniques have reported increases in maximal cardiac output following training in the range of 5–20% [54]. A meta-analysis of 104 patients reported a mean increase in maximal cardiac output of 2.5 L/min, corresponding to a 21% increase [42]. Whether this increase in cardiac output is a result of increases in maximal heart rate or stroke volume is unclear; studies have reported small improvements in both indices as well as no change [54]. When changes in maximal cardiac output do occur, they have been attributed to some combination of small changes in peak heart rate, stroke volume, and afterload reduction (due to enhanced endothelial-dependent vasodilation) [37, 38, 52–55].

Vascular Adaptations Numerous recent studies have characterized abnormal endothelial function in HF, and favorable adaptations in endothelial function have been consistently reported after rehabilitation programs [38, 52, 56, 57]. Exercise training decreases circulating catecholamine levels in patients with HF, has anti-inflammatory and antioxidative effects, reduces natriuretic peptide concentrations, and increases shear stress and nitric oxide bioavailability [56–61], all leading to reduced peripheral vasoconstriction, improved endothelial function, and enhanced endothelial repair [55, 57, 62, 63]. These adaptations result in better skeletal muscle perfusion during exercise. There have been dozens of such studies over the last two decades; the volume of work by Hambrecht and colleagues is particularly notable [63]. They reported that a regimen using handgrip exercise training six times per day significantly improved endothelial-dependent vasodilation after 4 weeks in patients with HF; the effects of training were similar to those of the potent vasodilator L-arginine. Circulating progenitor cells, which have the ability to differentiate and exhibit endothelial properties and enhance endothelial function, increase following training in HF [29, 55, 58, 63]. Numerous studies have reported that changes in endothelium-dependent peripheral blood flow after training are paralleled by improvements in peak VO_2 [38, 57, 63].

Skeletal Muscle Adaptations Metabolic changes in the skeletal muscle with aerobic training include increases in aerobic enzymes, increases in mitochondrial size and density, and increases in capillary density [37, 38, 56–60]. Muscle biopsy studies have demonstrated shifts from type II to type I muscle fibers after training [39]. Cytochrome c oxidase-positive mitochondria, an important rate-limiting enzyme in oxidative phosphorylation, was demonstrated to increase 41% after 6 months of training [40]. ^{31}P MRI spectroscopy has been used to document abnormalities in skeletal muscle metabolism in HF, including early intracellular acidification, accumulation of inorganic phosphate (Pi), accelerated utilization of phosphocreatine (PCr), and delayed PCr regeneration during recovery from exercise [64–68]. Exercise training has been demonstrated to partially reverse these abnormalities in oxidative metabolism measured by MRI and near-infrared spectroscopy techniques, including a slower increase in Pi, a decline in phosphocreatine, a decrease in Pi/CP versus power output, and faster recovery of O_2 stores after exercise [69, 70]. Regular exercise also reduces muscle wasting and helps restore the anabolic/catabolic imbalance that is common in HF [71, 72].

Ventilatory Adaptations Ventilatory inefficiency has been demonstrated to be strongly associated with morbidity and mortality in HF; in fact, studies performed over the last 20 years have shown that markers of ventilatory inefficiency, such as the VE/VCO_2 slope and oxygen uptake efficiency slope (OUES), are more powerful predictors of risk for adverse outcomes than many clinical and cardiopulmonary exercise test responses in HF [3, 5, 12]. Application of these indices for the identification of high-risk patients has been recommended in recent guidelines on the evaluation and management of HF [4, 7, 73], and the influence of training on these indices is therefore important to document. Excessive ventilation in patients with HF has been associated with ventilation/perfusion mismatching due to impaired cardiac output responses to exercise, early lactate accumulation (which stimulates ventilation through the buffering of lactate), and chemo- and muscle receptor hyperactivity [4, 5, 12, 73]. Improvements in abnormal ventilation after training involve some combination of hemodynamic changes (reduced pulmonary pressures or improved ventilation-perfusion matching), metabolic changes reflected by a delay in lactate accumulation, a change in ventilatory control, and a change in the ventilatory pattern that makes breathing more efficient. Recent studies have reported that these indices respond favorably to training [74, 75]. In addition, a growing number of studies have demonstrated that specific training of the respiratory muscles results in improved ventilatory dynamics and exercise performance [76, 77]. Improvements in the ventilatory response to exercise are a critically important mechanism underlying the enhanced functional capabilities and outcomes following training in patients with HF.

Studies have also identified a pathophysiologic mechanism unique to HF that underlies abnormal ventilation and that responds favorably to training. This mechanism involves specific ventilatory signals arising from the exercising muscle which are abnormally enhanced in HF (termed an "ergoreflex" contribution to ventilation) [78, 79]. These signals have been demonstrated to contribute to the abnormal hemodynamic, autonomic, and ventilatory responses to exercise that characterize HF. Afferent fibers present in the skeletal muscle (ergoreceptors) are sensitive to metabolic changes that occur during muscular work. These receptors, which appear to mediate circulatory adaptations occurring in the early stages of exercise, are stimulated by metabolic acidosis and are partially responsible for sympathetic vasoconstriction [78–80]. It has also been demonstrated that hypoxic chemosensitivity is increased in HF and that this heightened chemosensitivity is correlated with the VE/VCO$_2$ slope. The results of these enhanced ergoreflex and chemoreceptor responses are hyperventilation and heightened sympathetic outflow, which cause an increase in peripheral resistance and thus a decrease in muscle perfusion. These muscle receptors are less sensitive to stimulation after training. It has been demonstrated that after a 6-week forearm training protocol, the ergoreflex contribution to exercise ventilation was reduced by 58% [80]. These salutary effects on ventilatory control are an additional mechanism by which outcomes are improved with regular exercise in HF.

Cardiorespiratory Fitness and Incidence of HF

Recent studies have reported that higher CRF reduces the incidence of HF. This is important because while advances in treatment have led to a decline in most cardiovascular diseases, marked growth in the prevalence of HF has occurred over the last three decades [81, 82]. The growing prevalence of HF reflects a combination of increasing incidence, an aging population, and improvements in the treatment of both acute CVD and HF [82]. Older Americans are currently hospitalized for HF more than any other medical condition, and with the aging of the population, the impact of HF is expected to increase dramatically [82, 83]. Therefore, strategies to reduce the incidence of HF have important public health implications, including the considerable impact of HF on health-care costs and disability.

Four recent studies have addressed the association between CRF and incidence of HF. Berry et al. [84] reported an approximate 3.5-fold higher rate of hospitalization for HF in the least fit quartile of subjects versus the highest fit quartile among >20,000 subjects from the Cooper Center Longitudinal Study (CCLS). Each 1-MET increment in fitness was associated with an ≈20% lower risk for HF hospitalization after the age of 65 years in men and women. Khan et al. [85] studied 1873 men without HF at baseline and followed them for a mean of 21 years. Each 1-MET increment in fitness was associated with a 21% multivariable-adjusted lower risk of HF. Pandey et al. [86] assessed >19,000 adults and observed that higher fitness in midlife was associated with a significantly lower risk of hospitalization due to HF during follow-up; each 1-MET higher fitness level was associated with an 18% reduction in risk for incidence of HF. In a subgroup of 8683 participants who underwent a second fitness examination a mean of 4.2 years after the initial examination, each 1-MET improvement in fitness was associated with a 17% reduction in HF risk. Echouffo-Tcheugui and colleagues [87] developed a composite risk estimate from these studies in a meta-analysis and reported a random effect model estimate of 21% lower risk of HF for each 1-MET higher fitness level.

Our group assessed CRF in 21,080 subjects who were free of HF at baseline at the Veterans Affairs Medical Centers in Washington, DC, and Palo Alto, CA [88]. Subjects were classified by age-specific quintiles of CRF [89]. Multivariable Cox models were used to determine the association between HF incidence and clinical and exercise test variables. Reclassification characteristics of fitness relative to standard clinical risk factors were determined using the category-free net reclassification improvement index (NRI). During a mean follow-up of 12.3 ± 7.4 years, 1902 subjects developed HF. When CRF was considered as a binary variable (unfit/fit), low fitness was the strongest predictor of risk for HF among clinical and exercise test variables, with unfit subjects having nearly double the risk for developing HF. In a fully adjusted model with the least fit group as the reference, there was a graded and progressive reduction in risk for HF as fitness level was higher. Risks for developing HF were 36%, 41%, 67%, and 76% lower among increasing quintiles of fitness compared to the least fit subjects (Fig. 18.1, $p < 0.001$). Adding CRF to standard risk factors resulted in an NRI of 0.37 ($p < 0.001$). The results from the Veterans Affairs group are in general agreement with the studies mentioned above in that each 1-MET higher fitness level was associated with a 19% reduction in future HF risk. Collectively, these observations underscore the message that small increments in

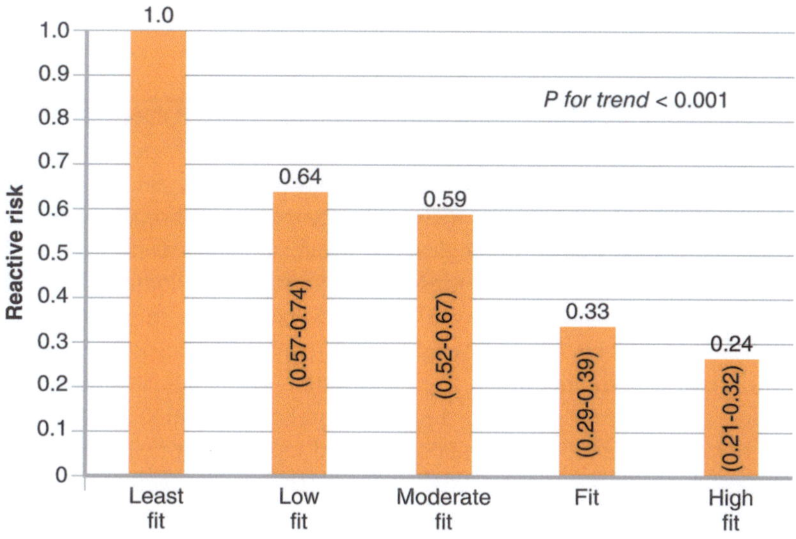

Fig. 18.1 Relative risks of heart failure incidence between quintiles of fitness, with the least fit group (<6 METs) as the referent group. Ninety-five percent confidence limits are in parentheses within each bar. *Adjusted for age, body mass index, ethnic origin, gender, β blockers, calcium channel blockers, angiotensin-converting enzymes, angiotensin receptor blockers, aspirin, diuretics, lipid-lowering agents, hypoglycemic agents, history of smoking, hypertension, diabetes mellitus, chronic kidney failure (stage < 4), and HIV/AIDS.* (Modified from Myers et al. [88])

exercise capacity yield considerable health outcome benefits in the context of HF prevention.

Potential Mechanisms for Lower HF Incidence Among Fitter Subjects There are a number of potential explanations for the lower HF incidence among more active or fitter subjects. Many of the risk factors for CAD and other forms of CVD are considered risk factors for HF, including hypertension, smoking, and diabetes. Individuals who are relatively fit have a lower risk factor burden when compared to those who are not fit [90, 91], and studies have generally observed lower fitness and a higher burden of chronic disease among individuals who develop HF. Fitter subjects have a marked attenuation in blood pressure trajectory with aging [92] which could potentially reduce the risk of future HF. Left ventricular compliance is reduced in older individuals, and this can contribute to the development of HF in the elderly [93, 94]. Elderly individuals who are physically active have higher ventricular compliance compared to sedentary individuals [93]. Brinker et al. [95] studied 2925 men and women from the Cooper Center Longitudinal Study and found that low fitness was associated with a higher prevalence of concentric remodeling and diastolic dysfunction, suggesting that regular exercise may lower HF risk through its favorable effects on cardiac remodeling and diastolic function. Regular exercise not only improves fitness but is associated with numerous other physiological benefits, including reduced blood pressure, improved insulin resistance, improved lipid profiles, and reduced obesity which collectively may contribute to a reduction in the incidence of HF. Endothelial dysfunction is associated with various forms of CVD, and favorable adaptations in endothelial function have been consistently reported after exercise training among individuals with and without HF [52, 96, 97].

Exercise Training and Clinical Outcomes in HF

In addition to studies on the physiologic effects of exercise training in HF, a growing number of studies have followed patients for long-term outcomes after exercise training programs. These studies have consistently shown that outcomes are improved among HF patients who have been randomized to exercise therapy compared to usual care. These analyses were influential in the recent US Centers for Medicare and Medicaid Services approval of coverage for phase 2 cardiac rehabilitation for Medicare beneficiaries with HFrEF. Beginning in the 1980s, numerous single-center studies were performed documenting improvements in exercise tolerance, quality of life, and other physiological benefits following various periods of exercise training [37, 38]. However, adoption of exercise training for patients with HF in clinical practice was limited due to lack of Medicare reimbursement, small sample sizes of the available trials, the lack of data from large multicenter trials, and limited data on safety.

The most ambitious effort to address these gaps in the literature was the Heart Failure: A Controlled Trial Investigating Outcomes of Exercise Training (HF-ACTION) study, designed and funded by the US National Heart, Lung, and Blood Institute (NHLBI). Investigators randomized 2331 patients with HFrEF to endurance exercise training or usual care [98]. Patients randomized to exercise participated in 3 months of supervised exercise training (3 days per week) and transitioned from supervised exercise to 5 days per week of home-based exercise training. Patients were provided a heart rate monitor to guide exercise intensity and a leg ergometer or treadmill for their home. Patients in the usual care group were provided secondary prevention education, including information on the importance of regular physical activity. Both groups were contacted every 2–4 weeks. The primary outcome was the composite endpoint of incident all-cause mortality or all-cause hospitalization.

The HF-ACTION investigators randomized patients from 82 sites in the United States, Canada, and France. In an intent-to-treat analysis, exercise training was associated with an 11% lower adjusted risk for all-cause mortality or hospitalization and a 15% lower adjusted risk for incidence of cardiovascular-related mortality or heart failure hospitalization. This effect was seen in spite of significant crossover between groups (22–28% of the patients in the usual care group self-reported regular exercise participation) and the fact that only 30% of the patients in the exercise group achieved the goal of 120 min per week of exercise. In a secondary analysis from HF-ACTION, Keteyian et al. [99] examined the dose-response relationship between the volume of exercise performed and clinical outcomes among patients randomized to the exercise group. An inverse relationship was observed between the volume of exercise performed (expressed as MET/hours) and adjusted risk for all-cause mortality or hospitalization as well as cardiovascular-related mortality or heart failure hospitalization. The lowest risk for both outcomes was observed among patients who performed 3–5 MET/h per week and 5–7 MET/h per week of exercise (>30% reduced risk) compared to patients who remained sedentary. A further secondary analysis from HF-ACTION suggested that, similar to patients with coronary artery disease, relatively small changes in fitness can have a significant impact on health outcomes in patients with HF. Swank et al. [47] studied 1620 participants enrolled in HF-ACTION at baseline and 3 months later and followed the subjects for all-cause and cardiovascular hospitalization and cardiovascular and all-cause mortality. They observed that every 6% increase in peak VO_2 (approximately 1 ml/kg/min), adjusted for other significant predictors, was associated with a 5% lower risk of all-cause mortality or hospitalization, a 4% lower risk of time to cardiovascular mortality or cardiovascular hospitalization, an 8% lower risk of cardiovascular mortality or heart failure hospitalization, and a 7% lower all-cause mortality.

Meta-Analyses Single-center trials have rarely been large enough to gain much insight into long-term health outcome benefits following exercise training in HF, but numerous meta-analyses over the last 10–15 years have been a major advance in this area. Among the first meta-analyses to focus on HF was the Exercise Training for Chronic Heart Failure (ExTraMatch) Collaborative group analysis in 2004 [100]. Combining 9 randomized controlled trials among 801 patients followed for a mean of

≈2 years, a 35% reduction in all-cause mortality and a 28% reduction in death or hospitalization were observed among subjects randomized to exercise training. In a follow-up analysis of the ExTraMatch Collaborative that included 23 randomized trials and >4000 patients, those randomized to exercise intervention had an 18% lower risk of all-cause mortality and an 11% reduced risk of hospitalization compared to usual care subjects [101].

In a recent review and meta-analysis using the Cochrane Library database, 33 randomized controlled trials and 4740 patients were included, largely with HFrEF [102]. All trials included a cardiopulmonary exercise training intervention, and in 11 of the studies, aerobic training was complemented by resistance training. Exercise training was delivered in either an exclusively center-based setting or a center-based setting in combination with home exercise sessions. Although there was no significant difference in pooled mortality up to 12-month follow-up between the exercise training and control groups, there was a trend toward a reduction in all-cause mortality when pooled across the longest follow-up point of the trials with more than 12-month follow-up. In addition, significant reductions were observed in both overall and heart failure-specific hospital admissions with exercise compared to control up to 12-month follow-up (15 trials, fixed-effect RR 0.75, 95% CI 0.62–0.92; $p = 0.005$) (Fig. 18.2a–c). Quality of life was determined using a variety of instruments, including the HF-specific Minnesota Living with Heart Failure Questionnaire and the Kansas City Cardiomyopathy Questionnaire, along with generic health-related quality of life tools including the EuroQoL, Short Form 36, Psychological General Well-Being Index, Patient's Global Assessment and improving quality of life, and Spritzer's Quality of Life Index. Across the 13 studies reporting the total Minnesota Living with Heart Failure Questionnaire score up to 12 months follow-up, there was a clinically important improvement among subjects randomized to exercise training compared to usual care. Pooling across all studies, regardless of outcome measure used, there was a significant improvement in quality of life with exercise training. Notably, a number of studies have observed improvements in quality of life without an improvement in exercise capacity [103, 104], suggesting that there are factors other than physiologic changes that may contribute to quality of life with exercise training.

Taken together, these results strongly support the concept that exercise intervention reduces mortality in HF, particularly in the longer term (>12 months) [102]. In addition, training programs appear to have consistent benefits in terms of reducing hospitalization and quality of life [105–107]. Home-based intervention appears to be similar to center-based exercise programs in terms of CRF changes and outcomes [108]. Moreover, improvements in exercise capacity, hospitalization, and health-related quality of life with exercise-based rehabilitation are consistent regardless of cardiac rehabilitation program characteristics (exercise training dose, program duration, exercise only vs. comprehensive rehabilitation, risk of bias, publication date) [106–109].

Recommendations/Conclusions

Similar to apparently healthy individuals and patients with other forms of cardiovascular disease, higher CRF is strongly associated with better outcomes in patients with HF. Over the last three decades, exercise training has evolved from a contraindicated treatment to one that is widely recognized to be an effective adjunct therapy in patients with HF. A major challenge going forward is to increase the referral and participation rates in cardiac rehabilitation for these patients. While the 2014 CMS approval for cardiac rehabilitation coverage for HF will continue to have an important impact on participation, recent evidence suggests that only a small fraction of eligible patients with HF receive the benefits of this important treatment [17, 110]. Work must be done to close the gap between the known benefits of rehabilitation for HF and the relatively small fraction of patients who receive them. In addition, patients with HFpEF, females, and elderly patients remain

a

Study or Subgroup	Experimental Events	Experimental Total	Control Events	Control Total	Weight	Risk ratio M-H,Fixed, 95% CI
Austin 2005	9	100	19	100	12.4%	0.47 [0.23, 1.00]
Bocalini 2008	0	22	3	20	2.4%	0.13 [0.01, 2.38]
Davidson 2010	23	53	36	52	23.7%	0.63 [0.44, 0.90]
Dracup 2007	35	87	37	86	24.3%	0.94 [0.66, 1.33]
Giannuzzi 2003	2	45	1	45	0.7%	2.00 [0.19, 21.28]
Gielen 2003	1	10	0	10	0.3%	3.00 [0.14, 65.90]
Hambrecht 1995	0	12	1	10	1.1%	0.28 [0.01, 6.25]
Jolly 2009	16	84	20	85	13.0%	0.81 [0.45, 1.45]
Jónsdóttir 2006	2	21	5	22	3.2%	0.42 [0.09, 1.93]
Keteyian 1996	0	21	1	19	1.0%	0.30 [0.01, 7.02]
Klecha 2007	0	25	0	25		Not estimable
Passino 2006	0	44	2	41	1.7%	0.19 [0.01, 3.78]
Witham 2005	10	41	11	41	7.2%	0.91 [0.43, 1.90]
Witham 2012	13	53	10	54	6.5%	1.32 [0.64, 2.75]
Yeh 2011	2	50	4	50	2.6%	0.50 [0.10, 2.61]
Total (95% CI)		**668**		**660**	**100.0%**	**0.75 [0.62, 0.92]**
Total events	113		150			

Heterogeneity: $Chi^2 = 11.71$, df = 13 (P = 0.55); $I^2 = 0\%$
Test for overall effect: Z = 2.79 (P = 0.005)

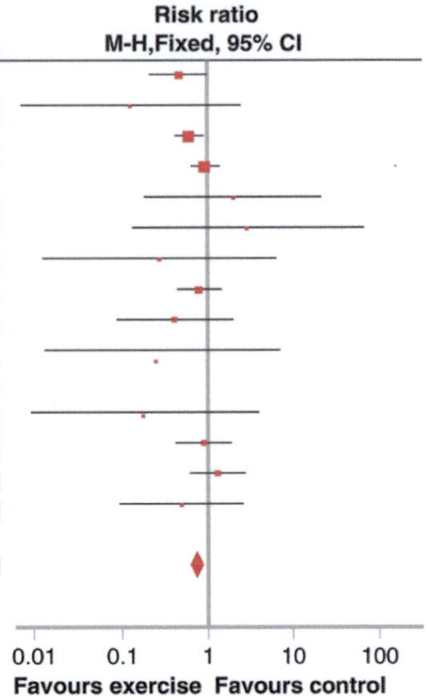

b

Study or Subgroup	Treatment Events	Treatment Total	Control Events	Control Total	Weight	Risk ratio M-H,Random, 95% CI
Austin 2005	53	100	38	100	31.0%	1.39 [1.02, 1.90]
Belardinelli 1999	5	50	14	49	9.7%	0.35 [0.14, 0.90]
HF ACTION 2009	729	1159	760	1171	41.9%	0.97 [0.91, 1.03]
Jónsdóttir 2006	7	21	11	22	13.9%	0.67 [0.32, 1.39]
Mueller 2007	2	25	3	25	3.5%	0.67 [0.12, 3.65]
Total (95% CI)		**1355**		**1367**	**100.0%**	**0.92 [0.66, 1.29]**
Total events	796		826			

Heterogeneity: $Tau^2 = 0.071$; $Chi^2 = 10.90$ df = 4 (P = 0.03); $I^2 = 63\%$
Test for overall effect: Z = 0.48 (P = 0.63)

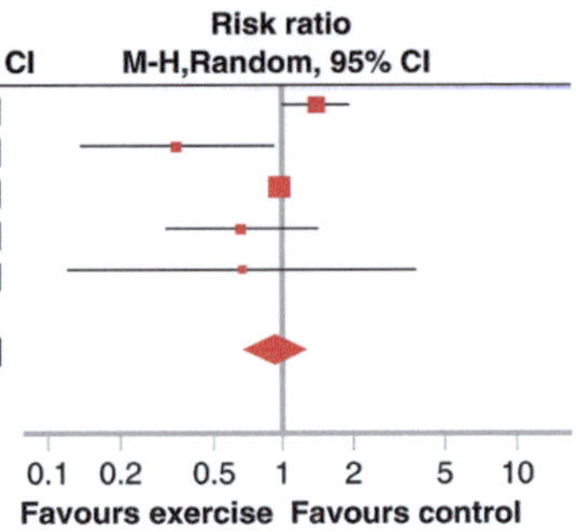

c

Study or Subgroup	Treatment Events	Treatment Total	Control Events	Control Total	Weight	Risk ratio M-H,Fixed, 95% CI
Belardinelli 1999	5	50	14	49	14.5%	0.35 [0.14, 0.90]
Belardinelli 2012	8	63	25	60	26.3%	0.30 [0.15, 0.62]
Dracup 2007	35	87	37	86	38.3%	0.94 [0.66, 1.33]
Giannuzzi 2003	2	45	1	45	1.0%	2.00 [0.19, 21.28]
Hambrecht 1995	0	12	1	10	1.7%	0.28 [0.01, 6.25]
Jolly 2009	4	84	2	85	2.0%	2.02 [0.38, 10.75]
Jónsdóttir 2006	0	21	3	22	3.5%	0.15 [0.01, 2.73]
Mueller 2007	2	25	3	25	3.1%	0.67 [0.12, 3.65]
Myers 2006	0	12	2	13	2.5%	0.22 [0.01, 4.08]
Passino 2006	0	44	2	41	2.7%	0.19 [0.01, 3.78]
Willenheimer 2001	0	23	3	27	3.3%	0.17 [0.01, 3.07]
Witham 2012	1	53	1	54	1.0%	1.02 [0.07, 15.87]
Total (95% CI)		**519**		**517**	**100.0%**	**0.61 [0.46, 0.80]**
Total events	57		94			

Heterogeneity: $Chi^2 = 16.70$, df = 11 (P = 0.12); $I^2 = 34\%$
Test for overall effect: Z = 3.52 (P = 0.0004)

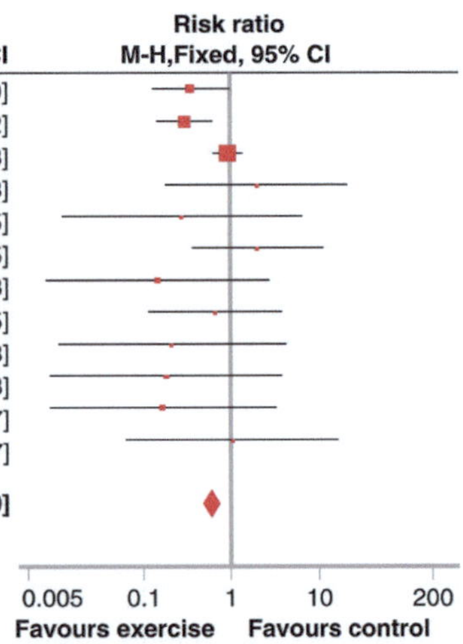

Fig. 18.2 (**a**) All hospital admissions up to 12-month follow-up. Two trials reported no deaths in either exercise CR or control arms (e16,e31). (**b**) All hospital admission more than 12-month follow-up. Two trials reported no deaths in either exercise CR or control arms (e16,e31). (**c**) Heart failure-related hospital admissions up to 12-month follow-up. (Modified from Taylor et al. [102])

underrepresented and warrant greater focus in future clinical trials. Future trials are also needed to explore strategies to enhance the long-term maintenance of cardiac rehabilitation for patients with HF and outcomes, costs, and cost-effectiveness of programs delivered exclusively in a home-based setting.

Clinical/Public Health Significance

A growing body of data, including single-center randomized trials and multicenter trials such as HF-ACTION, the ExTraMatch Collaborative, and other recent meta-analyses, have been influential in supporting exercise therapy for patients with HF. Simply improving fitness level by a small amount (1–2 ml $O_2 \bullet kg^{-1} \bullet min^{-1}$ measured peak VO_2) has a significant impact on reducing mortality and HF-related hospitalizations. The recent CMS approval for Medicare coverage will undoubtedly have a major impact on referral and participation in rehabilitation programs for patients with HF, which remains unacceptably low. Results from these randomized trials are important from a public health perspective given that HF is the one cardiovascular disease that continues to increase in prevalence. This increase in HF prevalence will represent a growing burden on health-care systems, but it also means that the pool of eligible patients who stand to benefit from rehabilitation will increase. A gap in understanding the value of exercise therapy for patients with HF remains across the medical community, and referral to rehabilitation programs in HF remains inadequate. Efforts should be made to inform both patients and clinicians regarding the benefits of being physically active, and the myth that exercise causes harm to the myocardium should be dispelled.

References

1. Smith TW, Braunwald E, Kelly RA. The management of heart failure. In: Braunwald E, editor. Heart disease. Philadelphia: W.B. Saunders; 1988. p. 485–543.
2. Kokkinos PF, Choucair W, Graves P, Papademetriou V, Ellahham S. Chronic heart failure and exercise. Am Heart J. 2000;140(1):21–8.
3. O'Connor CM, Whellan DJ, Lee KL, et al. Efficacy and safety of exercise training in patients with chronic heart failure: HF-ACTION randomized controlled trial. JAMA. 2009;301(14):1439–50.
4. Balady GJ, Arena R, Sietsema K, Myers J, Coke L, Fletcher GF, on behalf of the American Heart Association Exercise, Cardiac Rehabilitation, and Prevention Committee of the Council on Clinical Cardiology; Council on Epidemiology and Prevention; Council on Peripheral Vascular Disease; and Interdisciplinary Council on Quality of Care and Outcomes Research, et al. Clinicians guide to cardiopulmonary exercise testing in adults. Circulation. 2010;122:191–225.
5. Ingle L. Theoretical rationale and practical recommendations for cardiopulmonary exercise testing in patients with chronic heart failure. Heart Fail Rev. 2007;12:12–22.
6. Guazzi M, Adams V, Conraads V, Halle M, Mezzani M, Vanhees L, et al. EACPR/AHA scientific statement. Clinical recommendations for cardiopulmonary exercise testing data assessment in specific patient populations. A joint statement by the European Association of Cardiovascular Prevention and Rehabilitation and the American Heart Association. Circulation. 2012;126:2261–74.
7. Myers J. Essentials of cardiopulmonary exercise testing. Human Kinetics: Champaign; 1997.
8. Mancini DM, Eisen H, Kussmaul W, Mull R, Edmunds LH Jr, Wilson JR. Value of peak exercise oxygen consumption for optimal timing of cardiac transplantation in ambulatory patients with heart failure. Circulation. 1991;83:778–86.
9. Stelken AM, Younis LT, Jennison SH, Miller DD, Miller LW, Shaw LJ, et al. Prognostic value of cardiopulmonary exercise testing using percent achieved of predicted peak oxygen uptake for patients with ischemic and dilated cardiomyopathy. J Am Coll Cardiol. 1996;27:345–52.
10. Myers J, Gullestad L, Vagelos R, Do D, Bellin D, Ross H, et al. Clinical, hemodynamic, and cardiopulmonary exercise test determinants of survival in patients referred for evaluation of heart failure. Ann Intern Med. 1998;129(4):286–93.
11. Myers J, Gullestad L. The role of exercise testing and gas-exchange measurement in the prognostic assessment of patients with heart failure. Curr Opin Cardiol. 1998;13:145–55.
12. Arena R, Myers J, Guazzi M. The clinical and research applications of aerobic capacity and ventilatory efficiency in heart failure: an evidence-based review. Heart Fail Rev. 2008;13:245–69.
13. Myers J, Gullestad L, Vagelos R, Do D, Bellin D, Ross H, et al. Cardiopulmonary exercise testing and prognosis in severe heart failure: 14 mL/kg/min revisited. Am Heart J. 2000;139:78–84.

14. Roul G, Moulichon ME, Bareiss P, Gries P, Sacrez J, Germain P, et al. Exercise peak VO2 determination in chronic heart failure: is it still of value? Eur Heart J. 1994;4:495–502.
15. Piepoli MF, Corra U, Agostoni PG, Belardinelli R, Cohen-Solal A, Hambrecht R, et al. Statement on cardiopulmonary exercise testing in chronic heart failure due to left ventricular dysfunction: recommendations for performance and interpretation part III: interpretation of cardiopulmonary exercise testing in chronic heart failure and future applications. Eur J Cardiovasc Prev Rehabil. 2006;13:485–94.
16. American Thoracic Society; American College of Chest Physicians. ATS/ACCP statement on cardiopulmonary exercise testing. Am J Respir Crit Care Med. 2003;167(2):211–77.
17. Arena R, Williams M, Foreman D, Cahalin L, Coke L, Myers J, et al. Increasing referral and participation rates to outpatient cardiac rehabilitation: the valuable role of healthcare professionals in the acute care and home health settings. A scientific statement from the American Heart Association Council on exercise, prevention, and rehabilitation. Circulation. 2012;125:1–9.
18. Kotseva K, Wood D, De Backer G, De Bacqueur D. Use and effects of cardiac rehabilitation in patients with coronary heart disease: results from the EUROASPIRE III survey. Eur J Prevent Cardiol. 2013;20(5):817–26. https://doi.org/10.1177/2047487312449591.
19. Aragam KG, Dai D, Neely ML, Bhatt DL, Roe MT, Rumsfeld JS, et al. Gaps in referral to cardiac rehabilitation of patients undergoing percutaneous coronary intervention in the United States. J Am Coll Cardiol. 2015;65:2079–88.
20. Judgutt BI, Michorowski BL, Kappagoda CT. Exercise training after anterior Q-wave myocardial infarction: importance of regional left ventricular function and topography. J Am Coll Cardiol. 1988;12:363–72.
21. Oh BH, Ono S, Gilpin E, Ross J. Altered left ventricular remodeling with b-adrenergic blockade and exercise after coronary reperfusion in rats. Circulation. 1993;87:608–16.
22. Gaudron P, Hu K, Schamberger R, Budin M, Walter B, Ertl G. Effect of endurance training early or late after coronary artery occlusion on left ventricular remodeling, hemodynamics, and survival in rats with chronic transmural myocardial infarction. Circulation. 1994;89:402–12.
23. Oh BH, Ono S, Rockman HA, Ross J. Myocardial hypertrophy in the ischemic zone induced by exercise in rats after coronary reperfusion. Circulation. 1993;87:598–607.
24. Burch GW, Walsh JJ, Ferrans VJ, Hibbs R. Prolonged bed rest in the treatment of the dilated heart. Circulation. 1965;32:852–6.
25. Burch GE, McDonald CD. Prolonged bed rest in the treatment of ischemic cardiomyopathy. Chest. 1971;60:424–30.
26. McDonald CD, Burch GE, Walsh JJ. Prolonged bed rest in the treatment of idiopathic cardiomyopathy. Am J Med. 1972;52:41–50.
27. Abildgaard U, Aldershvile J, Ring-Larsen H, Falk J, Christensen NJ, Giese J, et al. Bed rest and increased diuretic treatment in chronic congestive heart failure. Eur Heart J. 1985;6(12):1040–6.
28. Dubach P, Myers J, Dzieken G, Goebbels U, Reinhart W, Vogt P, et al. Effect of exercise training on myocardial remodeling in patients with reduced left ventricular function after myocardial infarction; application of magnetic resonance imaging. Circulation. 1997;95:2060–7.
29. Giannuzzi P, Tavazzi L, Temporelli PL, et al. Long-term physical training and left ventricular remodeling after anterior myocardial infarction. Results of exercise in anterior myocardial infarction (EAMI) trial. J Am Coll Cardiol. 1993;22:1821–9.
30. Giannuzzi P, Corra U, Gattone M, Corra U, Imparato A, Gattone M, et al. Attenuation of unfavorable remodeling by exercise training in postinfarction patients with left ventricular dysfunction: results of exercise in left ventricular dysfunction (ELVD) trial. Circulation. 1997;96:1790–7.
31. Myers J, Goebbels U, Dziekan G, Dubach P. Influence of exercise training on myocardial remodeling in patients with reduced ventricular function: one year follow-up with magnetic resonance imaging. Am Heart J. 2000;139:252–61.
32. Cannistra LB, Davidoff R, Picard MH, Balady GJ. Moderate-high intensity exercise training after myocardial infarction: effect on left ventricular remodeling. J Cardpulm Rehabil. 1999;19:373–80.
33. Brum PC, Bacurau AVN, Medeiros A, Ferreira JCB, Vanzelli AS, Negrão CE. Aerobic exercise training in heart failure: impact on sympathetic hyperactivity and cardiac and skeletal muscle function. Braz J Med Biol Res. 2011;44(9):827–35.
34. Giannuzzi P, Temporelli PL, Corra U, Tavazzi L, for the ELVD-CHF Study Group. Antiremodeling effect of long-term exercise training in patients with stable chronic heart failure. Circulation. 2003;108:554–9.
35. Hambrecht R, Gielen S, Linke A, Fiehn E, Yu J, Walther C, et al. Effects of exercise training on left ventricular function and peripheral resistance in patients with chronic heart failure. JAMA. 2000;283:3095–101.
36. Haykowsky M, Scott J, Esch B, Schopflocher D, Myers J, Paterson I, et al. A meta-analysis of the efforts of exercise training on left ventricular remodeling following myocardial infarction: start early and go longer for greatest exercise benefits on remodeling. Trials. 2011;12:92.
37. Pina IL, Apstein CS, Balady GJ, Belardinelli R, Chaitman BR, Duscha BD, et al. Exercise and heart failure: a statement from the American Heart Association Committee on exercise, rehabilitation, and prevention. Circulation. 2003;107:1210–25.
38. Downing J, Balady GJ. The role of exercise training in heart failure. J Am Coll Cardiol. 2011;58:561–9.

39. Hambrecht R, Fiehn E, Yu J, Niebauer J, Weigl C, Hilbrich L, et al. Effects of endurance training on mitochondrial ultrastructure and fiber type distribution in skeletal muscle of patients with stable chronic heart failure. J Am Coll Cardiol. 1997;29:1067–73.
40. Hambrecht R, Niebauer J, Fiehn E, Kalberer B, Offner B, Hauer K, et al. Physical training in patients with stable chronic heart failure: effects on cardiorespiratory fitness and ultrastructural abnormalities of leg muscles. J Am Coll Cardiol. 1995;25:1239–49.
41. Myers J, Froelicher VF. Hemodynamic determinants of exercise capacity in chronic heart failure. Ann Intern Med. 1991;115:377–86.
42. Van Tol BA, Huijsmans RJ, Droon DW, Schothorst M, Kwakkel G. Effects of exercise training on cardiac performance, exercise capacity and quality of life in patients with heart failure: a meta-analysis. Eur J Heart Fail. 2006;8:841–50.
43. Flynn KE, Piña IL, Whellan DJ, Lin L, Blumenthal JA, Ellis SJ, Fine LJ, et al. HF-ACTION investigators. Effects of exercise training on health status in patients with chronic heart failure: HF-ACTION randomized controlled trial. JAMA. 2009;301:1451–9.
44. Sagar VA, Davies EJ, Briscoe S, Coats AJ, Dalal HM, Lough F, et al. Exercise-based rehabilitation for heart failure: systematic review and meta-analysis. Open Heart. 2015;2(1):e000163.
45. Myers J, Brawner CA, Haykowsky MJ, Taylor RS. Prognosis: does exercise training reduce adverse events in heart failure? Heart Fail Clin. 2015;11:59–72.
46. Williams MA, Pozehl B. Reasonable expectations: how much aerobic capacity, muscle strength, and quality of life can improve with exercise training in heart failure. Heart Fail Clin. 2015;11:37–57.
47. Swank AM, Horton J, Fleg JL, Fonarow GC, Keteyian S, Goldberg L, et al. Modest increase in peak VO2 is related to better clinical outcomes in chronic heart failure patients: results from heart failure and a controlled trial to investigate outcomes of exercise training (HF-ACTION). Circulation. 2012;5:579–85.
48. Tucker WJ, Lijauco CC, Hearon CM Jr, Angadi SS, Nelson MD, Sarma S, et al. Mechanisms of the improvement in peak VO2 with exercise training in heart failure with reduced or preserved ejection fraction. Heart Lung Circ. 2018;27:9–21.
49. Tucker WJ, Nelson MD, Beaudry RI, Halle M, Sarma S, Kitzman DW, et al. Impact of exercise training on peak oxygen uptake and its determinants in heart failure with preserved ejection fraction. Card Fail Rev. 2016;2:95–101.
50. Haykowsky MJ, Brubaker PH, Stewart KP, Morgan TM, Eggebeen J, Kitzman DW. Effect of endurance training on the determinants of peak exercise oxygen consumption in elderly patients with stable compensated heart failure and preserved ejection fraction. J Am Coll Cardiol. 2012;60:120–8.
51. Wisloff U, Stoylen A, Leonnenchen JP, Bruvold M, Rogmo O, Haram PM, et al. Superior cardiovascular effect of aerobic interval training versus moderate continuous training in heart failure patients: a randomized study. Circulation. 2007;115:3086–94.
52. Hambrecht R, Gielen S, Linke A, Fiehn E, Yu J, Walther C, et al. Effects of exercise training on left ventricular function and peripheral resistance in patients with chronic heart failure: a randomized trial. JAMA. 2000;283:3095–101.
53. Erbs S, Linke A, Gielen S, Fiehn E, Walther C, Yu J, et al. Exercise training in patients with severe chronic heart failure: impact on left ventricular performance and cardiac size. A retrospective analysis of the Leipzig heart failure training trial. Eur J Cardiovasc Prev Rehabil. 2003;10:336–44.
54. Mezzani A, Corra U, Gianuzzi P. Central adaptations to exercise training in patients with chronic heart failure. Heart Fail Rev. 2008;13:13–20.
55. Erbs S, Hollriegel R, Linke A, Beck EB, Adams V, Bielen S, et al. Exercise training in patients with advanced chronic heart failure (NYHA IIIb) promotes restoration of peripheral vasomotor function, induction of endogenous regeneration, and improvement of left ventricular function. Circ Heart Fail. 2010;3:486–94.
56. Piepoli MF, Guazzi M, Boriani G, Cicoira M, Corra U, Dalla Libera L, et al. Exercise intolerance in chronic heart failure: mechanisms and therapies. Part 1. Eur J Cardiovasc Prev Rehabil. 2010;17:637–42.
57. Duscha BD, Schulze PC, Robbins JL, Forman DE. Implications of chronic heart failure on peripheral vasculature and skeletal muscle before and after exercise training. Heart Fail Rev. 2008;13:21–37.
58. Gielen S, Schuler G, Adams V. Cardiovascular effects of exercise training: molecular mechanisms. Circulation. 2010;122:1221–38.
59. Gielen S, Adams V, Mobius-Winkler S, Linke A, Erbs S, Yu J, et al. Anti-inflammatory effects of exercise training in the skeletal muscle of patients with chronic heart failure. J Am Coll Cardiol. 2003;42:861–8.
60. Tabet J, Meurin P, Driss AB, Weber H, Renaud N, Grosdemouge A, et al. Benefits of exercise training in chronic heart failure. Arch Cardiovasc Dis. 2009;102:721–30.
61. Mendes-Ribeiro AC, Mann GE, Meirelles LR, Moss MB, Matsuura C, Brunini TMC. The role of exercise on L-arginine nitric oxide pathway in chronic heart failure. Open Biochem J. 2009;3:55–65.
62. Van Craenebroeck EM, Hoymans VY, Beckers PJ, Possemiers NM, Wuyts K, Paelinck BP, et al. Exercise training improves function of circulating angiogenic cells in patients with chronic heart failure. Basic Res Cardiol. 2010;105:665–76.
63. Hambrecht MD, Hillbrich L, Erbs S, Gielen S, Fiehn E, Schoene N, et al. Correction of endothelial dysfunction in chronic heart failure: additional effects of exercise training and oral L-arginine supplementation. J Am Coll Cardiol. 2000;35:706–13.
64. Kao W, Helpern JA, Goldstein S, Gheorghiade M, Levine B. Abnormalities of skeletal muscle

metabolism during nerve stimulation determined by 31P nuclear magnetic resonance spectroscopy in severe congestive heart failure. Am J Cardiol. 1995;76:606–9.
65. Van Der Ent M, Jeneson JA, Remme WJ, Berger R, Ciampricotti R, Visser F. A non-invasive selective assessment of type I fibre mitochondrial function using 31P NMR spectroscopy. Evidence for impaired oxidative phosphorylation rate in skeletal muscle in patients with chronic heart failure. Eur Heart J. 1998;19:124–31.
66. Stassijns G, Lysens R, Decramer M. Peripheral and respiratory muscles in chronic heart failure. Eur Respir J. 1996;9:2161–7.
67. Cohen-Solal A, Laperche T, Morvan D, Geneves M, Caviezel B, Gourgon R. Prolonged kinetics of recovery of oxygen consumption after maximal graded exercise in patients with chronic heart failure. Analysis with gas exchange measurements and NMR spectroscopy. Circulation. 1995;91:2924–32.
68. Belardinelli R, Barstow TJ, Nguyen P, Wasserman K. Skeletal muscle oxygenation and oxygen uptake kinetics following constant work rate exercise in chronic congestive heart failure. Am J Cardiol. 1997;80:1319–24.
69. Vasileiadis I, Kravari M, Terrovitis J, Gerovasili V, Drakos S, Ntaliannis A, et al. Interval exercise training improves tissue oxygenation in patients with chronic heart failure. World J Cardiovasc Dis. 2013;3:301–7.
70. Adamopoulos S, Coats AJS, Brunotte F, Arnolda L, Meyer T, Thompson CH, et al. Physical training improves skeletal muscle metabolism in patients with chronic heart failure. J Am Coll Cardiol. 1993;21:1101–6.
71. Gielen S, Sandri M, Kozarez I, Kratzsch J, Teupser D, Thiery J, et al. Exercise training attenuates MuRF-1 expression in the skeletal muscle of patients with chronic heart failure independent of age: the randomized Leipzig exercise intervention in chronic heart failure and aging catabolism study. Circulation. 2012;125:2716–27.
72. Adams V, Doring C, Schuler G. Impact of physical exercise on alterations in the skeletal muscle in patients with chronic heart failure. Front Biosci. 2008;13:302–11.
73. Corrà U, Agostoni PG, Anker SD, Coats AJS, Crespo Leiro MG, de Boer RA, et al. Role of cardiopulmonary exercise testing in clinical stratification in heart failure. A position paper from the Committee on Exercise Physiology and Training of the Heart Failure Association of the European Society of Cardiology. Eur J Heart Fail. 2017; https://doi.org/10.1002/ejhf.979.
74. Myers J, Gademan M, Brunner K, Kottman W, Boesch C, Dubach P. Effects of high-intensity training on indices of ventilatory efficiency in chronic heart failure. J Cardiopulm Rehabil Prev. 2012;32:9–16.
75. Gademan MG, Swenne CA, Verwey HF, van de Vooren H, Haest JC, van Exel HJ, et al. Exercise training increases oxygen uptake efficiency slope in chronic heart failure. Eur J Cardiovasc Prev Rehabil. 2008;15:140–4.
76. Cahalin LP, Semigran MJ, Dec GW. Inspiratory muscle training in patients with chronic heart failure awaiting cardiac transplantation: results of a pilot clinical trial. Phys Ther. 1997;77:830–8.
77. Lin S, McElfresh J, Hall B, Bloom R, Farrell K. Inspiratory muscle training in patients with heart failure: a systematic review. Cardiopulm Phys Ther J. 2012;23:29–36.
78. Clark AL, Piepoli M, Coats AJ. Skeletal muscle and the control of ventilation on exercise: evidence for metabolic receptors. Eur J Clin Investig. 1995;25:299–305.
79. Ponikowski PP, Chua TP, Francis DP, Capucci A, Coats AJ, Piepoli MF. Muscle ergoreceptor overactivity reflects deterioration in clinical status and cardiorespiratory reflex control in chronic heart failure. Circulation. 2001;104:2324–30.
80. Piepoli M, Clark AL, Volterrani M, Adamopoulos S, Sleight P, Coats AJ. Contribution of muscle afferents to the hemodynamic, autonomic, and ventilator responses to exercise in patients with chronic heart failure: effects of physical training. Circulation. 1996;93:940–52.
81. Roger VL. Epidemiology of heart failure. Circ Res. 2013;113:646–59.
82. Heidenreich PA, Albert NM, Allen LA, Bluemke DA, Butler J, Fonarow GC, American Heart Association Advocacy Coordinating Committee; Council on Arteriosclerosis, Thrombosis and Vascular Biology; Council on Cardiovascular Radiology and Intervention; Council on Clinical Cardiology; Council on Epidemiology and Prevention; Stroke Council, et al. Forecasting the impact of heart failure in the United States: a policy statement from the American Heart Association. Circ Heart Fail. 2013;6:606–19.
83. Mozaffarian D, Benjamin EJ, Go AS, Arnett DK, Blaha MJ, Cushman M, American Heart Association Statistics Committee and Stroke Statistics Subcommittee, et al. Heart disease and stroke statistics–2015 update: a report from the American Heart Association. Circulation. 2015;131:e29–322.
84. Berry JD, Pandey A, Gao A, Leonard D, Farzaneh-Far R, Ayers C, et al. Physical fitness and risk for heart failure and coronary artery disease. Circ Heart Fail. 2013;6:627–34.
85. Khan H, Kunutsor S, Rauramaa R, Savonen K, Kalogeropoulos AP, Georgiopoulou VV, et al. Cardiorespiratory fitness and risk of heart failure: a population-based follow-up study. Eur J Heart Fail. 2014;16:180–8.
86. Pandey A, Patel M, Gao A, Willis BL, Das SR, Leonard D, et al. Changes in mid-life fitness predicts heart failure risk at a later age independent of interval development of cardiac and noncardiac risk

factors: the Cooper Center Longitudinal Study. Am Heart J. 2015;169:290–7.
87. Echouffo-Tcheugui JB, Butler J, Yancy CW, Fonarow GC. Association of physical activity or fitness with incident heart failure: a systematic review and meta-analysis. Circ Heart Fail. 2015;8:853–61.
88. Myers J, Kokkinos P, Chan K, Dandekar E, Yilmaz B, Nagare A, et al. Cardiorespiratory fitness and reclassification of risk for incidence of heart failure: the Veterans Exercise Testing Study. Circ Heart Fail. 2017;28572213
89. Kokkinos P, Faselis C, Myers J, Sui X, Zhang J, Blair SN. Age-specific exercise capacity threshold for mortality risk assessment in male veterans. Circulation. 2014;130:653–8.
90. Katzmarzyk PT, Church TS, Blair SN. Cardiorespiratory fitness attenuates the effects of the metabolic syndrome on all-cause and cardiovascular disease mortality in men. Arch Intern Med. 2004;164:1092–7.
91. LaMonte MJ, Eisenman PA, Adams TD, Shultz BB, Ainsworth BE, Yanowitz FG. Cardiorespiratory fitness and coronary heart disease risk factors: the LDS Hospital Fitness Institute cohort. Circulation. 2000;102:1623–8.
92. Liu J, Sui X, Lavie CJ, Zhou H, Park YM, Cai B, et al. Effects of cardiorespiratory fitness on blood pressure trajectory with aging in a cohort of healthy men. J Am Coll Cardiol. 2014;64:1245–53.
93. Arbab-Zadeh A, Dijk E, Prasad A, Fu Q, Torres P, Zhang R, et al. Effect of aging and physical activity on left ventricular compliance. Circulation. 2004;110:1799–805. https://doi.org/10.1161/01.CIR.0000142863.71285.74.
94. Kitzman DW. Diastolic dysfunction in the elderly. Genesis and diagnostic and therapeutic implications. Cardiol Clin. 2000;18:597–617.
95. Brinker SK, Pandey A, Ayers CR, Barlow CE, DeFina LF, Willis BL, et al. Association of cardiorespiratory fitness with left ventricular remodeling and diastolic function: the Cooper Center Longitudinal Study. JACC Heart Fail. 2014;2:238–46. https://doi.org/10.1016/j.jchf.2014.01.004.
96. Duscha BD, Schulze PC, Robbins JL, Forman DE. Implications of chronic heart failure on peripheral vasculature and skeletal muscle before and after exercise training. Heart Fail Rev. 2008;13:21–37. https://doi.org/10.1007/s10741-007-9056-8.
97. Myers J, Brawner CA, Haykowsky MJ, Taylor RS. Prognosis: does exercise training reduce adverse events in heart failure? Heart Fail Clin. 2015;11:59–72. https://doi.org/10.1016/j.hfc.2014.08.012.
98. O'Connor CM, Whellan DJ, Lee KL, Keteyian SJ, Cooper LS, Ellis SJ, et al. Efficacy and safety of exercise training in patients with chronic heart failure: HF-ACTION randomized controlled trial. JAMA. 2009;301(14):1439–50.
99. Keteyian SJ, Leifer ES, Houston-Miller N, Kraus WE, Brawner CA, O'Connor CM, et al. Relation between volume of exercise and clinical outcomes in patients with heart failure. J Am Coll Cardiol. 2012;60(19):1899–905.
100. ExtraMATCH Investigators. Exercise training meta-analysis of trials in patients with chronic heart failure. Br Med J. 2004;328:189–96.
101. Taylor RS, Piepoli MF, Smart N, Coats AJ, Ellis S, Dalal H, ExTraMATCH II Collaborators, et al. Exercise training for chronic heart failure (ExTraMATCH II): protocol for an individual participant data meta-analysis. Int J Cardiol. 2014;174:683–7.
102. Taylor RS, Sagar VA, Davies EJ, Briscoe S, Coats AJ, Dalal H, et al. Exercise-based rehabilitation for heart failure. Cochrane Database Syst Rev. 2014;4:CD003331. https://doi.org/10.1002/14651858.CD003331.pub4.
103. Koch M, Douard H, Broustet JP. The benefit of graded physical exercise in chronic heart failure. Chest. 1992;101:231–5.
104. Oka RK, De Marco T, Haskell WL, Botvinick E, Dae MW, Bolen K, et al. Impact of a home-based walking and resistance training program on quality of life in patients with heart failure. Am J Cardiol. 2000;85:365–9.
105. Davies EJ, Moxham T, Rees K, Singh S, Coats AJ, Ebrahim S, et al. Exercise based rehabilitation for heart failure. Cochrane Database Syst Rev. 2010;4:CD003331.
106. Davies EJ, Moxham T, Rees K, Singh S, Coats AJS, Ebrahim S, et al. Exercise training for systolic heart failure: Cochrane systematic review and meta-analysis. Eur J Heart Fail. 2010;12:706–15.
107. Taylor RS, Sagar VA, Davies EJ, Briscoe S, Coats AJ, Dalal H, et al. Exercise-based rehabilitation for heart failure. Cochrane Database Syst Rev. 2014;14:CD003331. https://doi.org/10.1002/14651858.CD003331.pub4.
108. Anderson L, Sharp GA, Norton RJ, Dalal H, Dean SG, Jolly K, et al. Home-based versus Centre-based cardiac rehabilitation. Cochrane Database Syst Rev. 2017;6:CD007130. https://doi.org/10.1002/14651858.CD007130.pub4.
109. Sagar VA, Davies EJ, Briscoe S, Coats AJ, Dalal HM, Lough F, et al. Exercise-based rehabilitation for heart failure: systematic review and meta-analysis. Open Heart. 2015 Jan 28;2(1):e000163. https://doi.org/10.1136/openhrt-2014-000163.
110. Golwala H, Pandey A, Ju C, Butler J, Yancy C, et al. Temporal trends and factors associated with cardiac rehabilitation referral among patients hospitalized with heart failure. Findings from get with the guidelines - heart failure registry. J Am Coll Cardiol. 2015;2015(66):917–26.

19 Cardiorespiratory Fitness, Physical Activity, and Stroke

Steven P. Hooker and Michelle N. McDonnell

Introduction

Stroke continues to be a worldwide killer and disabler. In 2013, stroke was the second most common cause of death and third most common cause of disability globally after ischemic heart disease [1]. This translates to approximately 6.5 million stroke deaths, 113 million disability-adjusted life-years (DALYs), and 10.3 million new strokes. In addition, there are an estimated 25.7 million stroke survivors in the world.

In the United States alone, 795,000 people experience a stroke each year, which equates to 1 person every 40 s, and on average, someone in America dies of a stroke every 4 min [2]. An additional four million Americans will have a stroke by 2030 [3], and the incidence of stroke is increasing with a concurrent acceleration due to the aging of the population [4] and preponderance of modifiable cardiovascular risk factors in the population.

Interestingly, declines in both stroke mortality and DALYs rates have been observed globally since 1990 [1]. However, the absolute number of people who have died from stroke, remained disabled from stroke, suffered new strokes, or survived stroke has significantly increased over the same timeframe [1]. With greater scrutiny, it is recognized that there has not been any appreciable change in the proportional contribution of DALYs and deaths from stroke in developed countries but significant increases in developing countries (e.g., Russia, Eastern Europe, and East Asia). Furthermore, stroke should no longer be viewed as only a disease of the elderly as stroke in young and middle-aged adults is not declining (may actually be increasing) [5, 6] and two-thirds of all strokes befall those <70 years of age [1].

We echo the declaration that a majority of strokes are preventable [7]. As mentioned above, stroke is undeniably linked to modifiable cardiovascular risk factors such as hypertension, diabetes mellitus, dyslipidemia, obesity, tobacco use, and physical inactivity [8–10]. Independent of other risk factors, physical activity (PA) and cardiorespiratory fitness (CRF) have emerged as significant predictors of future risk of stroke incidence [8]. A renewed emphasis on stroke prevention has been recently trumpeted with major modifiable risk factors including physical inactivity being labeled as the most cost-effective means of prevention [1]. Thus, the purpose of this chapter is to (1) present a summary of PA and CRF terminology and measurement, (2) synthesize the results of prospective longitudinal cohort studies of PA and CRF and stroke risk, (3) discuss the biologic mechanisms by which PA

S. P. Hooker (✉)
College of Health and Human Services, San Diego, CA, USA
e-mail: shooker@sdsu.edu

M. N. McDonnell
School of Health Sciences, University of South Australia, Adelaide, SA, Australia

P. Kokkinos, P. Narayan (eds.), *Cardiorespiratory Fitness in Cardiometabolic Diseases*,
https://doi.org/10.1007/978-3-030-04816-7_19

and CRF exert their influence on stroke risk, (4) provide an overview of the strengths and weaknesses of the research to date, (5) clarify the clinical and public health significance of the findings, and (6) propose future research directions.

Terminology and Assessment of Physical Activity and Cardiorespiratory Fitness

Physical activity and exercise are complex behaviors and are difficult to measure in both epidemiological studies and from participants directly. The first challenge is terminology, for PA and exercise are often used interchangeably, which leads to confusion among participants and researchers. While PA and exercise do share common elements (bodily movement using skeletal muscles resulting in variable energy expenditure, positively correlated with physical fitness), the specific additional element related to exercise is that it is a planned, structured, and repetitive bodily movement designed to maintain or improve physical fitness [11]. Everyone performs some physical activity in their daily lives, and the commonly assessed categories relate to activities of daily living, household activities, commuting, occupational, and leisure-time PA which may be quantified in relation to intensity, frequency, and duration related to each activity. Exercise is subset of PA and due to the structured and preplanned nature may be easier to quantify through recall.

Physical fitness differs in that it refers to "a set of attributes that people have or achieve that relates to their ability to perform physical activity." With regard to health-related components of physical fitness, key aspects are cardiorespiratory and muscular endurance, muscular strength, body composition, and flexibility [11]. Physical fitness is generally easier to measure and is most frequently focused on CRF. This can be defined as "an objective, reproducible physiological measure that reflects the functional influences of physical activity habits, genetics, and disease status" [12]. CRF is commonly measured objectively with a maximal or submaximal performance test on an exercise bike or treadmill, with quantification of CRF through maximal oxygen consumption or maximal metabolic equivalents.

A limitation of most research related to the amount and intensity of PA required to prevent stroke and improve recovery from stroke centers around the quantification of PA. This often involves a structured questionnaire, asking about activities, intensity, and time spent across the past week/month. This method is affected by recall bias; people tend to overestimate their self-reported activity [13]. An alternative method to objectively record PA is using accelerometers, but there are only moderate to low correlations between self-reported and measured PA [14], possibly due to the issue of noncompliance and inaccurate wear time reporting [15]. In recent years there has been a considerable rise in consumer-level activity monitors, with 3.4 million devices of a single brand sold in only 3 months in late 2016 [16]. This method of activity monitoring may be incorporated more into future stroke prevention strategies. There are moderate correlations between these devices and research-grade accelerometers with regard to total daily energy expenditure and moderate to vigorous PA quantification [17]. This may address the limitations with accessibility and non-wear of research-grade accelerometers and help to establish minimum activity levels for stroke prevention.

Physical Activity and the Primary Prevention of Stroke

A considerable body of evidence from prospective, observational studies indicates that regular PA reduces the risk of stroke and decreases risk of mortality from stroke [8]. The evidence regarding the amount and intensity of PA to lower the risk of stroke incidence for men compared to women is inconsistent, with the overall evidence suggesting that vigorous physical activity reduces the risk of stroke in men

[18–22], but not women [19, 20]. In contrast, a number of women-only cohort studies found that those in the middle tertile for physical activity [23] or those who performed relatively modest amounts of PA obtained a significant reduction in risk of ischemic stroke in particular [24]. Two studies investigated walking in women, and both found that longer duration (≥2 hours per week) [25] and brisk walking compared to an easy pace afforded greater benefits [26] in risk reduction.

While prevalence of stroke is on the rise, mortality has been decreasing steadily over time [27]. PA influences mortality from stroke at all ages. Adults aged 40–69 in the Jichi Medical School Cohort in Japan who were most physically active had a significantly lower risk of death from cardiovascular disease, with the most powerful effect in the most active men (hazard ratio 0.40, 95% CI (confidence interval) 0.22–0.73), compared to women (hazard ratio 0.48, 95% CI 0.22–1.05) [28]. Similarly, the Nord-Trondelag Health Survey of women aged ≥50 in Norway has also shown lower stroke mortality in those undertaking high levels of PA, with regard to both intensity and duration [29]. Another high-intensity activity, running, has been shown to have a powerful protective effect. Participants from the Aerobics Center Longitudinal Study (mean age 44) who participated in running in the previous 3 months had 29% and 50% lower risks of all-cause and cardiovascular mortality, respectively, compared to non-runners [30].

Stroke incidence increases in older adults and in individuals with other cardiovascular risk factors. A study of elderly Japanese patients with diabetes (mean age 72) indicated that higher PA was protective against all cardiovascular events [31]. This is consistent with the findings in diabetic women in the Nurses' Health Study [24]. Older adults in the Cardiovascular Health Study (mean age 73) who walked briskly or walked greater distances had significantly reduced incidence and mortality from stroke [32]. For example, the greatest benefits were observed for those who walked at a pace above 3 miles per hour and/or walked a distance of ≥49 blocks per week. The protective effect on stroke mortality from high levels of PA (determined based on tertiles of self-reported frequency, intensity, and duration) was also found in women aged 81–100 years [29].

In adults after acute coronary syndromes, PA is more protective than changes in diet only for death from combined cardiovascular events in men and women, although the combination of both affords the greatest protection [33]. The large HUNT study in Norway investigated the protective effect of PA in people with clustering of known cardiovascular risk factors (diabetes, hypertension, and obesity) [34]. It was discovered that the most active people (based on a summary score derived from PA frequency, duration, and intensity) had a lower risk of mortality from stroke than inactive adults without this combination of risk factors.

Similar to the way that cardiovascular risk factors cluster together, healthy lifestyle factors may also cluster together with PA a key component of this constellation. A number of cohort studies have investigated the combination of lifestyle factors such as diet, PA, not smoking, and healthy body weight on stroke incidence. The combination of these four lifestyle factors and three medical factors, hypertension, blood glucose, and cholesterol, has been termed Life's Simple 7 and adopted by the American Heart Association (see Fig. 19.1) [35]. A simple point system can be used to quantify cardiovascular health, with 0 points allocated for poor, 1 for intermediate, and 2 for ideal health for these 7 medical and lifestyle factors for a total score of 14. A 1-point higher score on this 14-point scale has been associated with an 8% reduction in stroke risk in a large, population-based sample of US adults [36]. A number of other studies have used slightly different combinations of healthy lifestyle factors, always including PA, confirming the benefit of regular moderate to vigorous PA on stroke incidence [37–41]. Even in adults after stroke, the combination of routine PA and not smoking has been demonstrated to reduce all-cause and cardiovascular mortality in the NHANES study [42].

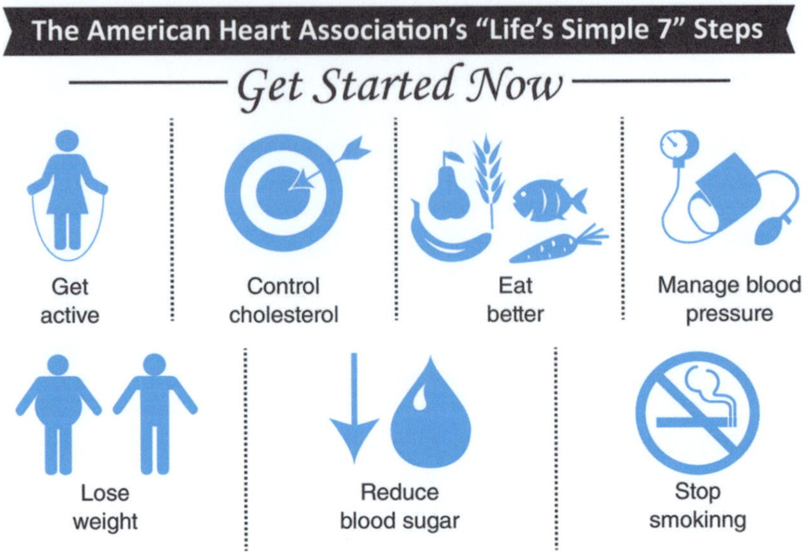

Fig. 19.1 The American Heart Association schematic encouraging physical activity as part of "Life's Simple 7" steps to better cardiovascular health. (Modified from: https://ahacharlotte.wordpress.com/2013/03/20/lifes-simple-7-may-help-to-reduce-cancer-risk/)

Cardiorespiratory Fitness and the Primary Prevention of Stroke

It is well documented that moderate- to vigorous-intensity aerobic activities improve CRF [43], and it is reasonable to assume that CRF is a good indicator of recent PA habits. Data from a number of sources estimate the genetic contribution to CRF is in the range of 25–40% of the variation in an individual's aerobic power. Thus, CRF is largely a function of habitual PA and to a lesser extent genetic influences. As mentioned earlier, because CRF can be objectively measured resulting in less exposure misclassification in analyses, it is preferable to self-reported PA in establishing risk reductions in epidemiological studies. Unfortunately, only a handful of studies have reported on the association between CRF and stroke risk. They do, however, make a valuable contribution to the literature and our understanding of how an active lifestyle may impact the future risk of a stroke-related event.

The earliest published paper on CRF and stroke was by Lee and Blair [44] who examined fatal stroke in 16,878 males in the Aerobic Center Longitudinal Study (ACLS). Although the study was limited to only 32 total deaths due to stroke during a 10-year follow-up, after adjustment for age and examination year, there was an inverse association between CRF (measured by maximal treadmill endurance) and stroke mortality ($P < 0.005$ for trend). This association remained after further adjustment for cigarette smoking, alcohol intake, body mass index, hypertension, diabetes mellitus, and parental history of coronary heart disease ($P < 0.02$ for trend). High-fit men (most fit 40%) had 68% (95% CI 0.12–0.82), and moderate-fit men had 63% (95% C: 0.17–0.83) lower risk of stroke mortality when compared with low-fit men (least fit 20%), respectively.

Kurl et al. [45] examined the relationship between CRF and stroke in 2011 Finnish men during an average of 11 years of follow-up. The age-adjusted risk of ischemic stroke in the 25% lowest-fit men was more than three times higher compared to the men in the highest 25% of CRF. The lower risk remained after adjustment for several stroke risk factors. Interestingly, the relative risk associated with the lowest level of CRF was similar to risks observed for obesity, smoking, systolic blood pressure, alcohol consumption, and low-density lipoprotein cholesterol.

These two early studies, however, did not provide separate risk estimates for fatal and nonfatal strokes, and neither included women. To evaluate the precise role of CRF in primary stroke prevention, it is important to determine whether CRF is also related to incident nonfatal events. It is also useful to determine whether greater CRF protects both women and men. To address these gaps, Hooker et al. [12] reported on fatal and nonfatal strokes in 46,405 men and 15,282 women from the ACLS who were followed for an average of 18 years. After adjusting for several covariates, there was a significant independent association between CRF and fatal and nonfatal stroke in men and nonfatal stroke in women. In women, the lack of a significant independent association between CRF and fatal stroke in the fully adjusted model may have been due to the small number of fatal stroke cases with only ten such events in the top 2 CRF quartiles.

The relative risk reduction in stroke mortality for ACLS men was 41–50% when comparing those in the highest two CRF quartiles with the lowest CRF quartile. This level of stroke protection is greater than that for self-reported occupational (36% lower risk) and leisure-time (20% to 25% lower risk) PA levels when comparing the most active and the least active men [46, 47]. In ACLS women in the highest two CRF quartiles compared with the lowest CRF quartile, the relative risk reduction in nonfatal and total stroke was 44% to 66% and 43% to 57% lower, respectively. This level of stroke protection associated with higher CRF is greater than that reported in cohort studies using self-reported PA (pooled risk reduction = 43%).

Of particular note in the findings reported by Hooker et al. [12], a dramatic reduction in the incidence of total stroke for both men and women was observed at a CRF level of 7–8 METs. Beyond this level of CRF, no further decreases in total stroke rate were noted for either men or women. Interestingly, in this ACLS cohort, some men and women in the lowest fitness quartile, and all of them in the next highest quartile of fitness, exhibited a CRF greater than 8 METs. This finding of an apparent CRF threshold adds insight into the relationship between CRF and stroke. A functional capacity of 7–8 METs is rated as a low to moderate level of CRF for men and women across the adult age spectrum. Most people can attain this level of CRF by participating in moderate- and/or vigorous-intensity physical activities for 150 min weekly.

Utilizing a subset of 19,815 participants from the ACLS, the Cooper Center Longitudinal Study (CCLS) sought to determine if there was a direct effect of CRF on stroke risk independent of established stroke risks factors of hypertension, diabetes mellitus (DM), and atrial fibrillation (AF) [48]. After 129,436 person-years of Medicare follow-up, there were significant differences in the observed stroke hospitalization rates among participants according to baseline CRF levels. Compared with the low-fit participants (quintile 1), moderate-fit (quintile 2–3) and high-fit (quintile 4–5) participants had a lower risk of stroke hospitalization. There was a definitive dose-dependent inverse association between midlife CRF and risk of stroke hospitalization later in life (see Fig. 19.2). Each 1-MET higher CRF was associated with 7% reduction in risk for stroke hospitalization (hazard ratio 0.93 (0.98–0.97 per MET)). In addition, the inverse association was independent of hypertension, DM, and AF and not different between men and women. In contrast to the results presented by Hooker et al. [12], these data indicated no apparent threshold effect or limit to the protective effects of CRF on long-term stroke risk.

In another study involving a Finnish population, Khan et al. [49] assessed baseline CRF and followed 2089 men for an average of 19 years while monitoring participants for the first major nonfatal cardiovascular event including stroke. After adjustment for several traditional risk factors, there was an inverse association between CRF and incident myocardial nonfatal infarction and heart failure rates, but not for nonfatal stroke rates. The hazard ratio per 1-MET increase in CRF was 0.94 (95% CI 0.87–1.01) for nonfatal stroke after full adjustment for potential confounders. Although nonsignificant, this 6% reduction in nonfatal stroke per 1-MET increase in CRF is similar to the 7% reduction on stroke hospitalization per 1-MET increase reported by Pandey et al. [48] in the CCLS cohort and the approximate 10% reduction in total stroke per 1-MET increase observed by Hooker et al. [12] in ACLS men and women.

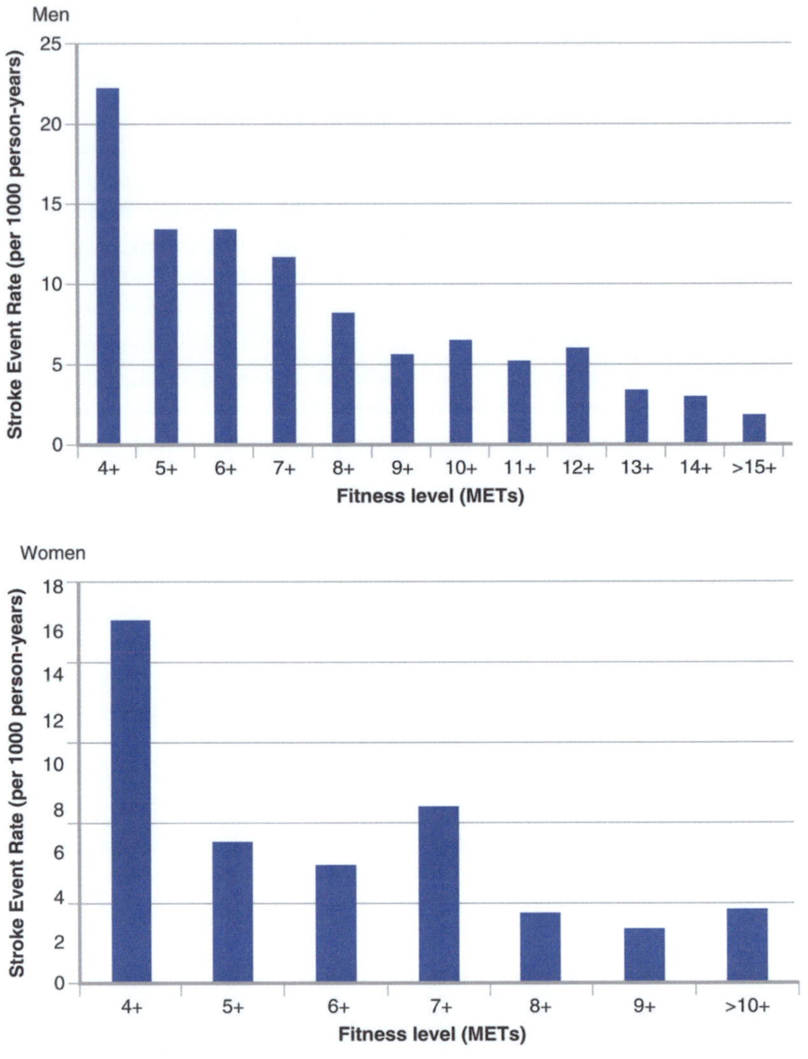

Fig. 19.2 Stroke hospitalization rate by midlife cardiorespiratory fitness (METs) among the Cooper Center Longitudinal Study participants. (Modified from: Pandey et al. [48]. http://stroke.ahajournals.org/content/47/7/1720)

Factors such as varying age, sex, and ethnic groups, follow-up periods, dietary habits, environmental contexts, and type and number of stroke-related outcomes may account for the differing results between studies. Regardless, as with the studies using PA as the predictor, research with CRF indicates that healthcare providers, public health practitioners, fitness professionals, and others should consider the potential independent cerebrovascular benefits of greater CRF and encourage their less active patients and clients to become more physically active and improve their CRF as a strategy to considerably reduce their stroke risk.

Physical Activity for Stroke Survivors

Regular participation in PA is a key lifestyle factor associated with better health and is particularly important for those who have already suffered a stroke. International clinical management guidelines for rehabilitation recommend that all stroke survivors undertake regular PA [50–52] to prevent stroke and minimize disability. At the time of their incident stroke, many patients have a cluster of risk factors such as hypertension and obesity and often have led a sedentary lifestyle. This pre-stroke inactivity is compounded by the disability from the stroke, leading to fitness levels much lower than their age-matched counterparts [53], and often so low that it impacts upon their abilities to carry out daily activities [54, 55].

The American Heart Association/American Stroke Association Scientific Statement *Physical Activity and Exercise Recommendations for Stroke Survivors* published in 2014 has reviewed the evidence for the benefits of PA for stroke survivors (see Fig. 19.3) [55]. The body of evidence supports PA and exercise to improve functional capacity and quality of life and reduce the risk of further cardiovascular events. There is also consistent evidence that regular cardiorespiratory training improves physical fitness, gait speed, and endurance [51]. There are some small studies suggesting that PA improves mood and cognition, but the evidence is inconsistent, and further research is needed to confirm the benefits of PA on psychological outcomes.

Despite substantial epidemiological evidence confirming that PA can reduce the risk of a first-ever stroke, less research has been conducted on reductions in stroke incidence in stroke survivors. Research conducted on the impact of a healthy lifestyle on mortality post-stroke found that people post-stroke who self-reported that they participated in PA at least three times a week had reduced all-cause mortality, independent of other variables [42]. There are no intervention studies that have followed large numbers of stroke survivors to confirm the reduced incidence of stroke with increasing PA. Small-scale

Setting/Mode of Exercise	Goals/Objectives	Prescriptive Guidelines: Frequency/Intensity/Time
Hospitalization and early convalescence (acute phase) • Low-level walking, self-care activities • Intermittent sitting or standing • Seated activities • Range of motion activities, motor challenges	• Prevent deconditioning, hypostatic pneumonia, orthostatic intolerance, and depression • Evaluate cognitive and motor deficits • Stimulate balance and coordination	• ~10- to 20-bpm increases in resting HR; RPF ≤11 (6-20 scale); frequency and duration as tolerated, using an interval or work-rest approach
Inpatient and outpatient exercise therapy or "rehabilitation"		
Aerobic • Large-muscle activities (eg, walking, graded walking, stationary cycle ergometry, arm ergometry, arm-leg ergometry, functional activities seated exercises, if appropriate	• Increase walking speed and efficiency • Improve exercise tolerance (functional capacity) • Increase independence in ADLs • Reduce motor impairment and improve cognition • Improve vascular health and induce other cardioprotective benefits (eg, vasomotor reactivity, decrease risk factor)	• 40-70% Vo_2 reserve or HR reserve; 55%-80% HR max; RPE 11-14 (6-20 scale) • 3-5 d/wk • 20-60 min/session (or multiple 10-min sessions) • 5-10 min of warm-up and cool-down activities • Complement with pedometers to increase lifestyle physical activity
Muscular strength/endurance • Resistance training of U/L extremities, trunk using free weights, weight-bearing or partial weight-bearing activities; elastic bands, spring coils, pulleys • Circuit training • Functional mobility	• Increase muscle strength and endurance • Increase ability to perform leisure-time and occupational activities and ADLs • Reduce cardiac demands (ie, RPP) during lifting or carrying objects by increasing muscular strength, thereby decreasing the % MVC that a given load now represents	• 1-3 sets of 10-15 repetitions of 8-10 exercises involving the major muscle groups at 50%-80% of 1RM • 2-3 d/wk • Resistance gradually increased over time as tolerance permits
Flexibility • Stretching (trunk, upper and lower extremities)	• Increase ROM of involved segments • Prevent contractures • Decrease risk of injury • Increase ADLs	• Static stretches: hold for 10-30 s • 2-3 d/wk (before or after aerobic or strength training)
Neuromuscular • Balance and coordination activities • Tai chi • Yoga • Recreational activities using padlles/sport balls to challenge hand-eye coordination • Activity-play video gaming and interactive computer games	• Improve balance, skill reacquistion, quality of life, and mobility • Decrease fear of falling • Improve level of safety during ADLs	• Use as a complement to aerobic, muscular strength/endurance training, and stretching activities • 2-3 d/wk

1 RM indicates 1 repetition maximum; ADLs, activities of daily living; HR, heart rate; MVC, maximal voluntary contraction; ROM, range of motion; RPE, rate of percieved exertion (6-20 category scale); RPP, rate-pressure product; U/L, upper/lower; and Vo_2, oxygen uptake.

Fig. 19.3 Summary of exercise/physical activity recommendations for stroke survivors. (Modified from: Stroke Foundation [51])

studies have examined a multimodal intervention, such as the cardiac rehabilitation model, and documented reduction in overall stroke risk [56] or individual risk factors such as low-density lipoprotein cholesterol [57]. A community exercise class for stroke survivors has also been shown to reduce blood pressure and cholesterol after a 19-week intervention [58], but without long-term follow-up, it is unclear whether these effects can be sustained.

In the absence of research data from randomized controlled trials, recommendations for secondary prevention following stroke extrapolate the benefits from primary prevention studies or follow expert consensus. It is clear that stroke survivors have additional barriers to participation in PA and need tailored interventions to break the cycle of reduced PA leading to lower functional capacity and increased risk of complications, cardiovascular and otherwise [50]. Some of the most common barriers are related to accessing exercise programs (cost, transport) [59, 60], but patient-related factors such as lack of interest are also common and often predate the stroke event [61]. To increase PA levels in stroke survivors, health professionals need to understand the barriers and facilitators to PA and work to increase exercise self-efficacy to ultimately change exercise behaviors [62].

Biologic Plausibility

It is well documented that moderate- to vigorous-intensity PA aerobic activities improve CRF [63]. Thus, it is reasonable to assume that CRF is a valid indicator of recent PA. With this in mind, it also supposed the biologic mechanisms by which PA and CRF modify the risk of stroke are the same. However, without conclusive findings from rigorous exercise intervention trials, the mechanistic pathways through which physical activity, physical training, and improved CRF reduce the risk of stroke remain to be fully elucidated.

It has been postulated that PA reduces the risk of stroke through the positive effect it has on other stroke risk factors such as hypertension, diabetes mellitus (DM), obesity, and atrial fibrillation. Hypertension is one of the most vital risk factors for stroke prevention [8], and regular moderate-intensity PA helps to control blood pressure [64, 65]. For those with DM, structured PA has positive effects on glycemic control, visceral adipose tissue, and plasma triglycerides [66]. Even in people with DM, stroke risk was reduced substantially in those who participated in daily brisk walking compared to those who remained inactive [67]. Although PA alone usually results in only modest weight loss (1–2 kg) [68], improvements are noted in body mass index, waist circumference, visceral adipose tissue, and overall body fat in those undertaking regular PA [69] particularly in those with DM [70]. Despite a lack of weight loss, PA also enhances lipid profiles by lowering low-density lipoprotein cholesterol and triglycerides and increasing high-density lipoprotein cholesterol [71].

Due to the positive changes with regular PA noted above, there is general consensus that PA reduces the risk of ischemic stroke by reducing the risk of developing atherosclerosis and thrombosis [72]. Ischemic stroke involves pathophysiology comparable to that of atherosclerotic disease, and arterial thrombosis develops similar to coronary artery disease. Thus, the benefits of regular PA on decreasing clotting risk, reducing blood lipids, and increasing high-density lipoprotein cholesterol could explain a reduction in the risk of developing ischemic cerebrovascular disease.

The protective effect of PA and CRF is proposed to go beyond risk factor modification. Previous research indicates that higher levels of physical activity and CRF favorably act on carotid artery distensibility, nitric oxide availability, and endothelial dysfunction [69, 73–76]. These biologic actions result in improvements in cerebrovascular function via increased cerebral blood flow and brain volume with a parallel delay in naturally declining cerebral tissue density [77–79].

PA may also provide anti-inflammatory effects. It has been established that inflammatory biomarkers, such as C-reactive protein and fibrinogen, are linked to cardiovascular disease risk. Regular PA and increasing levels of CRF have consistently been shown to be associated with reduced levels of C-reactive protein which could mediate the impact of PA and CRF on stroke risk [80–82].

It is also possible that regular PA and higher levels of CRF help protect against stroke mortality by limiting brain cell damage after a stroke [72]. Rodents undergoing voluntary running of moderate intensity exhibited positive neurotrophic effects on neurons in several brain regions [83]. Such biologic adaptations to regular PA could protect against ischemic stroke by upregulating nitric oxide synthase expression which would stimulate endothelium-dependent vasodilation in the brain [84] and diminish brain injury [85] and mortality rate [86] following stroke.

When the evidence from both animal and human studies is considered, it is clear that current PA guidelines recommending regular PA and improvements in CRF for prevention of cardiovascular and cerebrovascular disease are well justified. The precise biologic mechanisms undergirding the associations between PA and CRF and a reduced risk of stroke are beginning to be illuminated. However, more studies are required to determine the dose-response relationships between PA and CRF and various mechanistic pathways connected to stroke risk and brain health.

Impact on Public Health

Physical inactivity and low CRF contribute substantially to the economic burden of stroke, the leading cause of disability in the United States. The annual direct and indirect cost of stroke is $33.6 billion [10]. Globally, the annual cost of physical inactivity has been estimated at $53.8 billion, and $6.0 billion of the healthcare costs of inactivity was spent on stroke in 2013 [87]. Research is required to quantify the public health benefits from increasing population levels of activity and CRF.

Another consideration related to increasing PA and CRF is the potential for reduced burden of stroke. Evidence is emerging that patients who suffer a stroke, but were more physically active pre-stroke, may recover more quickly following stroke [88]. Combined with the benefits of PA for stroke survivors, as discussed above, there is compelling evidence that targeting PA would likely impact favorably on morbidity, mortality, hospitalization rates, productivity, and quality of life-years [55]. These economic evaluations are a priority for future research. The public health challenge for both primary and secondary prevention of stroke through increasing PA is to implement effective models of care. While individual studies have successfully increased fitness levels in stroke survivors with exercise interventions [89], it is likely that behavioral interventions are needed to achieve long-term changes. There is some evidence that multifaceted approaches with education, social support, and community involvement can assist with lifestyle modification, including PA, for stroke survivors [55]. In addition to reductions in disability and self-efficacy, incorporating PA as part of a comprehensive self-management intervention is also likely to improve quality of life [90].

Future Directions

Despite this vast literature confirming that PA reduces the risk of stroke incidence and decreases stroke mortality, there remain two important unanswered questions. Does PA also confer a reduced risk for hemorrhagic stroke? What dose of PA is required for optimal health benefits? The lower incidence of hemorrhagic stroke may contribute to the lack of significant inverse associations between PA and stroke incidence [20, 32, 91]; however, meta-analyses with significantly more hemorrhagic stroke events have established that increased PA is associated with reduced incidence [46, 47]. The issues related to measurement and quantification of PA, and the possibility of a sex interaction where men may benefit more from higher-intensity PA, are largely unresolved. Most studies investigated the benefits of moderate to vigorous PA, but several large cohorts divided participants into tertiles based on amount of any PA or dichotomized those who did any PA compared to none. This suggests that even low intensity and frequency of PA can be associated with health benefits. Future research is required to evaluate the health benefits obtained by those who increase their PA over time; recent research in older adults (>70 years) revealed that relatively small increases of PA (43 mins/week) resulted in clinically meaningful benefits in relation to physical function and preventing disability [92]. Increasing PA may have similar benefits in stroke risk reduction and reducing morbidity following stroke.

There are a multitude of other research avenues for future work in the area of CRF, PA, and stroke. Based on individual published papers, professional society consensus, and clinical recommendations, the topics listed below summarize additional scientific gaps:

- With the use of objectively measured PA, refinement of dose-response relationship between PA and stroke to help develop national guidelines.
- Studies on the influence of the total amount and patterns (including bouts and breaks) and types of sedentary behavior on incidence of stroke and/or cardiovascular biomarkers associated with stroke risk.
- Animal and human exercise intervention trials to help discover mechanistic pathways through which physical training and exercise could prevent or reduce the risk of stroke.
- Determine if there is an independent effect of PA/CRF on stroke risk above and beyond the modulation of risk factors
- Develop models or systems that integrate either objectively measured or predicted CRF to help screen patients who may benefit from exercise training to reduce their risk of stroke.
- More studies with varying populations based on age, sex, race/ethnicity, geographic location, and socioeconomic status.
- Evaluate the influence of PA and exercise training on reducing the occurrence of secondary events or outcomes related to the cardiovascular health (e.g., mortality, vascular risk factors) of stroke survivors.

References

1. Feigin VL, Norrving B, Mensah GA. Global burden of stroke. Circ Res. 2017;120(3):439–48.
2. Roger VL, Go AS, Lloyd-Jones DM, Benjamin EJ, Berry JD, Borden WB, et al. Heart disease and stroke statistics – 2012 update: a report from the American Heart Association. Circulation. 2012;125(1):e2–e220.
3. Heidenreich PA, Trogdon JG, Khavjou OA, Butler J, Dracup K, Ezekowitz MD, et al. Forecasting the future of cardiovascular disease in the United States: a policy statement from the American Heart Association. Circulation. 2011;123(8):933–44.
4. Go AS, Mozaffarian D, Roger VL, Benjamin EJ, Berry JD, Blaha MJ, et al. Heart disease and stroke statistics – 2014 update: a report from the American Heart Association. Circulation. 2014;129(3):e28–e292.
5. Giang KW, Bjorck L, Nielsen S, Novak M, Sandstrom TZ, Jern C, et al. Twenty-year trends in long-term mortality risk in 17,149 survivors of ischemic stroke less than 55 years of age. Stroke. 2013;44(12):3338–43.
6. Kissela BM, Khoury JC, Alwell K, Moomaw CJ, Woo D, Adeoye O, et al. Age at stroke: temporal trends in stroke incidence in a large, biracial population. Neurology. 2012;79(17):1781–7.
7. Howard VJ, McDonnell MN. Physical activity in primary stroke prevention: just do it! Stroke. 2015;46(6):1735–9.
8. Meschia JF, Bushnell C, Boden-Albala B, Braun LT, Bravata DM, Chaturvedi S, et al. Guidelines for the primary prevention of stroke: a statement for healthcare professionals from the American Heart Association/American Stroke Association. Stroke. 2014;45(12):3754–832.
9. O'Donnell MJ, Xavier D, Liu L, Zhang H, Chin SL, Rao-Melacini P, et al. Risk factors for ischaemic and intracerebral haemorrhagic stroke in 22 countries (the INTERSTROKE study): a case-control study. Lancet. 2010;376(9735):112–23.
10. Benjamin EJ, Blaha MJ, Chiuve SE, Cushman M, Das SR, Deo R, et al. Heart disease and stroke statistics-2017 update: a report from the American Heart Association. Circulation. 2017;135(10):e146–603.
11. Caspersen CJ, Powell KE, Christenson GM. Physical activity, exercise, and physical fitness: definitions and distinctions for health-related research. Public Health Rep. 1985;100(2):126–31.
12. Hooker SP, Sui X, Colabianchi N, Vena J, Laditka J, LaMonte MJ, et al. Cardiorespiratory fitness as a predictor of fatal and nonfatal stroke in asymptomatic women and men. Stroke. 2008;39(11):2950–7.
13. Banda JA, Hutto B, Feeney A, Pfeiffer KA, McIver K, Lamonte MJ, et al. Comparing physical activity measures in a diverse group of midlife and older adults. Med Sci Sports Exerc. 2010;42(12):2251–7.
14. Prince SA, Adamo KB, Hamel ME, Hardt J, Connor Gorber S, Tremblay M. A comparison of direct versus self-report measures for assessing physical activity

in adults: a systematic review. Int J Behav Nutr Phys Act. 2008;5:56.

15. Hutto B, Howard VJ, Blair SN, Colabianchi N, Vena JE, Rhodes D, et al. Identifying accelerometer non-wear and wear time in older adults. Int J Behav Nutr Phys Act. 2013;10:120.
16. Fitbit Reports $353M in Revenue, Sells 3.4M Devices in Q2'17, Up 14% Sequentially [press release]. 2017.
17. Ferguson T, Rowlands AV, Olds T, Maher C. The validity of consumer-level, activity monitors in healthy adults worn in free-living conditions: a cross-sectional study. Int J Behav Nutr Phys Act. 2015;12:42.
18. Glynn RJ, Rosner B. Comparison of risk factors for the competing risks of coronary heart disease, stroke, and venous thromboembolism. Am J Epidemiol. 2005;162(10):975–82.
19. Willey JZ, Moon YP, Paik MC, Boden-Albala B, Sacco RL, Elkind MS. Physical activity and risk of ischemic stroke in the Northern Manhattan Study. Neurology. 2009;73(21):1774–9.
20. McDonnell MN, Hillier SL, Hooker SP, Le A, Judd SE, Howard VJ. Physical activity frequency and risk of incident stroke in a national US study of blacks and whites. Stroke. 2013;44:2519–24.
21. Lee IM, Hennekens CH, Berger K, Buring JE, Manson JE. Exercise and risk of stroke in male physicians. Stroke. 1999;30(1):1–6.
22. Kiely DK, Wolf PA, Cupples LA, Beiser AS, Kannel WB. Physical activity and stroke risk: the Framingham Study. Am J Epidemiol. 1994;140(7):608–20.
23. Folsom AR, Prineas RJ, Kaye SA, Munger RG. Incidence of hypertension and stroke in relation to body fat distribution and other risk factors in older women. Stroke. 1990;21(5):701–6.
24. Hu FB, Stampfer MJ, Solomon C, Liu S, Colditz GA, Speizer FE, et al. Physical activity and risk for cardiovascular events in diabetic women. Ann Intern Med. 2001;134(2):96–105.
25. Sattelmair JR, Kurth T, Buring JE, Lee IM. Physical activity and risk of stroke in women. Stroke. 2010;41(6):1243–50.
26. Hu FB, Stampfer MJ, Colditz GA, Ascherio A, Rexrode KM, Willett WC, et al. Physical activity and risk of stroke in women. JAMA. 2000;283(22):2961–7.
27. Lackland DT, Roccella EJ, Deutsch AF, Fornage M, George MG, Howard G, et al. Factors influencing the decline in stroke mortality: a statement from the American Heart Association/American Stroke Association. Stroke. 2014;45(1):315–53.
28. Shibata Y, Hayasaka S, Yamada T, Goto Y, Ojima T, Ishikawa S, et al. Physical activity and cardiovascular disease in Japan: the Jichi Medical School Cohort Study. J Epidemiol. 2010;20(3):225–30.
29. Ellekjaer H, Holmen J, Ellekjaer E, Vatten L. Physical activity and stroke mortality in women. Ten-year follow-up of the Nord-Trondelag health survey, 1984–1986. Stroke. 2000;31(1):14–8.
30. Lee DC, Pate RR, Lavie CJ, Sui X, Church TS, Blair SN. Leisure-time running reduces all-cause and cardiovascular mortality risk. J Am Coll Cardiol. 2014;64(5):472–81.
31. Iijima K, Iimuro S, Shinozaki T, Ohashi Y, Sakurai T, Umegaki H, et al. Lower physical activity is a strong predictor of cardiovascular events in elderly patients with type 2 diabetes mellitus beyond traditional risk factors: the Japanese Elderly Diabetes Intervention Trial. Geriatr Gerontol Int. 2012;12(Suppl 1):77–87.
32. Soares-Miranda L, Siscovick DS, Psaty BM, Longstreth WT Jr, Mozaffarian D. Physical activity and risk of coronary heart disease and stroke in older adults: the Cardiovascular Health Study. Circulation. 2016;133(2):147–55.
33. Chow CK, Jolly S, Rao-Melacini P, Fox KA, Anand SS, Yusuf S. Association of diet, exercise, and smoking modification with risk of early cardiovascular events after acute coronary syndromes. Circulation. 2010;121(6):750–8.
34. Tjonna AE, Lund Nilsen TI, Slordahl SA, Vatten L, Wisloff U. The association of metabolic clustering and physical activity with cardiovascular mortality: the HUNT study in Norway. J Epidemiol Community Health. 2010;64(8):690–5.
35. Lloyd-Jones DM, Hong Y, Labarthe D, Mozaffarian D, Appel LJ, Van Horn L, et al. Defining and setting national goals for cardiovascular health promotion and disease reduction: the American Heart Association's strategic Impact Goal through 2020 and beyond. Circulation. 2010;121(4):586–613.
36. Kulshreshtha A, Vaccarino V, Judd SE, Howard VJ, McClellan WM, Muntner P, et al. Life's Simple 7 and risk of incident stroke: the reasons for geographic and racial differences in stroke study. Stroke. 2013;44(7):1909–14.
37. Chiuve SE, Rexrode KM, Spiegelman D, Logroscino G, Manson JE, Rimm EB. Primary prevention of stroke by healthy lifestyle. Circulation. 2008;118(9):947–54.
38. Tikk K, Sookthai D, Monni S, Gross ML, Lichy C, Kloss M, et al. Primary preventive potential for stroke by avoidance of major lifestyle risk factors: the European Prospective Investigation into Cancer and Nutrition-Heidelberg cohort. Stroke. 2014;45(7):2041–6.
39. Larsson SC, Akesson A, Wolk A. Healthy diet and lifestyle and risk of stroke in a prospective cohort of women. Neurology. 2014;83(19):1699–704.
40. Myint PK, Luben RN, Wareham NJ, Bingham SA, Khaw KT. Combined effect of health behaviours and risk of first ever stroke in 20,040 men and women over 11 years' follow-up in Norfolk cohort of European Prospective Investigation of Cancer (EPIC Norfolk): prospective population study. BMJ. 2009;338:b349.
41. Zhang Y, Tuomilehto J, Jousilahti P, Wang Y, Antikainen R, Hu G. Lifestyle factors on the risks of ischemic and hemorrhagic stroke. Arch Intern Med. 2011;171(20):1811–8.

42. Towfighi A, Markovic D, Ovbiagele B. Impact of a healthy lifestyle on all-cause and cardiovascular mortality after stroke in the USA. J Neurol Neurosurg Psychiatry. 2012;83(2):146–51.
43. American College of Sports Medicine. ACSM's resource manual for guidelines for exercise testing and prescription. Philadelphia: Lippincott Williams & Wilkins; 2014.
44. Lee CD, Blair SN. Cardiorespiratory fitness and stroke mortality in men. Med Sci Sports Exerc. 2002;34(4):592–5.
45. Kurl S, Laukkanen JA, Rauramaa R, Lakka TA, Sivenius J, Salonen JT. Cardiorespiratory fitness and the risk for stroke in men. Arch Intern Med. 2003;163(14):1682–8.
46. Wendel-Vos GC, Schuit AJ, Feskens EJ, Boshuizen HC, Verschuren WM, Saris WH, et al. Physical activity and stroke. A meta-analysis of observational data. Int J Epidemiol. 2004;33(4):787–98.
47. Lee CD, Folsom AR, Blair SN. Physical activity and stroke risk: a meta-analysis. Stroke. 2003;34(10):2475–81.
48. Pandey A, Patel MR, Willis B, Gao A, Leonard D, Das SR, et al. Association between midlife cardiorespiratory fitness and risk of stroke: the Cooper Center Longitudinal Study. Stroke. 2016;47(7):1720–6.
49. Khan H, Jaffar N, Rauramaa R, Kurl S, Savonen K, Laukkanen JA. Cardiorespiratory fitness and nonfatal cardiovascular events: a population-based follow-up study. Am Heart J. 2017;184:55–61.
50. Winstein CJ, Stein J, Arena R, Bates B, Cherney LR, Cramer SC, et al. Guidelines for adult stroke rehabilitation and recovery: a guideline for healthcare professionals from the American Heart Association/American Stroke Association. Stroke. 2016;47(6):e98–e169.
51. Stroke Foundation. Clinical guidelines for stroke management 2017. Melbourne: Stroke Foundation; 2017.
52. Lindsay MP, Gubitz G, Bayley M, Hill MD, Davies-Schinkel C, Singh S, et al. Canadian best practice recommendations for stroke care (update 2010). On behalf of the Canadian Stroke Strategy Best Practices and Standards Writing Group. Ottawa: Canadian Stroke Network; 2010.
53. Macko RF, Ivey FM, Forrester LW, Hanley D, Sorkin JD, Katzel LI, et al. Treadmill exercise rehabilitation improves ambulatory function and cardiovascular fitness in patients with chronic stroke: a randomized, controlled trial. Stroke. 2005;36(10):2206–11.
54. Shephard RJ. Maximal oxygen intake and independence in old age. Br J Sports Med. 2009;43(5):342–6.
55. Billinger SA, Arena R, Bernhardt J, Eng JJ, Franklin BA, Johnson CM, et al. Physical activity and exercise recommendations for stroke survivors: a statement for healthcare professionals from the American Heart Association/American Stroke Association. Stroke. 2014;45(8):2532–53.
56. Lennon O, Carey A, Gaffney N, Stephenson J, Blake C. A pilot randomized controlled trial to evaluate the benefit of the cardiac rehabilitation paradigm for the non-acute ischaemic stroke population. Clin Rehabil. 2008;22(2):125–33.
57. Olaiya MT, Cadilhac DA, Kim J, Nelson MR, Srikanth VK, Gerraty RP, et al. Community-based intervention to improve Cardiometabolic targets in patients with stroke: a randomized controlled trial. Stroke. 2017;48(9):2504–10.
58. Moore SA, Hallsworth K, Jakovljevic DG, Blamire AM, He J, Ford GA, et al. Effects of community exercise therapy on metabolic, brain, physical, and cognitive function following stroke: a randomized controlled pilot trial. Neurorehabil Neural Repair. 2015;29(7):623–35.
59. Nicholson S, Sniehotta FF, van Wijck F, Greig CA, Johnston M, McMurdo ME, et al. A systematic review of perceived barriers and motivators to physical activity after stroke. Int J Stroke. 2013;8(5):357–64.
60. Rimmer JH, Wang E, Smith D. Barriers associated with exercise and community access for individuals with stroke. J Rehabil Res Dev. 2008;45(2):315–22.
61. McDonnell MN, Esterman AJ, Williams RS, Walker J, Mackintosh SF. Physical activity habits and preferences in the month prior to a first-ever stroke. PeerJ. 2014;2:e489.
62. Shaughnessy M, Resnick BM. Using theory to develop an exercise intervention for patients post stroke. Top Stroke Rehabil. 2009;16(2):140–6.
63. Pescatello LS, Arena R, Riebe D, Thompson PD, editors. ACSM's guidelines for exercise testing and prescription. 9th ed. Philadelphia: Wolters Kluwer/Lippincott Williams & Wilkins; 2014.
64. James PA, Oparil S, Carter BL, Cushman WC, Dennison-Himmelfarb C, Handler J, et al. 2014 evidence-based guideline for the management of high blood pressure in adults: report from the panel members appointed to the Eighth Joint National Committee (JNC 8). JAMA. 2014;311(5):507–20.
65. Eckel RH, Jakicic JM, Ard JD, de Jesus JM, Houston Miller N, Hubbard VS, et al. 2013 AHA/ACC guideline on lifestyle management to reduce cardiovascular risk: a report of the American College of Cardiology/American Heart Association Task Force on Practice Guidelines. Circulation. 2014;129(25 Suppl 2):S76–99.
66. Thomas DE, Elliott EJ, Naughton GA. Exercise for type 2 diabetes mellitus. Cochrane Database Syst Rev. 2006;(3):CD002968.
67. Sone H, Tanaka S, Tanaka S, Suzuki S, Seino H, Hanyu O, et al. Leisure-time physical activity is a significant predictor of stroke and total mortality in Japanese patients with type 2 diabetes: analysis from the Japan Diabetes Complications Study (JDCS). Diabetologia. 2013;56(5):1021–30.
68. Marcus BH, Williams DM, Dubbert PM, Sallis JF, King AC, Yancey AK, et al. Physical activity intervention studies: what we know and what we need to know: a scientific statement from the American Heart Association Council on Nutrition, Physical Activity, and Metabolism (Subcommittee on Physical Activity); Council on Cardiovascular Disease in the

Young; and the Interdisciplinary Working Group on Quality of Care and Outcomes Research. Circulation. 2006;114(24):2739–52.

69. Pedersen MT, Blangsted AK, Andersen LL, Jorgensen MB, Hansen EA, Sjogaard G. The effect of worksite physical activity intervention on physical capacity, health, and productivity: a 1-year randomized controlled trial. J Occup Environ Med. 2009;51(7):759–70.
70. Motahari-Tabari N, Ahmad Shirvani M, Shirzad EAM, Yousefi-Abdolmaleki E, Teimourzadeh M. The effect of 8 weeks aerobic exercise on insulin resistance in type 2 diabetes: a randomized clinical trial. Global J Health Sci. 2015;7(1):34118.
71. Ahmed HM, Blaha MJ, Nasir K, Rivera JJ, Blumenthal RS. Effects of physical activity on cardiovascular disease. Am J Cardiol. 2012;109(2):288–95.
72. Dishman RD, Heath GW. Physical activity epidemiology. 2nd ed. Champaign: Human Kinetics; 2013.
73. Jae SY, Carnethon MR, Heffernan KS, Choi YH, Lee MK, Fernhall B. Association between cardiorespiratory fitness and prevalence of carotid atherosclerosis among men with hypertension. Am Heart J. 2007;153(6):1001–5.
74. Lee CD, Jae SY, Iribarren C, Pettee KK, Choi YH. Physical fitness and carotid atherosclerosis in men. Int J Sports Med. 2009;30(9):672–6.
75. Quan HL, Blizzard CL, Sharman JE, Magnussen CG, Dwyer T, Raitakari O, et al. Resting heart rate and the association of physical fitness with carotid artery stiffness. Am J Hypertens. 2014;27(1):65–71.
76. Taddei S, Galetta F, Virdis A, Ghiadoni L, Salvetti G, Franzoni F, et al. Physical activity prevents age-related impairment in nitric oxide availability in elderly athletes. Circulation. 2000;101(25):2896–901.
77. Ainslie PN, Cotter JD, George KP, Lucas S, Murrell C, Shave R, et al. Elevation in cerebral blood flow velocity with aerobic fitness throughout healthy human ageing. J Physiol. 2008;586(16):4005–10.
78. Clarkson P, Montgomery HE, Mullen MJ, Donald AE, Powe AJ, Bull T, et al. Exercise training enhances endothelial function in young men. J Am Coll Cardiol. 1999;33(5):1379–85.
79. Kramer AF, Hahn S, Cohen NJ, Banich MT, McAuley E, Harrison CR, et al. Ageing, fitness and neurocognitive function. Nature. 1999;400(6743):418–9.
80. Ford ES, Ajani UA, Croft JB, Critchley JA, Labarthe DR, Kottke TE, et al. Explaining the decrease in U.S. deaths from coronary disease, 1980–2000. N Engl J Med. 2007;356(23):2388–98.
81. Church TS, Barlow CE, Earnest CP, Kampert JB, Priest EL, Blair SN. Associations between cardiorespiratory fitness and C-reactive protein in men. Arterioscler Thromb Vasc Biol. 2002;22(11):1869–76.
82. Lin X, Zhang X, Guo J, Roberts CK, McKenzie S, Wu WC, et al. Effects of exercise training on cardiorespiratory fitness and biomarkers of cardiometabolic health: a systematic review and meta-analysis of randomized controlled trials. J Am Heart Assoc. 2015;4(7).
83. Cotman CW, Berchtold NC. Exercise: a behavioral intervention to enhance brain health and plasticity. Trends Neurosci. 2002;25(6):295–301.
84. Endres M, Gertz K, Lindauer U, Katchanov J, Schultze J, Schrock H, et al. Mechanisms of stroke protection by physical activity. Ann Neurol. 2003;54(5):582–90.
85. Wang RY, Yang YR, Yu SM. Protective effects of treadmill training on infarction in rats. Brain Res. 2001;922(1):140–3.
86. Ang ET, Wong PT, Moochhala S, Ng YK. Neuroprotection associated with running: is it a result of increased endogenous neurotrophic factors? Neuroscience. 2003;118(2):335–45.
87. Ding D, Lawson KD, Kolbe-Alexander TL, Finkelstein EA, Katzmarzyk PT, van Mechelen W, et al. The economic burden of physical inactivity: a global analysis of major non-communicable diseases. Lancet. 2016;388(10051):1311–24.
88. Stroud N, Mazwi TM, Case LD, Brown RD Jr, Brott TG, Worrall BB, et al. Prestroke physical activity and early functional status after stroke. J Neurol Neurosurg Psychiatry. 2009;80(9):1019–22.
89. Stoller O, de Bruin ED, Knols RH, Hunt KJ. Effects of cardiovascular exercise early after stroke: systematic review and meta-analysis. BMC Neurol. 2012;12:45.
90. Fryer CE, Luker JA, McDonnell MN, Hillier SL. Self management programmes for quality of life in people with stroke. Cochrane Database Syst Rev. 2016;8:CD010442.
91. Zhang Q, Zhou Y, Gao X, Wang C, Zhang S, Wang A, et al. Ideal cardiovascular health metrics and the risks of ischemic and intracerebral hemorrhagic stroke. Stroke. 2013;44(9):2451–6.
92. Fielding RA, Guralnik JM, King AC, Pahor M, McDermott MM, Tudor-Locke C, et al. Dose of physical activity, physical functioning and disability risk in mobility-limited older adults: results from the LIFE study randomized trial. PLoS One. 2017;12(8):e0182155.

20 Cardiorespiratory Fitness, Physical Activity, and Incidence of Atrial Fibrillation

Apostolos Tsimploulis, Andreas Pittaras, and Charles Faselis

Introduction

Atrial fibrillation (AF) is the most common cardiac arrhythmia, and it is associated with significant mortality and morbidity. Its incidence and prevalence have been progressively increasing despite the progress of medicine and the introduction of more sophisticated ways of management, e.g., with the use of catheter ablation. In addition, there has been a significant increase in mortality associated with AF from 1990 to 2010 [1]. AF has been linked to several risk factors including hypertension (HTN), type 2 diabetes mellitus (DM2), obesity, obstructive sleep apnea, thyroid disease, alcohol, and drugs [2] with at least one identifiable risk factor in approximately 56% of AF cases [3]. These Maybe These observations, along with the limitations of the definitive management of AF observations, along the limitations in the definitive management of AF, have increased interest in the modification of risk factors to prevent AF [4].

Cardiorespiratory fitness (CRF) is inversely associated with significantly lower incidence of several risk factors linked to AF, including HTN, DM2, and obesity, and protects against coronary artery diseases and heart failure [5–11]. However, the role of exercise in AF remains controversial. Several observational studies have reported increased incidence of AF in endurance athletes proportional to the duration of high-intensity exercise and the type of sport engagement [12–18]. In contrast, engaging in low-to-moderate-intensity physical activities is associated with decreased AF incidence, especially in middle-aged population [19–25]. The aforementioned reports, showing either positive or negative associations of exercise with AF, were mainly based on self-reported physical activity (PA) status using questionnaires, potentially over- or under-estimating the true impact of PA on AF incidence. Studies where CRF was assessed objectively and more accurately by standardized exercise protocols have also reported favorable cardiovascular outcomes [26–29] including significant reductions in AF incidence [30, 31]. This chapter will elucidate (1) the association between PA, CRF, and incident AF, (2) the pathophysiologic mechanisms involved, (3) the type of PA necessary that could potentially decrease the incidence of AF, and (4) the role of exercise in patients with AF.

A. Tsimploulis (✉)
Department of Cardiology, Stony Brook University Hospital, Stony Brook, NY, USA

A. Pittaras
Department of Cardiology, GW University, VAMC, Washington, DC, USA

C. Faselis
Veterans Affairs Medical Center, Washington, DC, USA

Pathophysiology of Atrial Fibrillation

AF is a supraventricular tachyarrhythmia with an unorganized and erratic atrial activation resulting

P. Kokkinos, P. Narayan (eds.), *Cardiorespiratory Fitness in Cardiometabolic Diseases*,
https://doi.org/10.1007/978-3-030-04816-7_20

in compromised atrial contractions [4, 32, 33]. Prerequisite for the onset of AF is the presence of several triggers which initiate the arrhythmia and the substrate to preserve it. Ultimately, AF is the result of a combination of electrophysiological and structural changes.

Several triggers have been associated with the generation of AF including sympathetic or parasympathetic stimulation, bradycardia, atrial premature beats, tachycardia, accessory AV pathways, acute atrial stretch, and ectopic foci occurring in "sleeves" of atrial tissue within the pulmonary veins or vena cava junctions [33–35]. Although the aforementioned triggers are important for the initiation of AF, the propagation and sustainability of the arrhythmia require the presence of atrial structural changes [36]. Atrial electrical abnormalities include increased heterogeneity, decreased conduction, shortening of action potential/refractoriness, increased automaticity, and abnormal intracellular calcium handling. Abnormalities in atrial architecture which are observed in cases of AF are hypertrophy of the cells, ischemia of the tissue, infiltrative processes, dilation, and increased atrial stretch. The common denominator and final result of the above changes are fibrosis of the atrial tissue [4]. All the common risk factors of AF like HTN, DM2, obesity, obstructive sleep apnea, thyroid disease, etc., have been shown to cause structural and electrophysiological abnormalities [33, 35]. These abnormalities create the necessary conditions for the two basic mechanisms responsible for the initiation of AF: reentry and focal ectopic activity [33, 34]. Reentry is caused by both electrophysiological changes, such as decreased refractory period, which allows the wavelength to find excitable tissue, and structural abnormalities, like tissue dilation and stretch, which increase the reentrant pathways and, as a result, create the conditions for proarrhythmic state [33].

Increased focal ectopic activity is another mechanism that contributes to AF. This is caused by rapidly firing foci, initially starting at the left atrium myocardial sleeves and propagating to the pulmonary veins [34–36]. This increased propensity for automaticity and arrythmogenicity can likely be explained by the electrophysiological and anatomic characteristics of the cells in the pulmonary veins and the atrial and pulmonary vein junction [37–39]. These include (1) pulmonary vein myocytes with relatively depolarized resting potential that promotes sodium channel inactivation and (2) shortened action potentials and refractoriness. Lastly, another plausible mechanism is triggered activity which is caused by delayed afterdepolarizations (DADs), DADs are spontaneous depolarizations after completed cellular repolarizations. They are caused by imbalance in cellular calcium ($Ca2^+$) and more specifically excess of it. When DADs reach the threshold potential, cell firing is caused, either as an isolated ectopic beat or as tachycardia. This rate-dependent entry of $Ca2^+$ can provoke DAD-related tachycardia and eventually AF [4, 36, 40].

Epidemiology

AF is the most common arrhythmia in the elderly affecting 1 in 10 individuals over the age of 80 years and approximately 33.5 million worldwide [2, 41]. AF can be asymptomatic or present with severe symptoms associated with increased and frequent hospitalizations, thromboembolic events, hemodynamic instability, and significant morbidity and mortality. In the United States, AF is the primary cause of admission in more than 497,000 cases annually and approximately 99,000 deaths [4, 36, 41]. Approximately six million US adults have AF, with an estimated healthcare cost of 26 billion. The number of AF patients is expected to double in the next 25 years as more than 50% of the patients will be older than 80 years of age [36, 41].

The most dreadful complication of AF is a thromboembolic event with the increase in the risk of stroke up to five times compared to the general population. Furthermore, given the pathophysiology of the embolic event and the involvement of larger arteries, strokes caused by AF are more fatal compared to other causes [4, 42, 43]. In addition to an increased risk of stroke, there is a significant association of AF with heart failure, decline in physical performance, cognitive ability, dementia, shorter disability-free survival, and eventually, higher mortality [44–51].

Despite the use of different approaches to manage AF, including pharmacologic and interventional treatments, a significant portion of

Table 20.1 Risk factors for AF and relative risk

Risk factors	Relative risk (95% CI)
Congestive heart failure	4.11 (2.1–8.03)
Male gender	2.68 (1.34–5.38)
Coronary artery disease	1.65 (1.23–2.14)
Hypertension	1.46 (1.29–1.65)
Left ventricular hypertrophy	1.35 (1.16–1.6)
Diabetes mellitus	1.22 (1.09–1.38)
Age (per year)	1.09 (1.07–1.1)
BMI (per unit)	1.07 (1.05–1.08)
Alcohol consumption	1.04 (1.0–1.70)

Adapted from: Lau et al. [35]

patients experience recurrences of AF and its detrimental complications. Thus, there have been significant efforts to study the predisposing factors that lead to AF and strategies to decrease its incidence. In this regard, several risk factors have been identified that independently contribute to AF, including increased age, male gender, HTN, heart failure, coronary artery disease, valvular heart disease, DM2, obesity, obstructive sleep apnea, thyroid disease, and alcohol or drug abuse [33, 48–57]. These risk factors contribute to electrophysiological and anatomical cardiac abnormalities and create conditions that foster the development of AF. Approximately 60% of the patients presenting with the AF have at least one identifiable risk factor [52]. The hierarchical, independent contribution of selective risk factors to AF is presented in Table 20.1.

Epidemiology of Exercise and Atrial Fibrillation

The efficacy of increased PA or structured exercise in positively modifying a number of risk factors related to AF is well-established [5–11]. However, the role of PA, exercise, and increased CRF in the incidence of AF is less clear. The participants included in most of the studies assessing the exercise-AF association were high-endurance athletes or military personnel. In studies reporting a positive correlation between PA and AF, physical activity status was self-reported in most, using mainly questionnaires [20–23, 25], and relatively few studies assessed CRF using standardized exercise test protocols. In contrast, when CRF was assessed by standardized exercise tests, certainly more objective than questionnaires, the association between CRF and AF was inverse and graded.

Collectively, the findings support that individuals who engage in high-intensity and volume endurance exercise are at increased risk for AF, whereas persons engaging in low-to-moderate-intensity exercise, as per AHA/ACSM recommendations for physical activity and exercise, are not at increased risk of AF.

Atrial Fibrillation Incidence on High-Endurance Individuals

One of the first studies to investigate the association of AF and exercise was conducted by Karjalainen et al. [13] This study included 300 middle-aged, high-ranked veteran orienteers (age ranging from 35 to 59) and 495 controls in the same age range. At the time of enrollment, participants in both groups completed questionnaires about the existence of any diseases and the amount of PA they were engaging in. After 11 years of follow-up, individuals in both groups again filled the same questionnaires. In addition, they were asked if their doctor had informed them that they had AF or atrial flutter. Positive answers were verified by examining the medical records of these patients. Although there was a significant decrease in mortality and other cardiovascular outcomes, AF was found in 5.3% of the veteran orienteers and 0.9% of the control group. These results were attributed to the increased vagal tone and the atrial structural changes which are expected to happen in the athletes.

Mont et al. [14] also reported an independent association between AF and engaging in moderate and heavy physical activities in 107 middle-aged patients (mean age 48 years) who presented at the hospital. Interestingly, the height of the individual and left atrial size were also risk factors for incident AF. Heidbüchel et al. [16] also reported that in patients who underwent an isthmus ablation for atrial flutter, a history of endurance sports or those who continued engaging in endurance exercise after the ablation was an independent and significant risk factor for incident AF after the ablation.

An even higher AF incidence has been reported by Molina et al. [17] The investigators retrospectively studied 252 marathon runners and compared them to 305 sedentary men. After a follow-up of approximately 10 years, medical records were reviewed, and the presence of AF was diagnosed based on the EKG recordings. After adjusting for age and blood pressure, the investigators reported that the AF risk in marathon runners was nearly ninefold higher (hazard ratio = 8.80; 95% confidence interval, 1.26–61.29) compared to sedentary controls. Similarly, a meta-analysis of six case-control studies also revealed a more than fivefold increased risk of AF in athletes compared to nonathletes (odds ratio, 5.29; 95% confidence interval, 3.57–7.85) [15].

Finally, in the Physicians' Health Study cohort, Aizer et al. [18] identified 16,921 male physicians with no medical history of AF. They were then categorized according to the frequency of vigorous exercise (0, <1, 1–2, 3–4, 5–7 days per week), the exercise intensity extrapolated from the question "Do you engage in a regular program of exercise vigorous enough to work up a sweat?" and, the duration of each exercise session (≤10 min; 11–24;25–40 and ≥41 min). The 3-year questionnaire asked, "What types of vigorous exercise do you engage in? (racquet sports, swimming, jogging/running, cycling, including indoor and others). During a 12-year follow-up, the investigators noted an incremental association between the engagement of vigorous exercise and incident AF. However, when variables potentially involved in the biologic pathway through which exercise influences AF risk were excluded, the risk was not significantly elevated. Furthermore, a subgroup analysis, this elevated risk was observed only in men below age 50 and joggers.

Collectively, the aforementioned findings suggest a direct association between AF and exercise volume and intensity of exercise performed. The participants in these studies were relatively young (<50 years of age) and were either athletes or participated in high-intensity physical activities. The increase in AF was attributed mainly to increased vagal tone, which is more common in athletes, sympathetic/parasympathetic mismatch, or structural changes (increased atrial dimensions). In contrast to these findings, Pelliccia et al. [19] reported that increased dimension of the left atrium, measured by echocardiograms, in men and women athletes participating in different competitive sports did not have increased prevalence of AF or other supraventricular tachycardia, compared to athletes who did not have increased LA dimensions.

The common denominator of the above studies was that exercise status was determined by questionnaires. Also, on several studies AF incidence was self-reported. The presence of AF was then verified by examining medical records. This raises several concerns regarding the accuracy of the findings. In addition, athletes or individuals who engage in higher-intensity physical activity may be more health-conscious and therefore more prone to identify and report symptoms suggestive of arrhythmia, ultimately leading to more reporting of AF compared to the control groups Table 20.2.

Table 20.2 AF risk with high-intensity exercise

Study	Participants	Physical activity level	Results/AF risk
Karjalainen et al. [13]	300 middle-aged veterans	High	Increased prevalence (5.3% in athletes vs 0.9% in non-athletes)
Mont et al. [14]	107 middle-aged patients	High	Increased AF incidence
Heidbüchel et al. [16]	137 post-atrial flutter ablation	High	Increased AF risk (multivariate HR = 1.81)
Molina et al. [17]	252 marathon runners	High	AF 8.8-fold higher than sedentary controls
Aizer et al. [18]	16,921 male physicians	High recreational	Increased AF in high-frequency exercise group (HR = 1.2)
Pelliccia et al. [19]	1777 competitive athletes	High	Increased LA dimension; no increase in AF

Low-to-Moderate-Intensity Physical Activity and Atrial Fibrillation

Several studies have also assessed the association between AF incidence and relatively low-to-moderate-intensity physical activity. In contrast to the findings reported by high-intensity exercises, the conclusions of these studies support the concept that engaging in low-to-moderate-intensity exercise or physical activities protects against the occurrence of AF. Mozaffarian et al. [20] followed 5446 participants in the Cardiovascular Health Study (CHS) (mean age 74 years), for a total of 12 years. Physical activity status was assessed by the Minnesota Leisure-Time Activities at baseline and then after 3 and 7 years, evaluating the frequency and duration of 15 different types of activities in the 2 prior weeks. Based on this information, they formed quintiles of fitness categories, ranging from no physical activity to high. AF was evaluated by assessing electrocardiograms (EKGs) yearly and by contacting the patients every 6 months. They found a significant decrease in incident AF ranging from 22% to 36% in the moderate-intensity leisure-time physical activity group, but this association lost significance for the high-intensity group, suggesting a U-shaped association between exercise and AF.

Drca et al. examined the association between physical activity and the incidence of AF in different age groups and gender differences [21, 22]. In the first study [21], 44,410 men with a mean age of 60 years were followed for 12 years. Physical activity was assessed by questionnaires completed at baseline. Participants reported retrospectively the time they spent on leisure-time exercise when they were 15, 30, and 50 years old. They reported that individuals who were engaging in physical activity (walking or bicycling) for more than 5 hours per week at the age of 30, compared to participants who were exercising for less than 1 hour per week, had 19% higher risk of developing AF. This association was even more prominent for individuals in the high activity group who quit exercising later in life. In contrast, the group of older men, with a mean age of 60, who were exercising more than 1 hour per week, had a 13% reduction in the incidence of AF. In their study, the investigators evaluated the incidence of AF in 36,513 women (median age of 60 years), followed for a total of 12 years [22]. PA was also assessed by questionnaires with participants reporting retrospectively the time spent on leisure exercise at the age of 30 and 50 years old. The investigators reported an inverse association between engaging in PA and decreased incidence of AF. Compared to women who reported no PA, AF was 15% lower in women exercising ≥4 hours per week and 19% for those exercising ≥40 minutes per day [22].

The association of PA and AF was also assessed in the Atherosclerosis Risk in Communities (ARIC) Study [23]. Investigators followed 14,219 individuals (mean age of 54 years), for a total of 12 years of follow-up. The modified Baecke questionnaire was used to assess physical activity in sports, leisure time, and at work. The questions were then converted to min/week using the American Heart Association (AHA) definition of PA; three groups were created accordingly: poor, intermediate, and ideal. Incident AF was evaluated based on EKGs conducted during clinic visits, on the presence of the ICD-9 diagnosis on the medical records and if AF was listed as a cause of death on a death certificate. The investigators reported a protective association of PA with a risk of AF that was of a similar magnitude for both men and women. Compared to those classified as having "poor" PA, those who reported having an ideal level of PA at baseline had 11% (95% CI, 0–21%) lower risk of AF after adjusting for relevant confounders. In a more recent study, the investigators examined the association between the ideal cardiovascular health metrics known as Life's Simple 7 (LS7), defined by the American Heart Association that includes PA status and incident AF in a biracial cohort of middle- and older-aged adults without known cardiovascular disease. The modified Baecke questionnaire was used to assess PA in sports, leisure time, and at work. The study included 13,182 ARIC participants (mean baseline age = 54 ± 5.7 years; 56% women; 25% black) free of AF and cardiovascular disease. An overall LS7 score was calculated as the sum of the LS7 component scores and classified as inadequate (0–4), average [5–9], or optimal [10–14] cardiovascular health. AF was identified primarily by ECG and hospital discharge coding of AF. Cox multivariable proportional hazard model was used to assess AF risk over a median follow-up of 25.1 years. Participants in the average ($n = 8629$) and optimal ($n = 3496$) LS7 categories each had a lower risk of developing AF (hazard ratio 0.59, 95% confidence interval 0.51–0.67 for average and hazard ratio 0.38, 95% confidence interval 0.32–0.44 for optimal). The AF risk was 12% lower for each 1-point-higher LS7 score when compared with the inadequate category (hazard ratio 0.88, 95% confidence interval 0.86–0.89; $n = 1057$) [24].

Azarbal et al. [25] assessed the role of obesity, PA, and their interaction with the risk of incident AF. They followed 81,317 women (mean age of 64 years) with no baseline AF for a total of 11.5 years. PA was assessed by self-reported questionnaires. PA was classified as low if individuals reported frequent walks outside the home for more than 10 min without stopping and engaged in recreational physical activity at levels that increased heart rate and produced sweating. Strenuous activity was classified if participants reported frequently engaging in strenuous or very hard exercise, resulting in sweating and fast heartbeat, such as aerobics, aerobic dancing, jogging, tennis, and swimming laps. Metabolic equivalents (METs) hours per week (MET-h/week) were estimated for each participant based on the activities reported, and the following four categories of physical activity were established: 0 MET-h/week, >0 to 3 MET-h/week, >3 to 9 MET-h/week, and >9 MET-h/week. AF was assessed by using medical records and by identifying the code of the disease (ICD-9). Multivariable adjustment individuals in the highest category of PA (>9 MET-h/week) had a significantly lower risk of incident AF (HR, 0.90; 95% CI, 0.85–0.96), compared to sedentary women. When the obesity-PA-AF interaction was assessed, the risk of incident AF was greater in the sedentary group (HR, 1.30; 95% CI, 1.17–1.45) than in the physically active group (HR, 1.16; 95% CI, 1.08–1.24).

Bapat et al. [58] also examined the association between PA (including everyday activities) and AF, using the Multi-Ethnic Study of Atherosclerosis (MESA) database of 5793 men and women (mean age of 62 years), followed for 7.7 years. PA was assessed using the MESA Typical Week Physical Activity Survey (TWPAS), completed at the baseline examination, which identifies the amount of time spent and the frequency of various physical activities during a typical week in the previous month (1, household chores; 2, lawn/yard/garden/farm; 3, care of children/adults; 4, transportation; 5, nonoccupational walking; 6, dancing and sport activities; 7, conditioning activities; 8, leisure activities; 9, work). Participants reported whether they participated in these activities, and, if applicable, they answered questions regarding the average number of days per week and time per day engaged in each activity. Where appropriate, the PA survey accounted for exercise intensity at three levels (heavy, moderate, or light), which was determined by the type of activity in any given category (i.e., sitting or standing versus pushing or lifting), and three groups were created. Minutes of activity were summed for each discrete activity type and multiplied by the METs. Overall, neither vigorous PA nor total intentional exercises were independently associated with incident AF after multivariable adjustment. However, in the group that reported any vigorous PA, there was a statistically significant inverse association between total intentional exercise and incident AF. Being in the top tertile, total intentional exercise was associated with a 54% lower risk of incident AF, compared with the group with no total intentional exercise in the fully adjusted model (HR 0.46, 95% CI 0.22–0.98). No subgroup of participants demonstrated an increased risk of incident AF with greater PA.

Collectively, the findings of the aforementioned studies support an inverse association between the level and intensity of PA and the risk

Table 20.3 AF risk in low-moderate-intensity exercise

Study	Participants	Level of activity	Results/AF risk
Mozaffarian et al. [20]	5446 older participants	Moderate	Decreased (22–36%)
Drca et al. [21]	44,410 men, mean age of 60 years	Moderate-low	Decreased 13%
Drca et al. [22]	36,513 women (median age of 60 years)	Leisure-time exercise	Decreased 15–19% with increasing levels of leisure-time exercise
ARIC study [23]	14,219 individuals (mean age of 54 years)	Leisure time	Decreased AF 11% on ideal vs poor PA groups
Azarbal et al. [25]	81,317 women (mean age of 64 years)	Leisure time/ sports	Decreased AF HR 0.90 high vs low PA group
Bapat et al. [58]	5793 participants (mean age of 62 years)	Leisure time/ sports	Decreased 54% on the higher activity group

of developing AF, regardless of gender or the type of PA performed. However, it is important to emphasize that PA in all studies was self-reported using questionnaires (Table 20.3).

Exercise and Cardiorespiratory Fitness

Several studies assessed cardiorespiratory fitness (CRF) more objectively using standardized exercise protocols. The first of these studies included 2014 healthy middle-aged men. The investigators assessed fitness by a standardized exercise protocol using a cycle ergometer [26]. Participants were followed for a total of 35 years, and AF was identified by examining the medical records. Increased risk for AF was observed only in men with low fitness, and the overall risk of AF was reduced by 23% in the fit men. Obesity was an independent risk factor for incident AF. Men with a baseline BMI of ≥28 kg/m^2 had a 68% higher risk (HR 1.68, 95% confidence interval 1.14–2.40) compared to those with BMI <28 kg/m^2.

Khan et al. [59] used data from the Kuopio Ischemic Heart Disease (KIHD) study to assess the AF-CRF association. Participants (n = 1950; mean age 52.6 years) were followed for a total of 19.5 years. Four CRF groups were formed based on maximal oxygen consumption ($VO_{2\ max}$) achieved at baseline exercise testing. The risk of developing AF was inversely associated with CRF. The incident rate varied from 11.5 (95% CI 9.4–14.0) for the first CRF to 9.1 (95% CI 7.4–11.2) for the second quartile, 5.7 (95% CI 4.4–7.4) for the third quartile, and 6.3 (95% CI 5.0–8.0) for the fourth quartile. After adjusting for age, there was still a significant decrease in AF incidence (hazard ratio 0.67, 95% CI 0.48–0.95) when comparing the least-fit group with the highest-fit.

The impact of CRF on AF incidence was also assessed in a larger study of 6,4561 middle-aged (mean age 54), predominantly white (64%), participants and a follow-up period of 5.4 years [30]. CRF was assessed by a standardized treadmill stress test at baseline (Bruce protocol). Four groups were formed according to the peak METs achieved: <6 METs, 6–9.9 METs; 10–11 METs and >11 METs. AF was determined by ICD-9 code. After adjustment for potential confounders, an incremental increase of 1 MET was associated with a 7% lower risk of incident AF (hazard ratio, 0.93; 95% confidence interval, 0.92–0.94; $P < 0.001$). When AF risk was examined across CRF categories, an inverse and graded association was noted. The risk of AF for individuals with an exercise capacity of 6–9 METs (CRF group the next to the least-fit) was 20% lower, compared to those in the least-fit group (hazard ratio 0.80 (0.74–0.86). For those in the next two CRF categories (10–11 and >11 METs), the risk was lower by 40% (HR 0.60; CI 0.54–0.65) and 56% (HR 0.44; CI, 0.39–0.50), respectively.

Similar and more impressive findings were reported by Faselis et al. [31]. The investigators examined the CRF-AF association in 5962 middle-aged US veterans with no evidence of AF prior to a maximal stress test using the Bruce protocol. Data were collected from 1987 to 2012 with a median follow-up of 8.3 years. Four fitness categories were established based on age-stratified quartiles of peak METs achieved: least fit (4.9 ± 1.10 METs; n = 1446), moderately fit (6.7 ± 1.0 METs; n = 1490), fit (7.9 ± 1.0 METs; n = 1585), and highly fit (9.3 ± 1.2 METs; n = 1441). Incident AF was determined using the ICD-9 code for diagnosis of AF in the medical records. Incident AF was significantly less common in the highly fit individuals. Compared with the least fit and after multivariable adjusting, hazard ratios were 0.80 (95% CI, 0.67–0.97) for moderately fit individuals, 0.55 (95% CI, 0.45–0.68) for fit individuals, and 0.37 (95% CI, 0.29–0.47) for highly fit individuals. Each 1 MET incremental increase in exercise capacity was associated with 21% lower risk for incident AF (hazard ratio, 0.79; 95% CI, 0.76–0.82). The above findings were particularly significant because they were derived from a population predominantly composed of African Americans and because of the equal access to care of all the participants independent of a patient's financial status.

In a recent review, Elliott AD et al. [60] sought to define the optimal dose and duration for the prevention and treatment of AF. In doing so, they reviewed the evidence that supports a decline in AF risk for those who achieve a weekly physical activity dose slightly above the current recommended guidelines of 150 min of moderate-intensity activity per week [61]. The investigators identified a CRF threshold of 8 METs (metabolic equivalents of task) or more during maximal exercise testing for reduced incidence of AF.

Collectively, the findings of the aforementioned studies support an independent, inverse, and graded association between moderate levels of exercise/physical activity and the incidence of AF. Importantly, no U-shaped association was observed, suggesting that increased exercise levels do not increase the incidence of AF. It is also noteworthy that only 1 MET increase in the CRF confers a significant decrease in incident AF ranging from 7% to 21%. The strength of the above studies as we have underscored is that CRF was assessed objectively using standardized exercise treadmill or bike test. It is important to note that CRF was based on one assessment at baseline in all studies, and CRF follow-up data on changes over time were not available, increasing the probability of regression dilution bias. However, CRF is more likely to decline with age. Therefore, it is reasonable to assume that the impact of CRF assessed at baseline on AF risk is likely to be underestimated rather than overestimated (Table 20.4).

Table 20.4 Atrial fibrillation and cardiorespiratory fitness

Study	Participants	Level of activity	Results/AF risk
Grundvold et al. [26]	2014 middle-aged men	Assessed using a cycle ergometer	AF risk was 23% in the fit compared to non-fit men
Khan et al. [59]	1950; mean age 52.6 years	METs quartiles	Progressive decrease in AF risk when compared to the least-fit group. The risk for those in the highest fitness category was 33% lower. Decreased AF with an HR 0.44 fit
Qureshi et al. [30]	64,561 middle-aged (mean age 54)	4 METs groups	Progressive decrease in AF risk when compared to the least-fit group. The risk for those in the highest fitness category was 56% lower
Faselis et al. [31]	5962 middle-aged veterans with a mean age of 56 years	METs quartiles	Progressive decrease in AF risk when compared to the least-fit group. The risk for those in the highest fitness category was 63% lower

Pathophysiologic Mechanisms of Atrial Fibrillation and Exercise

The available evidence supports that moderate exercise is associated with a protective effect against incident AF. There is also strong evidence supporting that high intensity and high volume of exercise endured by marathon runners and other high-endurance athletes can increase the rate of developing AF. The potential mechanisms involved in exercise-induced increase in AF risk are not completely elucidated, but several mechanisms have been proposed.

As mentioned earlier, prerequisite for AF is the presence of triggers to initiate it and the substrate to preserve it. High-endurance exercise is associated with structural changes leading to increased dimensions of both the atria [19]. There are several causes including increased height and left atria size in athletes and higher blood pressure at rest and peak exercise [19, 62–64], leading to a more concentric type of left ventricular remodeling. In addition, high-intensity exercise is associated with increased inflammation, oxidative stress, and eventually fibrosis of the atria [63].

Besides the pathological substrate, there should also be triggers which will initiate the arrhythmogenic cascade. High-endurance exercise has been associated with increased ectopy at the level of the atria [65]. This phenomenon in conjunction with the increased shifts in the sympathetic/parasympathetic balance [62, 66–69] could cause the electrophysiological abnormalities described above. Although increased parasympathetic tone commonly seen in athletes may be expected to potentially have a protective effect against AF, it seems that there is a vagal subtype of AF which presents in individuals with predominance of vagal tone [70]. Collectively, all these could explain the potential mechanisms of increased incidence of AF in high-endurance athletes as illustrated in Fig. 20.1.

On the other hand, there are several mechanisms which could explain the decrease in frequency of AF in individuals who engage in less competitive physical activity. Increased PA improves well-established risk factors which are related to AF like DM2, HTN, heart failure, obesity, CAD, etc. and decreases inflammation and oxidative stress [5–11]. Furthermore, exercise decreases the sympathetic tone with a predominance of vagal tone which, with the exception of a specific type of AF (see above), is related to decrease in incident AF [7].

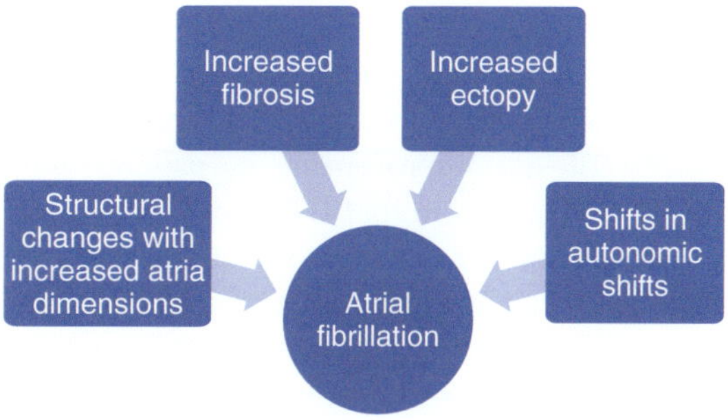

Fig. 20.1 Proposed mechanisms of atrial fibrillation in athletes

Exercise in Patients with Atrial Fibrillation

Relatively little is known about the impact of exercise in patients with established AF, paroxysmal, or permanent and if the prescription of PA in addition to the established treatment methods is beneficial. The beneficial effect of exercise in modifying multiple factors associated with AF is well described, but the direct effect of PA on AF is not well studied [62, 71].

In a large review study, Abdul-Aziz et al. [72] identified ten studies describing the effect of PA in patients with existing AF. The articles included one study on yoga, two studies on acupuncture, three studies that examined weight loss programs, and four studies that evaluated the impact of moderate physical activity. Yoga caused less symptomatic disease and improved the quality of life. Acupuncture decreased the episodes of AF, weight loss was associated with a significant reduction in AF occurrence and symptoms, and finally, moderate exercise resulted in a decrease in symptomatic disease and higher AF-free disease. The above findings though should be interpreted with caution, as the design of the studies was poor. In another Cochrane database review study, Risom et al. [73] concluded that there was not a clinically relevant effect of PA on health-related quality of life improvement in patients with AF. Pooled data from six RCTs showed a positive association on the outcome of exercise capacity, but due to the low number of participants and the quality of the evidence, the association of exercise and other outcomes (mortality and cardiovascular outcomes) could not be safely assessed.

In another study, Kato et al. [74] conducted a meta-analysis including five trials with a combined total of 379 participants. In AF patients, PA was associated with increased exercise capacity and improved left ventricular ejection fraction compared with the control (standardized mean difference (SMD), 0.91; 95% CI, 0.70–1.12; MD, 4.8%; 95% CIs, 1.56–8.03, respectively). Compared with the control, exercise training also significantly reduced BMI (SMD, −0.47 kg/m; 95% CIs, from −0.89 to −0.06) and improved the quality of life in some of the standardized questionnaires.

Only two randomized studies assessed the different intensities of PA and the effect on the AF burden in patients with paroxysmal or persistent AF. In the study by Skielboe et al. [75], 76 patients with paroxysmal/persistent atrial fibrillation were randomized to a 12-week low-intensity or high-intensity exercise program (50% and 80% of maximal perceived exertion, respectively). The primary outcome was burden of AF and the secondary outcome was change in $VO_{2\ max}$. There was no statistical difference in AF burden (incidence rate ratio 0.742, 95% CI 0.29–1.91, $p = 0.538$) or $VO_{2\ max}$ between high- and moderate-intensity groups. However, lack of significantly higher $VO_{2\ max}$ values for the high-intensity group suggests that the exercise intervention was not adequate to affect the primary outcome. In addition, the study lacked a control (non-exercising) group.

Malmo et al. [76] also randomly assigned 51 AF patients referred for catheter ablation to high-intensity aerobic interval training exercise over 12 weeks, or no exercise, and recorded AF burden from implantable loop recorders as the primary study outcome. A significant reduction in AF burden was noted in the exercise group, where the mean time in AF declined from 8.1% to 4.8%, with no significant change in the control group. Increased AF burden was more common in the control patients (64%) than in the exercise group (12%). A decline in the arrhythmia burden was noted in the exercise group, where 38% of patients experienced a decline in their arrhythmia compared to only 20% of the control group. The exercise group also experienced fewer and less severe symptoms following the intervention, with no concomitant change in the control group.

Conclusions

In conclusion, the current literature strongly suggests that long-term participation in exercise/physical activity of high intensity and/or volume is likely to predispose at least some individuals to increased incidence of AF. The threshold of exercise intensity and/or volume where the potentially deleterious effects of exercise occur has not been identified and is an issue of great interest for future studies. However, moderate levels of physical activity close to the guidelines recommended by the American Heart Association and the American College of Sports Medicine are likely to protect against the development of AF. The benefits of increased PA in such patients are at least, in part, attributed to the beneficial effect of PA on modifying risk factors which have shown to be related with increase in AF burden.

References

1. Chugh SS, Havmoller R, Narayanan K, Singh D, Rienstra M, Benjamin EJ, et al. Worldwide epidemiology of atrial fibrillation: a Global Burden of Disease 2010 Study. Circulation. 2014;129(8):837–47.
2. Go AS, Hylek EM, Phillips KA, Chang Y, Henault LE, Selby JV, et al. Prevalence of diagnosed atrial fibrillation in adults: national implications for rhythm management and stroke prevention: the AnTicoagulation and Risk Factors in Atrial Fibrillation (ATRIA) Study. JAMA. 2001;285(18):2370–5.
3. Huxley RR, Lopez FL, Folsom AR, Agarwal SK, Loehr LR, Soliman EZ, et al. Absolute and attributable risks of atrial fibrillation in relation to optimal and borderline risk factors: the Atherosclerosis

Risk in Communities (ARIC) study. Circulation. 2011;123:1501–8.
4. January CT, Wann LS, Alpert JS, et al. AHA/ACC/HRS guideline for the management of patients with atrial f. A report of the American College of Cardiology/American Heart Association Task Force on Practice Guidelines and the Heart Rhythm Society. J Am Coll Cardiol. 2014;64(21):2014. https://doi.org/10.1016/j.jacc.2014.03.022.
5. Kokkinos P, Myers J, Faselis C, Panagiotakos DB, Doumas M, Pittaras A, et al. Exercise capacity and mortality in older men: a 20-year follow-up study. Circulation. 2010;122(8):790–7.
6. Kokkinos P, Myers J. Exercise and physical activity: clinical outcomes and applications. Circulation. 2010;122(16):1637–48.
7. Faselis C, Doumas M, Pittaras A, Narayan P, Myers J, Tsimploulis A, et al. Exercise capacity and all-cause mortality in male veterans with hypertension aged 70 years. Hypertension. 2014;64(1):30–5.
8. Kokkinos PF, Faselis C, Myers J, Panagiotakos D, Doumas M. Interactive effects of fitness and statin treatment on mortality risk in veterans with dyslipidaemia: a cohort study. Lancet. 2013;381(9864):394–9.
9. Kokkinos P, Faselis C, Myers J, Narayan P, Sui X, Zhang J, et al. Cardiorespiratory fitness and incidence of major adverse cardiovascular events in US veterans: a cohort study. Mayo Clin Proc. 2017;92(1):39–48.
10. Myers J, Kokkinos P, Chan K, Dandekar E, Yilmaz B, Nagare A, et al. Cardiorespiratory fitness and reclassification of risk for incidence of heart failure: the Veterans Exercise Testing Study. Circ Heart Fail. 2017;10:e003780.
11. Kokkinos P, Myers J, Faselis C, Doumas M, Kheirbek R, Nylen E. BMI-mortality paradox and fitness in African-American and Caucasian men with type 2 diabetes. Diabetes Care. 2012;35(5):1021–7.
12. Baldesberger S, Bauersfeld U, Candinas R, Seifert B, Zuber M, Ritter M, et al. Sinus node disease and arrhythmias in the long-term follow-up of former professional cyclists. Eur Heart J. 2008;29(1):71–8.
13. Karjalainen J, Kujala UM, Kaprio J, Sarna S, Viitasalo M. Lone atrial fibrillation in vigorously exercising middle aged men: case-control study. BMJ. 1998;316(7147):1784–5.
14. Mont L, Tamborero D, Elosua R, Coll-Vinent B, Sitges M, Vidal B, et al., GIRAFA (Grup Integrat de Recerca en Fibril-lació Auricular) Investigators. Physical activity, height, and left atrial size are independent risk factors for lone atrial fibrillation in middle-aged healthy individuals. Europace. 2008;10(1):15–20.
15. Abdulla J, Nielsen JR. Is the risk of atrial fibrillation higher in athletes than in the general population? A systematic review and meta-analysis. Europace. 2009;11(9):1156–9.
16. Heidbüchel H, Anné W, Willems R, Adriaenssens B, Van de Werf F, Ector H. Endurance sports is a risk factor for atrial fibrillation after ablation for atrial flutter. Int J Cardiol. 2006;107(1):67–72.
17. Molina L, Mont L, Marrugat J, Berruezo A, Brugada J, Bruguera J, et al. Long-term endurance sport practice increases the incidence of lone atrial fibrillation in men: a follow-up study. Europace. 2008;10(5):618–23.
18. Aizer A, Gaziano JM, Cook NR, Manson JE, Buring JE, Albert CM. Relation of vigorous exercise to risk of atrial fibrillation. Am J Cardiol. 2009;103(11):1572–7.
19. Pelliccia A, Maron BJ, Di Paolo FM, Biffi A, Quattrini FM, Pisicchio C, et al. Prevalence and clinical significance of left atrial remodeling in competitive athletes. J Am Coll Cardiol. 2005;46(4):690–6.
20. Mozaffarian D, Furberg CD, Psaty BM, Siscovick D. Physical activity and incidence of atrial fibrillation in older adults: the Cardiovascular Health Study. Circulation. 2008;118:800–7.
21. Drca N, Wolk A, Jensen-Urstad M, Larsson SC. Atrial fibrillation is associated with different levels of physical activity levels at different ages in men. Heart. 2014;100:1037–42.
22. Drca N, Wolk A, Jensen-Urstad M, Larsson SC. Physical activity is associated with a reduced risk of atrial fibrillation in middle-aged and elderly women. Heart. 2015;101:1627–30.
23. Huxley RR, Misialek JR, Agarwal SK, Loehr LR, Soliman EZ, Chen LY, et al. Physical activity, obesity, weight change and risk of atrial fibrillation: the Atherosclerosis Risk in Communities (ARIC) Study. Circ Arrhythm Electrophysiol. 2014;7:620–5.
24. Garg PK, O'Neal WT, Chen LY, Loehr LR, Sotoodehnia N, Soliman EZ, et al. American Heart Association's life simple 7 and risk of atrial fibrillation in a population without known cardiovascular disease: the ARIC (Atherosclerosis Risk in Communities) Study. J Am Heart Assoc. 2018;7:e008424.
25. Azarbal F, Stefanick ML, Salmoirago-Blotcher E, Manson JE, Albert CM, LaMonte MJ, et al. Obesity, physical activity, and their interaction in incident atrial fibrillation in postmenopausal women. J Am Heart Assoc. 2014;3:17.
26. Grundvold I, Skretteberg PT, Liestøl K, Gjesdal K, Erikssen G, Kjeldsen SE, et al. Importance of physical fitness on predictive effect of body mass index and weight gain on incident atrial fibrillation in healthy imaged men. Am J Cardiol. 2012;110(3):425–32.
27. Myers J, Prakash M, Froelicher V, Do D, Partington S, Atwood JE. Exercise capacity and mortality among men referred for exercise testing. N Engl J Med. 2002;346:793–801.
28. Laukkanen JA, Kurl S, Salonen R, Rauramaa R, Salonen JT. The predictive value of cardiorespiratory fitness for cardiovascular events in men with various risk profiles: a prospective population-based cohort study. Eur Heart J. 2004;25:1428–37.
29. Lee D-C, Sui X, Artero EG, Lee I-M, Church TS, McAuley PA, et al. Long-term effects of changes in cardiorespiratory fitness and body mass index on all-cause and cardiovascular disease mortality in men: the Aerobics Center Longitudinal Study. Circulation. 2011;124:2483–90.

30. Qureshi WT, Alirhayim Z, Blaha MJ, Juraschek SP, Keteyian SJ, Brawner CA, et al. Cardiorespiratory fitness and risk of incident atrial fibrillation: results from the Henry Ford ExercIse Testing (FIT) Project. Circulation. 2015;131:1827–34.
31. Faselis C, Kokkinos P, Tsimploulis A, Pittaras A, Myers J, Lavie CJ, et al. Exercise capacity and atrial fibrillation risk in veterans: a cohort study. Mayo Clin Proc. 2016;91(5):558–66.
32. Camm AJ, Kirchhof P, Lip GY, European Heart Rhythm Association, European Association for Cardio-Thoracic Surgery, et al. Guidelines for the management of atrial fibrillation: the task force for the management of atrial fibrillation of the European Society of Cardiology (ESC). Eur Heart J. 2010;31(19):2369–429. https://doi.org/10.1093/eurheartj/ehq278.
33. Allessie MA, Boyden PA, Camm AJ, Kléber AG, Lab MJ, Legato MJ, et al. Pathophysiology and prevention of atrial fibrillation. Circulation. 2001;103(5):769–77.
34. Wakili R, Voigt N, Kaab S, Dobrev D, Nattel S. Recent advances in the molecular pathophysiology of atrial fibrillation. J Clin Invest. 2011;121:2955–68.
35. Lau DH, Nattel S, Kalman JM, Sanders P. Modifiable risk factors and atrial fibrillation. Circulation. 2017;136:583–96.
36. Nattel S, Burstein B, Dobrev D. Atrial remodeling and atrial fibrillation: mechanisms and implications. Circ Arrhythm Electrophysiol. 2008;1:62–73. https://doi.org/10.1161/CIRCEP.107.754564.
37. Haissaguerre M, Jais P, Shah DC, Takahashi A, Hocini M, Quiniou G, et al. Spontaneous initiation of atrial fibrillation by ectopic beats originating in the pulmonary veins. N Engl J Med. 1998;339:659.
38. Jais P, Haissaguerre M, Shah DC, Chouairi S, Gencel L, Hocini M, et al. A focal source of atrial fibrillation treated by discrete radiofrequency ablation. Circulation. 1997;95:572.
39. Scherf D, Romano FJ, Terranova R. Experimental studies on auricular flutter and auricular fibrillation. Am Heart J. 1948;36:241–51.
40. Ehrlich JR, Cha TJ, Zhang L, Chartier D, Melnyk P, Hohnloser SH, et al. Cellular electrophysiology of canine pulmonary vein cardiomyocytes: action potential and ionic current properties. J Physiol. 2003;551:801–13.
41. Lip GY, Brechin CM, Lane DA. The global burden of atrial fibrillation and stroke: a systematic review of the epidemiology of atrial fibrillation in regions outside North America and Europe. Chest. 2012;142:1489.
42. Go AS, Mozaffarian D, Roger VL, Benjamin EJ, Berry JD, Blaha MJ, et al. Heart disease and stroke statistics–2014 update: a report from the American Heart Association. Circulation. 2014;129:e28–292.
43. Kim MH, Johnston SS, Chu BC, Dalal MR, Schulman KL. Estimation of total incremental health care costs in patients with atrial fibrillation in the United States. Circ Cardiovasc Qual Outcomes. 2011;4:313–20.
44. Kannel WB, Wolf PA, Benjamin EJ, Levy D. Prevalence, incidence, prognosis, and predisposing conditions for atrial fibrillation: population-based estimates. Am J Cardiol. 1998;82:2N–9N.
45. Miller PS, Andersson FL, Kalra L. Are cost benefits of anticoagulation for stroke prevention in atrial fibrillation underestimated? Stroke. 2005;36:360–6.
46. Magnani JW, Wang N, Benjamin EJ, Garcia ME, Bauer DC, Butler J, et al. Atrial fibrillation and declining physical performance in older adults: the Health, Aging, and Body Composition Study. Circ Arrhythm Electrophysiol. 2016;9:e003525.
47. Santangeli P, Di Biase L, Bai R, Mohanty S, Pump A, Cereceda Brantes M, et al. Atrial fibrillation and the risk of incident dementia: a meta-analysis. Heart Rhythm. 2012;9(11):1761–8.
48. Wallace ER, Siscovick DS, Sitlani CM, Dublin S, Mitchell PH, Odden MC, et al. Incident atrial fibrillation and disability- free survival in the cardiovascular health study. J Am Geriatr Soc. 2016;64:838–43.
49. Benjamin EJ, Wolf PA, D'Agostino RB, Silbershatz H, Kannel WB, Levy D. Impact of atrial fibrillation on the risk of death: the Framingham Heart Study. Circulation. 1998;96:946–52.
50. Wang TJ, Larson MG, Levy D, Vasan RS, Leip EP, Wolf PA, et al. Temporal relations of atrial fibrillation and congestive heart failure and their joint influence on mortality: the Framingham Heart Study. Circulation. 2003;107:2920–5.
51. Krahn AD, Manfreda J, Tate RB, Mathewson FA, Cuddy TE. The natural history of atrial fibrillation: incidence, risk factors, and prognosis in the Manitoba Follow-Up Study. Am J Med. 1995;98:476–84.
52. Stewart S, Hart CL, Hole DJ, McMurray JJ. A population based study of the long-term risks associated with atrial fibrillation: 20-year follow-up of the Renfrew/Paisley study. Am J Med. 2002;113:359.
53. Ott A, Breteler MM, de Bruyne MC, van Harskamp F, Grobbee DE, Hofman A. Atrial fibrillation and dementia in a population-based study. The Rotterdam Study. Stroke. 1997;28:316–21.
54. Benjamin EJ, Levy D, Vaziri SM, D'Agostino RB, Belanger AJ, Wolf PA. Independent risk factors for atrial fibrillation in a population-based cohort. The Framingham Heart Study. JAMA. 1994;271:840–4.
55. Rangnekar G. The characterisation of risk factors, substrate and management strategies for atrial fibrillation [dissertation]. School of Medicine, The University of Adelaide; 2015.
56. Jamaly S, Carlsson L, Peltonen M, Jacobson P, Sjöström L, Karason K. Bariatric surgery and the risk of new-onset atrial fibrillation in Swedish obese subjects. J Am Coll Cardiol. 2016;68:2497–504.
57. Chamberlain AM, Agarwal SK, Ambrose M, Folsom AR, Soliman EZ, Alonso A. Metabolic syndrome and incidence of atrial fibrillation among blacks and whites in the Atherosclerosis Risk in Communities (ARIC) Study. Am Heart J. 2010;159(5):850–6. https://doi.org/10.1016/j.ahj.2010.02.005.
58. Bapat A, Zhang Y, Post WS, Guallar E, Soliman EZ, Heckbert SR, et al. Relation of physical activ-

ity and incident atrial fibrillation (from the Multi-Ethnic Study of Atherosclerosis). Am J Cardiol. 2015;116:883–8.

59. Khan H, Kella D, Rauramaa R, Savonen K, Lloyd MS, Laukkanen JA. Cardiorespiratory fitness and atrial fibrillation: a population-based follow-up study. Heart Rhythm. 2015;12:1424–30.
60. Elliott AD, Maatman B, Emery MS, Sanders P. The role of exercise in atrial fibrillation prevention and promotion: finding optimal ranges for health. Heart Rhythm. 2017;14:1713–20.
61. Haskell WL, Lee I-M, Pate RR, Powell KE, Blair SN, Franklin BA, et al. Physical activity and public health: updated recommendation for adults from the American College of Sports Medicine and the American Heart Association. Circulation. 2007;116:1081–93.
62. Kapa S, Asirvatham S. A MET a day keeps arrhythmia at bay: the association between exercise or cardiorespiratory fitness and atrial fibrillation. Mayo Clin Proc. 2016;91(5):545–50.
63. Geffken DF, Cushman M, Burke GL, Polak JF, Sakkinen PA. Tracy RP Association between physical activity and markers of inflammation in a healthy elderly population. Am J Epidemiol. 2001;153(3):242–50.
64. Grundvold I, Skretteberg PT, Liestøl K, Gjesdal K, Erikssen G, Kjeldsen SE, et al. Importance of physical fitness on predictive effect of body mass index and weight gain on incident atrial fibrillation in healthy middle-age men. Am J Cardiol. 2012;110(3):425–32.
65. Stiles MK, John B, Wong CX, Kuklik P, Brooks AG, Lau DH, et al. Paroxysmal lone atrial fibrillation is associated with an abnormal atrial substrate: characterizing the "second factor". J Am Coll Cardiol. 2009;53:1182–91.
66. Guasch E, Benito B, Qi X, Cifelli C, Naud P, Shi Y, et al. Atrial fibrillation promotion by endurance exercise: demonstration and mechanistic exploration in an animal model. J Am Coll Cardiol. 2013;62:68–77.
67. Winder WW, Hagberg JM, Hickson RC, Ehsani AA, McLane JA. Time course of sympathoadrenal adaptation to endurance exercise training in man. J Appl Physiol Respir Environ Exerc Physiol. 1978;45(3):370–4.
68. Chen PS, Chen LS, Fishbein MC, Lin SF, Nattel S. Role of the autonomic nervous system in atrial fibrillation: pathophysiology and therapy. Circ Res. 2014;114(9):1500–15.
69. Wilhelm M. Atrial fibrillation in endurance athletes. Eur J Prev Cardiol. 2014;21:1040–8.
70. Kapa S, Mears JA, Asirvatham SJ. The autonomic ether; emerging electrophysiologic associations. Indian Heart J. 2011;63(4):333–40.
71. Elliott AD, Mahajan R, Pathak RK, Lau DH, Sanders P. Exercise training and atrial fibrillation. Further evidence of the importance of lifestyle change. Circulation. 2016;133:457–9.
72. Abdul-Aziz AA, Altawil M, Lyon A, MacEachern M, Richardson CR, Rubenfire M, et al. Lifestyle therapy for the management of atrial fibrillation. Am J Cardiol. 2018;121(9):1112–7.
73. Risom SS, Zwisler AD, Johansen PP, Sibilitz K, Lindschou J, Gluud C, et al. Exercise-based cardiac rehabilitation for adults with atrial fibrillation. Cochrane Database Syst Rev. 2017;(2):CD011197.
74. Kato M, Kubo A, Nihei F, Ogano M, Takagi H. Effects of exercise training on exercise capacity, cardiac function, BMI, and quality of life in patients with atrial fibrillation: a meta-analysis of randomized-controlled trials. Int J Rehabil Res. 2017;40(3):193–201.
75. Skielboe AK, Bandholm TQ, Hakmann S, Mourier M, Kallemose T, Dixen U. Cardiovascular exercise and burden of arrhythmia in patients with atrial fibrillation – A randomized controlled trial. PLoS One. 2017;12(2):e0170060.
76. Malmo V, Nes BM, Amundsen BH, Tjonna AE, Stoylen A, Rossvoll O, et al. Aerobic interval training reduces the burden of atrial fibrillation in the short term: a randomized trial. Circulation. 2016;133:466–73.

21 Chronic Kidney Disease and Physical Activity

Anubhav Kumar, Puneet Narayan, and Peter Kokkinos

Abbreviations

AER	Albumin excretion rate
ACR	Albumin-to-creatinine ratio
BP	Blood pressure
CKD	Chronic kidney diseases
CRF	Cardiorespiratory fitness
CV	Cardiovascular
DM2	Type II diabetes mellitus
eGFR	Estimated glomerular filtration rate
ESRD	End-stage renal disease
GFR	Glomerular filtration rate
HF	Heart failure
hsCRP	High-sensitivity C-reactive protein
HTN	Hypertension
KDQOL-SF	Kidney Disease Quality of Life Short Form
LV	Left ventricular
METs	Metabolic equivalents
PA	Physical activity
UACR	Urine albumin-to-creatinine ratio
VO_2 max	Peak oxygen uptake
5STS	Five-times sit-to-stand test time
6MWD	6-minute walk distance

A. Kumar (✉) · P. Narayan
Clinical Research Institute of Northern Virginia, Burke, VA, USA

P. Kokkinos
Veterans Affairs Medical Center, Department of Cardiology, Washington, DC, USA

Georgetown University School of Medicine, Washington, DC, USA

Department of Kinesiology and Health, Rutgers University, New Brunswick, NJ, USA

George Washington University School of Medicine and Health Sciences, Washington, DC, USA

University of South Carolina, Department of Exercise Science, Arnold School of Public Health, Columbia, SC, USA
e-mail: peter.kokkinos@va.gov

Introduction

Chronic kidney diseases (CKD) are collectively characterized by an abnormal change in kidney function or structure that persists for at least 3 months [1, 2]. CKD are most commonly detected by measurement of serum creatinine, allowing for the calculation of estimated glomerular filtration rate (eGFR) by various formulae (such as Cockcroft-Gault, Modification of Diet in Renal Disease, and Chronic Kidney Disease-Epidemiology [CKD-EPI]), and the presence of albumin in the urine, indicating damage to the renal glomeruli. Kidney diseases are classified by etiology and staged by eGFR (Table 21.1) and degree of protein loss in the urine (Table 21.2).

P. Kokkinos, P. Narayan (eds.), *Cardiorespiratory Fitness in Cardiometabolic Diseases*,
https://doi.org/10.1007/978-3-030-04816-7_21

In the absence of kidney damage, neither GFR category G1 nor G2 fulfills the criteria for CKD.

With progressive loss of eGFR and increase in albuminuria, the risks of cardiovascular (CV) disease, mortality, further renal injury, and progression to dialysis dependency increase (Fig. 21.1) [1]. Stage 3 CKD represents the largest proportion of CKD patients in the United States, encompassing some 43% of the CKD population [3].

Table 21.1 GFR categories in CKD [1]

GFR category	GFR (mL/min/1.73 m^2)	Terms
G1	≥90	Normal or high
G2	60–89	Mildly decreased[a]
G3a	45–59	Mildly to moderately decreased
G3b	30–44	Moderately to severely decreased
G4	15–29	Severely decreased
G5	<15	Kidney failure

[a]Relative to young adult level

Table 21.2 Albuminuria categories in CKD [1]

Category	AER (mg/24 h)	ACR (approximate equivalent) (mg/mmol)	ACR (approximate equivalent) (mg/g)	Terms
A1	< 30	< 3	< 30	Normal to mildly increased
A2	30–300	3–30	30–300	Moderately increased[a]
A3	> 300	> 30	> 300	Severely increased[b]

Abbreviations: *AER* albumin excretion rate, *ACR* albumin-to-creatinine ratio

[a]Relative to young adult

[b]Including nephrotic syndrome (albumin excretion usually >200 mg/24 h [ACR > 2200 mg/g; > 220 mg/mmol])

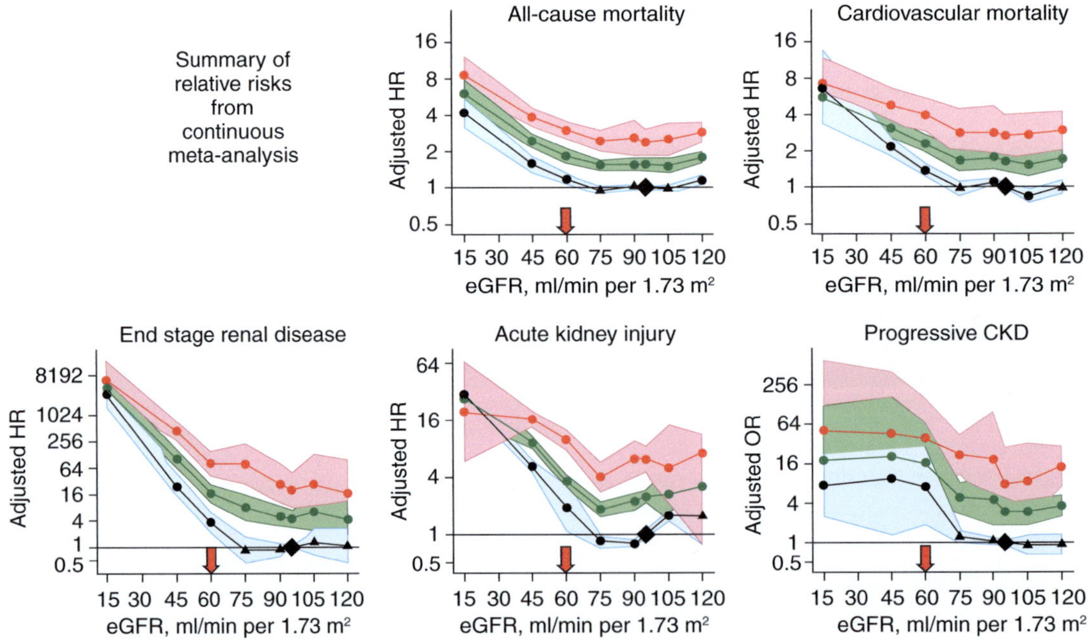

Fig. 21.1 Impact of albuminuria on the relative risk of various health-related outcomes. (Modified from Kidney Disease: Improving Global Outcomes [2])

Prevalence and Incidence

CKD is a growing concern, not just for its serious health consequences but for its increasing prevalence in the general population and vulnerable subpopulations. Approximately 14% of the general adult US population, or 1 in 7 adults, was estimated to have CKD based on 2015 data. The prevalence rose 2% between the periods of 1994–1998 and 1999–2004 [4]. Gender and racial disparities also exist; women are 3.8% more likely to have CKD stages 1–4, while African-Americans and Mexican-Americans are, respectively, 2.4% and 0.6% more likely to have CKD than Caucasian-Americans [5]. While a slight decline in kidney function may be inevitable with aging, possessing risk factors that predispose to chronic kidney disease accelerates the decline. However, even though some of the risk factors for getting kidney disease are non-modifiable (e.g., polycystic kidney disease or family history of genetic CKD), many of the other risk factors which are more commonly implicated in CKD, including but not limited to hypertension (HTN), type I and II (DM2) diabetes mellitus, dyslipidemia, heart disease, and obesity, are modifiable. About a third of diabetics and a fifth of hypertensives are at risk of developing CKD. Both HTN and DM2 are known risk factors for increased mortality and cardiovascular disease including coronary heart disease and strokes, and these risks are compounded further with the development of CKD [6, 7].

Similar to its associated risk factors, CKD can remain hidden for many years, with nonspecific symptoms such as fatigue, pruritis, fluid overload, nausea, and loss of appetite emerging only at moderate to severe stages. This insidiousness is alarming considering CKD can ultimately lead to end-stage renal disease (ESRD), rendering the patient dialysis dependent and in need of renal transplant. Men are more likely to progress to ESRD than women. Though the incidence of ESRD was slightly lower in the first three quarters of 2017 than in 2016 and 2015 (92,767 vs. 94,517 vs., 94,210, respectively), the prevalence of ESRD (Fig. 21.2) with its associated morbidity and mortality continues to rise. While there

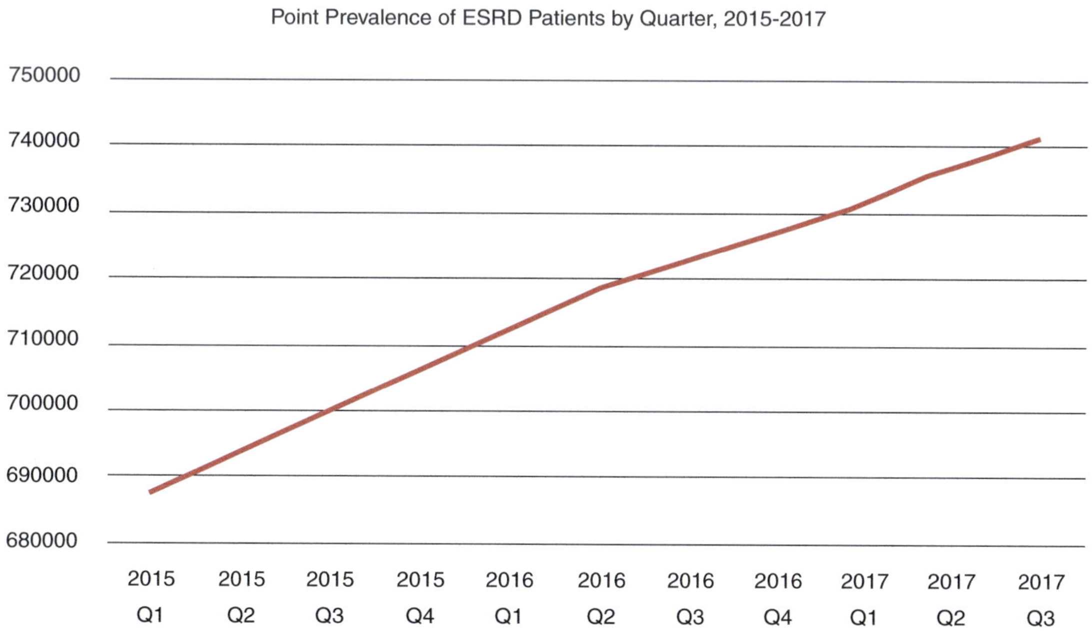

Fig. 21.2 Prevalence of ESRD from the first quarter 2015 to third quarter 2017. (Modified from ESRD Quarterly Update [8])

are numerous etiologies of kidney disease, including glomerulonephritides, urological disorders, and ischemic injury, hypertension and diabetes are the leading causes of ESRD, outnumbering all others by a 3:1 ratio from 2015 to 2017 [8].

Patient and Societal Impact of Chronic Kidney Diseases

The financial impact of CKD is staggering. In 2015, Medicare spending for all patients with CKD and ESRD was almost $100 billion, divided roughly in a 2:1 ratio; 20% of Medicare spending for patients aged 65 years and greater was devoted to the treatment of CKD alone. Annual spending per patient with CKD was $15,930, 54% higher than beneficiaries without CKD, DM, or heart failure (HF). If patients had concurrent diagnoses of diabetes and heart failure, their annual expenditure was 44% higher than those patients without CKD but with diabetes and heart failure [9]. Expenditures increased with CKD severity; the more severe the CKD stage, the higher the expenditure. For patients with ESRD receiving treatment via in-center hemodialysis, the annual Medicare expenditure is approximately $85,000 per annum [10].

In addition to the economic consequences of CKD, patients are at a significantly increased risk for developing cardiovascular (CV) disease, CV events, and other comorbidities resulting in frequent hospitalizations and a 15–30-fold higher mortality rate compared to an age-matched healthy population [11]. The presence of CKD has dramatic negative consequences for life expectancy. A systematic review and meta-analysis assessing the relationship between CKD and mortality was conducted by Tonelli et al., examining 39 trials totaling 1.37 million patients. In 38 of 41 cohorts, they found a statistically significant association with CKD progression and mortality risk, which increased exponentially with severity of CKD [12]. Large cohort studies have revealed that patients aged 30 years with stage 3B or 4 CKD, respectively, lose 17 and 25 years from their expected life expectancy compared to patients in the general population. Patients of the same age with stage 2 and 3 albuminuria have an associated reduction in life expectancy of 10 and 18 years, respectively. Declines in eGFR and increasing albuminuria were also associated with increased cardiovascular mortality; patients with CKD stages 3A and 3B are at higher risk of death from cardiovascular etiologies than kidney failure; this relationship is inverted when patients reach CKD stage 4 [13].

Some other less recognized but equally critical consequences of CKD are deterioration of quality of life, depression, and decline in muscular strength. Quality of life is low for patients across the CKD and ESRD spectrum [14]. Although early stages may be asymptomatic, progressive loss of renal function can lead to symptoms such as fatigue, loss of appetite, nausea, vomiting, and confusion. Prior to the onset of symptoms, laboratory abnormalities such as hyperkalemia and hyperphosphatemia can require the use of binding medications, increasing pill burdens. A 2009 assessment of 235 ESRD patients on chronic dialysis found that their median pill burden was 19 per day, with a quarter of the patient population taking over 25 pills per day [15].

Physical Activity and Exercise Habits of Patients with Chronic Kidney Diseases

In 2003, Stengel et al. reported an association between physical inactivity and risk of chronic kidney disease in the NHANES II dataset [16]. Since then, numerous studies have examined the association between physical activity status and renal outcomes in large cohorts. An international analysis of exercise habits of 20,920 chronic dialysis patients enrolled in the Dialysis Outcomes and Practice Patterns Study (DOPPS) revealed that 54% of patients exercised less than once a week, while 47.4% were regular exercisers defined ≥1 exercise session per week [17]. In a prospective study of 54 chronic dialysis patients followed over 1 year, physical activity declined 3.4% per month as measured by accelerometry and a validated questionnaire [18]. Others have also identified that CKD and ESRD patients have decreased aerobic exercise capacity with increased muscle atrophy and weakness, evident even in the early stages of CKD and progressively worsen as kidney function deteriorates, contributing to comorbidities and lowering quality of life [19, 20]. Cardiovascular response to exercise and the relationships between cardiorespiratory fitness (CRF) and CV burden were evaluated in 136 CKD patients with eGFR of 40 ± 9 ml/min/1.73 m^2 aged 59.7 ± 9.6 years. Fifty-five percent of them were males, 38% diabetic, 17% smokers, and 39% with established CV disease. Assessments included direct peak oxygen uptake (VO_2 max) PA level by a questionnaire, echocardiographic left ventricular parameters, central arterial stiffness by aortic pulse wave velocity, and LV afterload using augmentation index. The investigators reported that significantly the peak VO_2 and heart rate response to exercise were significantly impaired in these patients. This was more pronounced on the low-fit individuals, who tended to be older and obese and with higher prevalence of CV disease. The reduced cardiorespiratory fitness was also independently associated with increased aortic stiffness, increased left ventricle afterload, poor left ventricle function, and higher burden of cardiovascular risk [21].

Physiologic Limitations to Physical Activity in CKD and ESRD

Several factors limit exercise tolerance and promote deconditioning in the CKD/ESRD population. One such factor is anemia, a common issue in the CKD/ESRD population from loss of erythropoietin generation. When corrected, exercise capacity improves. However, in a prospective study of 9 patients with CKD stages 3a–4 with hemoglobin levels >12 g/dL without any prior treatment for anemia, VO_2 max declined with eGFR despite maintenance of hemoglobin levels during a follow-up period of 2 years or until dialysis initiation, suggesting additional responsible mechanisms for deconditioning [22].

Sarcopenia has also been studied as a contributing factor to low exercise capacity in CKD patients. Progressive kidney disease is associated with an elevated inflammatory state, leading to increased catabolism of protein, as well as decreased appetite from the buildup of uremic toxins. This milieu can develop as early as CKD stage 3a and worsens with the loss of renal function [23]. Further protein losses occur from the process of dialysis, as well as increased acidemia from the loss of renal buffering capacity with advanced CKD. Sarcopenia and CKD were shown to have a multivariate association by Foley et al. in 13,770 community living adults [24]. In 100 CKD patients not on dialysis, de Souza et al., using the European Working Group on Sarcopenia in Older People (EWGSOP) and the Foundation for the National Institutes of Health (FNIH) Sarcopenia Project diagnostic criteria, found that sarcopenia was present in 11.9% of CKD patients using the EWGSOP criteria and 28.7% using the FNIH criteria [25]. The prevalence of sarcopenia increased with worsening kidney functions, being present in 34.5% of CKD patients in stages 2 and 3A and 65.5% in stage 3B, 4, or 5. A reduced muscle mass was present in 44% of the patients, 9% had reduced muscle strength, and 69% had reduced muscle performance [26, 27]. Patients with sarcopenia had higher levels of high-sensitivity C-reactive protein (hsCRP) levels and lower levels of phosphorous and log of interleukin (log(IL)) [26].

Interventional Evidence of Physical Activity in Chronic Kidney Disease

One of the common denominators in managing the several risk factors and consequences of chronic kidney disease is lifestyle modification. Health benefits related to increased physical activity in patients with CV disease are well established, and several guidelines recommend improving lifestyle in patients with CKD. Kidney Disease: Improving Global Outcomes (KDIGO) guidelines recommend a minimum of 30-min exercise sessions 5 times per week. This is based on the beneficial effects of exercise on risk factors for CKD, even though specific effect of exercise on CKD is not fully elucidated. KDIGO exercise recommendations are the same for all stages of CKD, which may reflect an effort to facilitate physician counseling and patient compliance and the low level of evidence cited in the recommendation (a grade of D) [28]. More specific guidelines have been recommended in the Exercise & Sports Science Australia (ESSA) position statement, which recommends aerobic exercise at >60% of maximum capacity [29].

In a survey of DOPPS patients, ESRD patients on chronic dialysis, who exercised at least once a week, reported significantly higher quality of life scores, physical function, and sleep quality scores. Significantly fewer hospitalizations for fractures were observed in this group compared to the infrequent exercise cohort, though hospitalizations for cardiac events or amputations did not favor either group. Leisure-time physical activity was associated with lower mortality on a personal and facility-level, though this also correlated with socioeconomic factors [18]. In a meta-analysis of 24 studies totaling 879 CKD patients on chronic dialysis aged 18 or older, Smart et al. reported significant improvements in VO_2 max in the 10 trials where it was measured, as well as significant improvements in 6MWT in hemodialysis patients. Exercise was also associated with statistically significant decreases in reported depression symptoms on the Beck Depression Score [30].

Evidence supports that exercise need not be strenuous to confer health benefit. After 12 weeks of Tai Chi exercise in hemodialysis patients, Chang et al. reported improvements in kidney disease-related quality of life and physical functioning in Taiwanese patients [31]. The findings of a meta-analysis also suggest that combining aerobic and resistance exercises may confer greater health benefits than either exercise alone. A greater improvement in VO_2 max was noted in studies where aerobic and strength training were combined compared to aerobic training alone, though this was not a significant finding. Training on non-dialysis days also appears to have a greater increase in VO_2 max (30.8 ± 7.6%) versus training during dialysis days (17.8 ± 7.7%). Of note, hemodialysis facilities offering exercise programs were associated with a 38% higher odds ratio for having patients performing regular exercise [30]. Thus, offering exercise programs may lead to increased participation in leisure-time physical activity among in-center hemodialysis patients.

The effect of different types of exercises on clinical outcomes was evaluated in a meta-analysis of 41 randomized, controlled trials with 928 CKD patients [32]. Measured parameters varied by study, such as aerobic capacity, muscular functioning, CV function, walking capacity, and health-related quality of life. Most of the studies were in patients on dialysis and most used aerobic exercise for intervention. The overall conclusion was that exercise has a beneficial effect on several clinical outcomes including aerobic exercise capacity, muscle functioning, cardiovascular function, and health-related quality of life.

The role of exercise was also evaluated separately in patients with stage 2–5 CKD, patients on hemodialysis, and those with renal transplants. Overall, exercise-related health benefits were similar in all subgroups with no group-specific benefits noted for the different types of exercise [32]. An accompanying editorial highlighted some of the shortcomings of this meta-analysis. Poor quality of several studies and inadequate reporting of methodology and outcomes were factors mentioned that may explain the indeterminate results. Intention-to-treat analysis was not reported in 80% of the studies [33].

In the EXerCise Introduction To Enhance performance in dialysis patients (EXCITE) trial, a multicenter randomized trial was designed to assess the effect of walking over 6 months on 6-min walk distance (6MWD), five-times sit-to-stand test time (5STS), and cognitive and social interaction scores in the Kidney Disease Quality of Life Short Form (KDQOL-SF). A total of 296 chronic dialysis patients from 13 dialysis centers were randomized to normal physical activity (145 patients, control) or a home program modeled on a peripheral arterial disease rehabilitation program managed by dialysis staff (151 patients, intervention). The patients included both hemodialysis and continuous ambulatory peritoneal dialysis (CAPD) patients. Patients were matched for age, gender, type of dialysis, presence of DM2, heart failure, and tobacco use and biochemical parameters including kT/V (k, dialyzer clearance of urea; T, dialysis time; V, volume of distribution of urea). Systolic blood pressure (BP) in the intervention arm was somewhat higher compared to the control arm, but not statistically significant. At the end of 6 months, 91% of the intervention arm patients had documented their adherence, averaging 83% completion of the 144 sessions. Forty-six patients performed more than 144 sessions and 29 patients performed less. Reasons cited for low adherence included lack of interest, orthopedic issues, and problems with work. Neither group had any changes observed in BP, heart rate, serum creatinine, kT/V, albumin, phosphate, parathyroid hormone (PTH), triglycerides, or cholesterol. Significant improvements (Fig. 21.3) in the 6MWT were noted in the exercise group compared to the control group (+ 39 meters vs. +2 meters, $P < 0.001$), which was noted to correlate with adherence to the program, and correlated to a 23% reduction in mortality risk in 3.3-year follow-up. The number of patients who were unable to complete the 5STS trial at baseline decreased significantly in the intervention arm vs. the control arm ($p < 0.001$). Similar to 6MWD, the effect size increased with adherence to the intervention. Dialysis modality was not found to have a significant impact on the results of the tests. Although there was a trend to improvement in the intervention arm on the KDQOL-SF, this was not statistically significant when compared to the control arm. For patients who completed the trial, hospitalization-free survival was lower in the intervention arm compared to the control arm ($p = 0.04$). There was no difference in AV-fistula events between the two groups, a notable finding as many dialysis patients are counseled against vigorous use of their access arms for exercise for fear of provoking fistula morbidity [34].

For CKD patients not requiring dialysis, Narayan et al. reported on the relationship of cardiorespiratory fitness and risk for chronic kidney disease in a cohort of 5812 VAMC patients. They found that as cardiorespiratory fitness improved, the relative risk of progressive CKD decreased [35]. In the Seattle Kidney Study, 256 clinic patients with CKD stages G3a–4 were prospectively followed over a mean of 3.7 years. Patients were administered the Four-Week Physical Activity History Questionnaire (FWH) to self-report their leisure-time activity. Investigators reported that every 60-min increase in weekly physical activity was associated with a 0.5% decrease in the rate of renal decline, which was demonstrated when controlling for diabetes and coronary artery disease. There was a 2.8% percent difference between groups that did not participate in any leisure-time activity versus those who did more than 150 min per week [36]. The same group had previously examined 5888 patients 65 years and older enrolled in the Cardiovascular Health Study, finding that the decline in renal function was 16% in the group with the highest rate of physical activity and 30% in the group with the lowest [37]. Nylen et al. reported an improvement in GFR following a 12-week exercise program in 128 diabetic patients with mild CKD. Overall there was a 3.9% increase in eGFR, a 6% increase in patients with stage 2 CKD, and 12% in those with stage 3 CKD [38]. Other small interventional studies, however, have failed to find improvement in eGFR decline with exercise, further muddying the evidence [37].

Finally, there is epidemiologic evidence that increased cardiorespiratory fitness (CRF) decreases the risk for developing CKD. The association between CRF and CKD incidence was assessed in a recent study of 5812 US male veterans (mean age, 58.4 ± 11.5 years) with an estimated eGFR of ≥60 mL/min per 1.73 m^2 6 months before exercise testing and no evidence of CKD. During a median follow-up period of 7.9 years, the investigators reported an inverse and graded association between exercise capacity and CKD incidence. The adjusted risk was 22% lower for every 1 metabolic equivalent (MET) increase in exercise capacity. When the cohort was stratified by the exercise capacity (peak METs achieved), the risk across the CRF categories for developing CKD declined progressively

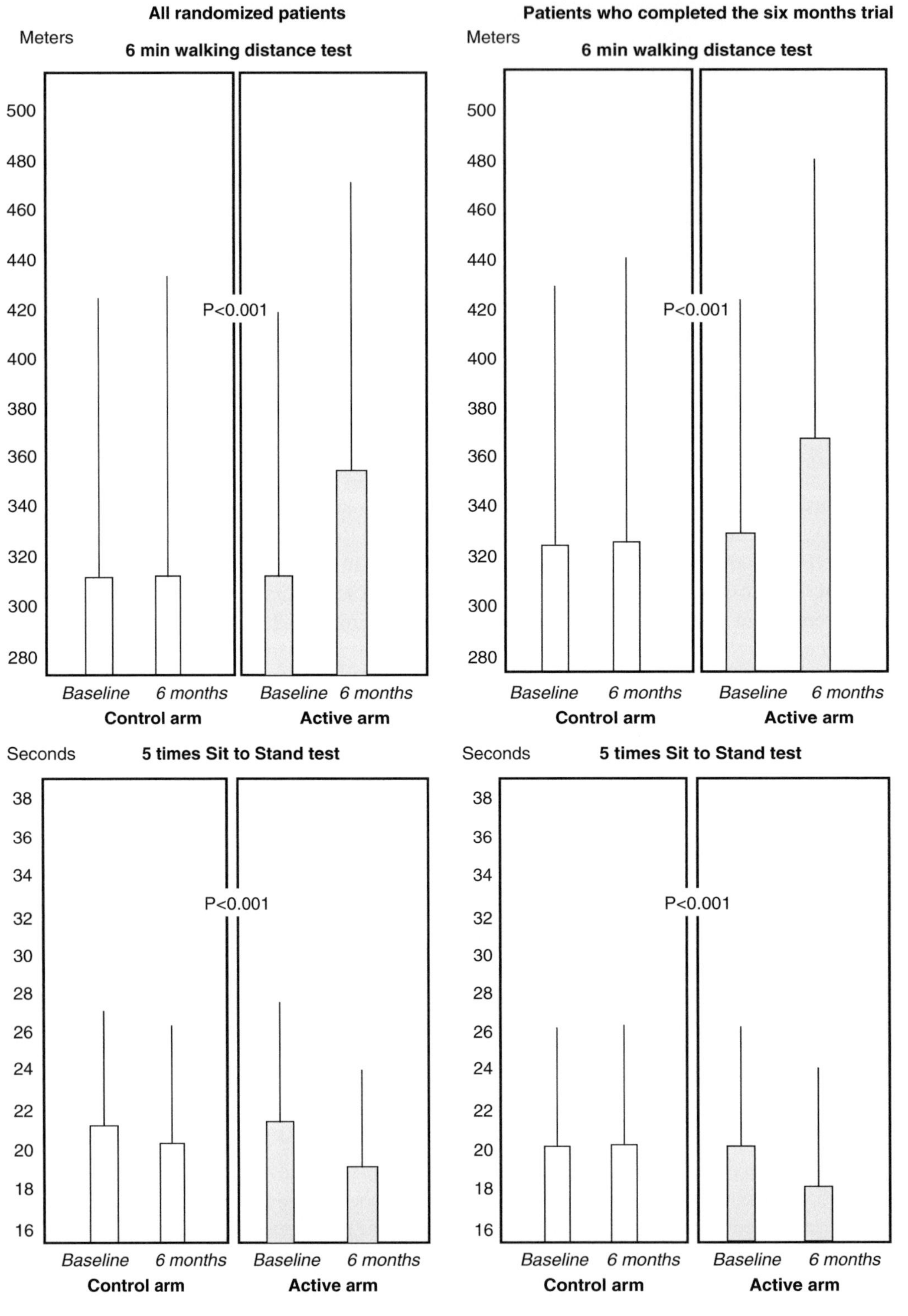

Fig. 21.3 Outcomes of the EXCITE study showing improvements in 6MWD and 5-times sit-to-stand test in the active arm compared to the control arm. (Reprinted with permission from Manfredini et al. [34])

with increased CRF. When compared with the least-fit individuals (reference group), the risk was 17% lower for individuals in the next CRF category, 45% lower for the moderate-fit, and 58% lower for the highest-fit individuals [39].

Conclusions

Progressive CKD is associated with declines in exercise capacity which can increase the risk of morbidity and mortality. Exercise programs can improve CRF though the data is based primarily on epidemiological data. More rigorous, prospective interventional evidence is needed to determine optimal exercise regimes and their effect on long-term outcomes in CKD patients and those at risk for developing renal disease.

References

1. Kidney Disease: Improving Global Outcomes. KDIGO 2012 Clinical practice guideline for the evaluation and management of chronic kidney disease. Kidney Int. 2013;3(1):S1–150.
2. Levey AS, Becker C, Inker LA. Glomerular filtration rate and albuminuria for detection and staging of acute and chronic kidney disease in adults: a systematic review. JAMA. 2015;313(8):837–46.
3. Hill NR, Fatoba ST, Oke JL, Hirst JA, O'Callaghan CA, Lasserson DS, FDR H. Global prevalence of chronic kidney disease – a systematic review and meta-analysis. PLoS One. 2016;11(7):e0158765. Published online 2016 Jul 6. https://doi.org/10.1371/journal.pone.0158765.
4. Kidney Disease Statistics for the United States [Internet]. Bethesda: National Institute of Diabetes and Digestive and Kidney Diseases. c2015 [cited 2018 June 1]. Available from https://www.niddk.nih.gov/health-information/health-statistics/kidney-disease.
5. Centers for Disease Control and Prevention. Age-adjusted prevalence of CKD Stages 1-4 by Gender 2013–2014. Chronic Kidney Disease (CKD) Surveillance Project website. https://nccd.cdc.gov. Accessed 5 June 2018.
6. Center for Disease Control and Prevention. National Chronic Kidney Disease Fact Sheet, 2017. Atlanta:US Department of Health and Human Services, Centers for Disease Control and Prevention; 2017.
7. Center for Disease Control and Prevention. Chronic kidney disease surveillance system – United States. Website, http://www.cdc.gov/ckd.
8. ESRD Quarterly Update – April 2018 – Incident and prevalent counts by quarter [Internet]. Ann Arbor (MI). United States Renal Data System. C2018 [cited 2018 June 4]. Available from.: https://www.usrds.org/qtr/default.aspx.
9. United States Renal Data System. 2017 USRDS Annual Data Report, Volume 1 – CKD in the United States, Chapter 6: Healthcare expenditures for persons with CKD. Ann Arbor (MI): 2017.
10. Wang V, Vilme H, Maciejewski M, Boulware L. The economic burden of chronic kidney disease and end-stage renal disease. Semin Nephrol. 2016;25(4):319–30.
11. Go AS, Chertow GM, Fan D, et al. Chronic kidney disease and the risks of death, cardiovascular events, and hospitalization. N Engl J Med. 2004;351:1296–305.
12. Toneli M, Wiebe N, Culleton B, House A, Rabbat C, Fok M, et al. CKD and mortality risk: a systematic review. JASN. 2006;17(7):2034–47.
13. Gansevoort RT, Correa-Rotter R, Hemmelgarn B, Tazeen J, Heerspink H, Mann J, et al. Chronic kidney disease and cardiovascular risk: epidemiology, mechanisms, and prevention. Lancet. 2013;382(9889):339–52.
14. Abdel-Kader K, Unruh M, Weisbord S. Symptom burden, depression, and quality of life in chronic and end-stage kidney disease. CJASN. 2009;4(6):1057–64.
15. Chiu Y, Teitelbaum I, Madhukar M, de Leon E, Adzize T, Mehrotra R. Pill burden, adherence, hyperphosphatemia, and quality of life in maintenance dialysis patients. CJASN. 2009;4(6):1089–96.
16. Stengel B, Tarver-Carr ME, Powe NR, Eberhardt MS, Brancati FL. Lifestyle factors, obesity, and the risk of chronic kidney disease. Epidemiology. 2003;14(4):479–87.
17. Tentori F, Elder SJ, Tuhmma J, Pisoni RL, Bommer J, Fissell RB, et al. Physical exercise among participants in the dialysis outcomes and practice patterns study (DOPPS): correlates and associated outcomes. Nephrol Dial Transplant. 2010;25:3050–62.
18. Johanesen KL, Kaysen GA, Young BS, Hung AM, DaSilva M, Chertow GM. Longitudinal study of nutritional status, body composition, and physical function in hemodialysis patients. Am J Clin Nutr. 2003;77(4):842–6.
19. Coresh J, Selvin E, Stevens LA, et al. Prevalence of chronic kidney disease in the United States. JAMA. 2007;298:2038–48.
20. Go AS, Chertow GM, Fan D, et al. Chronic kidney disease and the risks of death, cardiovascular events, and hospitalization. N Engl J Med. 2004;351:1296–305.
21. Howdena EJ, Westona K, Leano R, Sharman JE, Marwick T, Isbel NM, et al. Cardiorespiratory fitness and cardiovascular burden in chronic kidney disease. J Sci Med Sport. 2015;18(4):492–7.
22. Leikis MJ, MJ MK, Petersen AC, Kent AB, Mjurphy KT, Leppik JA, et al. Exercise performance falls over time in patients with chronic kidney disease despite

maintenance of hemoglobin concentration. CJASN. 2006;1(3):488–95.
23. Dukkipati R, Kopple J. Causes and prevention of protein-energy wasting in chronic kidney failure. Sem in Nephrology. 2009;29(1):39–49.
24. Foley RN, Wang C, Ishani A, Collins AJ, Murray AM. Kidney function and sarcopenia in the United States General Population: NHANES III. Am J Nephrol. 2007;27:279–86. https://doi.org/10.1159/000101827.
25. de Souza VA, Oliveira D, Barbosa SR, JOO C, FAB C, Mansur HN, NMA F, Bastos MG. Sarcopenia in patients with chronic kidney disease not yet on dialysis: analysis of the prevalence and associated factors. PLoS One. 2017;12(4):e0176230. PO 2017 Apr 27. https://doi.org/10.1371/journal.pone.0176230.
26. Cruz-Jentoft AJ, Baeyens JP, Bauer JM, Boirie Y, Cederholm T, Landi F, et al. Sarcopenia: European Consensus on definition and diagnosis: report of the European Working Group on Sarcopenia in older people. Age Ageing. 2010;39(4):412–23. https://doi.org/10.1093/ageing/afq034.
27. McLean RR, Kiel DP. Developing consensus criteria for Sarcopenia: an update. J Bone Miner Res. 2015;30(4):588–92. https://doi.org/10.1002/jbmr.2492.
28. Kidney Disease: Improving Global Outcomes. KDIGO clinical practice guideline for the management of blood pressure in chronic kidney disease. KI Supplements. 2012;2(5):337–414.
29. Smart NA, Williams AD, Levinger I, et al. Exercise & Sports Science Australia (ESSA) position statement on exercise and chronic kidney disease. J Sci Med Sport. 2013;16(5):406–11.
30. Smart N, McFarlane J, Cornelissen V. The effect of exercise therapy on physical function, biochemistry, and dialysis adequacy in haemodialysis patients: a systematic review and meta-analysis. Open J Nephrology. 2013;3(1):25–36.
31. Chang JH, Koo M, Wu SW, Chen CY. Effects of a 12-week program of Tai Chi exercise on the kidney disease quality of life and physical functioning of patients with end-stage renal disease on hemodialysis. Complement Ther Med. 2017;30:79–83.
32. Heiwe S, Jacobson SH. Exercise training in adults with CKD: a systematic review and meta-analysis. Am J Kidney Dis. 2014;64(3):383–93.
33. Williams AD, Fassett RG, Coombes JS. Exercise in CKD: Why is it important and how should it be delivered? Am J Kidney Dis. 2014;64(3):329–31.
34. Manfredini F, Mallamaci F, D'Arrigo G, Baggetta R, Bolignano D, Torino C, Lamberti N, et al. Exercise in patients on dialysis: a multicenter, randomized clinical trial. JASN. 2017;28(4):1259–68.
35. Narayan P, Faselis C, Myers J, Nylen E, Kumar A, Kokkinos P. Cardiorespiratory fitness and all-cause mortality in veterans with Stage II-IV chronic kidney disease American Diabetes Association - 77th Scientific Sessions. San Diego; 2017.
36. Robinson-Cohen C, Littman A, Duncan GE, Weiss NS, Sachs MC, Ruzinski J, Kundzins J, et al. Physical activity and change in estimated GFR among persons with CKD. JASN. 2014;25(2):399–406.
37. Robinson-Cohen C, Katz R, Mozaffarian D, Dairymple LS, de Boer I, Sarnak M, et al. Physical activity and rapid decline in kidney function among older adults. Arch Intern Med. 2009;169(22):2116–23.
38. Nylen E, Gandhi M, Kheirbek R, Kokkinos P. Enhanced fitness and renal function in Type 2 diabetes. Diabet Med. 2015;32:1342–5.
39. Kokkinos P, Faselis C, Myers J, Sui X, Zhang J, Tsimploulis A, et al. Exercise capacity and risk of chronic kidney disease in US Veterans: a cohort study. Mayo Clin Proc. 2015;90(4):461–8.

Physical Activity, Fitness, and Sexual Dysfunction

22

Konstantinos P. Imprialos, Konstantinos Stavropoulos, and Michael Doumas

Introduction

Sexual dysfunction is a public health problem that impairs the quality of life of affected individuals and their sexual partners [1]. The World Health Organization defines sexual dysfunction as "the various ways in which an individual is unable to participate in a sexual relationship as he or she would wish." For males, sexual dysfunction is defined as the persistent inability to attain and/or sustain penile erection for at least 3 months for sufficient time to achieve a successful intercourse [2]. For females, sexual dysfunction is defined as a persistent or recurring reduction in sexual desire and/or sexual arousal, dyspareunia, and inability or difficulty to achieve orgasm [3]. In this chapter, the terms "sexual dysfunction" will be used when referring to both genders, and "erectile dysfunction" [ED] will be used when referring to males.

A strong association between erectile dysfunction and cardiovascular (CV) risk is exemplified by the fact that ED is independently associated with an increased CV risk, and in men not yet diagnosed with CV disease, it precedes the development of overt CV disease by 3–5 years [4–7]. The pathophysiology of ED includes a variety of psychological, hormonal, and vascular causes. The management algorithm includes the implementation of exercise and other lifestyle interventions as the first step, and then physicians can proceed to targeted treatment based on the etiology of ED and/or administration of phosphodiesterase 5 (PDE-5) inhibitors [1, 5–9].

The purpose of this chapter is to summarize the prevalence and the pathophysiology of ED and its association with CV disease and critically discuss available data on the effects of exercise on sexual function.

Erectile Dysfunction

Prevalence of Erectile Dysfunction

The prevalence of ED varies and depends on age, comorbidities, and concomitant therapy, as well as the definition and the assessment methods used. Thus, studies offer a large variation in prevalence of ED. Age seems to be the major determinant with an increasing prevalence of ED from 2% in men younger than 40 years to 86% in men older than 80 years. In general, most studies have demonstrated that the prevalence of ED in the general adult population is approximately 15–20% [10–15].

The prevalence of ED seems to share a bidirectional relation with the presence of CV risk factors or disease. Patients with overt CV disease or CV risk factors more often have sexual

K. P. Imprialos · K. Stavropoulos · M. Doumas (✉)
2nd Propedeutic Department Internal Medicine, Hippokration Hospital, Thessaloniki, Greece

P. Kokkinos, P. Narayan (eds.), *Cardiorespiratory Fitness in Cardiometabolic Diseases*,
https://doi.org/10.1007/978-3-030-04816-7_22

dysfunction and vice versa. ED patients more commonly suffer from hypertension, diabetes, obesity, dyslipidemia, or other established CV risk factors, as well as CV disease [16].

The prevalence of ED is two times higher in hypertensive patients compared to subjects with normal blood pressure levels. Similarly, ED is more common in patients treated with antihypertensive medications, suggesting that medications contribute to ED. The type of antihypertensive medications used is a major determinant of the presence and the severity of ED. B-blockers (except for nebivolol) and diuretics are related with more severe erectile function, whereas calcium channel blockers and angiotensin-converting enzyme inhibitors seem to have a neutral effect on sexual activity. On the contrary angiotensin receptor blockers have a neutral and even beneficial effect on erectile function [16–18]. In patients with diabetes mellitus (DM), ED is more frequent, seems to present at earlier stages of the disease, and becomes more severe as the disease progresses [19–23]. An increased risk of ED is also supported by most studies in patients with high total and low-density lipoprotein cholesterol (LDL-C) and triglycerides, as well as in those with low high-density lipoprotein cholesterol (HDL-C) compared with patients without dyslipidemia [24–27]. Similarly, the prevalence of ED is 30–90% and twofold higher in patients with obesity and metabolic syndrome, respectively [28–30]. Lastly, ED is highly prevalent in patients with overt CV disease. Approximately 50% of patients with overt CAD (myocardial infarction, angioplasty or bypass grafting, stable or unstable angina) have ED. Furthermore, patients with heart failure have even higher rates of ED, reaching up to 90% [31–36].

Pathophysiology of ED

The pathogenesis of vasculogenic ED involves complex mechanisms that include androgen deficiency, subclinical inflammation, and vascular structural and functional damage. In the setting of CV disease or risk factors (hypertension, diabetes, dyslipidemia, smoking), the arterial tree is typically more sclerotic than in healthy individuals and involves vessels of all sizes, including the penile arterial tree. In addition, the development of atherosclerotic lesions further exaggerates the structural abnormalities and reduces the diameter of the vessels. Based on the "artery size" hypothesis, vessels of smaller diameter, like the penile artery, are usually affected first by such lesions. Therefore, ED might be one of the first manifestations of subclinical systematic vascular disease [37–47].

The mechanisms involved in ED are presented in Fig. 22.1. Endothelial function is commonly altered in patients with CV disease or CV risk factors. The endothelial cells are the primary source of nitric oxide (NO), a vital molecule involved in the regulation of vascular wall dilation. NO increases the levels of cyclic guanosine monophosphate (cGMP) in the penile smooth muscular cells, thus resulting in vasodilation. Several factors seem to decrease the bioavailability of NO in the altered endothelial function setting [48–50]. Oxidative stress is directly toxic to the endothelium and reduces the release of NO, while enhancing the aggregation of platelets and neutrophils that activate the release of several vasoconstrictor substances. Given the small diameter of the penile arteries, these changes result in significant reduction in arterial blood flow [51, 52], leading to a cascade of events all contributing to ED. First, the increased ROS production in the penile tissue has been shown to increase peroxynitrite formation, leading to lower NO concentrations [53]. Second, peroxynitrite and superoxide increase the apoptosis rate in the endothelium of cavernosal smooth cells, thus further exacerbating NO deficiency [54]. Third, reactive oxygen species seem to directly interact with NO, further reducing its bioavailability [55]. Finally, nicotinamide adenine dinucleotide phosphate (NADPH) is upregulated in patients with endothelial dysfunction and produces great amounts of superoxidase radicals leading to further endothelial damage [56].

Advanced glycation end products (AGEs) have also been implicated in the pathophysiology of vasculogenic ED. It has been suggested that in a cellular environment with increased AGEs concentrations, NO is unavailable to interact

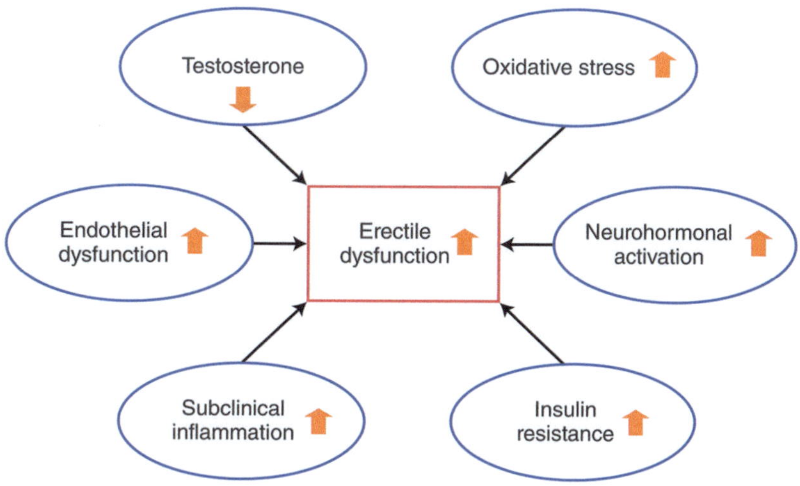

Fig. 22.1 Pathophysiology of erectile dysfunction

with guanylate cyclase. As a result, cGMP levels are decreased, and vasodilation cannot be sufficiently achieved. AGEs are found to be elevated in human penile tissues of diabetic patients, especially in the corpus cavernosum [57]. In addition, the receptors of AGEs seem to be involved in the production of endothelin 1, a strong vasoconstrictor substance, in penile tissue of rats [58]. It has also been shown that AGEs reduce NO production through direct alteration of endothelial NO synthase phosphorylation in diabetic rats, compared with controls [59]. Interestingly, inhibitors of AGEs formation were shown to prevent the development of several complications including ED in animals [60, 61].

ED and CV Disease

ED and CV disease are strongly associated. In a retrospective study of more than 12,800 patients, ED was associated with a twofold increase in risk of myocardial infarction [62]. Similarly, in a study of approximately 2500 patients, ED was associated with an increased 10-year risk of CAD (by 65%) and stroke (43%) [63]. In 300 patients with angiographically documented CAD, 50% had ED, and in approximately 70% ED preceded the onset of CAD by 3 years [34]. In another study, 19% and 24% of ED patients had angiographically documented CAD and positive exercise treadmill and/or stress echocardiography tests, respectively [64].

The Prostate Cancer Prevention Trial prospectively assessed the risk for CV events in patients with and without ED. After 5 years, ED was associated with a significant 25% increase in the risk for CV disease [65]. In another study of approximately 1250 CV disease-free male subjects, ED was associated with a significantly elevated risk of stroke, myocardial infarction, and sudden death after 6.3 years [66]. The risk for CV and all-cause death is also strongly related with the presence of ED, according to a study of 1300 ED patients showing an increased risk of 26% and 43%, respectively, after 15 years [67]. In addition, the severity of ED is strongly associated with the risk for CV events. In a prospective study of more than 95,000 patients, on follow-up CV disease-free subjects with severe ED had a 60%, 92%, and 35% risk increase for CAD, peripheral arterial disease, and any CV events, respectively, compared to subjects with normal sexual function, and even greater risks were found in patients with severe ED and overt CV disease [68].

Important information comes from post hoc analyses of randomized trials. A sub-analysis of the ADVANCE study found that ED among more than 6000 men was associated with a 36% increased risk for cerebrovascular disease, 35% increased risk for CAD, and 19% increased risk for any CV event [69]. The ONTARGET/

TRANSCEND trials demonstrated that ED was an independent predictor of the composite outcome of CV mortality, myocardial infarction, stroke, and hospitalization for heart failure (risk increase of 42%) and an 84% increased risk for all-cause death [70].

Confirming data come from 2 meta-analyses, 1 of more than 36,000 subjects in 12 prospective studies and the other of more than 92,000 participants in 14 studies. In the first one, ED was associated with increased risk for CAD (46%), stroke (35%), CV disease (48%), and all-cause death (19%) [71]. The second one found a 44%, 62%, 39%, and 25% risk increase for CV events, myocardial infarction, cerebrovascular disease, and all-cause death, respectively, in participants with ED compared with non-ED patients [72].

Exercise and Sexual Dysfunction: Epidemiological Data

Healthy Subjects and ED

Several data exist that support the existence of a close relation between exercise and ED in healthy participants. A study of healthy men aged 18–40 years evaluated the impact of physical exercise on sexual function. The sedentary group (lower than 1400 kilocalories expenditure per week) presented lower scores in several International Index of Erectile Function (IIEF) Questionnaire domains. Erectile function, intercourse satisfaction, and overall satisfaction were significantly lower in the sedentary compared to the active group. Sexual desire scores were similar across the two groups, while a trend for a decrease in the overall satisfaction domain was observed in the physically active compared with the sedentary group [73].

Exercise and ED in Patients of CV Risk Factors or Disease

CV disease and/or risk factors are strongly related with the presence of ED. Since increased physical activity and cardiorespiratory fitness (CRF) confer health benefits in healthy individuals and in patients with chronic disease [74], several studies have been devoted to also assess the association between physical activity and CRF in patients with ED. A population-based study of approximately 1000 high CV risk patients reported that more than half of the study population had ED. Among several lifestyle and socioeconomic parameters examined, high-intensity physical activity was associated with a 50% reduced risk for ED [75]. In a sub-analysis of the Action for Health in Diabetes (Look AHEAD trial) where patients with type 2 diabetes were evaluated for the impact of several factors on sexual function, CRF was found to be protective for ED (risk reduction of 24%). Improved levels of fitness were associated with a 40% reduction in the risk for ED compared with the lowest fitness levels, whereas self-reported ED was related with lower scores in the social functioning health index and depression scores. The protective role of CRF on erectile function remained significant even after adjustment for potential cofounders, including antihypertensive medications [76].

Another study examined the association of exercise with ED in approximately 300 patients. Study participants were predominantly obese (body mass index, 30.5 kg/m^2), 39% reported that they were diabetic, and 36% with CAD. The majority of the patients (44%) reported physical activity totaling less than three metabolic equivalents (MET) hours per week (sedentary). Compared to the sedentary group, those exercising ≥3–17.9 MET hours per week had better sexual function scores. However, not all sexual domains were shown to be significantly associated with these exercise levels. Patients who exercised ≥18 MET hours per week had significantly greater sexual function scores compared to those exercising <3 MET hours per week. It is important to emphasize that exercising ≥18 MET hours per week represents moderate levels of physical activity, achieved by a brisk walk 4–6 times per week, approximately 40–60 min per session. These physical activity levels are attainable by most middle-aged and older individuals [77]. Lastly, the prevalence of ED and its relation with several atherosclerotic markers were assessed in a relatively small study of 57 patients with metabolic syndrome and 48 physically active subjects without metabolic syndrome. The prevalence of ED was 63.2% and 27.1%, in the metabolic syndrome and physically active groups, respectively. In addition, the prevalence of ED was 88% lower in those engaging in physical activity requiring more than 400 kilocalories per day. Large arterial elasticity was lower, and fibrinogen and resting heart rate are higher in patients with metabolic syndrome compared to physically active subjects. Importantly, all these markers were significantly worse in patients with ED compared with non-ED patients. Of note, the lowest values of large arterial elasticity and the highest levels of fibrinogen and resting heart rate were observed among patients with both metabolic syndrome and ED [78].

ED was evaluated in 139 middle-aged men (60 ± 12 years old), admitted to an intensive cardiac rehabilitation program 13 days post-myocardial infarction. The exercise capacity of the participants was assessed by two 6-min walk tests (performed 2 weeks apart) and by a symptom-limited cardiopulmonary exercise test. Both the 6-min walk test and cardiopulmonary exercise were negatively related with the presence of ED and were associated with the degree of sexual dysfunction [79]. Furthermore, exercise seems to ameliorate premature ejaculation, an important parameter of sexual activity and satisfaction. In this setting, a population-based study evaluated the impact of exercise on premature ejaculation and found a significant negative relation between the level of physical exercise and premature ejaculation, which remained significant after adjustment for age, body mass index, alcohol intake, and erectile dysfunction [80].

Female Sexual Dysfunction and Exercise

A study of 2030 female married patients assessed the prevalence of female sexual dysfunction (FSD) with the use of the female sexual function score and examined potential association of FSD with sociodemographic and lifestyle parameters. The prevalence of FSD was 51% among this study population, and it was found that physical exercise was protective against FSD [81]. In a study of 1217 women (18–80 years old), the investigators evaluated the association between the existence of risk factors associated with FSD and urinary incontinence. Compared to sexually active women, female patients with sexual dysfunction were more likely to have a higher body mass index, less physical exercise, and a lower educational level [82]. In another study of 400 healthy women (18–58 years old), the prevalence of FSD was 72.8%, with anorgasmia, sexual insufficiency, vaginismus, dissatisfaction, non-sensuality, and avoidance of intercourse being the more prevalent among the parameters examined with the Golombok Rust Inventory of Sexual Satisfaction. Age, smoking, exercise, and marital and educational status failed to provide a significant relation with sexual dysfunction areas. Only alcohol intake was significantly associated with alteration of sexual activity [83]. In a cross-sectional study of more than 400 women, the authors reported that Female Sexual Function Index (FSFI) scores and scores of lubrication and pain domains were significantly better in women exercising compared with women who reported only walking as physical activity or women who did not report any type of exercise. Of note, every unit increase in weekly exercise was associated with an approximately 80% reduction in the risk for deterioration of sexual desire [84]. In 216 women with history of breast cancer, physical inactivity along with age and body mass index were unfavorably and independently related with sexual dysfunction and hypoactive sexual desire disorder [85]. In a cross-sectional study of approximately 300 patients with ovarian cancer, sedentary behavior was related with lower quality of life scores and sexual function [86]. However, in a small study of 59 diabetic female patients, sexual dysfunction along with diabetic neuropathy, hypertension, and CAD were not associated with exercise levels [87]. Collectively, conflicting data exist about the association of female sexual dysfunction with exercise. Further studies are needed to clarify this association and uncover the underlying mechanisms.

Exercise and Sexual Dysfunction: Interventional Data

ED and Exercise: Non-randomized Intervention Studies

Patients with ED appear to have a lower capacity for exercise. In 180 ED patients and 50 with normal erectile function, ED patients had a lower peak exercise time and thus reduced exercise capacity compared with non-ED subjects. The severity of ED was significantly and inversely related with the duration of exercise and peak overload, as well as with chronotropic parameters such as heart rate recovery in 2 min after exercise and chronotropic index (markers of autonomic dysfunction). In addition, flow-mediated dilatation of the brachial artery, a recognized marker of endothelial dysfunction, was found to be positively related with both chronotropic parameters [88].

As mentioned, ED is closely related with the presence of CV disease risk factors. Given the favorable health outcomes of exercise in patients with CV disease [74], several studies investigated the effect of exercise in CV disease patients with ED. In a study of patients with essential hypertension and ED, participants were instructed to stop their antihypertensive drug treatment for 1 week prior to study's initiation. Patients were then subdivided into the exercise and control group. Those in the exercise group ($n = 22$; 62 ± 5 years) engaged in interval exercise training for 8 weeks exercise intensity of 60–79% of heart rate max reserve for a duration of between 45 and 60 min per session. The age-matched control group ($n = 21$; 64 ± 5 years) remained sedentary during this period. The findings revealed that even a short duration of exercise (8 weeks) had a significant and favorable effect of on erectile function of hypertensive patients with ED ($P < 0.05$). In the exercise group, IIEF-5 scores increased significantly from 11.5 to 15.1; on the contrary, IIEF-5 scores were similar at the end of study compared with baseline values in the control group (8.1 vs 8.9 at the beginning vs end of study). It was concluded that adequate exercise program may be a possible effective noninvasive and nonpharmacological management of ED in male hypertensive patients [89, 90].

The effects of exercise on ED were also assessed in a 6-month rehabilitation program (that included cycle ergometers, general gym, or outdoor exercises and resistance training) on IIEF-5 scores in patients with ischemic heart disease. The mean IIEF-5 score increased in the intervention group (89 patients) from 13.15 to 15.36. These changes were not observed in the control group (35 patients; IIEF-5 score: 12.26 at baseline vs 12.43 at end of study). In addition, heart rate recovery was also greater in the intervention group, and its change from baseline was significantly related with the changes in the IIEF-5 scores in the intervention group. In another study, the same investigators also examined the impact of exercise intensity on changes in erectile function, in 150 men with ischemic heart disease. Of those, 115 underwent cardiac rehabilitation with endurance exercise for 6 months, and 35 patients served as controls (no exercise). Upon completion of the study, IIEF-5 scores were significantly greater in the intervention compared with the control group. However, parameters evaluating the intensity of the training program (initial, final, and mean training work and training work growth) were not associated with the noted changes in sexual function. In contrast, parameters evaluating the chronotropic response (peak heart rate and heart rate growth dynamics at beginning and end of program) were significantly related with the changes in IIEF-5 scores [91–93].

ED and Exercise: Randomized Intervention Studies

A few randomized studies have been conducted to assess the effect of exercise on ED. The impact of physical activity on ED was assessed in patients with recent myocardial infarction and ED, randomized to an unsupervised home-based outdoor walking program ($n = 41$) and usual care ($n = 45$). After 30 days, the investigators reported that ED increased by 9% in the control group and a significant 71% reduction in the walking group. The 6-min walk distance was significantly higher in the walking group compared with usual care, and this distance was negatively associated with ED [94]. Another study in patients with late-onset hypogonadism assessed the combination of testosterone replacement therapy (TRT) alone or in combination with exercise on sexual dysfunction. TRT was administrated for 12 weeks and then discontinued for 8 weeks. Patients were randomized in a sedentary and an exercise group. After 12 weeks, testosterone levels were significantly increased in both groups. However, testosterone levels were significantly higher in the exercise group compared with the sedentary one. Similarly, IIEF scores were improved in both groups but significantly greater in the exercise group at week 12. The sexual symptoms subscale of the Aging Males' Symptoms (AMS) questionnaire showed better symptomatology with exercise compared to the sedentary group at week 12, a difference that remained statistically significant even after the termination of TRT. Interestingly, exercise intensity was directly related to the degree of improvement in ED [95]. In another study 90 sedentary obese men were randomized to either low-volume (<150 min/week) or high-volume (200–300 min/week) exercise plus diet for 24 weeks. The group on the high-volume exercise program had significantly greater increases in the IIEF-5 scores and testosterone levels compared with the low-volume exercise group. Greater improvements in body weight and fat mass were also observed in the high- compared with the low-volume exercise group [96].

PDE-5 Inhibitors and Exercise

The combination of exercise with PDE-5 inhibitors to achieve improvements in erectile function compared to PDE-5 inhibitors administration alone has been evaluated in a few studies. A study of patients with ED and metabolic syndrome assessed the impact of tadalafil and exercise compared with tadalafil alone on sexual function. After 2 months, the double intervention group showed greater improvements in sexual function scores compared to the tadalafil group. Peak oxygen consumption during cardiopulmonary exercise testing was significantly related with the IIEF score changes in the group on a combination of both exercise program and tadalafil [97]. Lastly, in patients with late-onset hypogonadism and severe erectile dysfunction, exercise in combination with tadalafil was associated with significant improvements in IIEF scores. In addition, ultrasound parameters such as penile artery peak systolic velocity and end-diastolic velocity were ameliorated with exercise and PDE-5 inhibitor administration compared to baseline [98].

The promising data for the combination effect of PDE-5 inhibitors and exercise on sexual function have been confirmed from small randomized trials. Effect of sildenafil citrate on erectile function in type 2 diabetic ED patients on intensive glycemic control was compared with diet and exercise. Both interventions resulted in significantly greater IIEF-5 scores compared with baseline values. However, PDE-5 inhibitor use was associated with greater benefits compared with lifestyle modifications (change in IIEF-5 score: 5 vs 2.5 in the PDE-5 inhibitors and exercise groups, respectively) [99]. A randomized study of 60 patients with ED assessed the impact of PDE-5 inhibitors alone or in combination with aerobic physical activity on erectile function. Physical activity of 3.4 h per week resulted in restoration of ED in approximately 78% of patients in the group on the combined intervention. All IIEF-15 domains were better in the PDE-5 inhibitor plus physical activity group compared with group on the PDE-5 inhibitor alone, with the exception of the domain evaluating the extent of orgasm which did not reach statistical significance. Testosterone levels were also significantly improved in the double intervention group compared with baseline values. Lastly, physical activity was found to be an independent variable for normal erection and IIEF-15 scores and high sexual satisfaction [100].

Meta-analyses of Studies Assessing the Impact of Exercise on ED

A meta-analysis of 5 randomized studies of over 380 ED patients showed that aerobic exercise was associated with significant increases in IIEF scores from 13.91 to 16.74. On the contrary, the control group did not show such benefits (13.25 vs 13.61 in IIEF score at baseline vs end of study, respectively) [101]. Another meta-analysis of 7 studies and 478 patients assessed the impact of aerobic, pelvic, or combined exercise on ED. A significant increase in IIEF scores of 3.85 was found before and after the intervention. Of note, physical activity and exercise, alone or in combination with usual care, were associated with significant benefits. Similarly, short- and long-term physical interventions were found to provide significant improvements [102].

Female Sexual Dysfunction and Exercise

Relatively few interventional studies have assessed the effects of structured exercise programs on sexual dysfunction in women. In a small study of 34 healthy women, all domains in the FSFI questionnaire along with the overall score were significantly improved (total FSFI score: 25.9 vs 32.2 at baseline vs end of study, respectively) following 12 weeks of Pilates exercise [103]. In another study, 41 women with metabolic syndrome were randomized to a 12-week yoga exercise or no exercise. Yoga exercise was associated with improvements in sexual arousal and lubrication compared with the controls [104]. In yet another study, more than 220 menopausal women were provided with instructions for a 12-week program of lifestyle interventions with some subjects participating in face-to-face consultation meetings with nurses that provided help in implementing the lifestyle interventions. Sexual dysfunction was significantly improved in all women, compared with baseline scores, and women participating in nurse consultation showed greater benefits compared with women not participating in meetings [105].

The impact of exercise on sexual function has been examined in females with polycystic ovary syndrome as well. In a case-control study of 43 women with PCOS and 51 control ovulatory women, participants underwent a physical resistance training program for 16 weeks. Patients with polycystic ovary syndrome had a significant increase in the overall FSFI score and in the desire, excitement, and lubrication domains at end of study. In the control group, only the pain domain was significantly ameliorated with exercise [106].

Lastly, two studies investigated the impact of exercise on sexual function in women on antidepressant drugs. Female patients on selective serotonin reuptake inhibitors (implicated in sexual arousal impairment through reduction in sympathetic nervous system tone) or selective serotonin and norepinephrine reuptake inhibitors participated in three sessions with erotic film projections, in two of which they exercised before the projection. In both drug groups, exercise significantly increased sexual arousal before the stimuli. Of note, women with worse sexual function presented greater sexual arousal after exercise. In patients on selective serotonin receptor inhibitors, sexual arousal following exercise was associated with the activity of the sympathetic nervous system [107]. In a small randomized crossover study of women reporting antidepressant drug-related sexual dysfunction, women were randomized to exercise three times per week for 3 weeks either before intercourse or in time periods not relevant to the time of intercourse. Patients with sexual dysfunction at baseline and exercise prior to intercourse had significant amelioration of sexual activity. However, orgasm was increased only in the group on regular exercise, and in neither group satisfaction was improved [108].

Mechanisms: Pathophysiology and Experimental Data on the Benefits of Exercise on ED

The mechanisms involved in the exercise-induced improvement in ED are presented in Fig. 22.2. In diabetic and sedentary mice, superoxide dismutase was 53% lower compared with nondiabetic controls but was restored after exercise. In addition, relaxation responses were also reduced in diabetic rats and were also restored after training. Similarly, the impaired relax-

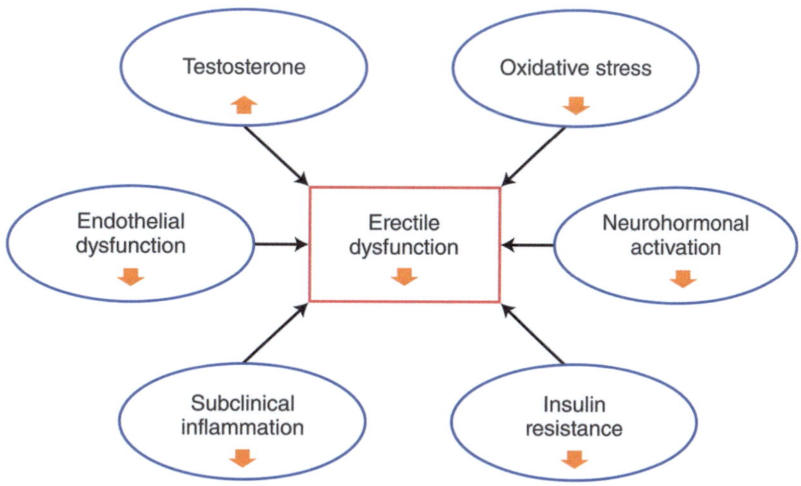

Fig. 22.2 Beneficial effects of exercise on erectile function

ation via electrical-field stimulation in diabetic animals was also restored after exercise [109]. The impact of exercise was also assessed on Western diet-associated erectile dysfunction. Erectile function improved significantly in sedentary rats on a 12-Western diet with exercise with improvements in mean arterial pressure and intracavernosal pressure. In addition, significant benefits were observed in parameters of endothelial function [110].

Evidence supports that the exercise-related improvements in ED are mainly mediated through increases in the bioavailability of NO increased testosterone levels in men. Physical activity increases systematic endothelial NO production via shear stress, secondary to the elevation of blood flow [111, 112]. In type 1 diabetic rats, exercise training was found to improve the erectile response and the intracavernous pressure changes to N-methyl-D-aspartic acid and sodium nitroprusside. Furthermore, an increase in the expression of neuronal NO synthase in the paraventricular nucleus of the hypothalamus was noted with exercise training [113]. Of note, the impact of exercise on NO might be affected by both the frequency and the intensity of exercise. Acute exercise was found to increase NO release for 48 h. On the contrary, daily exercise resulted in a fourfold elevation of NO levels that was maintained for 1 week [114]. Flow-mediated dilation, another marker of endothelial function, is improved with moderate exercise. Acute severe physical exercise, however, increases oxidative stress that in turn reduces flow-mediated dilation [115].

Circulating testosterone levels have also been shown to increase with exercise. An experimental study assessed the impact of exercise on age-related reduction in testosterone and on the activity of endothelial and neuronal NO synthase in rats. In the control group, the activity of both endothelial and neuronal NO synthase was reduced in aged compared with young animals. On the contrary, aged rats that exercised had significantly higher NO synthase activity compared with the control group without exercise. Similarly, testosterone levels were higher in young and trained aged rats compared with the controls [116].

Other potential erectile function-related beneficial mechanisms might include the exercise-induced secretions of myokines, adipokines, and hepatokines that might attenuate vascular alterations and result in functional benefits [117].

Recommendations/Conclusions

Large studies have shown that ED is strongly and independently related with increased CV risk. Lifestyle interventions are recommended in the management of patients with any CV risk factor or overt CV disease and are undoubtedly a vital intervention for the primary and secondary prevention of CV disease. Since ED shares common pathophysiological mechanisms with CV disease, lifestyle interventions are recommended by several experts and international guidelines for the management of ED patients, as well [118–123]. Several observational and interventional studies have shown benefits of exercise on ED in healthy subjects, patients with CV risk factors or overt CV disease, patients on treatment-induced ED, and other subgroups of patients. However, most of these studies were performed in rather small study populations, and their design was usually not optimal. Only a few randomized studies exist that also did not implement exercise intervention in a sufficient number of patients. Large randomized trials could verify the benefits noted in these studies. However, in the interim physicians should recommend exercise interventions in all patients with sexual dysfunction (men and women) to optimize their CV profile and potentially ameliorate their sexual dysfunction.

Clinical/Public Health Significance

Sexual dysfunction affects approximately one fifth of the general population, and its prevalence increases in patients with CV risk factors and disease by up to 90%. The early identification of ED is of major clinical significance since ED precedes the manifestation of overt CV disease by 3–5 years. However, physicians are unaware of the significance of ED in the prevention algorithm of CV disease and most often are not assessing sexual function in everyday clinical practice. Furthermore, given the sensitive nature of this subject, patients are unwilling to discuss the details of their sexual life [124–127].

Accumulating evidence suggests that SD impairs the quality of life of affected individuals. Patients feel nervous when initiating an intercourse and are afraid of sexual intimacy. SD exerts detrimental effects on self-esteem and self-confidence of patients that might trigger anxiety and depressive symptoms. In addition, impaired sexual function affects other aspects of life, such as daily life activities and work performance. Importantly, the presence of SD negatively affects the sexual health and total well-being of the sexual partners of the affected patients [126, 128–133]. On the contrary, improved erectile function is related with better self-esteem and quality of life of both SD patients and their partners [134, 135].

Nevertheless, ED has been associated with lower adherence to therapeutic treatment. The most common cause for treatment discontinuation is drug side effects. Antihypertensive treatment has been related with increased incidence of ED. It has been noted that ED compromises medication adherence and results in treatment self-termination. On the other hand, PDE-5 inhibitors use has been found to improve antihypertensive treatment adherence and thus might reduce the risk for CV events [136].

Collectively, sexual dysfunction affects a variety of aspects of patient's life. Therefore, the management of SD is of paramount importance to improve patients' quality of life and increase treatment adherence to optimize their CV profile. Exercise interventions could have a significant role in management of SD, based on the abovementioned studies reporting improvements in sexual function in both men and women. Larger studies are needed to verify these findings and to reinforce the significant role of exercise in the routine management of patients with sexual dysfunction.

References

1. Manolis A, Doumas M. Sexual dysfunction: the 'prima ballerina' of hypertension-related quality-of-life complications. J Hypertens. 2008;26(11):2074–84.
2. NIH Consensus Conference. Impotence. NIH Consensus Development Panel on Impotence. JAMA. 1993;270(1):83–90.
3. Bachman GA, Avci D. Evaluation and management of female sexual dysfunction. Endocrinologist. 2004;14:337–45.
4. Gandaglia G, Briganti A, Montorsi P, Montorsi F, Vlachopoulos C. Erectile dysfunction in coronary artery disease and heart failure. In: Viigimaa M, Vlachopoulos C, Doumas M, editors. Erectile dysfunction in hypertension and cardiovascular disease. Springer International Publishing: Switzerland; 2015. p. 59–71.

5. Jackson G, Boon N, Eardley I, Kirby M, Dean J, Hackett G, et al. Erectile dysfunction and coronary artery disease prediction: evidence-based guidance and consensus. Int J Clin Pract. 2010;64(7):848–57.
6. Vlachopoulos C, Jackson G, Stefanadis C, Montorsi P. Erectile dysfunction in the cardiovascular patient. Eur Heart J. 2013;34(27):2034–46.
7. Viigimaa M, Vlachopoulos C, Lazaridis A, Doumas M. Management of erectile dysfunction in hypertension: tips and tricks. World J Cardiol. 2014;6(9):908–15.
8. Menezes A, Artham S, Lavie CJ, Milani RV, O'Keefe J. Erectile dysfunction and cardiovascular disease. Postgrad Med. 2011;123(3):7–16.
9. Manolis A, Doumas M. Antihypertensive treatment and sexual dysfunction. Curr Hypertens Rep. 2012;14(4):285–92.
10. Johannes CB, Araujo AB, Feldman HA, Derby CA, Kleinman KP, McKinlay JB. Incidence of erectile dysfunction in men 40 to 69 year old: longitudinal results from the Massachusetts male aging study. J Urol. 2000;163(2):460–3.
11. Prins J, Blanker MH, Bohnen AM, Thomas S, Bosch JL. Prevalence of erectile dysfunction: a systematic review of population-based studies. Int J Impot Res. 2002;14(6):422–32.
12. Shabsigh R, Perelman MA, Laumann EO, Lockhart DC. Drivers and barriers to seeking treatment for erectile dysfunction: a comparison of six countries. BJU Int. 2004;94(7):1055–65.
13. McKinlay JB. The worldwide prevalence and epidemiology of erectile dysfunction. Int J Impot Res. 2000;12(Suppl 4):S6–S11.
14. Laumann EO, Nicolosi A, Glasser DB, Paik A, Gingell C, Moreira E, et al. Sexual problems among women and men aged 40-80 y: prevalence and correlates identified in the Global Study of Sexual Attitudes and Behaviors. Int J Impot Res. 2005;17(1):39–57.
15. Rosen RC, Fisher WA, Eardley I, Niederberger C, Nadel A, Sand M. The multinational Men's Attitudes to Life Events and Sexuality (MALES) study: I. Prevalence of erectile dysfunction and related health concerns in the general population. Curr Med Res Opin. 2004;20(5):607–17.
16. Imprialos KP, Stavropoulos K, Doumas M, Tziomalos K, Karagiannis A, Athyros VG. Sexual dysfunction, cardiovascular risk and effects of pharmacotherapy. Curr Vasc Pharmacol. 2017; https://doi.org/10.2174/1570161115666170609101502.
17. Doumas M, Tsakiris A, Douma S, Grigorakis A, Papadopoulos A, Hounta A, et al. Factors affecting the increased prevalence of erectile dysfunction in Greek hypertensive compared with normotensive subjects. J Androl. 2006;27(3):469–77.
18. Doumas M, Douma S. Sexual dysfunction in essential hypertension: myth or reality? J Clin Hypertens. 2006;8(4):269–74.
19. Burke JP, Jacobson DJ, McGree ME, Nehra A, Roberts RO, Girman CJ, et al. Diabetes and sexual dysfunction: results from the Olmsted County study of urinary symptoms and health status among men. J Urol. 2007;177(4):1438–42.
20. Bacon CG, Hu FB, Giovannucci E, Glasser DB, Mittleman MA, Rimm EB. Association of type and duration of diabetes with erectile dysfunction in a large cohort of men. Diabetes Care. 2002;25(8):1458–63.
21. Penson DF, Latini DM, Lubeck DP, Wallace KL, Henning JM, Lue TF. Do impotent men with diabetes have more severe erectile dysfunction and worse quality of life than the general population of impotent patients? Results from the ExCEED database. Diabetes Care. 2003;26(4):1093–9.
22. Goldstein I, Lue TF, Padma-Nathan H, Rosen RC, Steers WD, Wicker PA. Oral sildenafil in the treatment of erectile dysfunction. N Engl J Med. 1998;338(10):1397–404.
23. Nikolaidou B, Nouris C, Lazaridis A, Sampanis C, Doumas M. Diabetes mellitus and erectile dysfunction. In: Viigimaa M, Vlachopoulos C, Doumas M, editors. Erectile dysfunction in hypertension and cardiovascular disease. Springer International Publishing: Switzerland; 2015. p. 119–28.
24. Smith NJ, Sak SC, Baldo O, Eardley I. The prevalence of newly diagnosed hyperlipidaemia in men with erectile dysfunction. BJU Int. 2007;100(2):357–61.
25. Gunduz MI, Gumus BH, Sekuri C. Relationship between metabolic syndrome and erectile dysfunction. Asian J Androl. 2004;6(4):355–8.
26. Vrentzos GE, Paraskevas KI, Mikhailidis DP. Dyslipidemia as a risk factor for erectile dysfunction. Curr Med Chem. 2007;14(6):1765–70.
27. Pittaras A, Avranas K, Imprialos K, Faselis C, Kokkinos P. The association between dyslipidemia and its treatment with erectile dysfunction. In: Viigimaa M, Vlachopoulos C, Doumas M, editors. Erectile dysfunction in hypertension and cardiovascular disease. Springer International Publishing: Switzerland; 2015. p. 129–38.
28. Kaya E, Sikka SC, Gur S. A comprehensive review of metabolic syndrome affecting erectile dysfunction. J Sex Med. 2015;12(4):856–75.
29. Esposito K, Giugliano F, Ciotola M, et al. Obesity and sexual dysfunction, male and female. Int J Impot Res. 2008;20:358–65.
30. Diaz-Arjonilla M, Schwartz M, Swerdloff RS, Wang C. Obesity, low testosterone levels and erectile dysfunction. Int J Impot Res. 2009;21(2):89–98.
31. Kloner RA, Mullin SH, Shook T, Matthews R, Mayeda G, Burstein S. Erectile dysfunction in the cardiac patient: How common and should we treat? J Urol. 2003;170(2Pt2):S46–50.
32. Montorsi P, Ravagnani PM, Galli S, Rotatori F, Veglia F, Briganti A. Association between erectile dysfunction and coronary artery disease. Role of coronary clinical presentation and extent of coronary vessels involvement: the COBRA trial. Eur Heart J. 2006;27(22):2632–9.
33. Gandaglia G, Briganti A, Jackson G, Kloner RA, Montorsi F, Montorsi P, et al. A systematic review of the association between erectile dysfunction and cardiovascular disease. Eur Urol. 2014;65(5):968–78.

34. Montorsi F, Briganti A, Salonia A, Rigatti P, Margonato A, Macchi A, et al. Erectile dysfunction prevalence, time of onset and association with risk factors in 300 consecutive patients with acute chest pain and angiographically documented coronary artery disease. Eur Urol. 2003;44(3):360–4.
35. Alberti L, Torlasco C, Lauretta L, Loffi M, Maranta F, Salonia A, et al. Erectile dysfunction in heart failure patients: a critical reappraisal. Andrology. 2013;1(2):177–91.
36. Apostolo A, Vignati C, Brusoni D, Cattadori G, Contini M, Veglia F, et al. Erectile dysfunction in heart failure: correlation with severity, exercise performance, comorbidities, and heart failure treatment. J Sex Med. 2009;6(1):2795–805.
37. Dean RC, Lue TF. Physiology of penile erection and pathophysiology of erectile dysfunction Urol. Clin North Am. 2005;32(4):379–95.
38. Moreland RB, Traish A, MA MM, Smith B, Goldstein I, Saenz de Tejada I. PGE1 suppresses the induction of collagen synthesis by transforming growth factor-beta 1 in human corpus cavernosum smooth muscle. J Urol. 1995;153(3Pt1):826–34.
39. Nehra A, Gettman MT, Nugent M, Bostwick DG, Barrett DM, Goldstein I, et al. Transforming growth factor-beta1 (TGF-beta1) is sufficient to induce fibrosis of rabbit corpus cavernosum in vivo. J Urol. 1999;162(3Pt1):910–5.
40. Saenz de Tejada I, Moroukian P, Tessier J, Kim JJ, Goldstein I, Frohrib D. Trabecular smooth muscle modulates the capacitor function of the penis. Studies on a rabbit model. Am J Physiol. 1991;260(5Pt2):H1590–5.
41. Nehra A, Azadzoi KM, Moreland RB, Pabby A, Siroky MB, Krane RJ, et al. Cavernosal expandability is an erectile tissue mechanical property which predicts trabecular histology in an animal model of vasculogenic erectile dysfunction. J Urol. 1998;159(6):2229–36.
42. Mulvany MJ. Small artery remodeling in hypertension. Curr Hypertens Rep. 2002;4:49.
43. Okabe H, Hale TM, Kumon H, Heaton JP, Adams MA. The penis is not protected--in hypertension there are vascular changes in the penis which are similar to those in other vascular beds. Int J Impot Res. 1999;11(3):133.
44. Toblli JE, Stella I, Inserra F, Ferder L, Zeller F, Mazza ON. Morphological changes in cavernous tissue in spontaneously hypertensive rats. Am J Hypertens. 2000;13(6Pt1):686–92.
45. Hale TM, Okabe H, Heaton JP, Adams MA. Antihypertensive drugs induce structural remodeling of the penile vasculature. J Urol. 2001;166(2):739.
46. Norman RA Jr, Dzielak DJ. Immunological dysfunction and enhanced sympathetic activity contribute to the pathogenesis of spontaneous hypertension. J Hypertens Suppl. 1986;4(3):S437–9.
47. Montorsi P, Ravagnani PM, Galli S, Rotatori F, Briganti A, Salonia A, et al. The artery size hypothesis: a macrovascular link between erectile dysfunction and coronary artery disease. Am J Cardiol. 2005;96(12B):19M–23M.
48. Sattar AA, Salpigides G, Vanderhaeghen JJ, Schulman CC, Wespes E. Cavernous oxygen tension and smooth muscle fibers: relation and function. J Urol. 1995;154(5):1736–9.
49. Leite R, Giachini FR, Carneiro FS, Nunes KP, Tostes RC, Webb RC. Targets for the treatment of erectile dysfunction: is NO/cGMP still the answer? Recent Pat Cardiovasc Drug Discov. 2007;2(2):119–32.
50. Toda N, Ayajiki K, Okamura T. Nitric oxide and penile erectile function. Pharmacol Ther. 2005;106(2):233–66.
51. Jeremy JY, Angelini GD, Khan M, Mikhailidis DP, Morgan RJ, Thompson CS. Platelets, oxidant stress and erectile dysfunction: an hypothesis. Cardiovasc Res. 2000;46(1):50–4.
52. Jones RW, Rees RW, Minhas S, Ralph D, Persad RA, Jeremy JY. Oxygen free radicals and the penis. Expert Opin Pharmacother. 2002;3(7):889–97.
53. Prieto D, Kaminski PM, Bagi Z, Ahmad M, Wolin MS. Hypoxic relaxation of penile arteries: involvement of endothelial nitric oxide and modulation by reactive oxygen species. Am J Physiol Heart Circ Physiol. 2010;299(3):H915–24.
54. Khan MA, Thompson CS, Mumtaz FH, Mikhailidis DP, Morgan RJ, Bruckdorfer RK, et al. The effect of nitric oxide and peroxynitrite on rabbit cavernosal smooth muscle relaxation. World J Urol. 2001;19(3):220–4.
55. Zalba G, Beaumont J, San Jose G, Fortuno A, Fortuno MA, Diez J. Vascular oxidant stress: molecular mechanisms and pathophysiological implications. J Physiol Biochem. 2000;56(1):57–64.
56. Warnholtz A, Nickenig G, Schulz E, Macharzina R, Bräsen JH, Skatchkov M, et al. Increased NADH-oxidase-mediated superoxide production in the early stages of atherosclerosis: evidence for involvement of the renin-angiotensin system. Circulation. 1999;99(15):2027–33.
57. Seftel AD, Vaziri ND, Ni Z, Razmjouei K, Fogarty J, Hampel N. Advanced glycation end products in human penis: elevation in diabetic tissue, site of deposition, and possible effect through iNOS or eNOS. Urology. 1997;50(6):1016–26.
58. Chen D, Shan YX, Dai YT. Advanced glycation end products and their receptors elevate the activity of endothelin-1 in rat cavernosum. Zhonghua Nan KeXue. 2008;14(2):110–5.
59. Musicki B, Kramer MF, Becker RE, Burnett AL. Inactivation of phosphorylated endothelial nitric oxide synthase (Ser-1177) by O-GlcNAc in diabetes-associated erectile dysfunction. Proc Natl Acad Sci U S A. 2005;102(33):11870–5.
60. Usta MF, Bivalacqua TJ, Yang DY, et al. The protective effect of aminoguanidine on erectile function in streptozotocin diabetic rats. J Urol. 2003;170(4Pt1):1437–42.
61. Usta MF, Kendirci M, Gur S, Ramanitharan A, Sell DR, Viswanathan A. The breakdown of preformed

advanced glycation end products reverses erectile dysfunction in streptozotocin-induced diabetic rats: preventive versus curative treatment. J Sex Med. 2006;3:242–50. discussion 50–2.
62. Blumentals WA, Gomez-Caminero A, Joo S, Vannappagari V. Should erectile dysfunction be considered as a marker for acute myocardial infarction? Results from a retrospective cohort study. Int J Impot Res. 2004;16(4):350–3.
63. Ponholzer A, Temml C, Obermayr R, Wehrberger C, Madersbacher S. Is erectile dysfunction an indicator for increased risk of coronary heart disease and stroke? Eur Urol. 2005;48(3):512–8.
64. Vlachopoulos C, Rokkas K, Ioakeimidis N, Aggeli C, Michaelides A, Roussakis G, et al. Prevalence of asymptomatic coronary artery disease in men with vasculogenic erectile dysfunction: a prospective angiographic study. Eur Urol. 2005;48(6):996–1003.
65. Thompson IM, Tangen CM, Goodman PJ, Probstfield JL, Moinpour CM, Coltman CA. Erectile dysfunction and subsequent cardiovascular disease. JAMA. 2005;294(23):2996–3002.
66. Schouten BW, Bohnen AM, Bosch JL, Bernsen RM, Deckers JW, Dohle GR, et al. Erectile dysfunction prospectively associated with cardiovascular disease in the Dutch general population: results from the Krimpen Study. Int J Impot Res. 2008;20(1):92–9.
67. Araujo AB, Travison TG, Ganz P, Chiu GR, Kupelian V, Rosen RC, et al. Erectile dysfunction and mortality. J Sex Med. 2009;6(9):2445–54.
68. Banks E, Joshy G, Abhayaratna WP, Kritharides L, Macdonald PS, Korda RJ, et al. Erectile dysfunction severity as a risk marker for cardiovascular disease hospitalization and all-cause mortality: a prospective cohort study. PLoS Med. 2013;10(1):e1001372.
69. Batty GD, Li Q, Czernichow S, Neal B, Zoungas S, Huxley R, et al. Erectile dysfunction and later cardiovascular disease in men with type 2 diabetes: prospective cohort study based on the ADVANCE (Action in Diabetes and Vascular Disease: Preterax and Diamicron Modified-Release Controlled Evaluation) trial. J Am Coll Cardiol. 2010;56(23):1908–13.
70. Bohm M, Baumhakel M, Teo K, Sleight P, Probstfield J, Gao P, et al. Erectile dysfunction predicts cardiovascular events in high-risk patients receiving telmisartan, ramipril, or both: the ONgoing Telmisartan Alone and in combination with Ramipril Global Endpoint Trial/Telmisartan Randomized AssessmeNt Study in ACE iN tolerant subjects with cardiovascular Disease (ONTARGET/TRANSCEND) Trials. Circulation. 2010;121(12):1439–46.
71. Dong JY, Zhang YH, Qin LQ. Erectile dysfunction and risk of cardiovascular disease: meta-analysis of prospective cohort studies. J Am Coll Cardiol. 2011;58(13):1378–85.
72. Vlachopoulos CV, Terentes-Printzios DG, Ioakeimidis NK, Aznaouridis KA, Stefanadis CI. Prediction of cardiovascular events and all-cause mortality with erectile dysfunction: a systematic review and meta-analysis of cohort studies. CircCardiovasc Qual Outcomes. 2013;6(1):99–109.
73. Hsiao W, Shrewsberry AB, Moses KA, Johnson TV, Cai AW, Stuhldreher P, et al. Exercise is associated with better erectile function in men under 40 as evaluated by the International Index of Erectile Function. J Sex Med. 2012;9(2):524–30.
74. Kokkinos P, Myers J. Exercise and physical activity: clinical outcomes and applications. Circulation. 2010;122(16):1637–48.
75. Ettala OO, Syvänen KT, Korhonen PE, Kaipia AJ, Vahlberg TJ, Boström PJ, et al. High-intensity physical activity, stable relationship, and high education level associate with decreasing risk of erectile dysfunction in 1,000 apparently healthy cardiovascular risk subjects. J Sex Med. 2014;11(9):2277–84.
76. Rosen RC, Wing RR, Schneider S, Wadden TA, Foster GD, West DS, et al. Erectile dysfunction in type 2 diabetic men: relationship to exercise fitness and cardiovascular risk factors in the Look AHEAD trial. J Sex Med. 2009;6(5):1414–22.
77. Simon RM, Howard L, Zapata D, Frank J, Freedland SJ, Vidal AC. The association of exercise with both erectile and sexual function in black and white men. J Sex Med. 2015;12(5):1202–10.
78. Pohjantähti-Maaroos H, Palomäki A, Hartikainen J. Erectile dysfunction, physical activity and metabolic syndrome: differences in markers of atherosclerosis. BMC Cardiovasc Disord. 2011;11:36.
79. Compostella L, Compostella C, Truong LV, Russo N, Setzu T, Iliceto S, et al. History of erectile dysfunction as a predictor of poor physical performance after an acute myocardial infarction. Eur J Prev Cardiol. 2017;24(5):460–7.
80. Ventus D, Jern P. Lifestyle factors and premature ejaculation: are physical exercise, alcohol consumption, and body mass index associated with premature ejaculation and comorbid erectile problems? J Sex Med. 2016;13(10):1482–7.
81. Yang YQ, Xu Q, Tong WJ, Gao CL, Li HM. Sexual dysfunction among Chinese nurses: prevalence and predictors. Biomed Environ Sci. 2017;30(3):229–34.
82. Çayan S, Yaman Ö, Orhan İ, Usta M, Başar M, Resim S, et al. Prevalence of sexual dysfunction and urinary incontinence and associated risk factors in Turkish women. Eur J Obstet Gynecol Reprod Biol. 2016;203:303–8.
83. Amidu N, Owiredu WK, Woode E, Addai-Mensah O, Quaye L, Alhassan A, et al. Incidence of sexual dysfunction: a prospective survey in Ghanaian females. Reprod Biol Endocrinol. 2010;8:106.
84. Nazarpour S, Simbar M, Ramezani Tehrani F, AlaviMajd H. Sexual function and exercise in postmenopausal women residing in Chalous and Nowshahr, Northern Iran. Iran Red Crescent Med J. 2016;18(5):e30120.
85. Paiva CE, Rezende FF, Paiva BS, Mauad EC, Zucca-Matthes G, Carneseca EC, et al. Associations of body mass index and physical activity with sexual

dysfunction in breast cancer survivors. Arch Sex Behav. 2016;45(8):2057–68.
86. Smits A, Smits E, Lopes A, Das N, Hughes G, Talaat A, et al. Body mass index, physical activity and quality of life of ovarian cancer survivors: time to get moving? Gynecol Oncol. 2015;139(1):148–54.
87. Vafaeimanesh J, Raei M, Hosseinzadeh F, Parham M. Evaluation of sexual dysfunction in women with type 2 diabetes. Indian J Endocrinol Metab. 2014;18(2):175–9.
88. Ioakeimidis N, Samentzas A, Vlachopoulos C, Aggelis A, Stefanadis C, Tousoulis D. Chronotropic incompetence and dynamic postexercise autonomic dysfunction are associated with the presence and severity of erectile dysfunction. Ann Noninvasive Electrocardiol. 2016;21(3):256–62.
89. Lamina S, Okoye CG, Dagogo TT. Therapeutic effect of an interval exercise training program in the management of erectile dysfunction in hypertensive patients. J ClinHypertens (Greenwich). 2009;11(3):125–9.
90. Lamina S, Okoye CG, Dagogo TT. Managing erectile dysfunction in hypertension: the effects of a continuous training programme on biomarker of inflammation. BJU Int. 2009;103(9):1218–21.
91. Kałka D, Domagała Z, Rusiecki L, Karpiński Ł, Gebala J, Kolęda P, et al. Heart rate recovery, cardiac rehabilitation and erectile dysfunction in males with ischaemic heart disease. Anatol J Cardiol. 2016;16(4):256–63.
92. Kalka D, Domagala ZA, Kowalewski P, Rusiecki L, Koleda P, Marciniak W, et al. Effect of endurance cardiovascular training intensity on erectile dysfunction severity in men with ischemic heart disease. Am J Mens Health. 2015;9(5):360–9.
93. Kałka D, Domagała Z, Dworak J, Womperski K, Rusiecki L, Marciniak W, et al. Association between physical exercise and quality of erection in men with ischaemic heart disease and erectile dysfunction subjected to physical training. Kardiol Pol. 2013;71(6):573–80.
94. Begot I, Peixoto TC, Gonzaga LR, Bolzan DW, Papa V, Carvalho AC, et al. A home-based walking program improves erectile dysfunction in men with an acute myocardial infarction. Am J Cardiol. 2015;115(5):571–5.
95. Cho DY, Yeo JK, Cho SI, Jung JE, Yang SJ, Kong DH, et al. Exercise improves the effects of testosterone replacement therapy and the durability of response after cessation of treatment: a pilot randomized controlled trial. Asian J Androl. 2017;19(5):602–7.
96. Khoo J, Tian HH, Tan B, Chew K, Ng CS, Leong D, et al. Comparing effects of low- and high-volume moderate-intensity exercise on sexual function and testosterone in obese men. J Sex Med. 2013;10(7):1823–32.
97. Maresca L, D'Agostino M, Castaldo L, Vitelli A, Mancini M, Torella G, et al. Exercise training improves erectile dysfunction (ED) in patients with metabolic syndrome on phosphodiesterase-5 (PDE-5) inhibitors. Monaldi Arch Chest Dis. 2013;80(4):177–83.
98. Condorelli RA, Calogero AE, Di Mauro M, Mongioì LM, Russo GI, Morgia G, et al. Effects of tadalafil treatment combined with physical activity in patients with low onset hypogonadism: results from a not-randomized single arm phase 2 study. Aging Male. 2016;19(3):155–60.
99. Kirilmaz U, Guzel O, Aslan Y, Balci M, Tuncel A, Atan A. The effect of lifestyle modification and glycemic control on the efficiency of sildenafil citrate in patients with erectile dysfunction due to type-2 diabetes mellitus. Aging Male. 2015;18(4):244–8.
100. Maio G, Saraeb S, Marchiori A. Physical activity and PDE5 inhibitors in the treatment of erectile dysfunction: results of a randomized controlled study. J Sex Med. 2010;7(6):2201–8.
101. Lamina S, Agbanusi E, Nwacha RC. Effects of aerobic exercise in the management of erectile dysfunction: a meta-analysis study on randomized controlled trials. Ethiop J Health Sci. 2011;21(3):195–201.
102. Silva AB, Sousa N, Azevedo LF, Martins C. Physical activity and exercise for erectile dysfunction: systematic review and meta-analysis. Br J Sports Med. 2017;51(19):1419–24.
103. Halis F, Yildirim P, Kocaaslan R, Cecen K, Gokce A. Pilates for better sex: changes in sexual functioning in healthy Turkish women after pilates exercise. J Sex Marital Ther. 2016;42(4):302–8.
104. Kim HN, Ryu J, Kim KS, Song SW. Effects of yoga on sexual function in women with metabolic syndrome: a randomized controlled trial. J Sex Med. 2013;10(11):2741–51.
105. Anderson D, Seib C, McGuire A, Porter-Steele J. Decreasing menopausal symptoms in women undertaking a web-based multi-modal lifestyle intervention: the Women's Wellness Program. Maturitas. 2015;81(1):69–75.
106. Lara LA, Ramos FK, Kogure GS, Costa RS, Silva de Sá MF, Ferriani RA, et al. Impact of physical resistance training on the sexual function of women with polycystic ovary syndrome. J Sex Med. 2015;12(7):1584–90.
107. Lorenz TA, Meston CM. Acute exercise improves physical sexual arousal in women taking antidepressants. Ann Behav Med. 2012;43(3):352–61.
108. Lorenz TA, Meston CM. Exercise improves sexual function in women taking antidepressants: results from a randomized crossover trial. Depress Anxiety. 2014;31(3):188–95.
109. Claudino MA, Delbin MA, Franco-Penteado CF, Priviero FB, De Nucci G, Antunes E, et al. Exercise training ameliorates the impairment of endothelial and nitrergic corpus cavernosum responses in diabetic rats. Life Sci. 2011;88(5–6):272–7.
110. La Favor JD, Anderson EJ, Dawkins JT, Hickner RC, Wingard CJ. Exercise prevents Western diet-associated erectile dysfunction and coronary artery endothelial dysfunction: response to acute apocynin

and sepiapterin treatment. Am J Physiol Regul Integr Comp Physiol. 2013;305(4):R423–34.
111. Meldrum DR, Gambone JC, Morris MA, Meldrum DAN, Esposito K, Ignarro LJ. The link between erectile and cardiovascular health: the canary in the coal mine. Am J Cardiol. 2011;108(4):599–606.
112. Buga GM, Gold ME, Fukuto JM, Ignarro LJ. Shear stress-induced release of nitric oxide from endothelial cells grown on beads. Hypertension. 1991;17(2):187–93.
113. Zheng H, Mayhan WG, Patel KP. Exercise training improves the defective centrally mediated erectile responses in rats with type I diabetes. J Sex Med. 2011;8(11):3086–97.
114. Haram PM, Adams V, Kemi OJ, Brubakk AO, Hambrecht R, Ellingsen O, et al. Time-course of endothelial adaptation following acute and regular exercise. Eur J Cardiovasc Prev Rehab. 2006;13(4):585–91.
115. Ignarro LJ, Balestrieri ML, Napoli C. Nutrition, physical activity and cardiovascular disease: an update. Cardiovasc Res. 2007;73(3):326–40.
116. Ozbek E, Tasci AI, Ilbey YO, Simsek A, Somay A, Metin G. The effect of regular exercise on penile nitric oxide synthase expression in rats. Int J Androl. 2010;33(4):623–8.
117. Booth FW, Roberts CK, Laye MJ. Lack of exercise is a major cause of chronic diseases. Compr Physiol. 2012;2(2):1143–211.
118. Nehra A, Jackson G, Miner M, Billups KL, Burnett AL, Buvat J, et al. The Princeton III Consensus recommendations for the management of erectile dysfunction and cardiovascular disease. Mayo Clin Proc. 2012;87(8):766–78.
119. Viigimaa M, Doumas M, Vlachopoulos C, Anyfanti P, Wolf J, Narkiewicz K, et al. Hypertension and sexual dysfunction: time to act. J Hypertens. 2011;29(2):403–7.
120. Manolis AJ, Doumas M, Viigimaa M, Narkiewitz K. Hypertension and sexual dysfunction. European Society of Hypertension Scientific Newsletter: Update on Hypertension Management. 2007;8
121. Mancia G, De Backer G, Dominiczak A, Cifkova R, Fagard R, Germano G, et al. Management of arterial hypertension of the European Society of Hypertension; European Society of Cardiology. 2007 Guidelines for the Management of Arterial Hypertension: The Task Force for the Management of Arterial Hypertension of the European Society of Hypertension (ESH) and of the European Society of Cardiology (ESC). J Hypertens. 2007;25:1105–87.
122. Mancia G, Laurent S, Agabiti-Rosei E, Ambrosioni E, Burnier M, Caulfield MJ, et al. Reappraisal of European guidelines on hypertension management: a European Society of Hypertension Task Force document. J Hypertens. 2009;27:2121–58.
123. Mancia G, Fagard R, Narkiewicz K, et al. 2013 ESH/ESC guidelines for the management of arterial hypertension: the Task Force for the management of arterial hypertension of the European Society of Hypertension (ESH) and of the European Society of Cardiology (ESC). Eur Heart J. 2013;34:2159–219.
124. Sánchez-Cruz JJ, Cabrera-León A, Martín-Morales A, Fernández A, Burgos R, Rejas J. Male erectile dysfunction and health-related quality of life. Eur Urol. 2003;44(2):245–53.
125. Fujisawa M, Sawada K, Okada H, Arakawa S, Saito S, Kamidono S. Evaluation of health-related quality of life in patients treated for erectile dysfunction with viagra (sildenafil citrate) using SF-36 score. Arch Androl. 2002;48(1):15–21.
126. Litwin MS, Nied RJ, Dhanani N. Health-related quality of life in men with erectile dysfunction. J Gen Intern Med. 1998;13(3):159–66.
127. Intili H, Nier D. Self-esteem and depression in men who present with erectile dysfunction. Urol Nurs. 1998;18(3):185–7. 208.
128. Pozzo MJ, Mociulsky J, Martinez ET, Senatore G, Farias JM, Sapetti A, et al. Diabetes and quality of life: initial approach to depression, physical activity, and sexual dysfunction. Am J Ther. 2016;23(1):e159–71.
129. Jønler M, Moon T, Brannan W, Stone NN, Heisey D, Bruskewitz RC. The effect of age, ethnicity and geographical location on impotence and quality of life. Br J Urol. 1995;75(5):651–5.
130. Shabsigh R, Klein LT, Seidman S, Kaplan SA, Lehrhoff BJ, Ritter JS. Increased incidence of depressive symptoms in men with erectile dysfunction. Urology. 1998;52(5):848–52.
131. Müller MJ, Ruof J, Graf-Morgenstern M, Porst H, Benkert O. Quality of partnership in patients with erectile dysfunction after sildenafil treatment. Pharmacopsychiatry. 2001;34(3):91–5.
132. Fisher WA, Rosen RC, Eardley I, Sand M, Goldstein I. Sexual experience of female partners of men with erectile dysfunction: The female experience of men's attitudes to life events and sexuality (FEMALES) study. J Sex Med. 2005;2(5):675–84.
133. Öberg K, Fugl-Meyer KS. On Swedish women's distressing sexual dysfunctions: some concomitant conditions and life satisfaction. J Sex Med. 2005;2(2):169–80.
134. Seidman SN, Roose SP, Menza MA, Shabsigh R, Rosen RC. Treatment of erectile dysfunction in men with depressive symptoms: Results of a placebo-controlled trial with sildenafil citrate. Am J Psychiatry. 2001;158(10):1623–30.
135. Moncada I, Martinez-Jabaloyas JM, Rodriguez-Vela L, Gutierrez PR, Giuliano F, Koskimaki J, et al. Emotional changes in men treated with sildenafil citrate for erectile dysfunction: A double-blind, placebo-controlled clinical trial. J Sex Med. 2009;6(12):3469–77.
136. McLaughlin T, Harnett J, Burhani S, Scott B. Evaluation of erectile dysfunction therapy in patients previously nonadherent to long-term medications: a retrospective analysis of prescription claims. Am J Ther. 2005;12(6):605–11.

Cardiorespiratory Fitness in the Context of Cardiac Rehabilitation

23

Jonathan K. Ehrman

Introduction

Cardiac rehabilitation (CR) is a medically supervised exercise and lifestyle education program designed for patients who have had a recent cardiac event. The focus of CR is to return a patient to an optimal physical, spiritual, sexual social, vocational, and emotional well-being. There is strong evidence that CR results in a reduction of morbidity and mortality for many cardiac-related diagnoses and comorbid conditions [7, 37, 47, 49, 59, 70]. Combined with an ever-improving public insurance and clinical environment, cardiac rehabilitation referral and participation have become an important part of the overall treatment model. For instance, in the United States, the Centers for Medicare and Medicaid Services (CMS) has expanded cardiac rehabilitation covered diagnoses twice over the past 10 years, and most third-party insurers have followed this lead. Additionally, CR referral following a qualifying cardiac event is a secondary preventive performance measure as stipulated by the American Heart Association (AHA) and the American College of Cardiology (ACC) [71]. Also, many centers are beginning to add CR to their post-hospitalization disease management processes, including for heart failure. Finally, in 2017, the CMS released a decision memo allowing for supervised exercise training in those with symptomatic peripheral arterial disease and suggested the CR setting as appropriate for implementation.

Although multifaceted, a primary goal of CR is to improve the cardiorespiratory fitness (CRF) of those who attend. A typical outpatient (aka phase 2) CR program consists of a 5–10-min warm-up using aerobic exercise equipment (e.g., treadmill, stationary cycle, seated or upright stepping machine, upper body ergometer, elliptical, etc.), followed by 30–45 min of aerobic exercise training, and a 5–10-min cooldown. The objective of this training is to increase exercise duration and intensity to promote a positive effect of the exercise training on CRF. Although exercise is the primary deliverable component of CR, most CR programs also provide education focused on lifestyle-related risk factors associated with cardiovascular disease progression and future cardiac events. Interestingly, all of the studies prior to the year 2000 that have found CR to reduce morbidity and mortality have only focused on the delivery of exercise training, but not the educational component. More recently studies using CR as a research intervention have also included a variety of non-exercise strategies aimed at reducing risk factors including providing individualized education, stress management, behavioral health support, smoking cessation, and other lifestyle strategies in addition to exercise training [67].

J. K. Ehrman (✉)
Department of Internal Medicine, Division of Cardiovascular Medicine, Preventive Cardiology, Henry Ford Medical Group, Detroit, MI, USA
e-mail: jehrman1@hfhs.org

P. Kokkinos, P. Narayan (eds.), *Cardiorespiratory Fitness in Cardiometabolic Diseases*,
https://doi.org/10.1007/978-3-030-04816-7_23

CRF is considered the most important targeted therapeutic outcome for those who participate in CR. There is ample evidence associating a higher CRF level with a reduced incidence of cardiovascular disease risk factors including hypertension, diabetes, obesity, and metabolic syndrome [68]. Based on the importance of exercise regarding CR, outlined in the preceding paragraph, it is rational to assume that CRF will also be connected to secondary prevention. The method used to assess CRF or changes in CRF after an exercise intervention program should also be considered. Typically, CRF is estimated based on the peak speed and grade of the treadmill or the workload when using a leg or arm ergometer and is expressed in metabolic equivalents of task (METs). One MET is considered to be equivalent to the amount of oxygen (O_2) consumed at rest (approximately 3.5 mL · kg^{-1} · min^{-1}). A more accurate assessment of CRF is achieved by a direct assessment of maximal or peak oxygen uptake (VO_2 max or VO_2 peak), performed by the open-circuit spirometry method during a standard symptom-limited exercise test, and is considered the "gold standard" of CRF assessment. Surrogate estimates of CRF also include the 6-min walk test (6MWT), and a crude estimate of change in CRF is determined by calculating the METs during exercise training in the first week of CR versus the final week. This chapter will focus on the effects of CR on CRF and how this is related to outcome in participating patients.

Box 23.1 Eligible Diagnoses for Cardiac Rehabilitation

- Acute myocardial infarction within the preceding 12 months
- Coronary artery bypass surgery
- Current stable angina pectoris
- Heart valve repair or replacement (open surgery or via catheterization lab, e.g., TAVR, TMVR)
- Percutaneous transluminal coronary angioplasty (PTCA) or coronary stenting
- Heart or heart/lung transplant
- Stable chronic heart failure with reduced ejection fraction (HFrEF, EF ≤ 35%)

Pathophysiology

Eligible diagnoses for CR participation as designated by the Centers for Medicare and Medicaid Services (CMS) are presented in Box 23.1. These diagnoses result from both the presence of atherosclerotic disease and nonspecific origins. For instance, myocardial infarction, bypass surgery, coronary artery stenting, and stable angina are associated with obstructive coronary artery disease. Heart failure may develop initially from ischemic coronary artery disease (e.g., causing a myocardial infarction which may lead to heart failure) or may have a non-ischemic origin due to factors such as uncontrolled hypertension, valvular disorders, toxic substance abuse (e.g., alcohol, illicit drugs), cancer treatment, and viral infection, or the cause may be unknown (i.e., idiopathic dilated cardiomyopathy) in up to 50% of the cases.

In addition patients with the comorbid diseases of diabetes, pulmonary arterial hypertension, and congenital heart disease are also included in CR and secondary prevention programs. TAVR = transcatheter aortic valve replacement; TMVR = transcatheter mitral valve replacement; HFrEF = heart failure reduced ejection fraction.

Epidemiological Evidence of the Scope of the Disease

As noted in the previous section, eligibility for participation in CR may or may not involve atherosclerotic disease. Although CR participation has been shown to improve functional capacity in all eligible populations, improvements in morbidity and mortality have not been demonstrated in some of these diagnoses [52]. The total number of Americans that are eligible for CR participation annually is relatively large. More than 900,000 people each year have a new or recurrent myocardial infarction [24], and approximately 400,000 coronary-artery bypass grafting surgeries are performed annually, although this number has declined by about 30% over the past decade [3]. Yet despite the known benefits of CR, participation occurs in less than 30% of eligible patient's post-myocardial infarction and ~30% post-coronary artery bypass surgery who are referred to a CR program [65]. Participation is even lower in eligible Medicare beneficiaries where the overall participation rate for all eligible diagnoses is between 19% and 34%, depending on US regional location, diagnosis, and age of the patient [1]. Additionally, there are more than 100,000 open valve surgeries (primarily mitral and aortic) and more than 50,000 transcatheter valve procedures performed annually in the United States [26]. Estimates of up to 1.25 million Americans are eligible for CR each year [53]. Note that this estimate does not include heart failure patients with reduced ejection fraction (HFrEF). Approximately 550,000 new cases of heart failure are diagnosed annually [17]. Some of these patients are likely to be included in the other eligible diagnoses (e.g., myocardial infarction or valve disease leading to heart failure).

More than 800,000 Americans die each year from a cardiovascular disease [12]. The Million Hearts Initiative has proposed an increase of CR participation to 70% of eligible patients in the next several years. It is estimated that this will save 25,000 lives and decrease 180,000 hospitalizations annually in the United States [1]. While the source of these anticipated benefits is likely multifactorial (i.e., exercise, lifestyle changes, improved medication adherence, three times weekly clinical surveillance, etc.), the increase in daily physical activity and intentional exercise and subsequent improvement in CRF likely play a significant role. However, if CR participation approached just 50% of all eligible patients, the current capacity to service those referred may not be sufficient [53].

Epidemiologic Association Between Cardiorespiratory Fitness and Disease Baseline Fitness

As previously stated, CRF can be assessed directly and expressed as peak oxygen consumption (peak VO_2) or indirectly (peak METs), as is often the method used in CR settings. The following section provides information on both measured peak VO_2 (via gas exchange analysis) and estimated peak METs for those entering CR. This information is also segmented, where possible, by both diagnosis and sex to account for the sex-specific and varying degrees of baseline CRF differences. Regarding sex, in 2896 male ($n = 2081$) and female ($n = 815$) patients of similar age and mixed cardiac diagnoses who were entering two separate CR centers in Vermont and Michigan, Ades et al. reported peak VO_2 values of 19.3 ± 6.1 mL · kg^{-1} · min^{-1} for men and 14.5 ± 3.9 mL · kg^{-1} · min^{-1} for women [18]. They also noted a greater age-related decline of peak VO_2 in men than women (−2.42 vs. −1.16 mL · kg^{-1} · min^{-1} per decade; $p < 0.01$, respectively).

Percutaneous Coronary Intervention, Myocardial Infarction, and Coronary Bypass

Specific to diagnosis, Ades et al. [2] reported that peak VO_2 was 3.5–6 mL · kg^{-1} · min^{-1} higher in male compared to female patients who had a previous percutaneous coronary intervention, a myocardial infarction, or a coronary artery bypass surgery (CABG) or who were treated medically for unstable angina (Table 23.1). Note that for each diagnosis, the peak VO_2 for males was 3.5–6 mL · kg^{-1} · min^{-1} higher than for females.

Beckie et al. also reported even lower MET levels in 232 women entering CR without considering the initial diagnosis [11]. The group consisted of 50% who had undergone a PCI, 33% CABG, 12% with stable angina, and 5% who had

Table 23.1 Baseline peak VO_2 by cardiac diagnosis of patients enrolling in cardiac rehabilitation [2]

	Peak VO_2, mL · kg^{-1} · min^{-1}	
Cardiac diagnosis	Women[a]	Men[b]
PCI, no MI	15.1 ± 4.1	21.2 ± 7.2
MI	14.7 ± 4.2	20.4 ± 6.6
Med Rx (unstable angina)	14.7 ± 3.8	18.3 ± 5.8
CABG	13.5 ± 3.4	17.8 ± 4.8

Modified from Ades et al. [2]
PCI percutaneous coronary intervention, *MI* myocardial infarction, *Med* medical, *Rx* prescription, *CABG* coronary artery bypass graft
Raw data are presented. Statistical analysis adjusts for age
[a]CABG significantly lower than PCI without MI
[b]CABG lower than MI. PCI without MI higher than MI

an MI. Peak estimated METs for the cohort were 5.8 ± 2.5. Similarly, relatively low MET levels were reported by Balady et al. [9] on a cohort of 558 men and 220 women (45% MI, 26% CABG, 10% PCI, 13% angina, 6% others) enrolled in CR program. At baseline, the peak MET level for men was 8.6 ± 3.4 and for women 6.0 ± 2.6 METs. As expected the peak MET values were highest for the youngest overall grouping (<65 years =8.9 ± 3.4; 65–75 years = 6.6 ± 2.6; >75 years =5.7 ± 2.9 METs). Exercise capacity improved significantly for men and women of every age group including those older than 75 years. The improvements were more pronounced among those with an initial peak MET level <5 (Fig. 23.1). The investigators concluded that referral to CR programs should be advocated for both men and women and should not be limited by age.

Kavanagh et al. reported on 12,169 men (aged 55.0 ± 9.6 years) with either a previous MI or CABG, who were diagnosed with ischemic heart disease and who were referred to a single-site CR program with peak VO_2 measured prior to participation [32]. The investigators stratified the cohort into three groups based on peak VO_2 values at baseline: <15, 15–22, and >22 mL · kg^{-1} · min^{-1}. After a median follow-up of 7.9 years, there were 1336 cardiac and 2352 all-cause deaths. The investigators reported a graded reduction in cardiac and all-cause death with increased CRF. A 9% reduction in death risk was noted for each 1 mL · kg^{-1} · min^{-1} incremental increase in VO_2. Similar findings were reported by the same group in 2380 women referred to CR [33]. For these women, each 1 mL · kg^{-1} · min^{-1} higher baseline peak VO_2 was associated with a 10% lower cardiac mortality risk. The investigators concluded that baseline peak VO_2 was a strong predictor of mortality in CR patients and that even small increments in peak VO_2 might significantly reduce the risk of death.

Aortic Valve Replacement/Implantation

Peak VO_2 values have been reported for patients entering a CR program who had either a transcatheter (TAVR or TAVI) or a traditional surgical aortic valve replacement/implantation [58]. Peak VO_2 was not different between patients in the TAVR group of 12.5 ± 3.6 mL · kg^{-1} · min^{-1} versus 13.9 ± 2.7 mL · kg^{-1} · min^{-1} for the surgical group. Note that 32% in the TAVR group were male versus 50% in the surgical group. The higher percent of males in the TAVR group, along with the usually higher-risk patients undergoing TAVR procedures, might explain, in part, the slightly higher peak VO_2 in the surgical group.

Heart Failure

The HF-ACTION trial randomized reduced ejection fraction heart failure patients (HFrEF) to

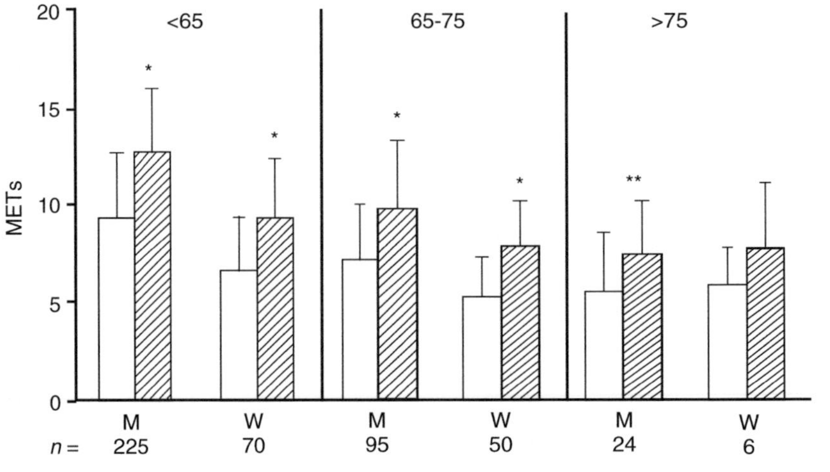

Fig. 23.1 Baseline and changes in peak estimated MET level, by age, in male and female cardiac rehabilitation participants. *Significantly different from baseline. (Modified from Balady et al. [9])

usual care or usual care plus CR [47]. In 2016 Keteyian et al. reported on baseline cardiopulmonary exercise test results in the HF-ACTION cohort of 2100 (71% male). Baseline peak VO_2 values for men and women were 15.2 (8.7–24.3 for 5th and 95th percentiles) and 13.4 (7.7–21.0) $mL \cdot kg^{-1} \cdot min^{-1}$, respectively [36]. The absolute mean values were 1.45 and 1.11 L min^{-1} which represented 57% and 68%, respectively, of the age- and sex-predicted peak VO_2 for the men and women. Guazzi et al. reported that baseline peak VO_2 values in a group of 34 HFrEF and 34 preserved ejection fraction heart failure patients (HFpEF) were not different (14.3 ± 5.0 vs. 14.3 ± 5.6 $mL \cdot kg^{-1} \cdot min^{-1}$, respectively; $p = 0.2$) [27]. Of note, each group had an identical representation of males (76%) and females (24%). One point of interest is that the HF-ACTION patients were all tested on a treadmill (standard in the U.S.) and the Guazzi group were all tested on leg cycle ergometers (standard in Europe). Cycle modalities are associated with a 10–15% lower peak VO_2 when compared to a treadmill [57].

Myers et al. reported on 41 male patients with HFrEF (68.3 ± 12 y, EF = 33 ± 9%) who performed a maximal exercise test on a treadmill using an individualized ramp protocol where the increase in walking speed and treadmill grade was adjusted to result in a test duration of approximately 10 min [43]. Peak oxygen consumption was measured at 16.1 ± 6.2 $mL \cdot kg^{-1} \cdot min^{-1}$, equivalent to 4.5 ± 1.8 METs. However, estimated METs were measured at 5.4 ± 2.2, indicating a discrepancy between measured and estimated peak METs. This issue is addressed later in this section.

Left Ventricular Assist Device (LVAD)

Kerrigan et al. assessed peak VO_2 in 26 patients (27% female; mean age 55 ± 13 years) who had an LVAD implanted more than 6 weeks prior [34]. The peak VO_2 for the entire group was 12.9 ± 3.1 $mL \cdot kg^{-1} \cdot min^{-1}$ (13.4 ± 3.5) for men and 11.3 ± 2.4 $mL \cdot kg^{-1} \cdot min^{-1}$ for women. In a comparison of peak VO_2 values between a group of HFrEF patients not yet eligible for LVAD placement and those with an implanted LVAD, Nahumi et al. found a significantly higher peak VO_2 in the HFrEF, group (15.0 vs. 12.4 $mL \cdot kg^{-1} \cdot min^{-1}$; $p < 0.001$) [44]. This difference is not surprising since a lower peak VO_2 is a criterion for LVAD placement [41]. Despite this, they reported that the LVAD group had a better submaximal exercise capacity as evidenced by a greater 6-min walk test distance. It is unclear how LVAD implantation affects peak VO_2, but the authors concluded that peak VO_2 might not be the best measure to assess functional changes after LVAD placement.

Cardiac Transplant

A peak VO_2 of 17.5 ± 0.9 $mL \cdot kg^{-1} \cdot min^{-1}$ (peak RER = 1.25 ± 0.01) was reported by Ehrman et al. in 16 orthotopic heart transplant recipients (45 ± 1.9 years of age) who performed a maximal exercise treadmill test at 3 months after surgery using a low-level protocol [22]. A substantially higher peak VO_2 was reported by Schmid et al. in 17 heart transplant recipients using a cycle ergometer cardiopulmonary exercise test (20.9 ± 5.2 $mL \cdot kg^{-1} \cdot min^{-1}$) [64]. Carter et al. reported on the natural course of posttransplant peak VO_2 and that the percent of age- and sex-predicted peak VO_2 increased from 41.3 ± 2.2% at pre-transplant evaluation to 48.6 ± 1.7% at 1-year posttransplant [18], with no further change at 5 years postoperative. Salyer et al. reported a measured peak VO_2 of 18.7 ± 4.7 $mL \cdot kg^{-1} \cdot min^{-1}$ and an estimated peak MET level of 7.8 ± 2.0 METs (actual measured METs = 5.3) at a mean of 68 ± 32 days post-surgery in 24 patients (age 26 ± 11 years, 9 women and 15 men) who underwent cardiac transplantation [60].

Measured and Estimated Functional Capacity Discrepancies

The information in the preceding sections, where available, demonstrates a consistent disconnect between measured peak VO_2 and predicted peak METs during a maximal symptom-limited graded exercise test. For instance, the cardiac transplant

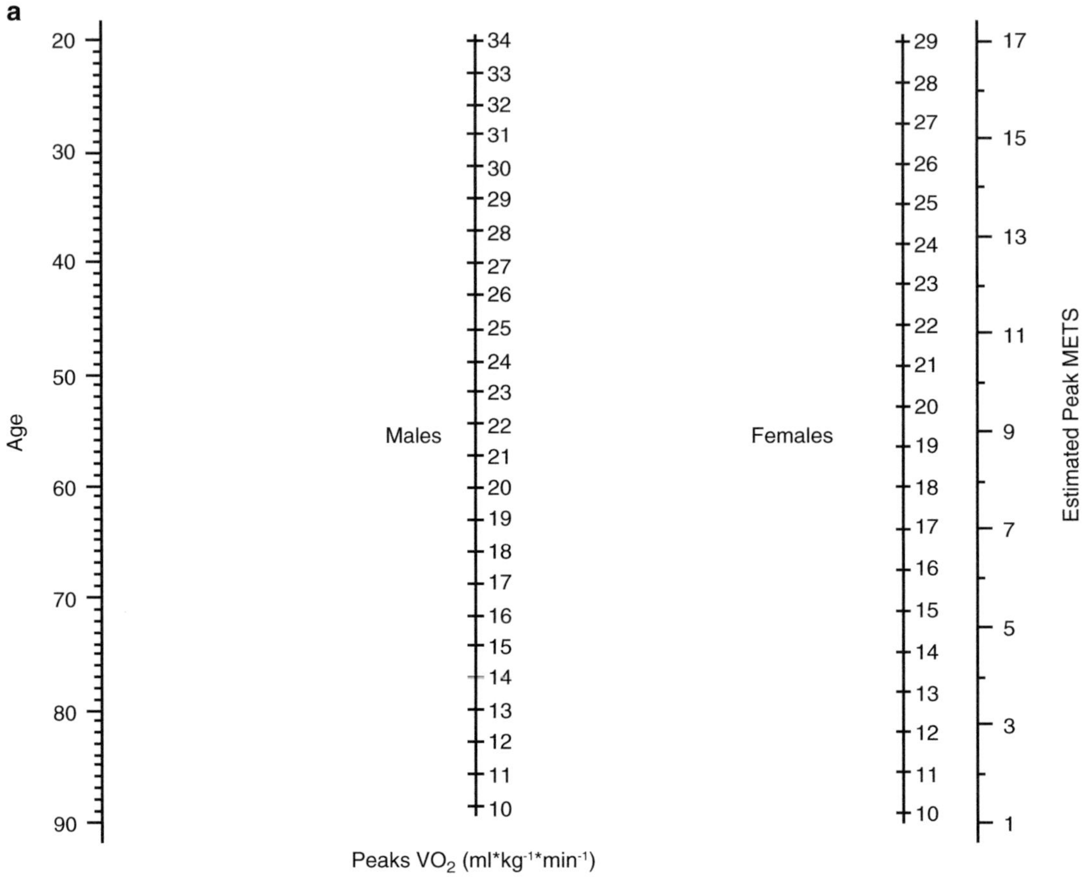

Fig. 23.2 Nomogram to convert estimated METs to peak VO_2 [2]

section presented data with a measured peak MET level of 5.3 (18.7 ± 4.7 mL · kg^{-1} · min^{-1}) and an estimated MET value of 7.8 [60]. This is a 32% difference. And a 17% overestimation of METs was noted in data presented in the heart failure section [43]. This type of overestimation is a consistent finding among all clinical populations and must be considered when addressing issues such a prognosis, an insurance company-mandated MET level to determine the number of approved CR sessions, and an individual patient response to treatment.

Ades et al. noted that the American College of Sports Medicine's (ACSM) equation for determining peak MET level during treadmill walking systematically overestimated peak METs in CR patients [2]. For men, Ades et al. reported the overestimation was 30%; and for women, it was 23% [2]. They provided a correlation coefficient of 0.48 (moderately weak) between the estimated and measured peak METs. They also noted that the correlation was stronger in women than men ($R = 0.66$ vs. 0.39; $p < 0.001$), but did not provide specific percent measurement differences between the groups. It is important to note that the ACSM equations were developed to estimate energy expenditure at submaximal rather than maximal workloads [57]. Based on this finding, Ades et al. developed a nomogram (Fig. 23.2) to correct the overestimation of METs by the ACSM formula.

Epidemiologic Association Between Fitness and Chronic Disease

It is well established that physical inactivity resulting in a low CRF is a risk factor for the

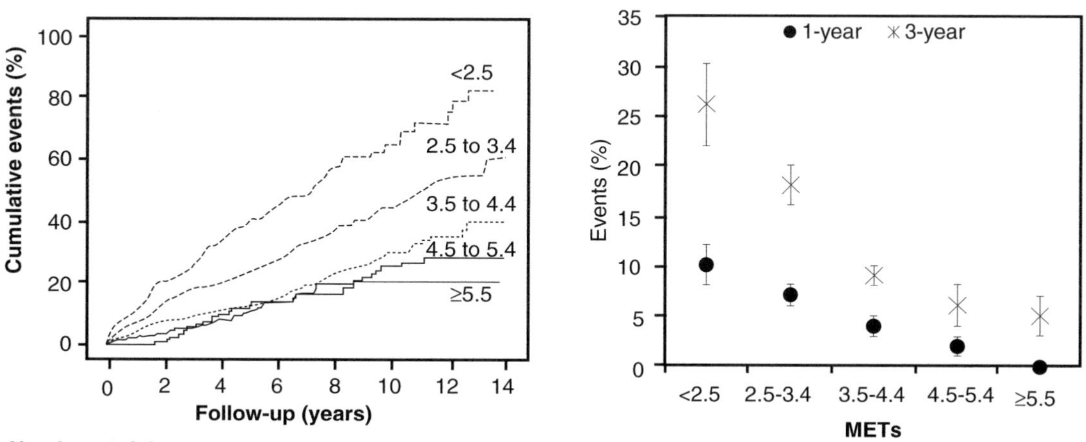

Number at risk

METs	2 YR	4 YR	6 YR	8 YR	10 YR	12 YR	14 YR
<2.5	174	113	86	60	31	15	7
2.5 to 3.4	621	475	389	333	233	135	74
3.5 to 4.4	504	403	355	265	170	101	40
4.5 to 5.4	278	235	194	142	93	61	32
≥5.5	149	131	100	75	46	27	13

Fig. 23.3 All-cause mortality, nonfatal MI, or HF hospitalization

cardiovascular disease and all-cause mortality [13, 14, 38]. Additionally, *sedentary behavior* is independently related to the risk of developing cardiovascular disease [23]. Specific to CR, there is evidence that CRF at baseline and upon completion of a CR program are each independently related to mortality risk [15, 39]. In a cohort of 5641 patients (76% male), stratified based on estimated peak METs at baseline as low (<5 METs), moderate (5–8 METs), and high fitness (>8 METs), mortality risk was associated 46% and 78% lower in the moderate and high fitness categories, respectively [39]. The improvement of CRF following CR participation was also associated with a 13% reduction in mortality risk per 1 MET increase in exercise capacity (hazard ratio [HR], 0.87; 95% CI, 0.79–0.96; $p < 0.001$).

In a study of 1726 patients (36% female) who completed 9–15 sessions of CR, Brawner et al. reported a 40–50% lower risk of a composite end point (all-cause mortality, nonfatal MI, or heart failure hospitalization) per MET at baseline and 32–37% lower risk, after completing the program [15]. METs achieved following training were a stronger predictor of the composite outcome and all-cause mortality compared to METs at baseline (Fig. 23.3).

Chronic Disease and Physical Activity Prevalence

The volume of physical activity performed is relatively low among those with an established chronic disease [16]. Using data from the 2014 National Health Interview Survey (NHIS), Brawner et al. reported that among those with a myocardial infarction, only 40% stated they performed at least 150 min per week of leisure-time aerobic physical activity as compared to about 55% among those with no known chronic disease (Fig. 23.4) [16]. Additionally, they reported that with each additional chronic disease within an individual, there was a 17% (OR = 0.83; 95% CI, 0.81–0.85; $P < 0.001$) lower likelihood of achieving 150 min per week of leisure-time aerobic physical activity [16].

Similar findings were reported by Evenson et al. in the National Health and Nutrition Examination Survey (NHANES). Participation in at least 150 min per week of moderate-intensity physical

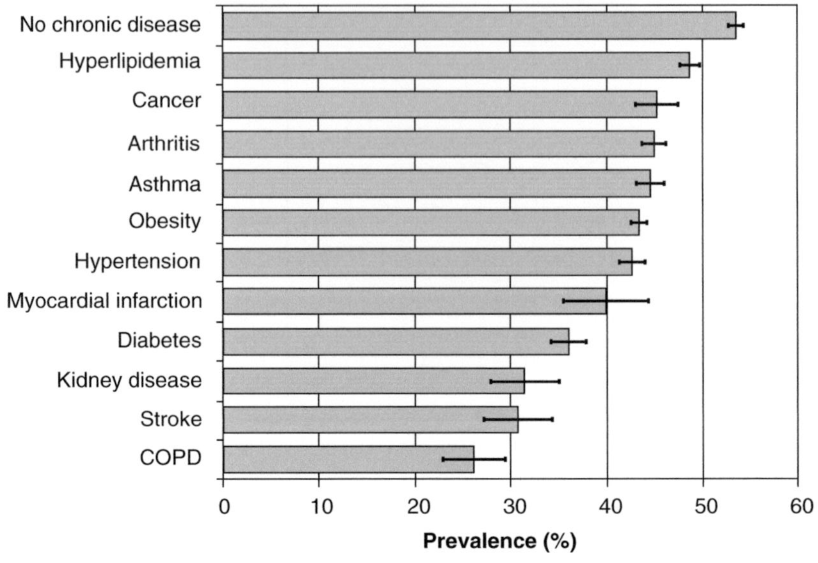

Fig. 23.4 Prevalence of adults reporting >150 min per week leisure-time physical activity

activity in chronic heart failure patients was 40% and 54% in patients with coronary heart disease. Both of these groups also had higher sedentary behavior than noted in those without disease.

Schairer et al. assessed the physical activity levels of 104 CR maintenance program participants (32% CABG, 22% MI, 16% PCI, 14% angina, 7% HF) using the Paffenbarger Physical Activity Questionnaire [63]. The total weekly exercise duration was 292 ± 188 min of which 174 ± 86 min was accumulated in CR. Thus, CR participation alone met the US physical activity recommendation of at least 150 min per week. The average weekly caloric expenditure in CR was 830 ± 428 kcals, and another 675 ± 659 kcals was expended during non-CR leisure-time physical activity for a total of 1504 ± 830 kcals expended per week during all physical activity/exercise training combined. Although activity intensity was not reported, this amount of energy expenditure is nearly the amount recommended to slow the progression of coronary artery disease (~1533 kcal per week) and improve CRF [29].

Because of the high prevalence of low physical activity volume and sedentary behavior in those with cardiovascular disease, CR programs provide an important tool to increase physical activity levels in patients with cardiovascular disease.

Interventional Evidence: Cardiac Rehabilitation

Change in CRF following CR participation is best assessed by an exercise test performed before and following the program, by a direct assessment of peak VO_2 (open-circuit spirometry method) rather than estimating METs based on the workload achieved. However, direct assessment of peak VO_2 requires specialized equipment and trained personnel and is costly, limiting a widespread application. Thus, estimated METs have been extrapolated based on treadmill speed and elevation (workloads) or cycle ergometry (work rate). Although estimated peak METs overestimate measured peak VO_2 [45], functional capacity estimated by peak METs is acceptable. The following sections review studies that have assessed change in functional capacity following CR participation.

Almodhy et al. studied the effects of CR on 117 patients who performed a shuttle walk performance test either once (n = 58) or twice (n = 59) a week for 6 weeks [4]. Both groups improved peak MET capacity by ~0.3 METs, with no difference between the groups. The authors reported that this change was well below typical improvement which range between 1.2 and 1.8 METs. They suggested that the training stimulus was too low for maximal MET improvement.

Percutaneous Coronary Intervention, Myocardial Infarction, and Coronary Artery Bypass Surgery

Armstrong et al. reported on a group of diabetic (n = 1546) and nondiabetic (n = 7036) patients who attended CR between 1996 and 2010 [8]. Approximately 50% of patients had a previous myocardial infarction, 60% percutaneous coronary intervention, 30% coronary artery bypass surgery, and about 10% heart failure. Participants completed an exercise test, and peak METs were estimated at baseline and at the end of the CR program (12 weeks). Data were analyzed in those who completed the program (85% of nondiabetic and 80% diabetic). The diabetic group had a significantly lower baseline peak MET level (by 1.0 in men and 0.5 METs in women) compared to the nondiabetics. Both groups significantly improved their peak MET levels with the nondiabetic group having a significantly larger increase (0.95 vs. 0.8 MET, $p < 0.001$). Interestingly, at 1-year follow-up, nondiabetic patients retained their gains in peak METs resulting from exercise training, while diabetic patients did not.

Lower baseline CRF levels in CR patients with type 2 diabetes (DM2) compared to nondiabetics have also been reported by Banzer et al. [10]. Baseline MET levels for diabetics (n = 250; age 62 ± 10 years) and 7.0 ± 2.6 for nondiabetics (n = 702; age 61 ± 11 years). The greater percentage of males in the nondiabetic group (64% vs. 53%) may have contributed some of this difference in baseline METs. Significant improvement in peak METs was noted in both diabetics and nondiabetics who completed the program (26% and 27%, respectively; $p < 0.001$). Similar findings were reported by Hindman et al. in 292 patients enrolled in a CR program. Baseline MET levels in DM2 patients were 5.7 ± 2.3 CRF and 7.3 ± 2.4 following CR participation of at least 7 weeks of three times per week. MET levels for the nondiabetic participants (n = 1213) were 7.1 ± 2.6 MET at baseline and increased to 8.9 ± 2.7 METs after CR participation. Similar findings have been reported by Keteyian et al. in 8319 patients (31% female) who participated in CR and completed at least nine sessions [35]. Peak MET levels increase by 1.3 ± 1.1 and 0.9 ± 0.7 in men and women, respectively.

Recently, high-intensity interval training (HIIT) has been advocated as an alternative method of increasing aerobic capacity in those with limited time to commit to a traditional CR program. In this regard, Currie et al. assessed CRF improvements in MI, PCI, and CABG patients (n = 22) randomly assigned to low-volume high-intensity interval training (HIIT) versus moderate-intensity steady-state training for 12 weeks, two times per week [19]. Training volume in the HIIT group was approximately 2.5 times less than the moderate-intensity endurance trained group. Both groups improved similarly (18.7 ± 5.7 vs. 22.3 ± 6.1 $mL \cdot kg^{-1} \cdot min^{-1}$ for the moderate-intensity program and 19.8 ± 3.7 vs. 24.5 ± 4.5 $mL \cdot kg^{-1} \cdot min^{-1}$, $p < 0.001$, for pre- vs. post-training) for the HIIT program. The finding suggest that HIIT may provide a viable, alternative method to improve CRF, requiring less time to perform for those struggling with the time commitment to participate in CR.

Aortic Valve Replacement/Implantation

Aortic valve replacement does not appear to improve exercise capacity or function in patients [42]. However, improvements in CRF and function have been noted in just 3 weeks of CR program participation in 76 patients following transcatheter aortic valve implantation (TAVI) and 366 following surgical aortic valve replacement [72]. Both groups improved in 6-min walk distance (28 vs. 46 m), with the surgical group improving significantly more ($p < 0.001$). Part of this difference may have been due to the older age of the TAVI group (80 ± 6 vs. 68 ± 11 years, $p < 0.001$).

Russo et al. also reported a 60.4 ± 46.4 m significant ($p < 0.001$) improvement from baseline in 78 patients who had a TAVI procedure after participation in CR [58]. Similar improvements were also noted in the group of 80 surgical aortic valve replacement patients (±72.3 ± 57.3 m). Similar improvements in peak VO_2 were also noted in both groups following CR (12.5 ± 3.6 and 13.9 ± 2.7 mL · kg^{-1} · min^{-1} for the TAVI and surgical groups, respectively; $p = 0.16$).

To date there have not been any studies reporting on the change in variables associated with CRF and morbidity or mortality in patients following aortic valve replacement. Additionally, there does not appear to be a survival advantage from participating in CR for patients who have had aortic (or mitral) valve disease or surgery [52].

Heart Failure

Prominent among recent investigations is the HF-ACTION study, which assessed the efficacy of 12 weeks of supervised training in the CR setting followed by an 18-month at-home exercise program in 2331 patients with systolic heart failure and left ventricular ejection fraction <35% [40]. Over a median follow-up period of 2.5 years, subgroup analysis demonstrated that patients receiving exercise training had a lower incidence of cardiovascular mortality and hospital admissions for heart failure. Several other subgroup analyses of this study have been published, on outcomes in patients with heart failure and diabetes, COPD, cancer, and different gender and ethnicities [46–50]. In general, comorbidities appeared to reduce the efficacy of exercise therapy, while female sex or self-identification as black race did not. Thus the HF-ACTION study supports a broad role for exercise in patients with systolic heart failure, with caveats for those with significant comorbidities.

Left Ventricular Assist Device

The literature is not robust for those with an LVAD, with only two studies available. Kerrigan et al. assessed 23 patients who had LVAD implantation ($n = 26$; 7 women; age 55 ± 13 years; ejection fraction 21 ± 8%) and who either were randomized to participate in 18 sessions of CR ($n = 16$) or to usual care ($n = 7$). The CR group had a significant increase in their peak VO_2 as compared to the usual care group (13.6 ± 3.3 to 15.3 ± 4.4 vs. 11.2 ± 2.0 to 11.8 ± 2.0 mL · kg^{-1} · min^{-1}; $p < 0.05$). The training group also had a significantly greater increase in 6-min walk test distance.

Marko et al. reported on 41 LVAD recipients who participated in CR within 48 ± 38 days after implantation. Exercise training included lower limb resistance training exercises, cycle ergometry, walking, and gymnastic movements. They reported an increase of peak VO_2 in a subgroup who underwent pre- and post-program testing (11.3 ± 4.1 to 14.5 ± 5.2 mL · kg^{-1} · min^{-1}; $p = 0.007$). To date there has been no report on the effect of change in CRF following exercise training on all-cause or cardiovascular morbidity or mortality in those who have had LVAD implantation.

Cardiac Transplantation

A Cochrane review from 2017 evaluated 10 randomized controlled trials involving 300 cardiac transplant patients (mean age 54.4 years; 25% female), who participated in CR [5]. They reported a median improvement of 2.49 mL · kg^{-1} · min^{-1} for peak VO_2 (95% CI 1.63 to 3.36; $N = 284$; studies = 9; moderate quality evidence) and concluded that there was moderate evidence that exercise-based CR improves exercise capacity as measured using peak VO_2.

Despite the ten trials using CR in those with a cardiac transplant, a recent paper is the only one that assessed the association between participation in CR and survival in those with a cardiac transplantation. Rosembaum et al. reported that participating in CR was associated with an improved survival in a group of 201 patients who participated between 2000 and 2013. Peak VO_2 was reported over 10 years in a subgroup who performed cardiopulmonary exercise testing. They reported a significant increase from prior to transplant to after (~14–17.5 mL · kg^{-1} · min^{-1}) with no further change thereafter. And although CR participation was associated with improved survival, change in peak VO_2 was not.

Mechanisms of Exercise-Induced Changes

The improvements in CRF noted following participation in CR exercise training programs are a result of multiple physiologic changes. Notably, skeletal muscle changes have been observed. These include histochemical (myoglobin increases, enhanced aerobic glycolysis enzymes and proteins, increased mitochondrial density) and histological (fiber size increases, enhanced capillary density, changes in muscle fiber type concentration). Adaptations of the cardiovascular system have also been reported. These include potential increases in left ventricular wall size and thickness which leads to an improved stroke volume. Additionally, increases in total blood volume, hemoglobin, and arteriovenous oxygen difference (a-vO_2 difference) have been reported resulting in more oxygen availability to and extraction by the working muscles. Collectively, these changes result to an increase in aerobic capacity of the patient. Although there are no known pulmonary improvements that occur with aerobic exercise training with respect to lung volumes, the accessory muscles oft used during ventilation may improve their functional ability and allow for enhanced tidal volumes, respiratory rates, and other volumes at a reduced physiologic cost.

The health benefits of improved CRF in apparently healthy and chronic disease populations are well-accepted and the mechanisms involved have also been elucidated. Some have suggested a systemic effect on the vasculature (aka "vascular conditioning") [25] that may involve a reduced rate or reversal of atherosclerotic progression [51], improved vascular function (i.e., reactivity, endothelial function), or functional changes in vascular structure (e.g., enhanced nitric oxide production). A possible link between improved CRF and a vascular effect was demonstrated by Hambrecht et al. [30]. In their study, patients with a cardiac lesion amenable to stenting were randomized to either percutaneous angioplasty or exercise training at 70% of their maximal heart rate. Heart rate and CRF were measured during a symptom-limited cycle ergometer exercise test performed prior to and following aerobic exercise training. The exercise training was performed daily over 12 months for 20 min plus a once-per-week, 60-min group exercise session. Measured peak VO_2 levels improved significantly in the exercise-trained group, but not in the stent group (22.6 to 26.2 vs. 22.3 to 22.8 mL · kg^{-1} · min^{-1}; $p < 0.001$). After 12 months, the exercise-trained patients had a significantly higher event-free survival (88% vs. 70%) than the stented group (OR 0.33, 95% CI 0.12–0.90, $P < 0.023$). These results suggest that exercise training may positively affect the vasculature of diseased vessels to a greater degree than placing a stent.

There is also ample evidence of an inverse relationship between CRF and atrial arrhythmia. Qureshi et al. [56] reported on over 64,000 adults who had a stress test between 1991 and 2009. They noted that each 1-MET increase in exercise capacity was associated with the 7% lower risk of atrial fibrillation. In the CARDIO-FIT study [55] that included 308 obese patients with a history of atrial fibrillation, the authors reported that those who increased their CRF by ≥2 METs had a significantly better arrhythmia-free survival (i.e., less atrial fibrillation recurrence) than a group who improved by <2 METs ($p < 0.001$). In a cohort of 5962 US Veterans (mean age, 56.8 ± 11.0 years), Faselis et al. reported an inverse association between CRF (peak METs) and the incidence of atrial fibrillation, during a median follow-up period of 8.3 years. Exercise capacity was inversely related to AF incidence. The risk was 21% lower (hazard ratio, 0.79; 95% CI, 0.76–0.82) for each 1 MET increase in exercise capacity. When the cohort was stratified according to fitness categories, the risk of AF declined progressively with increased fitness. Specifically, the AF risk was 20% lower in the moderate fit, 45% in the fit, and 63% lower in the highly fit individuals, compared with the least fit individuals. Similar trends were observed in those younger than 65 years and those 65 years or older [73].

There is very little direct evidence of an association of CRF and ventricular arrhythmias in humans. In a cohort of 2328 Japanese men, Hagnas et al. [28] reported that those categorized as low CRF (< 8 METs) and ST-segment depression, indicating cardiac ischemia, had a 4.8-fold higher risk of sudden cardiac death (defined as a death occurring within 1 hour of the onset of the symptoms) than those with a higher fitness level and no ST-segment depression (95% CI, 2.9–7.9). More importantly, the risk of sudden death in those with a high CRF level and ST-segment depression was similar to those with a high CRF level and no ST-segment depression, possibly indicating a protective effect of high CRF. There is ample evidence from animal model research supporting the protective effects of CRF on ventricular tachycardia and fibrillation. Dor-Haim [21] used a myocardial infarcted rat model and exposed them to either sedentary living or bouts of intensive aerobic exercise training. Exercise resulted in a significant increase in CRF compared to the sedentary rats ($p > 0.05$). In isolated hearts following sacrifice, they found a significantly lower risk of ventricular tachycardia and fibrillation in the exercise-trained group (4.5 ± 0.8% to 1.6 ± 0.2%; $p < 0.05$). They also assessed heart rate variability and noted an increase in electrical organization of excitation (i.e., coupling interval dispersion) and ventricular fibrillation dominant frequencies, both protective against arrhythmias.

Clinical Relevance

The importance of CR as a part of the treatment paradigm for many cardiac diagnoses is well established. Interestingly, the meta-analyses that assessed the effect of CR on morbidity and mortality only assessed the effects of exercise training and not lifestyle education aimed at reducing modifiable risk factors [6, 31, 48, 50, 70]. The strong correlation between CRF and mortality as noted in some disease states in this chapter reflects the importance of focusing on improving fitness during CR participation. However, CR is greatly underutilized. It is reported that less than 20% of eligible Medicare patients in the United States participate in at least one session of CR [1, 65]. Based on known data of mortality reduction, it is estimated that simply increasing CR participation threefold would save 25,000 lives and reduce annual hospitalizations by 180,000 in the United States.

Suaya et al. [66] reported a dose-response relationship between the number of CR sessions attended and mortality in a propensity-based matching analysis. This finding is corroborated by a meta-analysis of 31 studies (n = 3827) performed by Sandercock et al. [61] in which they reported a mean 1.55 (95% CI 1.21–1.89) MET improvement and fitness gains were greatest in those who completed at least 36 sessions. Interestingly, change in fitness was not related to whether a program offered exercise only or added an educational component. Thus, assuming more CR sessions attended are related to the amount of improvement in CRF, it would be prudent to design CR programs with a goal of maximally increasing peak oxygen consumption or estimated peak METs. The current literature suggests that this is best achieved by program adherence to as many CR sessions as possible.

Conclusions

There is abundant evidence that improvement in CRF is achievable during CR program participation. This most certainly leads to improved functional capacity in all patients referred to a program. And in some patients, it may lead to improved outcomes, including reduced hospitalizations and deaths. Because of this, it is very important to refer all eligible patients to CR and to improve their functional capacity to the greatest amount possible.

Recommendations: Key Points/Future Directions

While we know much about the relationship of CRF and patient health outcomes, we need to expand our understanding in certain areas. For instance, the current data on the adherence/exercise dose-response and risk is scant. Suaya et al. [66] reported a 19% reduced relative risk of death over the ensuing 5 years in those who attended 25 or more exercise sessions versus those who attended <25 sessions. Santiago et al. also reported a dose-response association in a meta-analysis of 33 studies [62]. Those attending more sessions had a lower risk of all-cause death, but not cardiovascular death. Although these studies suggest a dose-response association based on the number of sessions attended, there is no information on the independent and synergistic effect of exercise duration, intensity, or exercise volume and cardiovascular events. Thus a randomized trial is warranted to further our understanding.

There also is little data on the mortality and morbidity effects of CRF on several disease populations eligible for CR. These include valve replacement/repair, percutaneous coronary intervention, heart and heart/lung transplantation, and coronary artery bypass surgery. These conditions were approved for CR participation solely based on its effect on improving CRF. It is unlikely that the National Institutes of Health would fund a study to evaluate these conditions such as the HF-ACTION study. The HF-ACTION study was responsible for the approval of systolic heart failure as a covered diagnosis in the United States for CR based on both the functional improvement noted and the morbidity and mortality reductions [46]. Additionally, little is understood about the relationship of a generally lower CRF level in black versus white CR patients and the clinical significance [69].

The exercise training as implemented in the CR model has been efficacious for other chronic diseases. For instance, Dolan et al. presented outcomes of 152 subjects with female breast cancer survivors [20]. They performed one time weekly supervised CR sessions for 22 weeks, and their CRF level improved by 14% (21 ± 6 to 24 ± 7 $mL \cdot kg^{-1} \cdot min^{-1}$, $p < 0.001$). And with the recently approved Medicare coverage in the United States for supervised exercise training for those with peripheral artery disease, many of these patients will be performing their training in a CR setting (although this is not required). A meta-analysis by Parmenter et al. assessed 41 randomized controlled trials of those with symptomatic peripheral artery disease who performed exercise training [54]. In addition to the traditionally reported improvement in pain free and total walking distances as a result of exercise training, there is also a significant improvement in CRF as measured by peak VO_2. However, no studies have assessed improvement in CRF in these patient populations and clinical outcomes.

Finally, a recent training style that has received attention in the traditional CR setting is high-intensity interval training (HIIT). In a systematic review and meta-analysis of 17 studies (953 total participants), Hannan et al. reported significant improvements in CRF as measured by oxygen consumption using HIIT (±0.34 $mL \cdot kg^{-1} \cdot min^{-1}$) versus moderate-intensity continuous training. Improvements were optimized in programs longer than 6-week duration, and the high-intensity training was as safe as the moderate-intensity training. Despite these findings, there have been no studies investigating the effects of high-intensity interval versus moderate-intensity continuous training on morbidity and mortality in any CR population. Collectively, the evidence presented supports a strong argument for future research in the aforementioned areas.

References

1. Ades PA, Keteyian SJ, Wright JS, et al. Increasing cardiac rehabilitation participation from 20% to 70%: a road map from the million hearts cardiac rehabilitation collaborative. Mayo Clin Proc. 2017;92:234–42.
2. Ades PA, Savage PD, Brawner CA, et al. Aerobic capacity in patients entering cardiac rehabilitation. Circulation. 2006;113(23):2706–12.
3. Alexander JH, Smith PK. Coronary-artery bypass grafting. N Engl J Med. 2016;374(20):1954–64.
4. Almodhy MY, Sandercock GR, Richards L. Changes in cardiorespiratory fitness in patients receiving supervised outpatient cardiac rehabilitation either once or twice a week. Int J Cardiol. 2012;160(3):215–6.
5. Anderson L, Nguyen TT, Dall CH, Burgess L, Bridges C, Taylor RS. Exercise-based cardiac rehabilitation in heart transplant recipients. Cochrane Database Syst Rev. 2017;4:CD012264.
6. Anderson L, Oldridge N, Thompson DR, et al. Exercise-based cardiac rehabilitation for coronary heart disease: cochrane systematic review and meta-analysis. J Am Coll Cardiol. 2016;67(1):1–12.
7. Anderson L, Taylor RS. Cardiac rehabilitation for people with heart disease: an overview of Cochrane systematic reviews. Cochrane Database Syst Rev. 2014;(12):CD011273.

8. Armstrong MJ, Martin BJ, Arena R, et al. Patients with diabetes in cardiac rehabilitation: attendance and exercise capacity. Med Sci Sports Exerc. 2014;46(5):845–50.
9. Balady GJ, Jette D, Scheer J, Downing J. Changes in exercise capacity following cardiac rehabilitation in patients stratified according to age and gender. Results of the Massachusetts Association of Cardiovascular and Pulmonary Rehabilitation Multicenter Database. J Cardpulm Rehabil. 1996;16(1):38–46.
10. Banzer JAMT, Kennedy CM, O'Malley CJ, Balady GJ. Results of cardiac rehabilitation in patients with diabetes mellitus. Am J Cardiol. 2004;93:81–4.
11. Beckie TM, Beckstead JW, Kip K, Fletcher G. Physiological and exercise capacity improvements in women completing cardiac rehabilitation. J Cardiopulm Rehabil Prev. 2013;33(1):16–25.
12. Benjamin EJ, Blaha MJ, Chiuve SE, et al. Heart disease and stroke statistics-2017 update: a report from the American Heart Association. Circulation. 2017;135(10):e146–603.
13. Blair SN, Kampert JB, Kohl HW 3rd, et al. Influences of cardiorespiratory fitness and other precursors on cardiovascular disease and all-cause mortality in men and women. JAMA. 1996;276(3):205–10.
14. Blair SN, Kohl HW 3rd, Paffenbarger RS Jr, Clark DG, Cooper KH, Gibbons LW. Physical fitness and all-cause mortality. A prospective study of healthy men and women. JAMA. 1989;262(17):2395–401.
15. Brawner CA, Abdul-Nour K, Lewis B, et al. Relationship between exercise workload during cardiac rehabilitation and outcomes in patients with coronary heart disease. Am J Cardiol. 2016;117(8):1236–41.
16. Brawner CA, Churilla JR, Keteyian SJ. Prevalence of physical activity is lower among individuals with chronic disease. Med Sci Sports Exerc. 2016;48(6):1062–7.
17. Bui AL, Horwich TB, Fonarow GC. Epidemiology and risk profile of heart failure. Nat Rev Cardiol. 2011;8(1):30–41.
18. Carter R, Al-Rawas OA, Stevenson A, McDonagh T, Stevenson RD. Exercise responses following heart transplantation: 5 year follow-up. Scott Med J. 2006;51(3):6–14.
19. Currie KD, Dubberley JB, McKelvie RS, MacDonald MJ. Low-volume, high-intensity interval training in patients with CAD. Med Sci Sports Exerc. 2013;45(8):1436–42.
20. Dolan LB, Barry D, Petrella T, et al. The cardiac rehabilitation model improves fitness, quality of life, and depression in breast cancer survivors. J Cardiopulm Rehabil Prev. 2018;38:246–52.
21. Dor-Haim HLC, Horowitz M, Swissa M. Intensive exercise training improves cardiac electrical stability in myocardial-infarcted rats. J Am Heart Assoc. 2017;6:e005989.
22. Ehrman J, Keteyian S, Fedel F, Rhoads K, Levine TB, Shepard R. Cardiovascular responses of heart transplant recipients to graded exercise testing. J Appl Physiol (1985). 1992;73(1):260–4.
23. Ford ES, Caspersen CJ. Sedentary behaviour and cardiovascular disease: a review of prospective studies. Int J Epidemiol. 2012;41(5):1338–53.
24. Go AS, Mozaffarian D, Roger VL, et al. Heart disease and stroke statistics--2013 update: a report from the American Heart Association. Circulation. 2013;127(1):e6–e245.
25. Green DJ, O'Driscoll G, Joyner MJ, Cable NT. Exercise and cardiovascular risk reduction: time to update the rationale for exercise? *J Appl Physiol (1985)*. 2008;105(2):766–8.
26. Grover FL, Vemulapalli S, Carroll JD, et al. 2016 Annual report of the Society of Thoracic Surgeons/American College of Cardiology Transcatheter Valve Therapy Registry. J Am Coll Cardiol. 2017;69(10):1215–30.
27. Guazzi M, Labate V, Cahalin LP, Arena R. Cardiopulmonary exercise testing reflects similar pathophysiology and disease severity in heart failure patients with reduced and preserved ejection fraction. Eur J Prev Cardiol. 2013;21(7):847–54.
28. Hagnas MJ, Lakka TA, Kurl S, et al. Cardiorespiratory fitness and exercise-induced ST segment depression in assessing the risk of sudden cardiac death in men. Heart. 2017;103(5):383–9.
29. Hambrecht R, Niebauer J, Marburger C, et al. Various intensities of leisure time physical activity in patients with coronary artery disease: effects on cardiorespiratory fitness and progression of coronary atherosclerotic lesions. J Am Coll Cardiol. 1993;22(2):468–77.
30. Hambrecht R, Walther C, Mobius-Winkler S, Gielen S, Linke A, Conradi K, Erbs S, Luge R, Kendziorra K, Sabri O, Sick P, Schuler G. Percutaneous coronary angioplasty compared with exercise training in patients with stable coronary artery disease: a randomized trial. Circulation. 2004;109:1371–8.
31. Jolliffe JA, Rees K, Taylor RS, Thompson D, Oldridge N, Ebrahim S. Exercise-based rehabilitation for coronary heart disease. Cochrane Database Syst Rev. 2001;(1):CD001800.
32. Kavanagh T, Mertens DJ, Hamm LF, et al. Prediction of long-term prognosis in 12 169 men referred for cardiac rehabilitation. Circulation. 2002;106(6):666–71.
33. Kavanagh T, Mertens DJ, Hamm LF, et al. Peak oxygen intake and cardiac mortality in women referred for cardiac rehabilitation. J Am Coll Cardiol. 2003;42(12):2139–43.
34. Kerrigan DJ, Williams CT, Ehrman JK, et al. Cardiac rehabilitation improves functional capacity and patient-reported health status in patients with continuous-flow left ventricular assist devices: the Rehab-VAD randomized controlled trial. *JACC Heart Fail*. 2014;2(6):653–9.
35. Keteyian SJ, Kerrigan DJ, Ehrman JK, Brawner CA. Exercise training workloads upon exit from cardiac rehabilitation in men and women: THE HENRY FORD HOSPITAL EXPERIENCE. J Cardiopulm Rehabil Prev. 2017;37(4):257–61.
36. Keteyian SJ, Patel M, Kraus WE, et al. Variables measured during cardiopulmonary exercise testing as pre-

dictors of mortality in chronic systolic heart failure. J Am Coll Cardiol. 2016;67(7):780–9.
37. Lawler PR, Filion KB, Eisenberg MJ. Efficacy of exercise-based cardiac rehabilitation post-myocardial infarction: a systematic review and meta-analysis of randomized controlled trials. Am Heart J. 2011;162(4):571–84. e2
38. Li J, Loerbroks A, Angerer P. Physical activity and risk of cardiovascular disease: what does the new epidemiological evidence show? Curr Opin Cardiol. 2013;28(5):575–83.
39. Martin BJ, Arena R, Haykowsky M, et al. Cardiovascular fitness and mortality after contemporary cardiac rehabilitation. Mayo Clin Proc. 2013;88(5):455–63.
40. Mehanna E, Hamik A, Josephson RA. Cardiorespiratory fitness and atherosclerosis: recent data and future directions. Curr Atheroscler Rep. 2016;18(5):26.
41. Mehra MR, Canter CE, Hannan MM, et al. The 2016 International Society for Heart Lung Transplantation listing criteria for heart transplantation: a 10-year update. J Heart Lung Transplant. 2016;35(1):1–23.
42. Munt BI, Legget ME, Healy NL, Fujioka M, Schwaegler R, Otto CM. Effects of aortic valve replacement on exercise duration and functional status in adults with valvular aortic stenosis. Can J Cardiol. 1997;13(4):346–50.
43. Myers J, Zaheer N, Quaglietti S, Madhavan R, Froelicher V, Heidenreich P. Association of functional and health status measures in heart failure. J Card Fail. 2006;12(6):439–45.
44. Nahumi N, Morrison KA, Garan AR, Uriel N, Jorde UP. Peak exercise capacity is a poor indicator of functional capacity for patients supported by a continuous-flow left ventricular assist device. J Heart Lung Transplant. 2014;33(2):213–5.
45. Nichols S, Gleadall-Siddall DO, Antony R, et al. Estimated peak functional capacity: an accurate method for assessing change in peak oxygen consumption after cardiac rehabilitation? Clin Physiol Funct Imaging. 2018;38:681–8.
46. O'Connor CM, Whellan DJ, Lee KL, et al. Efficacy and safety of exercise training in patients with chronic heart failure: HF-ACTION randomized controlled trial. JAMA. 2009;301(14):1439–50.
47. O'Connor CM, Whellan DJ, Wojdyla D, et al. Factors related to morbidity and mortality in patients with chronic heart failure with systolic dysfunction: the HF-ACTION predictive risk score model. Circ Heart Fail. 2012;5(1):63–71.
48. O'Connor GT, Buring JE, Yusuf S, et al. An overview of randomized trials of rehabilitation with exercise after myocardial infarction. Circulation. 1989;80(2):234–44.
49. Oldridge N. Cardiac rehabilitation after myocardial InfarctionCombined experience of randomized clinical trials. JAMA. 1988;260(7):945–50.
50. Oldridge NB, Guyatt GH, Fischer ME, Rimm AA. Cardiac rehabilitation after myocardial infarction. Combined experience of randomized clinical trials. JAMA. 1988;260(7):945–50.
51. Ornish D, Brown SE, Scherwitz LW, et al. Can lifestyle changes reverse coronary heart disease? The lifestyle heart trial. *Lancet*. 1990;336(8708):129–33.
52. Pack QR, Lahr BD, Squires RW, et al. Survey reported participation in cardiac rehabilitation and survival after mitral or aortic valve surgery. Am J Cardiol. 2016;117(12):1985–91.
53. Pack QR, Squires RW, Lopez-Jimenez F, et al. The current and potential capacity for cardiac rehabilitation utilization in the United States. J Cardiopulm Rehabil Prev. 2014;34(5):318–26.
54. Parmenter BJ, Dieberg G, Smart NA. Exercise training for management of peripheral arterial disease: a systematic review and meta-analysis. *Sports Med*. 2015;45(2):231–44.
55. Pathak RK, Elliott A, Middeldorp ME, et al. Impact of CARDIOrespiratory FITness on arrhythmia recurrence in obese individuals with atrial fibrillation: the CARDIO-FIT study. J Am Coll Cardiol. 2015;66(9):985–96.
56. Qureshi WT, Alirhayim Z, Blaha MJ, et al. Cardiorespiratory fitness and risk of incident atrial fibrillation: results from the Henry Ford exercise testing (FIT) project. Circulation. 2015;131(21):1827–34.
57. Riebe DEJ, Liguori G, Magal M. ACSM's guidelines for exercise testing and prescription. 10th ed. Philadelphia: Wolters Kluwer; 2018, 472 p.
58. Russo N, Compostella L, Tarantini G, et al. Cardiac rehabilitation after transcatheter versus surgical prosthetic valve implantation for aortic stenosis in the elderly. Eur J Prev Cardiol. 2014;21(11):1341–8.
59. Rutledge T, Redwine LS, Linke SE, Mills PJ. A meta-analysis of mental health treatments and cardiac rehabilitation for improving clinical outcomes and depression among patients with coronary heart disease. Psychosom Med. 2013;75(4):335–49.
60. Salyer J, Jewell DV, Quigg RJ. Predictors of early post-cardiac transplant exercise capacity. J Cardpulm Rehabil. 1999;19(6):381–8.
61. Sandercock G, Hurtado V, Cardoso F. Changes in cardiorespiratory fitness in cardiac rehabilitation patients: a meta-analysis. Int J Cardiol. 2013;167(3):894–902.
62. Santiago de Araujo Pio C, Marzolini S, Pakosh M, Grace SL. Effect of cardiac rehabilitation dose on mortality and morbidity: a systematic review and meta-regression analysis. Mayo Clin Proc. 2017;92(11):1644–59.
63. Schairer JR, Keteyian SJ, Ehrman JK, Brawner CA, Berkebile ND. Leisure time physical activity of patients in maintenance cardiac rehabilitation. J Cardpulm Rehabil. 2003;23(4):260–5.
64. Schmid JP, Gaillet R, Noveanu M, Mohacsi P, Saner H, Hullin R. Influence of the exercise protocol on peak VO2 in patients after heart transplantation. J Heart Lung Transplant. 2005;24(11):1751–6.
65. Suaya JA, Shepard DS, Normand SL, Ades PA, Prottas J, Stason WB. Use of cardiac rehabilitation by Medicare beneficiaries after myocardial

infarction or coronary bypass surgery. Circulation. 2007;116(15):1653–62.
66. Suaya JA, Stason WB, Ades PA, Normand SL, Shepard DS. Cardiac rehabilitation and survival in older coronary patients. J Am Coll Cardiol. 2009;54(1):25–33.
67. Sumner J, Harrison A, Doherty P. The effectiveness of modern cardiac rehabilitation: a systematic review of recent observational studies in non-attenders versus attenders. PLoS One. 2017;12(5):e0177658.
68. Swift DL, Lavie CJ, Johannsen NM, et al. Physical activity, cardiorespiratory fitness, and exercise training in primary and secondary coronary prevention. Circ J. 2013;77(2):281–92.
69. Swift DL, Staiano AE, Johannsen NM, et al. Low cardiorespiratory fitness in African Americans: a health disparity risk factor? *Sports Med.* 2013;43(12):1301–13.
70. Taylor RS, Brown A, Ebrahim S, et al. Exercise-based rehabilitation for patients with coronary heart disease: systematic review and meta-analysis of randomized controlled trials. Am J Med. 2004;116(10):682–92.
71. Thomas RJ, King M, Lui K, Oldridge N, Pina IL, Spertus J, AACVPR/ACCF/AHA. Update: performance measures on cardiac rehabilitation for referral to cardiac rehabilitation/secondary prevention services endorsed by the American College of Chest Physicians, the American College of Sports Medicine, the American Physical Therapy Association, the Canadian Association of Cardiac Rehabilitation, the Clinical Exercise Physiology Association, the European Association for Cardiovascular Prevention and Rehabilitation, the Inter-American Heart Foundation, the National Association of Clinical Nurse Specialists, the Preventive Cardiovascular Nurses Association, and the Society of Thoracic Surgeons. J Am Coll Cardiol. 2010;56(14):1159–67.
72. Voller H, Salzwedel A, Nitardy A, Buhlert H, Treszl A, Wegscheider K. Effect of cardiac rehabilitation on functional and emotional status in patients after transcatheter aortic-valve implantation. Eur J Prev Cardiol. 2015;22(5):568–74.
73. Faselis C, Kokkinos P, Tsimploulis A, Pittaras A, Myers J, Lavie CJ, Kyritsi F, Lovic D, Karasik P, Moore H. Exercise capacity and atrial fibrillation risk in veterans. A Cohort Study Mayo Clin Proc. 2016;91(5):558–66.

24 Physical Activity and Cardiometabolic Health Benefits in Children

Konstantinos D. Tambalis and Labros S. Sidossis

Introduction

Physical activity is any activity that gets children and adolescents moving, resulting in adequate increases in heart rate and breathing rate. This wide definition includes all contexts of physical activity, i.e., leisure-time physical activity (including sports activities and dancing), school-related physical activity, occupational physical activity, physical activity at or near the home, and physical activity connected with transport. Physical activity and exercise are at times used interchangeably. However, it is important to make the distinction that exercise is a form of physical activity that is planned, structured, repetitive, and performed with the aim of improving health or fitness.

Physical activity, health, and quality of life are strongly interrelated. According to Hippocrates (ancient Greek doctor and philosopher), the human body was designed to move, and therefore regular physical activity is needed in order to function optimally and prevent illness and disease. It is now well-documented that physical inactivity is a major risk factor for developing health conditions and chronic diseases, including coronary heart disease, type 2 diabetes mellitus (T2DM), and obesity [1]. The incidence of these diseases is directly linked to lifestyle changes, specifically physical activity behaviors, eating habits, and smoking, present not only in adults but also in young children [2, 3]. These behaviors, including a sedentary lifestyle, start in childhood and are perpetuated by the attitudes and habits of the social environment (family members, friends, teachers) and media. In spite of the fact that children and adolescents don't usually develop chronic diseases, such as heart disease, hypertension, T2DM, or osteoporosis, data suggest that physically inactive children are more likely to possess risk factors for these diseases such as relatively lower levels of high-density lipoprotein cholesterol (HDL-C), higher blood pressure, increased serum insulin levels, and excess fat than physically active children [1, 4, 5]. Given that pathogenicity has its roots in childhood, and the likelihood that physical activity will attenuate the incidence of the aforementioned risk factors, the need for interventions during childhood is of great importance. Therefore, efforts to promote and foster a healthy lifestyle that includes increased physical activity and proper nutrition during childhood are essential in the prevention of chronic illness in adulthood.

K. D. Tambalis (✉)
Department of Nutrition and Dietetics, Harokopio University, Athens, Kalithea, Greece

L. S. Sidossis
Department of Kinesiology and Health, Rutgers University, New Brunswick, NJ, USA

P. Kokkinos, P. Narayan (eds.), *Cardiorespiratory Fitness in Cardiometabolic Diseases*,
https://doi.org/10.1007/978-3-030-04816-7_24

Physical Activity Level in Children and Adolescents

In the United States, only 25% of children and adolescents (6–15 years old) meet the 2008 Physical Activity Guidelines for Americans recommendation of at least 60 min of moderate-to-vigorous physical activity (MVPA) per day [6, 7]. Most recent data, from the combined 2012 NHANES and NHANES National Youth Fitness Survey, confirmed that 24.8% of adolescents 12–15 years of age reported 60 min of MVPA daily [8]. Meeting the recommendations differs by age, gender, and ethnicity, with males, younger children, and nonwhite ethnicities being more physically active than their female, older, and white ethnicity counterparts [9]. Moreover, on average, 20% of children in the Organisation for Economic Co-operation and Development countries participate in MVPA daily [10]. It has been speculated that at the onset of the twenty-first century, children expend for physical activity almost 600 kcal/day fewer than their counterparts 50 years ago [5]. Possible reasons for this include:

1. More sedentary recreational pursuits such as Internet/computer games and television viewing, which have replaced outdoor play time
2. Decreased opportunities for active recreational pursuits
3. Fewer physical education time in schools
4. Decreased active transportation to school (e.g., walking, cycling)
5. Towns and cities unfamiliar to physical activity opportunities without safe active transport
6. Overprotective parents with disproportionate worry about children's outdoor play
7. A family (e.g., inactive parents) and social environment (school, society) that does not support physical activity

The main limitations and benefits reported by children and adolescents associated with physical activity are presented in Table 24.1.

Table 24.1 Benefits and limitations reported by children and adolescents in relation to physical activity

Limitations	Benefits
Preference for in-house activities (TV, video, computer, books, music, etc.)	Social benefits (fun/enjoyment, socializing with friends, enjoying teamwork)
Low levels of energy (feeling tired, lack of energy, eating fast food)	Improvement of psychological characteristics (self-confidence, pride, discipline development, reduction of guilt)
Limited time (reading, extracurricular)	Improving body sensation (energy, fatigue reduction, feeling of increased physical strength, endurance, fitness, improved sleep)
Social factors (influence from a social pressure group, e.g., friends, lack of parental support, criticism from others)	Improving athletic performance (skill development, reflex improvement, flexibility, coordination, agility, endurance, strength)
Mobilization (nonrecurring benefits from exercise)	Cognitive benefits (improved concentration and brain function, good memory)
	Response strategies (stress relief, relaxation, diminished frustration and anger)

Adapted from O'Dea [11]

Physical Activity and Health Benefits in Children and Adolescents

The health benefits of physical activity for children and adolescents have been observed in several health domains and can be generally placed into three categories: (1) mental, social, and physical health benefits, (2) health benefits of childhood physical activity that carry over to adulthood, and (3) physical activity behaviors "tracked" from childhood to adulthood (Fig. 24.1).

Children and adolescents with low physical activity levels have a higher prevalence of psychological and emotional distress. Physical inactivity also contributes to increased incidence of

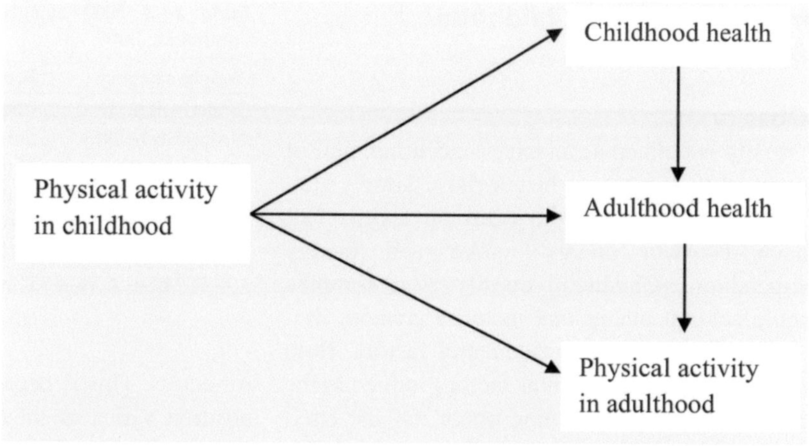

Fig. 24.1 Interrelationships of children and adolescent physical activity and health. (Adapted from Blair et al. [12])

obesity, insulin resistance, disordered lipid profile, and elevated blood pressure in children. This cardiometabolic profile is likely contributing to the increasing prevalence of T2DM in children and adolescents, a disease that until recently was found in overweight and obese adults [13]. The population impact of this development for the next generation is of great concern.

In contrast, increasing physical activity provides an important medium for children and adolescent to improve self-esteem, social well-being, and a healthy self-perception of body image and competence. Children that engage in adequate physical activity and maintain aerobic fitness are more likely to have better cognitive function and a wide range of health benefits [14]. These include maintenance of energy balance and consequently a healthy weight and healthy growth, healthy development of the cardiorespiratory and musculoskeletal system, avoidance of cardiovascular disease risk factors (e.g., hypertension, dyslipidemia, T2DM), and the opportunity for social interaction, academic achievement, and psychological well-being [14, 15]. The above health benefits are similar in children of all weight classes (normal, overweight, and obese) and are independent of gender, age, and health status (Table 24.2) [12].

Table 24.2 Important health benefits of physical activity in children and adolescents

1. Health benefits in childhood/adolescence
Maintains energy balance and prevents overweight/obesity
Reduces risk factors for:
Cardiovascular disease (e.g., obesity)
Type 2 diabetes
Hypertension
Dyslipidemia
Promotes management of type 1 diabetes
Promotes healthy growth and development of the musculoskeletal system
Develops a healthy cardiorespiratory system
Develops neuromuscular awareness
Improves mental health and psychological well-being through:
Decreasing anxiety, stress, and depression
Promoting self-esteem
Improving cognitive function and academic performance
Improving sleep
Improving social interaction
2. Health benefits of childhood physical activity that carry over to adulthood
Decreased probability of overweight/obesity during adulthood
Decreased probability of morbidity from cardiovascular disease during adulthood
Increased bone mass/strength reduces likelihood of osteoporosis in adulthood
3. Physical activity "track" from childhood to adulthood
Increased probability of becoming a physically active adult

Health Benefits in Childhood/Adolescence

Obesity

Obesity is defined as an excess accumulation of body fat that increases health risks. Simply stating it, obesity results from a chronic positive balance between energy intake and energy expenditure. Childhood obesity is a complex multifactorial matter that includes genetic, lifestyle, cultural, and environmental factors. Both genetic and environmental factors influence the predisposition to becoming obese. Of the environmental factors, lifestyle preferences and cultural environment are the most significant contributors to childhood obesity. They are also modifiable. Both physical activity and caloric intake must be considered to modulate body composition. Changes in the nutritional habits of children undoubtedly contributed to increasing global levels of childhood overweight/obesity. However, decreased physical activity is believed to be one of the main contributors and a critical factor in determining whether children can maintain a healthy body mass or lose excess body fat [16]. The International Obesity Taskforce (IOTF) stated that the most significant social habits contributing to the current childhood obesity epidemic are (a) the reduction in active transportation to school, (b) decreased opportunities for recreational physical activity, and (c) increased sedentary recreation and screen time [17]. Consequently, lack of sufficient physical activity level is of great concern to the rising problem of obesity in youth, globally [18].

Several methods are available to assess body fat, including magnetic resonance imaging or dual-energy X-ray absorptiometry, hydrostatic weighing, and measurement of subcutaneous fat. However, these methods are cost-prohibitive for they require expensive apparatus and trained personnel. Thus, body mass index (BMI; weight [kg]/height [m^2]) has been adopted as a surrogate for estimating body composition in large cohorts and for epidemiologic studies.

A child's weight status is determined using an age- and sex-specific percentile for BMI (Table 24.3) rather than the BMI categories used for adults. This is because children's body composition varies as they age and varies between boys and girls. Therefore, BMI levels among children and teens need to be expressed relative to other children of the same age and sex. BMI at or above the 85th percentile is considered overweight and at or above the 95th percentile is considered obese for children and teens of the same age and sex.

Table 24.3 BMI categories terminology by Expert Committee, 2007

Weight category	Percentile range
Underweight	<5th percentile
Normal or healthy weight	5th percentile to less than the 85th percentile
Overweight	85th to less than the 95th percentile
Obese	95th percentile or greater

Adapted from Barlow SE and the Expert Committee [19]

The prevalence of obesity in children and adolescents has reached a global epidemic. In 2012, 16.9% of 2- to 19-year-old children and adolescents in the United States were obese [20]. Similar statistics have been reported for the European Union. According to estimates from the WHO's Childhood Obesity Surveillance Initiative (COSI), 1 in 3 children in the European Union aged 6–9 years old were overweight or obese in 2010. This represents a considerable increase compared to 2008, when 1 in 4 children were overweight or obese [World Health Organization. European Childhood Obesity Surveillance Initiative, COSI, round 2008]. More than 300,000 children are becoming obese every year [21]. The rise in the prevalence of overweight and obesity in children and young people has a highly negative impact on health and quality of life and may overwhelm the healthcare systems in the near future.

Epidemiological Studies

The association between physical inactivity and overweight or obesity in school-aged children and adolescents has been extensively studied. In a review of 31 observational studies, where overweight and obesity were classified using age- and gender-specific BMI criteria, the authors reported the least physically active group was 1.33 times as likely to be obese than the most physically active group [22]. Moreover, studies that assessed MVPA alone were more strongly and consistently related to obesity compared to the studies that included low-intensity physical activities, suggesting a dose-response relationship [23]. In studies that physical activity was assessed objectively via accelerometers, the result indicated a stronger and significant relationship between physical activity and overweight/obesity. The association was stronger in males than in females [23].

Interventional Studies

A review of 24 intervention studies (17 randomized control trials, RCTs), ranging from 4 weeks to 2 years, reported significant decreases in BMI, total fat, and/or abdominal fat in response to engaging in 17–30 min of aerobic physical activity per day [22]. Similarly, a decrease in total body and visceral adiposity was reported in overweight children and adolescents (both genders) engaging in systematic physical activity interventions of moderate intensity, 30–60 min in duration, 3–7 days per week. Furthermore, a consistent and negative association between walking and adiposity was reported in studies that used pedometers to quantify physical activity [24]. Finally, a meta-analysis of 34 intervention trials (median exercise 3 times/week, 50 min/session over a 12-week period) reported significant reductions in BMI for aerobic activities and combined aerobic and strength, but not strength alone activities [25].

Mechanisms of Exercise-Induced Changes

The exercise-related mechanisms involved in body fat reduction are not well understood. A simplistic view is that increased physical activity results in a concomitant increase in energy expenditure. If caloric intake does not compensate for the exercise-related energy expenditure, a chronic and sustained energy deficit is achieved, ultimately resulting in body fat losses [22]. Exercise is one of the most significant contributors to the physiological stimuli for lipolysis. Several factors related to obesity, such as gender, body fat mass, size, and distribution of adipose cells, contribute to the response to exercise training. Moreover, several cardiometabolic adaptive responses occur with exercise training, ultimately favoring greater utilization of FFA by the working muscles at an absolute workload, instead of carbohydrates [26].

Clinical, Public Health Significance and Conclusions

The public health significance of physical activity on childhood obesity is that physical activity could reverse some of the negative consequences of obesity (physiological and psychosocial). For instance, it is of great concern that obese children and adolescents become targets of discrimination and tend to develop a negative self-image, while participation in sports improves their self-esteem. Specifically, physical activity could positively influence numerous health complications of childhood obesity such as disturbances in blood lipids, glucose intolerance, hypertension, sleep problems, and orthopedic complications [27].

In conclusion, childhood obesity presents a major public health concern. Proper dietary habits and increased levels of physical activity should be the foremost focus of strategies aimed at preventing and treating overweight/obesity in children and adolescents.

Type 2 Diabetes Mellitus: Prevalence and Incidence

Diabetes is a chronic metabolic disease characterized by total or partial insulin deficiency resulting in hyperglycemia [28, 29]. About three decades ago, type 2 diabetes mellitus was a rare occurrence in children and adolescents. However, in the mid-1990s, an increasing incidence of type 2 diabetes mellitus was observed particularly in the United States but also worldwide [1, 2].

Childhood T2DM is a disease that affects children who (a) are typically overweight or obese (BMI ≥85th–94th and >95th percentile for age and gender, respectively), (b) have a strong family history of T2DM, (c) have substantial residual insulin secretory capacity at diagnosis, (d) have insidious onset of disease, (e) demonstrate insulin resistance, and (f) lack evidence for diabetic autoimmunity [30]. According to the American

Diabetes Association, diabetes is defined as (1) HbA1c ≥6.5%, (2) fasting plasma glucose ≥126 mg/dL, (3) 2-h plasma glucose ≥200 mg/dL during an oral glucose tolerance test, or (4) a random plasma glucose ≥200 mg/dL with symptoms of hyperglycemia. Individuals with T2DM have an increased risk of developing complications in microcirculation such as retinopathy, nephropathy, as well as major vascular diseases of the nervous system.

Epidemiological evidence suggests that the emergence and increasing prevalence of T2DM in children and adolescents are linked to the increased prevalence of obesity in these age groups. The admission rate for obesity in hospitals in the United Kingdom for individuals 18 years and younger increased by 63.5% from 1996 to 2004, and the admission rate for T2DM rose to 44.4% during the same time period [31]. Currently, in the United States, almost one in three new cases of T2DM diagnosed in youth are among children and adolescents, 10–18 years old [30].

This increasing trend is occurring internationally, and it is estimated that by the year 2030, an expected 366 million people worldwide will have T2DM [32, 33].

Epidemiological Studies

Physical activity and cardiorespiratory fitness (CRF) in youth are directly associated with insulin sensitivity independent of adiposity [34]. Moreover, the results of a meta-analysis of studies in children and adolescents have shown that exercise training is a moderate predictor of T2DM incidence. Specifically, fasting insulin and HOMA-IR improved by 11.4 U/mL [95% CI, 5.2–17.5] and 2.0 [95% CI, 0.4–3.6], respectively, providing support to the belief that exercise is efficient in reducing fasting insulin and enhancing insulin sensitivity in children and adolescents [35].

Interventional Studies

Although physical activity plays an essential role in weight management, there is a scarcity of available data regarding physical activity and weight management for the prevention and treatment of T2DM in children and adolescents. It has been shown that physical activity is inversely related to insulin resistance and positively associated with insulin sensitivity in children [36, 37]. In a review of eight interventional studies (four aerobic training and four resistance training), exercise ranging from 6 to 40 weeks, 10–30 min/day, and 3–5 days/week resulted in favorable changes on fasting insulin and insulin resistance among overweight/obese children. Interestingly, all of the aerobic exercise studies reported significant improvements in at least one of the insulin variables examined. However, only one of the four resistance exercise studies reported favorable findings in insulin sensitivity (increased 45.1+/−7.3% in the training group vs. −0.9+/−12.9% in controls, $p < 0.01$) [23].

Mechanisms of Exercise-Induced Changes

The favorable effect of exercise/physical activity on T2DM has been documented by a plethora of studies. However, the mechanisms involved in the exercise-induced modulation of glucose metabolism are not well understood and are briefly presented here. It is well-accepted that exercise improves insulin sensitivity and increases glucose uptake by the contracting muscle. Potential mechanisms involving aerobic exercises include (a) higher postreceptor insulin signaling, (b) increased glucose transporter (GLUT4) mRNA, (c) improved activity of glycogen synthesis, (d) decreased release and increased clearance of free fatty acids, and (e) improved transport of glucose to the exercising muscles owing to an increased blood flow and muscle capillary network. Resistance exercise training also increased insulin-mediated glucose uptake, GLUT4 protein content, and insulin signaling in skeletal muscles [38].

Clinical, Public Health Significance and Conclusions

Sustained lifestyle changes such as diet and physical activity have a favorable impact in the prevention of T2DM in children and adolescents. There is also evidence that physical activity could prevent or delay many of the complications of T2DM, particularly for the control of weight gain, blood glucose, blood pressure, and blood lipids [27, 34, 38].

Thus, increased physical activity should be strongly recommended to children and adolescents as a component of a healthy lifestyle designed at preventing and managing T2DM.

Type 1 Diabetes Mellitus (T1DM)

Type 1 diabetes mellitus, also known as "insulin-dependent diabetes mellitus," is considered to have an autoimmune etiology. T1DM occurs as a consequence of the organ-specific immune damage of the insulin-producing β-cells in the islets of Langerhans within the pancreas. The β-cells regulate blood glucose levels by sensing glucose and releasing insulin to maintain physiologic glucose levels. Once these cells are destroyed, as is the case in patients with T1DM, glucose regulation is compromised. This leads to acute conditions related to blood glucose levels (e.g., ketoacidosis and severe hypoglycemia) and secondary complications (such as heart disease, blindness, and kidney failure). This form of diabetes usually strikes children and young adults, although disease onset can occur at any age. Risk factors for T1DM may be genetic, autoimmune, or environmental [39].

Type 1 diabetes mellitus is the most frequent type of diabetes in children and adolescents with a prevalence of about 5% of people with diabetes (an estimated 23.1 million people) in the United States. According to the US Diabetes Surveillance System, the estimated annual number of newly diagnosed cases in the United States during 2011–2012 included 17,900 children and adolescents younger than age 20 years with T1DM [40].

Epidemiological Studies

Epidemiological findings in children and adolescents with T1DM concluded that 90% had poor glycemic control and 80% had low physical activity levels. Also, fasting blood glucose was significantly correlated with physical activity levels and sedentary time. Differences in HbA1c, fasting blood glucose, duration of disease, and insulin dose were observed among the three groups of physical activity levels (insufficient, moderate, and active) [41]. Studies examining the relationship between physical activity and glycemic control in subjects with T1DM revealed that physical exercise had a positive influence on long-term glycemic control in these patients. Nevertheless results were contradictory with respect to insulin sensitivity and fasting glucose [42].

Interventional Studies

Meta-analysis of 26 physical activity/exercise interventions studies in children and adolescents with T1DM reported at least one favorable health outcome at follow-up. Specifically, results showed potential benefits of physical activity/exercise on HbA1c (standardized mean difference −0.52, 95% CI −0.97 to −0.07; corresponds to a reduction of 8.5 mmol/mol), BMI (standardized mean difference −0.41, 95% CI −0.70 to −0.12), and triglycerides (mean difference −0.70, 95% CI −1.25 to −0.14; corresponds to a reduction of almost 22 mg/dl). The largest reduction was observed for total cholesterol (standardized mean difference −0.91, 95% CI −1.66 to −0.17; corresponds to a reduction of almost 22 mg/dl). Moreover, the authors reported that physical activity interventions improved cardiovascular fitness and increase physical activity levels [43].

Mechanisms of Exercise-Induced Changes

In patients with T1DM, physical activities, both aerobic and anaerobic (resistance exercises), improve glucose uptake by the working muscle. In addition, both aerobic and anaerobic activities have a favorable effect on skeletal muscle endothelial cell function, inflammation, and insulin sensitivity. In children, total cholesterol in the blood appears to be a risk factor for the development of atherosclerosis, a precursor of cardiovascular diseases, which is the leading cause of mortality in patients with T1DM. On the other hand, physical activity improves lipid composition in blood [38, 44].

Clinical, Public Health Significance and Conclusions

Children with T1DM have twice the risk of developing cardiovascular disease in comparison with those without the disease. In children with diabetes, cardiovascular disease risk factors (i.e., endothelial dysfunction) can develop as early as preadolescence [44]. The findings support significant beneficial effects of physical activity in BMI, HbA1c, triglycerides, and total cholesterol in children and adolescents and on the development of complications later in life [43, 45].

In conclusion, physical activity is essential for the management of T1DM in children and adolescents and has the potential to protect against or delay the development of cardiovascular disease.

Dyslipidemia

Lipids are fats that are either synthesized by the liver or absorbed from ingested meals. Although all lipids are physiologically important, abnormal triglyceride (TG) and low-density lipoprotein cholesterol (LDL-C) metabolism may contribute to the development of metabolic diseases. A number of environmental, genetic, and pathological factors can alter cholesterol and triglyceride metabolism. Some of these factors are gender, age, fat distribution, diet, inheritance, and physical activity [46]. Combined dyslipidemia is considered the predominant dyslipidemic pattern in childhood, characterized by elevated triglycerides and non-high-density lipoprotein cholesterol, small increase in LDL-C, and reduced high-density lipoprotein cholesterol (HDL-C). Normal values for lipids for children and adolescents are defined according to population levels [47].

According to the National Health and Nutrition Examination Survey in the United States, in 2011–2012 dyslipidemia was present in approximately 20.2% of children and adolescents. Between 1999–2000 and 2011–2012, the prevalence of TC, HDL-C, and non-HDL-C concentrations decreased from 10.6% to 7.8% ($p = 0.006$), 17.9% to 12.8% ($p = 0.003$), and 13.6% to 8.4% ($p < 0.001$), respectively [48].

Epidemiological Studies

A systematic review of epidemiologic studies suggested that relationships between physical activity and TC, HDL-C, LDL-C, and TG levels are generally weak in observational studies. Increased physical activity was associated favorably with HDL-C and TG levels, but did not consistently affect TC or LDL-C, in nonobese and obese children and adolescents [23]. A study on a representative sample of 12- to 19-year-old US adolescents indicated that unfit girls were 1.89 and boys were 3.68 times more likely to have high TC compared to moderately and highly fit boys and girls [49].

Interventional Studies

A review of 38 RCTs reported that lifestyle interventions (including physical activity) on blood lipids in overweight or/and obese children resulted in significant reductions in TC (−3.5 mg/dL), LDL-C (−11.6 mg/dL), and TG (−13.3 mg/dL), but a nonsignificant improvement in HDL-C (+3.9 mg/dL) [50]. In another review, aerobic physical activity had a significant and favorable effect on LDL-C (−0.49 mg/dL) and TG (−0.55 mg/dL) [51]. Moreover, a review study of RCTs to children and adolescents with high cholesterol levels or obesity concluded that aerobic activities had a beneficial effect on HDL-C and TG levels, but not on total cholesterol or LDL-C levels [23]. Finally, a meta-analysis of intervention studies concluded that 70% of studies had a beneficial effect on blood lipids. Compared with control, intervention with physical activity alone or with diet improved lipid measures in children, with a mean reduction of −6.06 mg/dL in LDL-C, an increase of 1.87 mg/dL in HDL-C, and nonsignificant reductions in TC and TG [52].

Mechanisms of Exercise-Induced Changes

Exercise-induced favorable effects on lipid metabolism are attributed to the increased capacity of skeletal muscles to utilize free fatty acids for its energy demands that increase during aerobic exercise. This is achieved by activation of several enzymes in the muscle needed for lipid turnover. Aerobic exercise improves TG and HDL-C through its effect on lipoprotein lipase expression and activity, resulting in more TG hydrolysis [53]. In addition to the traditional mechanisms previously described, it was proposed that upregulation of Liver X receptor, a transcription factor that has a significant function in liver cholesterol metabolism, increased ATP-binding cassette transporter expression in macrophages, leading to enhanced reverse cholesterol transport to the liver through HDL-C. In addition, it is proposed that exercise may affect LDL-C by modulating PCSK9, a biomarker of LDL clearance. Thus, less PCSK9 potentially could result in more LDL-C absorbed and excreted by the liver [53].

Clinical, Public Health Significance and Conclusions

Dyslipidemia is a significant modifiable risk factor for cardiovascular diseases. Serum lipid concentrations in childhood and adolescence (e.g., TC and LDL-C) are linked to serum lipid concentrations in adulthood. There is an agreement that physical activity attenuates the development of cardiovascular diseases by modulating several risk factors including dyslipidemia.

In conclusion, the findings of the aforementioned studies support that increased aerobic activity in children has a favorable effect on the lipid profile of children and adolescents. The amount of activity required for favorable changes and the existence of a dose-response relationship between physical activity/exercise and blood lipids have not been well defined [47].

High Blood Pressure

Hypertension in children and adolescents is a crucial health problem in the developed world. Primary hypertension is becoming the most common form seen in childhood and mainly attributed to vascular, renal, or endocrine causes. The obesity epidemic is strongly associated with increasing prevalence rates of elevated blood pressure. The assessment of high blood pressure in children and adolescents is more involved than in adults and is aimed both at identifying secondary causes and identifying other comorbidities of cardiovascular risk. Appropriate emphasis should be given in the treatment of high blood pressure in childhood and adolescence to reduce cardiovascular risk [54, 55].

The prevalence of elevated blood pressure (diastolic blood pressure ≥90th percentile or systolic blood pressure/diastolic blood pressure ≥120/80 mmHg) increased considerably from 1988–1994 to 1998–2008 (NHANES; boys, 15.8–19.2%; girls, 8.2–12.6%) [55].

Epidemiological Studies

Observational studies in children and adolescents suggest an inverse association between PA (measured with accelerometers) and blood pressure [4, 23, 56]. Specifically, in adjusting for several potential confounders, the results suggested moderate but significant reductions in systolic blood pressure (ranging from 2.0 to 4.6 mmHg) and diastolic blood pressure (ranging from 1.6 to 2.0 mmHg). However, studies used self-reported questionnaire responses did not provide consistent results [56]. Review study proposed a dose-response association (stronger in overweight children) between aerobic fitness and blood pressure, but no association between self-reported sports participation and blood pressure [57].

Interventional Studies

There is a consensus that physical activity or structured exercise does not decrease blood pressure in normotensive youth [24, 58]. However, experimental studies in children and adolescents with high blood pressure or obesity reported significant decreases in systolic blood pressure, between 5.8 and 8.2 mmHg, in response to three exercise sessions per week, each lasting >60 min [24, 59–61]. In addition, a further decrease in diastolic blood pressure by almost 2.0 mmHg was achieved when the frequency of exercise was greater than three times per week. Furthermore, 8 months of aerobic physical activity in hypertensive and normotensive overweight children resulted in a decrease in systolic and diastolic blood pressures in the exercising subgroups of 6.5 and 4.1 mmHg, respectively, in the normotensive, and 4.9 and 3.8 mmHg, respectively, in the hypertensive group [24, 59, 60]. Resistance exercise has also been reported to have moderate but significant antihypertensive effects (−4.0 mmHg) on systolic blood pressure of obese children [23, 62]. Collectively, these findings suggest that a physical activity intervention lasting at least 30 min, three times per week, could reduce blood pressure in youth with mild essential hypertension.

Mechanisms of Exercise-Induced Changes

The mechanisms for the exercise-induced changes in blood pressure in children are multifactorial and independent of weight loss. Physical activity of adequate intensity duration and volume is likely to act on several factors that contribute to chronic increases in blood pressure. Such factors include improved insulin sensitivity and beneficial adaptation of the cardiovascular system (reduction in sympathetic tone, reduction in arterial stiffness, and reduction in endothelial dysfunction). In addition to the independent effects of exercise-induced BP reduction, body weight changes, as a result of exercise, can act synergistically to lower BP even further. Significant BP reductions have been reported with any weight loss at least in adults [60].

Clinical, Public Health Significance and Conclusions

The prevention and treatment of primary hypertension in children and adolescents is based on an interventional strategy on modifiable risk factors. These include body weight, salt intake, sedentary behavior, and bad sleep quality. Physical activity may exert a potentially favorable effect on overweight, sodium balance, and quality of sleep and therefore indirectly affect the metabolic mechanisms involved in the development and maintenance of blood pressure. These factors include deposition and distribution of the fat mass, insulin resistance, activation of the sympathetic nervous system, the renin-angiotensin system, sodium homeostasis, and regulation of vascular function [60].

In conclusion, the data suggests that physical activity with duration of at least 30 min, three times a week, and intensity sufficient to improve aerobic fitness can be effective in reducing blood pressure in children with hypertension.

Musculoskeletal System

Bone and muscle are two intricately related tissue types; however, factors such as sex, maturation, and physical activity/exercise can modify this relationship. Physical activity helps children promote muscle mass and bone mass, which can extent to adulthood and reduce weight-related wear to joints [63]. The forces associated with muscular contractions during weight-bearing physical activities such as strength/resistance training have a favorable influence on skeletal tissue [23]. An adequate level of physical activity during growth was associated with greater bone mass and bone development [64, 65]. Prospective studies indicated significant influence of physical activity on skeletal health (e.g., muscular strength and endurance) [23]. In children, strength training can increase muscle strength, power, and endurance and is now recommended as safe and appropriate for enhancing physical health and function [66, 67]. Studies suggest that 10 min of moderate-to-high-intensity weight-bearing physical activity performed 2–3 days/week can increase bone mineral density in both genders [22, 23].

Skeletal muscles have long been recognized as a main source of anabolic mechanical stimuli for bone tissue. According to the "mechanostat" theory, survival of the skeleton (as all other tissues, such as fibrous tissue, hyaline cartilage, fibrocartilage, cementum, or dentin) requires the functional coordination of modeling and remodeling. Modeling is an adaptive response to bone overloads, by enhancing additions of new bone and by changing bone architecture. Conversely, remodeling is an adaptive response to bone underloads, by removing bone next to marrow and conserving normally used bone. Habitual loads to bone are derived essentially from gravity. Above and beyond biomechanical function, the endocrine properties of bone and muscle may take effect to sense and transduce biomechanical signals such as loading, exercise, or systemic hormonal stimuli into biochemical signals [68, 69]. Adaptations of resistance exercise training are due to muscle fiber hypertrophy and neural adaptations.

Clinical, Public Health Significance and Conclusions

Muscle contractions during heavy exercise deliver up to ten times the gravity force, resulting in modeling beyond that provided by the gravitational force. Thus, habitual physical activity that generates relatively high-intensity loading forces may decrease osteoporosis-related fracture risk by improving muscle strength, flexibility, coordination, and balance, by enhancing bone mineral accrual during development, by enhancing bone strength, and by decreasing the risk of falls [70, 71]. Finally, it is reasonable to propose that habitual exercises or a physically active lifestyle that begins in childhood may result in lasting structural changes that may contribute to increased bone and muscle strength.

Mental Health (Anxiety, Stress, and Depression)

Mental disorders are a serious public health issue. It is estimated that up to 15% of US schoolchildren have a diagnosable mental health disorder [72, 73]. Observational studies have recognized the relationship between physical activity and mental health but are unable to clarify the direction of that association [22, 23]. Experimental studies observed significant improvements in at least one symptom of depression in response to 8- to 12-week aerobic exercise programs [22]. Cross-sectional studies suggest weak-to-moderate-positive influences of physical activity on anxiety and depression symptoms [23]. Finally, physical activity has been shown to improve mood and sleep and to prevent the onset of depression and anxiety [72, 74, 75].

Mechanisms of Exercise-Induced Changes

Both physiological and psychological mechanisms modify the association of physical activity with mental health [76]. One potential mechanism may be that physical activity elevates the synaptic transmission of monoamines and stimulates the release of endorphins, which have an inhibitory effect on the central nervous system, creating a sense of calm and improved mood [38, 73].

Clinical, Public Health Significance and Conclusions

Physical activity is associated with improved life satisfaction, physical health, and cognitive functioning, while physical inactivity seems to be related with the development of psychological disorders [77, 78]. Thus, physical activity can improve mental health by lessening and preventing conditions such as anxiety, stress, and depression, as well as improving mood and other aspects of well-being.

Health Benefits of Childhood Physical Activity that Carry Over to Adulthood

Physical activity in childhood can influence adult health status [79]. Childhood obesity tracks into adulthood, and it is of concern that obese children have twice the risk of being obese as adults compared to nonobese children [80, 81]. Low CRF or the decrease of CRF during childhood is connected to increased cardiovascular disease risk at this period of life [82]. It is proposed that maintaining adequate levels of CRF and physical activity during childhood reduces the risk of cardiovascular disease in adulthood [83]. Weight-bearing activities during growth result in the attainment of greater bone mass and are protective against osteoporosis in old age [84]. Studies of predictors of adult obesity proposed that there was suggestive evidence for a protective role of physical activity in childhood on adult fatness [85–88]. Risk factors for T2DM maintained from childhood to adulthood predict T2DM in young adulthood [89, 90]. Many studies have suggested that T2DM can be eliminated through balanced diet and adequate physical activity and by reducing sedentary behaviors [91]. On the other hand, several studies proposed that there is only a weak relationship between physical activity in childhood and cardiovascular disease risk factors in adulthood [91–93].

Detecting relationships between childhood physical activity and adult health is quite difficult. Decreasing sedentary behaviors and increasing physical activity levels may be an efficient strategy for the management of obesity in children and the prevention of health consequences in adulthood. Physical activity should be encouraged among children as one factor of lifestyle aimed at preventing T2DM, cardiovascular disease risk factors, and bone health [13, 88, 91, 93, 94].

In conclusion, there is accumulated scientific evidence suggesting that childhood physical activity influences health in adulthood.

Physical Activity "Track" from Childhood to Adulthood

Several public health interventions focused on children and adolescents are based on the principle that healthy behaviors established in childhood and adolescence will persist later in life [79]. There is a growing body of scientific evidence suggesting that physical activity habits established during childhood and adolescence tend to track into later life [95–97]. Children who emerge from their first years of life feeling confident about their physical skills and have had encouraging experiences of physical activity have a better chance of being physically active through adulthood. Negative attitudes toward physical activity during childhood may persist into adulthood and affect people's willingness to participate in physical activities [98]. The association between childhood physical activity and adult health is to be expected, as numerous health outcomes linked with physical activity (e.g., BMI) track from childhood into adulthood [79, 93, 99].

A study that examined the tracking of physical activity between adolescence and adulthood in a cohort followed at 3-year intervals (for 9–12 years to 21, 24, 27, and 30 years) reported moderate correlations, with the highest correlation for 3-year intervals declining as the intervals increased [96]. Several reviews examining tracking of physical activity suggested that tracking through childhood appears relatively good; however, there was only a weak relationship between childhood and adolescent physical activity and health and adult physical activity and health [78, 100, 101]. Another systematic review of adolescent physical activity and health reported a consistent effect of physical activity during adolescence on adult physical activity; however, the extent of this association was also moderate [92]. Finally, several studies reported stronger associations between physical activity in childhood and physical activity in adulthood when the quality of the physical activity in childhood, rather than the quantity, was taken into consideration [95, 98, 102].

The above findings support the importance of the type and quality of physical activity as factors determining the probability of tracking into adulthood.

In conclusion, it is strongly suggested that promotion of increased physical activity, especially in the school setting, is likely to result in children engaging in physical activity in adulthood [13, 79, 93, 99, 103].

Physical Activity Recommendations for Children and Adolescents

The referred guidelines have been adopted by governmental public health bodies in several countries including the United States (Centers for Disease Control and Prevention, American Center of Sports Medicine), the United Kingdom (Department of Health), and Australia (Department of Health and Ageing) [104–106]. The current recommendations are:

> Children and adolescents should accumulate at least 60 min of moderate-to-vigorous intensity physical activity, daily.

> Activities to improve bone health and muscle strength should be included at least 3 days per week.

> In children's physical activity, most of the 60 or more minutes per day should be either moderate- or vigorous-intensity aerobic physical activity.

> To achieve additional health benefits, children should engage in more activity – up to several hours per day.

> Children's daily physical activity does not have to be done all in one go. The 60 min can be accumulated with shorter bouts throughout the day.

Types of Activity

The guidelines for children and adolescents spotlight on three types of physical activity: aerobic, muscle-strengthening, and bone-strengthening. Each type has significant and partly different health benefits. Specifically:

- Aerobic physical activities are those in which children rhythmically move their large muscles and increase CRF. Walking, running, jogging, bicycling, skipping, jumping rope, swimming, and dancing are all examples of aerobic activities. Most of games and sports are considered aerobic.
- Muscle-strengthening physical activities are those that force muscles to work intensely (overload) than usual and strengthen the muscles. Muscle-strengthening activities can be structured such as lifting weights (own weight or partner's weight) or working with resistance bands and unstructured, such as climbing trees, playing on playground equipment, etc.
- Bone-strengthening physical activities generate a force on the bones that enhances bone strength and growth. Physical activities, such as running, jumping rope, basketball, tennis, etc., constitute examples of bone-strengthening activities. Bone-strengthening activities could be aerobic and/or muscle-strengthening activities, also.

Intensity

Though all physical activity offers health benefits in children and adolescents, the current guidelines recommend moderate-to-vigorous intensity physical activities.

- Moderate-intensity physical activities are defined as those activities requiring some effort, although children can carry a conversation easily while performing such activities. Such activities include fast walking, bicycle riding, volleyball, active play, etc.
- Vigorous-intensity physical activities require more effort, increasing the breathing rate of children and the feeling of fatigue. Such activities include running, chasing and playing tag, organized sports (e.g., soccer, basketball), jumping rope, etc.

Duration and Frequency

Children and adolescents should engage in at least 60 min of MVPA every day. This daily time of 60 min can be accumulated with shorter bouts (e.g., bouts of 15 min) throughout the day.

Table 24.4 presents examples of the types of physical activity recommended in the guidelines according to the type and level of intensity (aerobic), in children and adolescents.

It is important that children are encouraged to participate in physical activities that are appropriate for their age, enjoyable, and offer variety. It is also important to keep in mind that progressive increases in physical activity, beyond the minimum guidelines proposed, are likely to result in greater health benefits and therefore are highly recommended for most children and adolescents. Children can meet the 60-min per day target through the accumulation of bouts of activity of varying durations and types during the entire day. This can include short intermittent bouts of physical activity or longer bouts of play during breaks at school, walking to and from school, and programmed activities such as physical education, sports, or games. Activities should include aerobic in nature to improve CRF and resistance exercise, for improvements in muscular strength and bone health.

For bone health, it is crucial that children engage in bouts of bone-strengthening activities that impose a relatively high demand on the bones and joints (e.g., running, jumping, skipping, ball games, and gymnastics). To develop and maintain muscular fitness and flexibility,

Table 24.4 Types of physical activities by level of intensity in children and adolescents

Type of physical activity	Children	Adolescents
Aerobic moderate-intensity	Active recreation (e.g., hiking, skateboarding)Brisk walking Bicycle riding Games (e.g., volleyball)	Brisk walkingBicycle riding Active recreation (e.g., rollerblading, hiking, skateboarding) Housework and yard work Games involving catching and throwing (e.g., baseball, softball)
Aerobic vigorous-intensity	Games involving running and chasing (e.g., tag) Jumping rope Bicycle riding Martial arts (e.g., judo, karate) Running Sports such as soccer, basketball, tennis, swimming	Games involving running and chasing (e.g., flag, football) Jumping rope Bicycle riding Martial arts (e.g., judo, karate) Running Sports such as soccer, basketball, tennis, swimming Vigorous dancing
Muscle-strengthening	Resistance exercise with children's own weight (e.g., climbing) Resistance exercise with the weight of a partner Sit-ups (curl-ups or crunches) Swinging on playground equipment/bars Resistance exercise with activities such as throwing a ball, rowing, carrying things, etc.	Games like tug-of-war Push-ups, pull-ups, sit-ups (curl-ups or crunches) Resistance exercises with exercise bands, weight machines, handheld weights Climbing wall Sit-ups (curl-ups or crunches)
Bone-strengthening	Running Jumping rope Skipping, jumping, hopping Games such as hopscotch Sports like basketball, volleyball, tennis Gymnastics	Hopping, skipping, jumping Jumping rope Running Sports like basketball, volleyball, tennis Gymnastics

children should participate in active play involving carrying and climbing or in sports, as a wide range of different modes and intensities of physical activity can provide optimum health benefits across all body systems. Adolescents are likely to meet the recommended physical activity levels through a different range of activities, such as walking to and from school, organized sports and games, exercise classes in school, and recreational activities. With the aim of making lifetime physical activity attractive to children and adolescents, it is important that educational programs offer an extensive range of activities designed to foster an enjoyable experience, make them feel confident about their bodies, and appreciate the benefits of physical activity for health.

Table 24.5 proposes five "levels" of physical activity, the physical activity pattern needed to achieve that level, and the health benefits that each level may incur. For each physical activity pattern, the resultant "level" is a combined measure of type, frequency, intensity, and time spent in the various activities.

Overall Summary and Conclusions

The current available scientific data supports that physical activity confers significant health benefits for children and adolescents. The most documented health benefits include healthy growth and development of the musculoskeletal and cardiorespiratory systems; decreased body fatness; favorable cardiovascular and metabolic disease risk profiles (T2DM, blood pressure, and lipid); reduced symptoms of anxiety, depression, and stress and increased opportunity for social interaction; and academic achievement.

Table 24.5 Levels of physical activity and health benefits

Level	Descriptor	Physical activity pattern	Health benefits
1	Inactive	No active transportation to school Does very little physical education or active play at school Spends a lot of time on sedentary activities (e.g., watching TV, Internet, playing video games) No active recreation	None
2	Slightly active	Participate in one or more of: Some active transportation to school by foot or bike Some physical education or active play at school (<1 h/day) Some home activities (e.g., sweeping, cleaning) or garden activities Some active recreation at light intensity (<1 h/day)	Some protection against chronic diseases
3	Moderately active	Participate in one or more of: Regular active transportation school by foot or bike Active in physical education classes or school playtime (>1 h/day) Regular household or garden physical activities Regular active recreation or sports at moderate intensity	Adequate/high level of protection against chronic diseases
4	Very active	Participate in most of: Regular active transportation to school by foot or bike Very active in physical education classes or school playtime (>1 h/day) Regular household or garden physical activities Regular active recreation or sports at vigorous intensity	Maximal protection against chronic diseases
5	Highly active	Exercise intensely and for extended periods during the day or very vigorous sports training	Maximal protection against chronic diseases but increased risk of injury

Source: Adapted from [105]

Moreover, it seems that adequate physical activity level in childhood is likely to carry favorable behavioral and biological effects into later life, while physical activity behaviors track from childhood to adulthood, although at relatively low levels. The amounts and types of physical activity required incurring health benefits vary, and the limited available scientific data does not allow for definitive conclusions relating the optimal doses of physical activity needed to confer specific health benefits. Nonetheless, current recommendations propose that significant health benefits can be expected for most children and adolescents who participate in 60 or more minutes of moderate-to-vigorous physical activity every day. Participation in muscle-strengthening physical activity is expected to improve muscular strength and enhance bone health. Vigorous aerobic physical activity ≥3days per week for 60 min or more per day is likely to promote CRF, and cardiovascular health, by modulating established cardiometabolic risk factors. It is of great public health importance that children are encouraged to participate in physical activity that lead to long-lasting health benefits and promote a lifelong physically active lifestyle.

References

1. Booth FW, Roberts CK, Laye MJ. Lack of exercise is a major cause of chronic diseases. Compr Physiol. 2012;2(2):1143–211. Review.
2. Tremblay MS, LeBlanc AG, Kho ME, Saunders TJ, Larouche R, Colley RC, et al. Systematic review of

sedentary behaviour and health indicators in school-aged children and youth. Int J Behav Nutr Phys Act. 2011;8:98. Review.
3. Seppala T, Hankonen N, Korkiakangas E, Ruusuvuori J, Laitinen J. National policies for the promotion of physical activity and healthy nutrition in the workplace context: a behaviour change wheel guided content analysis of policy papers in Finland. BMC Public Health. 2017;18(1):87.
4. Andersen LB, Harro M, Sardinha LB, Froberg K, Ekelund U, Brage S, Anderssen SA. Physical activity and clustered cardiovascular risk in children: a cross-sectional study (The European Youth Heart Study). Lancet. 2006;368:299–304.
5. Boreham C, Riddoch C. The physical activity, fitness and health of children. J Sports Sci. 2001;19(12):915–29.
6. Song M, Carroll DD, Fulton JE. Meeting the 2008 physical activity guidelines for Americans among U.S. youth. Am J Prev Med. 2013;44(3):216–22.
7. Troiano RP, Berrigan D, Dodd KW, Masse LC, Tilert T, McDowell M. Physical activity in the United States measured by accelerometer. Med Sci Sports Exerc. 2008;40(1):181–8.
8. Fakhouri TH, Hughes JP, Burt VL, Song M, Fulton JE, Ogden CL. Physical activity in U.S. youth aged 12-15 years, 2012. NCHS Data Brief. 2014;141:1–8.
9. Belcher BR, Berrigan D, Dodd KW, Emken BA, Chou CP, Spruijt-Metz D. Physical activity in US youth: effect of race/ethnicity, age, gender, and weight status. Med Sci Sports Exerc. 2010;42(12):2211–21.
10. System YRBS. Centers for Disease Control and Prevention, National Center for HIV/AIDS, Viral Hepatitis, STD, and TB Prevention (CDC/NCHHSTP) 2014.
11. O'Dea JA. Why do kids eat healthful food? Perceived benefits of and barriers to healthful eating and physical activity among children and adolescents. J Am Diet Assoc. 2003;103(4):497–501.
12. Blair SN, Clark DG, Cureton KJ, Powell KE. Exercise and fitness in childhood: implications for a lifetime of health. In: Perspectives in Exercise Science and Sports Medicine, vol. 2: Youth, Exercise, and Sport. Indianapolis: Benchmark Press; 1989. p. 401–30.
13. Rush E, Simmons D. Physical activity in children: prevention of obesity and type 2 diabetes. Med Sport Sci. 2014;60:113–21.
14. Loprinzi PD, Cardinal BJ, Loprinzi KL, Lee H. Benefits and environmental determinants of physical activity in children and adolescents. Obes Facts. 2012;5(4):597–610.
15. Khan NA, Hillman CH. The relation of childhood physical activity and aerobic fitness to brain function and cognition: a review. Pediatr Exerc Sci. 2014;26(2):138–46.
16. Brown CL, Halvorson EE, Cohen GM, Lazorick S, Skelton JA. Addressing childhood obesity: opportunities for prevention. Pediatr Clin North Am. 2015;62(5):1241–61.
17. Lobstein T, Baur L, Uauy R, TaskForce IIO. Obesity in children and young people: a crisis in public health. Obes Rev. 2004;5(Suppl 1):4–104.
18. Janssen I, Katzmarzyk PT, Boyce WF, Vereecken C, Mulvihill C, Roberts C, et al. Comparison of overweight and obesity prevalence in school-aged youth from 34 countries and their relationships with physical activity and dietary patterns. Obes Rev. 2005;6(2):123–32.
19. Barlow SE, the Expert Committee. Expert committee recommendations regarding the prevention, assessment, and treatment of child and adolescent overweight and obesity: summary report. Pediatrics. 2007;120(Supplement):S164–92.
20. Ogden CL, Carroll MD, Kit BK, Flegal KM. Prevalence of childhood and adult obesity in the United States, 2011–2012. JAMA. 2014;311(8):806–14.
21. Kosti RI, Panagiotakos DB. The epidemic of obesity in children and adolescents in the world. Cent Eur J Public Health. 2006;14(4):151–9.
22. Janssen I, Leblanc AG. Systematic review of the health benefits of physical activity and fitness in school-aged children and youth. Int J Behav Nutr Phys Act. 2010;7:40.
23. Strong WB, Malina RM, Blimkie CJ, Daniels SR, Dishman RK, Gutin B, et al. Evidence based physical activity for school-age youth. J Pediatr. 2005;146(6):732–7.
24. Miguel-Berges ML, Reilly JJ, Moreno Aznar LA, Jimenez-Pavon D. Associations between pedometer-determined physical activity and adiposity in children and adolescents: systematic review. Clin J Sport Med. 2018;28(1):64–75.
25. Kelley GA, Kelley KS, Pate RR. Exercise and BMI z-score in overweight and obese children and adolescents: a systematic review and network meta-analysis of randomized trials. J Evid Based Med. 2017;10(2):108–28.
26. Poirier P, Després JP. Exercise in weight management of obesity. Cardiol Clin. 2001;19(3):459–70. Review.
27. Maffeis C. Physical activity in the prevention and treatment of childhood obesity: physio-pathologic evidence and promising experiences. Int J Pediatr Obes. 2008;3(2):29–32.
28. Arslanian S. Type 2 diabetes in children: clinical aspects and risk factors. Horm Res. 2002;57(Suppl 1):19–28.
29. Rodriguez BL, Fujimoto WY, Mayer-Davis EJ, Imperatore G, Williams DE, Bell RA, et al. Prevalence of cardiovascular disease risk factors in U.S. children and adolescents with diabetes: the SEARCH for diabetes in youth study. Diabetes Care. 2006;29:1891–6.
30. Copeland KC, Silverstein J, Moore KR, Prazar GE, Raymer T, Shiffman RN, et al. Management of newly diagnosed type 2 Diabetes Mellitus (T2DM) in children and adolescents. Pediatrics. 2013;131(2):364–82.
31. Aylin P, Williams S, Bottle A. Obesity and type 2 diabetes in children, 1996-7 to 2003-4. BMJ. 2005;331(7526):1167.

32. Narayan KM, Williams R. Diabetes–a global problem needing global solutions. Prim Care Diabetes. 2009;3(1):3–4.
33. Wild S, Roglic G, Green A, Sicree R, King H. Global prevalence of diabetes: estimates for the year 2000 and projections for 2030. Diabetes Care. 2004;27(5):1047–53.
34. Berman LJ, Weigensberg MJ, Spruijt-Metz D. Physical activity is related to insulin sensitivity in children and adolescents, independent of adiposity: a review of the literature. Diabetes Metab Res Rev. 2012;28(5):395–408.
35. Fedewa MV, Gist NH, Evans EM, Dishman RK. Exercise and insulin resistance in youth: a meta-analysis. Pediatrics. 2014;133(1):e163–74.
36. Imperatore G, Cheng YJ, Williams DE, Fulton J, Gregg EW. Physical activity, cardiovascular fitness, and insulin sensitivity among U.S. adolescents: the National Health and Nutrition Examination Survey, 1999–2002. Diabetes Care. 2006;29(7):1567–72.
37. Kasa-Vubu JZ, Lee CC, Rosenthal A, Singer K, Halter JB. Cardiovascular fitness and exercise as determinants of insulin resistance in postpubertal adolescent females. J Clin Endocrinol Metab. 2005;90(2):849–54.
38. Pedersen BK, Saltin B. Exercise as medicine – evidence for prescribing exercise as therapy in 26 different chronic diseases. Scand J Med Sci Sports. 2015;25(Suppl 3):1–72.
39. Bluestone JA, Herold K, Eisenbarth G. Genetics, pathogenesis and clinical interventions in type 1 diabetes. Nature. 2010;464:1293–300.
40. National Diabetes Statistics Report. 2017. Estimates of Diabetes and Its Burden in the United States. https://www.cdc.gov/diabetes/pdfs/data/statistics/national-diabetes-statistics-report.pdf. Assessed 27 Nov 2017.
41. Miculis CP, De Campos W, da Silva Boguszweski MC. Correlation between glycemic control and physical activity level in adolescents and children with type 1 diabetes. J Phys Act Health. 2015;12(2):232–7.
42. Lopes Souto D, Paes de Miranda M. Physical exercises on glycemic control in type 1 diabetes mellitus. Nutr Hosp. 2011;26(3):425–9.
43. Quirk H, Blake H, Tennyson R, Randell TL, Glazebrook C. Physical activity interventions in children and young people with Type 1 diabetes mellitus: a systematic review with meta-analysis. Diabet Med. 2014;31(10):1163–73.
44. Babar GS, Zidan H, Widlansky ME, Das E, Hoffmann RG, Daoud M, et al. Impaired endothelial function in preadolescent children with type 1 diabetes. Diabetes Care. 2011;34(3):681–5.
45. Kriska AM, LaPorte RE, Patrick SL, Kuller LH, Orchard TJ. The association of physical activity and diabetic complications in individuals with insulin-dependent diabetes mellitus: the Epidemiology of Diabetes Complications Study--VII. J Clin Epidemiol. 1991;44(11):1207–14.
46. Kraus WE, Houmard JA, Duscha BD, Knetzger KJ, Wharton MB, McCartney JS, et al. Effects of the amount and intensity of exercise on plasma lipoproteins. N Engl J Med. 2002;347(19):1483–92.
47. Kavey RE. Combined dyslipidemia in childhood. J Clin Lipidol. 2015;9(5):S41–56.
48. Kit BK, Kuklina E, Carroll MD, Ostchega Y, Freedman DS, Ogden CL. Prevalence of and trends in dyslipidemia and blood pressure among US children and adolescents, 1999-2012. JAMA Pediatr. 2015;169(3):272–9.
49. Carnethon MR, Gulati M, Greenland P. Prevalence and cardiovascular disease correlates of low cardiorespiratory fitness in adolescents and adults. JAMA. 2005;294(23):2981–8.
50. Ho M, Garnett SP, Baur L, Burrows T, Stewart L, Neve M, et al. Effectiveness of lifestyle interventions in child obesity: systematic review with meta-analysis. Pediatrics. 2012;130(6):e1647–71.
51. Escalante Y, Saavedra JM, Garcia-Hermoso A, Dominguez AM. Improvement of the lipid profile with exercise in obese children: a systematic review. Prev Med. 2012;54(5):293–301.
52. Cai L, Wu Y, Cheskin LJ, Wilson RF, Wang Y. Effect of childhood obesity prevention programmes on blood lipids: a systematic review and meta-analysis. Obes Rev. 2014;15(12):933–44.
53. Wang Y, Xu D. Effects of aerobic exercise on lipids and lipoproteins. Lipids Health Dis. 2017;16(1):132.
54. Samuels J, Bell C, Samuel J, Swinford R. Management of hypertension in children and adolescents. Curr Cardiol Rep. 2015;17(12):107.
55. Rosner B, Cook NR, Daniels S, Falkner B. Childhood blood pressure trends and risk factors for high blood pressure: The NHANES experience 1988-2008. Hypertension. 2013;62(2):247–54.
56. Leary SD, Ness AR, Smith GD, Mattocks C, Deere K, Blair SN, Riddoch C. Physical activity and blood pressure in childhood: findings from a population-based study. Hypertension. 2008;51(1):92–8.
57. Andersen LB, Riddoch C, Kriemler S, Hills AP, Hills A. Physical activity and cardiovascular risk factors in children. Br J Sports Med. 2001;45(11):871–6.
58. Kelley GA, Kelley KS, Tran ZV. The effects of exercise on resting blood pressure in children and adolescents: a meta-analysis of randomized controlled trials. Prev Cardiol. 2003;6(1):8–16.
59. Hansen HS, Froberg K, Hyldebrandt N, Nielsen JR. A controlled study of eight months of physical training and reduction of blood pressure in children: the Odense schoolchild study. BMJ. 1991;303(6804):682–5.
60. Strambi M, Giussani M, Ambruzzi MA, Brambilla P, Corrado C, Giordano U, et al. Novelty in hypertension in children and adolescents: focus on hypertension during the first year of life, use and interpretation of ambulatory blood pressure monitoring, role of physical activity in prevention and treatment, simple carbohydrates and uric acid as risk factors. Ital J Pediatr. 2016;42(1):69.

61. García-Hermoso A, Saavedra JM, Escalante Y. Effects of exercise on resting blood pressure in obese children: a meta-analysis of randomized controlled trials. Obes Rev. 2013;14(11):919–28.
62. Naylor LH, Watts K, Sharpe JA, Jones TW, Davis EA, Thompson A, et al. Resistance training and diastolic myocardial tissue velocities in obese children. Med Sci Sports Exerc. 2008;40:2027–32.
63. Weaver CM, Gordon CM, Janz KF, Kalkwarf HJ, Lappe JM, Lewis R, et al. The National Osteoporosis Foundation's position statement on peak bone mass development and lifestyle factors: a systematic review and implementation recommendations. Osteoporos Int. 2016;27(4):1281–386.
64. Bielemann RM, Martinez-Mesa J, Gigante DP. Physical activity during life course and bone mass: a systematic review of methods and findings from cohort studies with young adults. BMC Musculoskelet Disord. 2013;14:77. Review.
65. Ondrak KS, Morgan DW. Physical activity, calcium intake and bone health in children and adolescents. Sports Med. 2007;37(7):587–600.
66. Behringer M, Vom Heede A, Yue Z, Mester J. Effects of resistance training in children and adolescents: a meta-analysis. Pediatrics. 2010;126(5):e1199–210.
67. Bernhardt DT, Gomez J, Johnson MD, Martin TJ, Rowland TW, Small E, et al. Strength training by children and adolescents. Pediatrics. 2001;107(6):1470–2.
68. Cianferotti L, Brandi ML. Muscle-bone interactions: basic and clinical aspects. Endocrine. 2014;45(2):165–77.
69. Tyrovola JB. The "Mechanostat" Principle and the Osteoprotegerin-OPG/RANKL/RANK System PART II. The Role of the Hypothalamic-Pituitary Axis. J Cell Biochem. 2017;118(5):962–6.
70. Kohrt WM, Bloomfield SA, Little KD, Nelson ME, Yingling VR, American College of Sports M. American College of Sports Medicine Position Stand: physical activity and bone health. Med Sci Sports Exerc. 2004;36(11):1985–96.
71. Turner CH, Robling AG. Designing exercise regimens to increase bone strength. Exerc Sport Sci Rev. 2003;31(1):45–50.
72. Biddle SJ, Asare M. Physical activity and mental health in children and adolescents: a review of reviews. Br J Sports Med. 2011;45(11):886–95.
73. Ahn S, Fedewa AL. A meta-analysis of the relationship between children's physical activity and mental health. J Pediatr Psychol. 2011;36(4):385–97.
74. Penedo FJ, Dahn JR. Exercise and well-being: a review of mental and physical health benefits associated with physical activity. Curr Opin Psychiatry. 2005;18(2):189–93.
75. Dishman RK, Hales DP, Pfeiffer KA, Felton GA, Saunders R, Ward DS, et al. Physical self-concept and self-esteem mediate cross-sectional relations of physical activity and sport participation with depression symptoms among adolescent girls. Health Psychol. 2006;25(3):396–407.
76. Peluso MA, Guerra de Andrade LH. Physical activity and mental health: the association between exercise and mood. Clinics (Sao Paulo). 2005;60(1):61–70.
77. Carek PJ, Laibstain SE, Carek SM. Exercise for the treatment of depression and anxiety. Int J Psychiatry Med. 2011;41(1):15–28.
78. Donnelly JE, Hillman CH, Castelli D, Etnier JL, Lee S, Tomporowski P, et al. physical activity, fitness, cognitive function, and academic achievement in children: a systematic review. Med Sci Sports Exerc. 2016;48(6):1223–4.
79. Malina RM. Physical activity and fitness: pathways from childhood to adulthood. Am J Hum Biol. 2001;13(2):162–72.
80. Serdula MK, Ivery D, Coates RJ, Freedman DS, Williamson DF, Byers T. Do obese children become obese adults? A review of the literature. Prev Med. 1993;22(2):167–77.
81. Ruiz JR, Castro-Piñero J, Artero EG, Ortega FB, Sjöström M, Suni J, et al. Predictive validity of health-related fitness in youth: a systematic review. Br J Sports Med. 2009;43(12):909–23.
82. Castro-Piñero J, Perez-Bey A, Segura-Jiménez V, Aparicio VA, Gómez-Martínez S, Izquierdo-Gomez R, et al. Cardiorespiratory fitness cutoff points for early detection of present and future cardiovascular risk in children: a 2-year follow-up study. Mayo Clin Proc. 2017;92(12):1753–62.
83. Boreham C, Twisk J, Neville C, Savage M, Murray L, Gallagher A. Associations between physical fitness and activity patterns during adolescence and cardiovascular risk factors in young adulthood: the Northern Ireland Young Hearts Project. Int J Sports Med. 2002;23(Suppl 1):S22–6.
84. Bass SL. The prepubertal years: a uniquely opportune stage of growth when the skeleton is most responsive to exercise? Sports Med. 2000;30(2):73–8.
85. Kimm SY, Glynn NW, Obarzanek E, Kriska AM, Daniels SR, Barton BA, et al. Relation between the changes in physical activity and body-mass index during adolescence: a multicentre longitudinal study. Lancet. 2005;366(9482):301–7.
86. Yang X, Telama R, Viikari J, Raitakari OT. Risk of obesity in relation to physical activity tracking from youth to adulthood. Med Sci Sports Exerc. 2006;38(5):919–25.
87. Parsons TJ, Power C, Logan S, Summerbell CD. Childhood predictors of adult obesity: a systematic review. Int J Obes Relat Metab Disord. 1999;23(Suppl 8):S1–107.
88. Wareham N. Physical activity and obesity prevention. Obes Rev. 2007;8(Suppl 1):109–14.
89. Morrison JA, Glueck CJ, Woo JG, Wang P. Risk factors for cardiovascular disease and type 2 diabetes retained from childhood to adulthood predict adult outcomes: the Princeton LRC Follow-up Study. Int J Pediatr Endocrinol. 2012;2012(1):6.
90. King A, Fuster V. Children are key to CVD prevention. Nat Rev Cardiol. 2010;7(6):297.

91. Schulze MB, Hu FB. Primary prevention of diabetes: what can be done and how much can be prevented? Annu Rev Public Health. 2005;26:445–67.
92. Ferreira I, Twisk JW, van Mechelen W, Kemper HC, Stehouwer CD. Development of fatness, fitness, and lifestyle from adolescence to the age of 36 years: determinants of the metabolic syndrome in young adults: the amsterdam growth and health longitudinal study. Arch Intern Med. 2005;165(1):42–8.
93. Hallal PC, Victora CG, Azevedo MR, Wells JC. Adolescent physical activity and health: a systematic review. Sports Med. 2006;36(12):1019–30.
94. Brill PA, Burkhalter HE, Kohl HW, Blair SN, Goodyear NN. The impact of previous athleticism on exercise habits, physical fitness, and coronary heart disease risk factors in middle-aged men. Res Q Exerc Sport. 1989;60(3):209–15.
95. Janz KF, Dawson JD, Mahoney LT. Tracking physical fitness and physical activity from childhood to adolescence: the muscatine study. Med Sci Sports Exerc. 2000;32(7):1250–7.
96. Telama R, Yang X, Viikari J, Valimaki I, Wanne O, Raitakari O. Physical activity from childhood to adulthood: a 21-year tracking study. Am J Prev Med. 2005;28(3):267–73.
97. Trudeau F, Laurencelle L, Shephard RJ. Tracking of physical activity from childhood to adulthood. Med Sci Sports Exerc. 2004;36(11):1937–43.
98. Taylor WC, Blair SN, Cummings SS, Wun CC, Malina RM. Childhood and adolescent physical activity patterns and adult physical activity. Med Sci Sports Exerc. 1999;31(1):118–23.
99. Telama R, Yang X, Laakso L, Viikari J. Physical activity in childhood and adolescence as predictor of physical activity in young adulthood. Am J Prev Med. 1997;13(4):317–23.
100. Jones RA, Hinkley T, Okely AD, Salmon J. Tracking physical activity and sedentary behavior in childhood: a systematic review. Am J Prev Med. 2013;44(6):651–8.
101. Telama R. Tracking of physical activity from childhood to adulthood: a review. Obes Facts. 2009;2(3):187–95.
102. Engstrom H, Briand A. Puerperium. Health is an overview over one's own life. Interview by Jens Rossen. Sygeplejersken. 1991;91(10):8–9.
103. Baquet G, van Praagh E, Berthoin S. Endurance training and aerobic fitness in young people. Sports Med. 2003;33(15):1127–43.
104. American College of Sports M. Physical Activity in Children and Adolescents. 2015.
105. Department of Health Physical Activity HIaP. At least five a week: evidence on the impact of physical activity and its relationship with health. a report from the Chief Medical Officer. London: Department of Health; 2004.
106. Health AGDo. Australia's Physical Activity and Sedentary Behaviour Guidelines. 2014.

Association Between Cardiorespiratory Fitness and Healthcare Costs

25

Jonathan Myers and Peter Kokkinos

Introduction

Chronic illnesses are increasing in the USA in part because of the aging of the population, but an important contributing factor is increasing trends in unhealthy lifestyle behaviors including lack of physical activity [1, 2]. In the current era of rising healthcare costs, many healthcare systems have directed a greater emphasis toward promoting health behaviors that reduce the incidence of disability and disease [3, 4]. Despite the widely recognized observation that more physically active individuals have fewer health problems and lower overall health costs, surveys show that the majority of Americans do not meet the minimal recommendations for physical activity [5]. An abundance of data has been published in recent years suggesting that modulating fitness, physical activity patterns, or both have a profound effect on healthcare utilization [1, 2, 6, 7]. Indeed, numerous recent studies have reported that individuals who are comparatively sedentary have higher overall healthcare costs, which has been attributed to factors including greater illness, hospitalization, and disability [3, 5–9].

A great deal of epidemiologic evidence has also been published in recent years demonstrating a strong inverse association between level of cardiorespiratory fitness (CRF) and adverse health outcomes [1, 2, 10–20]. Relative to highly fit or moderately fit individuals, low-fit individuals are particularly susceptible not only to higher mortality but also to higher rates of cardiovascular events, type 2 diabetes, stroke, hypertension, particular forms of cancer, and other conditions [1, 2, 10–20]. In a growing number of studies, fitness has been reported to be a stronger predictor of risk for mortality and cardiovascular events than traditional risk factors including hyperlipidemia, hypertension, and smoking [1, 10, 12, 13, 17]. These observations have led many national and international health organizations to advocate strategies to improve fitness by promoting physical activity [13, 18, 21]. In addition, a great deal of research in recent years has been devoted to the economic consequences of physical inactivity [3, 6–9]. These studies have evolved from the assessment of physical activity patterns from

J. Myers (✉)
Department of Cardiology, VA Palo Alto Health Care System/Stanford University, Palo Alto, CA, USA

P. Kokkinos (✉)
Veterans Affairs Medical Center, Department of Cardiology, Washington, DC, USA

Georgetown University School of Medicine, Washington, DC, USA

Department of Kinesiology and Health, Rutgers University, New Brunswick, NJ, USA

George Washington University School of Medicine and Health Sciences, Washington, DC, USA

University of South Carolina, Department of Exercise Science, Arnold School of Public Health, Columbia, SC, USA
e-mail: peter.kokkinos@va.gov

P. Kokkinos, P. Narayan (eds.), *Cardiorespiratory Fitness in Cardiometabolic Diseases*,
https://doi.org/10.1007/978-3-030-04816-7_25

observational cohorts [7, 22], and a growing number of studies have evaluated the economic benefits of worksite wellness programs [4, 7, 23–25]. However, surprisingly few data are available regarding the association between objective measures of CRF and healthcare costs.

Physical activity patterns are often employed as a surrogate for CRF [19, 26], in part because direct measures of fitness require an exercise test and are frequently not available. However, quantifying physical activity patterns in epidemiologic studies typically relies on self-report, and self-reported physical activity can be unreliable [27, 28]. There remains a need for studies on the association between healthcare costs and CRF using objective measures. The demonstration of such an association provides an objective, economic rationale for employers, healthcare professionals, and professional organizations to promote physical activity. The purpose of this chapter is to provide an overview of the available evidence related to the impact of CRF on healthcare costs.

Previous Studies on the Association Between CRF and Healthcare Costs

Despite the current increase in the prevalence of chronic illnesses and heightened interest in limiting the unsustainable rise in healthcare costs, there are surprisingly few studies that have been performed on the impact of CRF on healthcare costs. This is likely due to the vicissitudes of healthcare costs, the difficulty obtaining them in a valid fashion, and the fact that CRF is underappreciated as a risk factor [1, 13]. An outline of the key studies is presented in Table 25.1, and an overview is provided in the following.

Table 25.1 Summary of studies assessing association between healthcare costs and cardiorespiratory fitness

Author	Year	Number	Type of subjects	Type of costs	Key findings
Weiss et al.	2004	881	Veterans Affairs patients referred for a clinical exercise test	Inpatient and outpatient costs expressed in relative cost units	Costs were incrementally lower by an average of 5.4% per higher MET
Grune de Souza e Silva et al.	2018	9789	Referred male veterans assessed over 7-year period	Total costs (inpatient, outpatient)	Each 1-MET improvement in fitness level associated with annual cost savings per person (USD) of $1346, $1823, and $2745 for normal-weight, overweight, and obese subjects, respectively
Myers et al.	2018	9942	Subjects undergoing a maximal exercise test for clinical reasons	Total and annualized healthcare costs	Each 1-MET increase in fitness was associated with a $1592 annual reduction in healthcare cost (5.6% lower cost per MET)
Bachmann et al.	2015	19,571	Healthy individuals in the Cooper Center Longitudinal Study undergoing fitness assessment	Average annual healthcare costs obtained from Medicare	Each 1-MET increase in fitness associated with 6.8% and 6.7% reduced annual healthcare costs a mean 22 years later in life among men and women, respectively
Mitchell et al.	2004	6679	Healthy male subjects undergoing medical exams on two occasions (including maximal ETT)	Incidence of medical treatments during a 1-year period before each of two exams	High-fit subjects had fewer hospital visits and overnight hospital stays vs. low-fit subjects; low-fit men at baseline who became fit during follow-up had reduced hospital stays
Pronk et al.	1999	8822	Employees enrolled in a worksite health promotion program	Annualized healthcare costs incurred over a period of 33 months	Low-fit subjects had 10% higher healthcare costs vs. high-fit subjects

Mitchell and colleagues [29] studied 6679 participants in the Aerobics Center Longitudinal Study and observed an inverse relation between fitness level (expressed in quartiles) and the number of office visits and hospitalizations over a 1-year period. Subjects who exhibited improved fitness on a second examination had a decreased number of hospital stays compared to those who remained classified as unfit. While direct costs were not available in the Mitchell et al. study [29], the comparison between the fittest subjects and the least fit amounted to a 53% reduction in costs based on overnight hospital stays. Weiss et al. [30] quantified inpatient and outpatient costs following a maximal exercise test among 881 veteran subjects and reported that among clinical, demographic, and exercise test variables, exercise capacity was the strongest predictor of healthcare costs during the year subsequent to the exercise test. Costs were incrementally lower by an average of 5.4% per metabolic equivalent (MET) achieved. Bachmann and colleagues [31] studied 19,571 individuals who underwent a baseline fitness assessment at a mean age of 49 years and who received Medicare coverage between 1999 and 2009. They observed that annual healthcare costs were significantly lower for participants with high midlife fitness compared to low midlife fitness (\$7559 vs. \$12,811 in men, $p < 0.001$, and \$6065 vs. \$10,029 in women, $p < 0.001$). The reductions in annual healthcare costs per MET achieved were 6.8 and 6.7% in men and women, respectively. Pronk et al. [32] studied >8800 employees enrolled in a managed care worksite health program and quantified health behaviors, risk factors, and healthcare costs over a period of 3 years. CRF, expressed as predicted VO_2 max, was not determined directly but was estimated using demographic variables, body mass, and weekly strenuous exercise habits ($R^2 = 0.78$ versus measured VO_2 max) [33]. After controlling for the presence of disease and demographic characteristics, annualized healthcare costs were 10% higher for participants with low vs. high predicted VO_2 max.

Our group recently studied 9942 subjects (mean 59 ± 11 years) who underwent a maximal exercise test for clinical reasons between January 2005 and December 2012 [34]. CRF, expressed as a percentage of age-predicted peak METs achieved, was categorized in quartiles. Total and annualized healthcare costs were derived from the VA Allocation Resource Center and were compared using multiple regression models, controlling for demographic and clinical characteristics. A gradient for reduced healthcare costs was observed as CRF increased, with subjects in the least-fit quartile having approximately \$14,662 higher overall costs per patient/year compared to

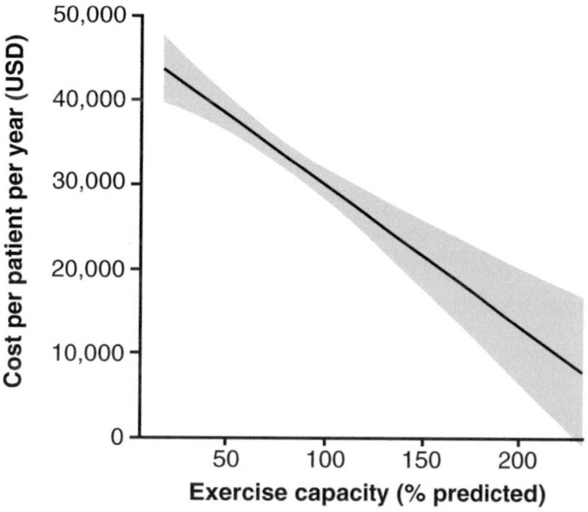

Fig. 25.1 The association between costs per patient per year (USD) and exercise capacity (% predicted). (Modified from: Myers et al. [34]; PMID 29195922)

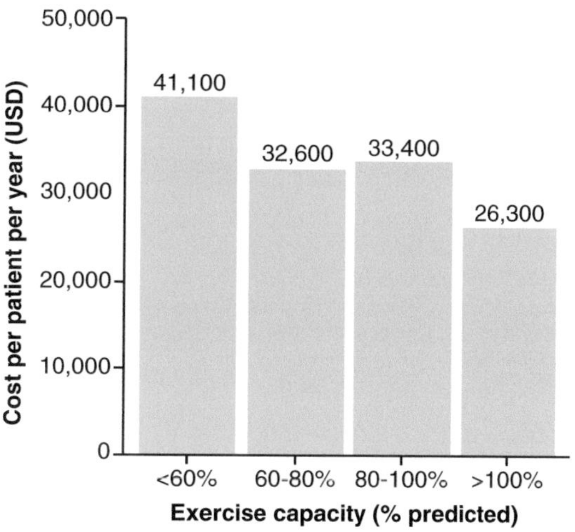

Fig. 25.2 Mean annual costs (USD) by category of exercise capacity. (Modified from: Myers et al. [34]; PMID 29195922)

those in the fittest quartile, after controlling for potential confounding variables ($p < 0.001$) (Fig. 25.1). Each 1-MET higher increment in fitness was associated with a $1592 annual reduction in healthcare costs. Similar to the Weiss et al. [30] and Bachmann et al. [31 studies, a 5.6% lower cost per MET was observed. Most notably, each higher quartile of fitness was associated with a $4163 annual cost reduction (USD) per patient (Fig. 25.2). The effect of CRF was more pronounced among subjects without cardiovascular disease (CVD), suggesting that the results were not driven by the possibility that less fit individuals had greater CVD. In a model including historical, clinical, and exercise test responses, heart failure was the strongest predictor of healthcare costs, followed by CRF ($p < 0.01$).

An ancillary observation in the latter study was the fact that cost savings related to higher CRF were most pronounced among overweight and obese subjects. This issue was therefore recently addressed in more detail among 2043 normal-weight, 4046 overweight, and 3700 obese veterans [35]. Total healthcare costs were quantified over a 7-year period. For each 1-MET improvement in CRF, annual cost savings per person (USD) were $1346, $1823, and $2745 for normal-weight, overweight, and obese subjects, respectively. Normal-weight, overweight, and obese subjects in the highest quartile of CRF had annual costs that were $2890, $12,059, and $16,379 lower, respectively, than subjects in the lowest quartile of fitness ($p < 0.01$). Thus, cost savings with higher fitness were far more evident among overweight and obese individuals. The association between annual healthcare costs per person and exercise capacity is shown in Fig. 25.3, in which the inverse association between costs and CRF was steeper among overweight and obese subjects compared to normal-weight subjects. The observation that cost savings associated with higher CRF were particularly apparent among

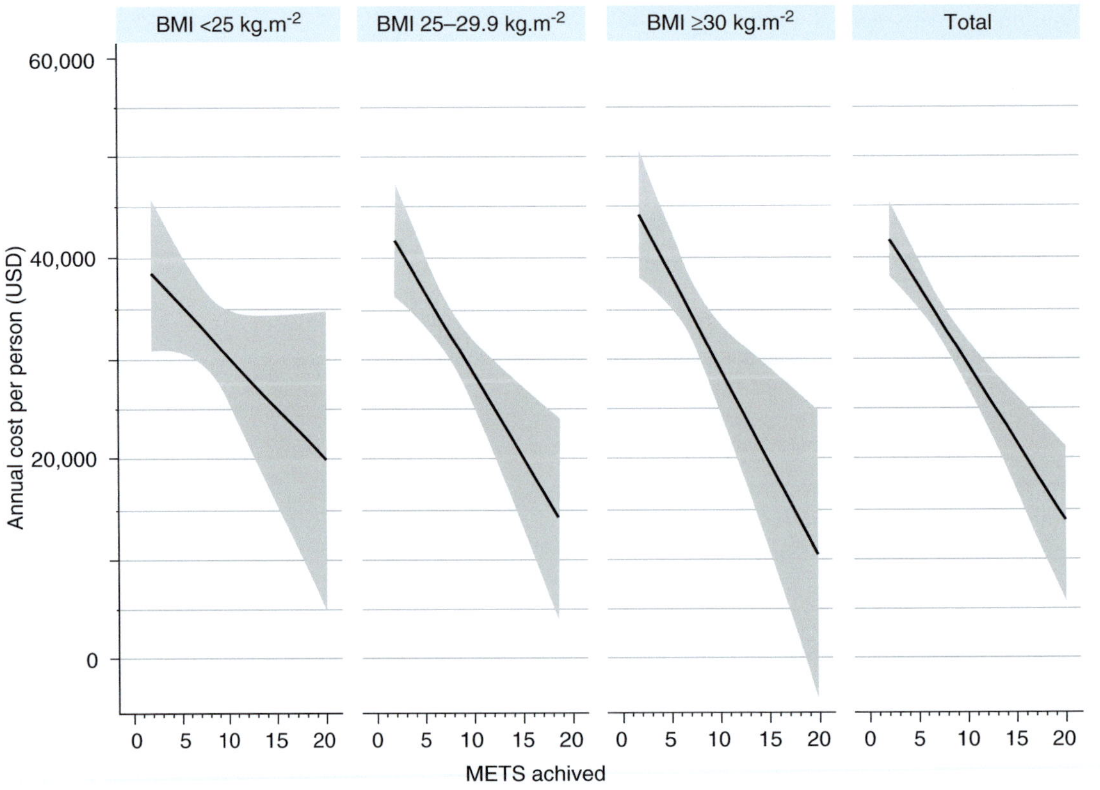

Fig. 25.3 Linear regression line and 95% confidence intervals between annual costs per person and exercise capacity according to body mass index (BMI). (Modified from: Grüne de Souza de Silva et al. [35])

overweight and obese subjects is provocative and suggests that the considerable economic burden of obesity [36] may be reduced through interventions that target improvements in CRF.

Limitations

It should be noted that the number of studies on the association between objective measures of CRF and healthcare costs remains limited; most of the results come from men, and little is known regarding types of costs (e.g., inpatient/outpatient, effect of particular illnesses). While the Mitchell et al. study [29] quantified hospital stays with serial measures of CRF, no studies are available to our knowledge on serial testing and *direct* healthcare costs; such data would be valuable in order to determine the influence of *changes* in CRF on healthcare costs. Fitness is a complex attribute that is influenced by many factors in addition to physical activity patterns, and it is not possible to account for all of them. For example, fitter subjects may engage in other healthy behaviors such as a better diet, regular physician visits, or better medication adherence. Additional observational studies are required to evaluate the impact of lifestyle factors in addition to CRF. Finally, the estimation of healthcare costs is a difficult undertaking under the best of circumstances; different healthcare systems use different processes to estimate costs, and private and Medicare costs and services are often poorly integrated, may vary considerably, and may not accurately reflect true healthcare costs [31, 32]. Additional studies are needed to better define the extent to which healthcare costs are influenced by CRF.

Clinical Implications and Conclusions

Collectively, the findings from these studies suggest that level of fitness is inversely related to overall healthcare costs among subjects in whom CRF has been objectively determined with a maximal exercise test. Total healthcare costs are consistently lower per MET achieved (in the range of 5–7%), are consistent when adjusted for potentially confounding factors, and, in at least one study, are not altered appreciably after excluding patients without cardiovascular disease or who died within 1 year of follow-up. Cost savings with higher CRF appear to be more pronounced among overweight and obese subjects [35], although this requires confirmation from other prospective cohort studies. CRF appears to be a powerful *predictor* of healthcare costs (surpassed only by heart failure [30, 34]). The latter finding is noteworthy given the spectrum of risk factors and chronic conditions that have been associated with rising healthcare costs and the fact that CRF has not generally been considered when assessing overall risk or healthcare costs [1, 12, 13].

Recent findings on the impact of CRF on healthcare costs extend the many recent studies showing lower mortality among individuals with higher versus lower CRF [1, 11–18]. Moreover, they support studies demonstrating that healthcare expenditures are considerably lower among more active individuals [3, 7–10, 22–25, 36] and the concept that programs designed to increase worksite physical activity participation have a positive economic impact [1, 4, 7–10]. These studies also support the recent case for "fitness as a vital sign" [12, 13], in which CRF should be routinely determined clinically along with traditional risk factors such as blood pressure, weight, and lipid levels. Finally, results from these studies provide an *economic-based* impetus for healthcare providers and health organizations to recommend moderate physical activity to their patients in order to improve CRF [1, 4, 12, 13, 22–25, 29–35].

References

1. Myers J, McAuley P, Lavie C, et al. Physical activity and cardiorespiratory fitness as major markers of cardiovascular risk: their independent and interwoven importance to health status. Prog Cardiovasc Dis. 2015;57(4):306–14.
2. Booth FW, Roberts CK, Laye MJ. Lack of exercise is a major cause of chronic diseases. Compr Physiol. 2012;2(2):1143–211.
3. Ding D, Lawson KD, Kolbe-Alexander TL, et al. Physical activity series 2 executive committee. The economic burden of physical inactivity: a global anal-

ysis of major non-communicable diseases. Lancet. 2016;388(10051):1311–24.

4. Cahalin LP, Myers J, Kaminsky L, et al. Current trends in reducing cardiovascular risk factors in the United States: focus on worksite health and wellness. Prog Cardiovasc Dis. 2014;56(5):476–83.
5. Centers for Disease Control and Prevention. One in 5 adults meet overall physical activity guidelines. www.cdc.gov/media/releases/2013/p0502-physical-activity.html. Accessed 3/8/2018.
6. Barr VJ, Robinson S, Marin-Link B, et al. The expanded chronic care model: an integration of concepts and strategies from population health promotion and the chronic care model. Healthc Q. 2003; 7(1):73–82.
7. Carlson SA, Fulton JE, Pratt M, et al. Inadequate physical activity and health care expenditures in the United States. Prog Cardiovasc Dis. 2015;57(4):315–23.
8. Burton WN, Chen CY, Li X, et al. The association of self-reported employee physical activity with metabolic syndrome, health care costs, absenteeism, and presenteeism. J Occup Environ Med. 2014;56(9):919–26.
9. Anderson LH, Martinson BC, Crain AL, et al. Health care changes associated with physical inactivity, overweight, and obesity. Prev Chronic Dis. 2005;2(4):A09.
10. Rosenberg D, Cook A, Gell N, et al. Relationships between sitting time and health indicators, costs, and utilization in older adults. Prev Med Rep. 2015;2: 247–9.
11. Kodama S, Saito K, Tanaka S, et al. Cardiorespiratory fitness as a quantitative predictor of all-cause mortality and cardiovascular events in healthy men and women: a meta-analysis. JAMA. 2009;301(19):2024–35.
12. Després JP. Physical activity, sedentary behaviours, and cardiovascular health: when will cardiorespiratory fitness become a vital sign? Can J Cardiol. 2016;32:505–13.
13. Ross R, Blair S, Arena R, et al. Importance of assessing cardiorespiratory fitness in clinical practice: a case for fitness as a clinical vital sign. An American Heart Association Scientific Statement from the Committee on Physical Activity and the Council on Lifestyle and cardiometabolic Health. Circulation. 2016;134(24):e653–99.
14. Kokkinos PF, Faselis C, Myers JN, et al. Cardiorespiratory fitness and incidence of major adverse cardiovascular events in US veterans: a cohort study. Mayo Clinic Proc. 2017;92(1):39–48.
15. Nauman J, Nes BM, Lavie CJ. Prediction of cardiovascular mortality by estimated cardiorespiratory fitness independent of traditional risk factors: the HUNT study. Mayo Clin Proc. 2017;92(2):218–27.
16. Jimenez-Pavon D, Artero EG, Lee D, et al. Cardiorespiratory fitness and risk of sudden cardiac death in men and women in the United States. Mayo Clin Proc. 2016;91(7):849–57.
17. Kokkinos P, Myers J. Physical activity: clinical outcomes and applications. Circulation. 2010;122(16):1637–48.
18. Kaminsky LA, Arena R, Beckie TM, et al. The importance of cardiorespiratory fitness in the United States: the need for a national registry. A Policy Statement from the American Heart Association. Circulation. 2013;127(5):652–62.
19. Defina LF, Haskell WL, Willis BL, et al. Physical activity versus cardiorespiratory fitness: two (partly) distinct components of cardiovascular health? Prog Cardiovascular Dis. 2015;57(4):324–9.
20. Myers J, Kokkinos P, Chan K, Dandekar E, Yilmaz B, Nagare A, Faselis C, Soofi M. Cardiorespiratory fitness and reclassification of risk for incidence of heart failure: The Veterans Exercise Testing Study. Circulation Heart Fail. 2017; PMID 28572213.
21. EU Working Group "Sport and Health". EU physical activity guidelines. 2008. Available at: http://ec.europa.eu/sport/what-we-do/doc/health/pa_guidelines_4th_consolidated_draft_en.pdf. Accessed 3/15/2017.
22. Wang F, McDonald T, Reffitt B, Edington DW. BMI, physical activity, and health care utilization among Medicare retirees. Obesity. 2005;13:1450–7.
23. Milani RV, Lavie CJ. Impact of worksite wellness intervention on cardiac risk factors and one-year health costs. Am J Cardiol. 2009;104:1389–92.
24. Naydeck BL, Pearson JA, Ozminkowski RJ, Day BT, Goetzel RZ. The impact of the Highmark employee wellness programs on 4-year health costs. J Occup Environ Med. 2008;50:146–56.
25. Fonarow GC, Calitz C, Arena R, et al. Workplace wellness recognition for optimizing workplace health. A Presidential Advisory from the American Heart Association. Circulation. 2015;131(20):e480–97.
26. Haskell WL, Lee IM, Pate RR, et al. Physical activity and public health. Updated recommendation for adults from the American College of Sports Medicine and the American Heart Association. Circulation. 2007;116(9):1081–93.
27. Hendrik JF, Helmerhorst HJF, Brage S, Warren J, Besson H, Ekelund U. Systematic review of reliability and objective criterion-related validity of physical activity questionnaires. Int J Behav Nutr Phys Act. 2012;9:103.
28. Ainsworth B, Cahalin L, Buman M, Ross R. The current state of physical activity assessment tools. Prog Cardiovasc Dis. 2015;57(4):387–95.
29. Mitchell TL, Gibbons LW, Devers SM, Earnest CP. Effects of cardiorespiratory fitness on healthcare utilization. Med Sci Sports Exerc. 2004;36:2088–92.
30. Weiss P, Froelicher V, Myers J, et al. Health care costs and exercise capacity. Chest. 2004;126(2):608–13.
31. Bachman JM, DeFina LF, Franzini L, et al. Cardiorespiratory fitness in middle age and health care costs in later life. J Am Coll Cardiol. 2015;66(17):1876–85.
32. Pronk NP, Tan AWH, O'Connor P. Obesity, fitness, willingness to communicate and health care costs. Med Sci Sports Exerc. 1999;31:1535–43.
33. Ainsworth BE, Richardson MT, Jacobs DR, Leon AS. Prediction of cardiorespiratory fitness using

physical activity questionnaire data. Med Exerc Nutr Health. 1992;1:75–82.

34. Myers J, Doom R, King R, Fonda H, Abella J, Froelicher V, Chan K, Kokkinos P. Higher fitness is associated with lower heath care costs: The Veterans Exercise Testing Study. Mayo Clin Proc. 2018;93:48–55.
35. Grüne de Souza de Silva C, Kokkinos P, Doom R, Loganathan D, Fonda H, Chan K, Soares de Araújo CG, Myers J. Association between cardiorespiratory fitness, obesity, and health care costs: The Veterans Exercise Testing Study. Submitted; 2018. https://doi.org/10.1038/s41366-018-0257-0
36. Kent S, Fusco F, Gray A, Jebb SA, Cairns BJ, Mihaylove B. Body mass index and healthcare costs: a systematic review of individual participant data studies. Obes Rev. 2017;18:869–79.

Index

P. Kokkinos, P. Narayan (eds.), *Cardiorespiratory Fitness in Cardiometabolic Diseases*,
https://doi.org/10.1007/978-3-030-04816-7

I

U

V

W

MIX
Papier aus verantwortungsvollen Quellen
Paper from responsible sources
FSC® C105338

If you have any concerns about our products,
you can contact us on
ProductSafety@springernature.com

In case Publisher is established outside the EU,
the EU authorized representative is:
Springer Nature Customer Service Center GmbH
Europaplatz 3, 69115 Heidelberg, Germany

Printed by Libri Plureos GmbH
in Hamburg, Germany